Handbook of
Children's Coping
Linking Theory and Intervention

Issues in Clinical Child Psychology

Series Editors: **Michael C. Roberts,** *University of Kansas–Lawrence, Kansas*
Lizette Peterson, *University of Missouri–Columbia, Missouri*

A Continuation Order Plan is available for this series. A continuation order will bring
delivery of each new volume immediately upon publication. Volumes are billed only
upon actual shipment. For further information please contact the publisher.

Handbook of
Children's Coping
Linking Theory and Intervention

Edited by

Sharlene A. Wolchik and
Irwin N. Sandler

*Arizona State University
Tempe, Arizona*

Plenum Press • New York and London

Library of Congress Cataloging in Publication Data

Handbook of children's coping: linking theory and intervention / edited by Sharlene A. Wolchik and Irwin N. Sandler.
    p.   cm.—(Issues in clinical child psychology)
    Includes bibliographical references and index.
    ISBN 0-306-45536-6
    1. Stress in children. 2. Adjustment disorders in children. 3. Adjustment (Psychology) in children. 4. Resilience (Personality trait) in children. 5. Mental illness—Prevention. I. Wolchik, Sharlene A. II. Sandler, Irwin N. III. Series.
    [DNLM: 1. Stress, Psychological—in infancy & childhood. 2. Adaptation, Psychological—in infancy & childhood. 3. Crisis Intervention—in infancy & childhood. WS 350 H23585 1997]
RJ507.S77H36 1997
155.4'18—dc21
DNLM/DLC   97-16901
for Library of Congress   CIP

ISBN 0-306-45536-6

© 1997 Plenum Press, New York
A Division of Plenum Publishing Corporation
233 Spring Street, New York, N. Y. 10013

http://www.plenum.com

10 9 8 7 6 5 4 3 2 1

Printed in the United States of America

We dedicate this volume to our families.

To Philip G. Poirier, my spouse and best friend;
and to our wonderful children, Katie Blair and Lauren Ann

—Sharlene A. Wolchik

To Linda Sandler, my spouse, friend, and life partner;
and to our truly terrific children, Jennifer and Deborah

—Irwin N. Sandler

Contributors

Tim S. Ayers, Department of Psychology and Program for Prevention Research, Arizona State University, Tempe, Arizona 85287-1108

Manuel Barrera, Jr., Department of Psychology, Arizona State University, Tempe, Arizona 85287-1104

Alicia Barr, Department of Psychology, Arizona State University, Tempe, Arizona 85287-1104

Ronald Belter, Department of Psychology, University of West Florida, Pensacola, Florida 32514

Rosemary Calderon, Department of Psychiatry, Children's Hospital Medical Center, (CHMC), Seattle, Washington 98195

Laurie Chassin, Department of Psychology, Arizona State University, Tempe, Arizona 85287-1104

John Coie, Department of Psychology, Duke University, Durham, North Carolina 27708

Bruce E. Compas, Department of Psychology, University of Vermont, Burlington, Vermont 05405

Nancy Eisenberg, Department of Psychology, Arizona State University, Tempe, Arizona 85287-1104

Sydney Ey, Department of Psychology, University of Memphis, Memphis, Tennessee 38152

Richard A. Fabes, Department of Family Resources and Human Development, Arizona State University, Tempe, Arizona 85287-1108

Margaret M. Feerick, Department of Human Development and Family Studies, Cornell University, Ithaca, New York 14853

Frank D. Fincham, Department of Psychology, University of Wales, Cardiff CF1 3YG, Great Britain

Nancy A. Gonzales, Department of Psychology, Arizona State University, Tempe, Arizona 85287-1104

Mark T. Greenberg, Human Development and Family Studies, Penn State University, University Park, Pennsylvania 16802

John H. Grych, Department of Psychology, Marquette University, Milwaukee, Wisconsin 53233

Nancy G. Guerra, Department of Psychology, University of Illinois at Chicago, Chicago, Illinois 60680

Ivanna K. Guthrie, Department of Psychology, Arizona State University, Tempe, Arizona 85287-1104

Constance Hammen, Department of Psychology, University of California, Los Angeles, Los Angeles, California 90095

Jeffrey J. Haugaard, Department of Human Development and Family Studies, Cornell University, Ithaca, New York 14853

Marlene Jacobs, Department of Psychology, Duke University, Durham, North Carolina 27708

Lauren S. Kim, Department of Psychology, Arizona State University, Tempe, Arizona 85287-1104

Wendy Kliewer, Department of Psychology, Virginia Commonwealth University, Richmond, Virginia 23284

Paul A. Langfield, Rocky Mountain Neuropsychological Sciences, P.C., Ft. Collins, Colorado 80524

Liliana J. Lengua, Department of Psychology, University of Washington, Seattle, Washington 98195

Janelle R. Lutzke, Department of Psychology, Arizona State University, Tempe, Arizona 85287-1104

David MacKinnon, Department of Psychology and Program for Prevention Research, Arizona State University, Tempe, Arizona 85287-1108

Luisa R. Montaini-Klovdahl, Department of Psychiatry, University of California at San Francisco, San Francisco, California 94560

Heather Montgomery, Department of Psychology, Arizona State University, Tempe, Arizona 85287-1104

Krista K. Oliver, Department of Psychology, University of Missouri at Columbia, Columbia, Missouri 65211

Kay Pasley, Human Development and Family Studies, University of North Carolina, Greensboro, Greensboro, North Carolina 27412

Lizette Peterson, Department of Psychology, University of Missouri at Columbia, Columbia, Missouri 65211

N. Dickon Reppucci, Department of Psychology, University of Virginia, Charlottesville, Virginia 22903

Mark W. Roosa, Department of Family Resources and Human Development and Program for Prevention Research, Arizona State University, Tempe, Arizona 85287-1108

Lisa Saldana, Department of Psychology, University of Missouri at Columbia, Columbia, Missouri 65211

Irwin N. Sandler, Department of Psychology and Program for Prevention Research, Arizona State University, Tempe, Arizona 85287-1108

Conway F. Saylor, Department of Psychology, The Citadel, Charleston, South Carolina 29409

Ellen A. Skinner, Department of Psychology, Portland State University, Portland, Oregon 97207

Sherri J. Stokes, New Hope Treatment Center, Charleston, South Carolina 29483

Patrick H. Tolan, Departments of Psychiatry and Psychology, University of Illinois at Chicago Medical School, Chicago, Illinois 60612

James G. Wellborn, Tennessee Christian Medical Center, Madison, Tennessee 37221

Sharlene A. Wolchik, Department of Psychology and Program for Prevention Research, Arizona State University, Tempe, Arizona 85287-1108

Nancy L. Worsham, Department of Psychology, Gonzaga University, Spokane, Washington 99258

Audrey Zakriski, E. P. Bradley Hospital, Brown University School of Medicine, East Providence, Rhode Island 02916

Preface

Many of today's children and adolescents are exposed to serious environmental stressors that present significant challenges to their healthy development. Growing up in inner-city neighborhoods, experiencing multiple transitions in family structure, and living with alcoholic or depressed parents are increasingly common aspects of growing up in America. Over the past couple of decades, a substantial amount of research has accrued on the mental health sequelae of such experiences. It is now well established that the experience of these stressful situations elevates the risk of serious mental health problems, academic difficulties, and drug and alcohol problems. Researchers have also repeatedly documented that many children are resilient and escape the negative mental health effects of these stressful situations. An exciting field of inquiry has developed to understand resilience, and this volume is intended to bring together some of the best thinking on this issue as it pertains to children's adaptation to 15 different stressful situations. The guiding vision is that increased knowledge will facilitate the design of effective theory-based interventions that build resilience when it does not naturally occur.

Until recently, little was known about why some children "sink" and others "swim" when faced with these stressors. Within the last few years, researchers have devoted significant attention to the critical issue of understanding variability in children's response to major stressors. Some researchers have begun to "unpack" the risk situations to identify those aspects of the stressor that are critical determinants of maladaptive outcomes. Others have focused on the role that children's cognitions, personality variables, and coping efforts play. Researchers have also identified aspects of social environments that promote healthy adaptation to these stressors. Concurrent with this growth in basic research on risk and protective factors, there has been an increase in the number of preventive interventions designed to promote healthy adaptation to these stressful situations. Results from experimental evaluations of several of these programs provide exciting evidence of positive effects. The findings are encouraging that we can promote healthy adaptation to major stressful conditions and, by so doing, prevent a wide range of mental health problems. However, for many stressful situations, there is little or no evidence of effective interventions, and even for areas where there are effective interventions, major questions remain about how they work, for whom they are effective, and their long-term consequences.

The purpose of this volume is to review the state of current knowledge about factors that affect children's adaptation to major stressful situations and to consider the implications of this knowledge for the design and evaluation of preventive interventions. The authors followed a common outline. First, they present evidence on the number of children who experience the stressor and critically evaluate the research on the short- and long-term effects of the stressful situation on mental health outcomes. Next, they discuss the literatures on the most stressful components of these situations and the relations between coping, social environmental resources, and children's adjustment. Then, they critically review the literature on preventive interventions, giving particular attention to the strength of empirical support for program efficacy and linkage between the basic and intervention research. Finally, they articulate important directions for future research.

Some of the stressors are time limited, whereas others involve a series of ongoing challenges for children and their families. Many of the stressors are family-level stressors, but a few are more circumscribed in their impact. Most represent stressors over which children have little direct control. Inclusion of a range of stressors allows the identification of unique as well as common aspects of children's responses, risk and protective factors, and preventive efforts.

For the past 15 years, we have been actively involved in building theory-based programs to enhance resilience in children who face stressful situations. We have no illusions that this is easy work. It requires a team with expertise in theory, program design, methodology, program evaluation, and implementation of programs collaboratively with communities. It is a long-term, iterative process involving multiple feedback loops between theory and intervention. This research is exciting work, which we believe will lead to better theory and, more importantly, healthier futures for children who grapple with these problems in their everyday lives.

This volume is addressed to professionals and students in a wide range of disciplines who share an interest in fostering the healthy development of our youth. It should be beneficial to researchers and mental health practitioners, as well as those involved in the design and evaluation of preventive interventions and public policies that affect children and their families.

There are many people who provided invaluable assistance and support. Sincere appreciation is extended to all the contributors for sharing our commitment to produce a volume that would advance the field. We acknowledge the time they took from their busy schedules to accomplish this goal. We thank the series editors, Lizette Peterson and Michael Roberts, for inviting us to edit this book. We also acknowledge Mariclaire Cloutier at Plenum Publishing Corporation. Her assistance, support, patience, and good humor helped to make this project an enjoyable one. Ernest Fairchild and Betty Barwegen at the Arizona State University (ASU) Program for Prevention are thanked for their secretarial help. We also thank LaVaun Habegger at the ASU Psychology Department for her assistance. We acknowledge the support provided by a grant from the National Institute of Mental Health (P50MH39246). We also thank the many children and families who, through participation in our research projects, have taught us much about thriving in spite of adversity.

Contents

Part V. Conclusion

I

Conceptual Issues in Studying Children's Coping

1

Developing Linkages between Theory and Intervention in Stress and Coping Processes

IRWIN N. SANDLER, SHARLENE A. WOLCHIK, DAVID MacKINNON, TIM S. AYERS, and MARK W. ROOSA

The constructs of stress and coping have held an important role in theories about the development of problems of childhood and adolescents and in intervention models about how to prevent the occurrence of such problems (Haggerty, Sherrod, Garmezy, & Rutter, 1994; Rolf, Masten, Cicchetti, Nuechterlein, & Weintraub, 1990; Cowen, 1980; Mrazek & Haggerty, 1994; Hetherington & Blechman, 1996). Stress has been implicated in the development of a wide range of problems, and a rich literature has developed on factors that enable children to be resilient against the negative effects of stress (Gore & Eckenrode, 1994). In a parallel fashion, improving child and adolescent adaptation to stress has been identified as one of the most promising approaches to preventing the development of problems of childhood and adolescence (Compas, Phares, & Ledoux, 1989; Cowen, 1985; Bloom, 1990). For example, in their comprehensive annotated bibliography of primary prevention programs between 1983 and 1991, Trickett, Dahiyal, and Selby (1994) identified 169 citations concerning prevention programs under the headings of stressful life events, social support, and crisis intervention. Many of these stress-based preventive interventions have been empirically evaluated and found to have beneficial effects (Mrazek &

IRWIN N. SANDLER, SHARLENE A. WOLCHIK, DAVID MacKINNON, and TIM S. AYERS • Department of Psychology and Program for Prevention Research, Arizona State University, Tempe, Arizona 85287-1108.   MARK W. ROOSA • Department of Family Resources and Human Development and Program for Prevention Research, Arizona State University, Tempe, Arizona 85287-1108.

Handbook of Children's Coping: Linking Theory and Intervention, edited by Wolchik and Sandler. Plenum Press, New York, 1997.

Haggerty, 1994; Price, Cowen, Lorion, & Ramos-McKay, 1988). Unfortunately, however, the links between the theoretical and intervention research literatures are not strong. Relatively few interventions have been designed specifically to change processes that have been empirically supported as protective against the negative effects of stress, and the evaluations of the interventions are rarely designed to assess the theoretical mechanisms by which they affect problematic outcomes.

In the prevention research literature wide support has developed for a model of program development whereby theoretical research identifies potentially modifiable mediators of the development of problems and intervention research tests whether changing those potential mediators reduces the onset of problems (Cowen, 1980; Price, 1983; Mrazek & Haggerty, 1994; National Institute of Mental Health, 1995). Coie et al. (1993) propose that "prevention trials should be guided initially by developmental theory and yield results that reflexively inform and revise the original theory" (p. 1017). While models exist for the development of theoretically based interventions (Caplan, Vinokur, Price, & van Ryn, 1989; Sandler et al., 1992; Wolchik et al., 1993), conceptual and methodological issues in linking research on stress theory and intervention have not been well articulated.

This chapter addresses issues in developing theoretically based interventions to prevent the problems that result from poor adaptation to stress and in testing the theoretical mechanisms by which such interventions work. The chapter first provides an overview of the impact of children's stressful experiences on their mental health. We then articulate a transactional model of adaptation to stress (Sameroff & Seifer, 1990) and discuss three domains of variables involved in adaptation: environmental stress, appraisal and coping variables, and social support. Each section discusses conceptual and measurement issues, briefly reviews evidence concerning how these concepts affect the development of problematic outcomes, and discusses implications for intervention design. Finally, we discuss four issues in the design and evaluation of theory-based interventions for children in stressful situations: use of theory to design interventions, design of experimental trials to evaluate the effects of the interventions, analysis and interpretation of the result, and use of the findings to strengthen interventions and enhance dissemination.

PUBLIC HEALTH IMPACT OF CHILDREN'S EXPOSURE TO STRESSFUL SITUATIONS

Exposure to serious stressful situations is a common aspect of growing up in America. Illustratively, 40% of children experience the divorce of their parents (Cherlin, 1992), 22% of children live in poverty (Knitzer & Aber, 1995), 5 to 15% of children live with a parent who suffers a serious medical condition (Worsham, Compas, and Ey, Chapter 7, this volume), 19% of children experience a chronic illness or physical disability (Nowachek & Stoddard, 1994), 3.4% of children experience the death of a parent (US Bureau of the Census, 1994), and 6.6 million children live with an alcoholic parent (Russell, Henderson, & Blume, 1985). A critical question for prevention researchers is what is the impact of these stressors on children's psychological health and well-being? What proportion of problems in the population would be prevented if the effects of these stressors were completely counteracted?

Attributable risk is one very useful way of estimating the potential public health benefit of an intervention with any risk factor. Attributable risk refers to the maximum proportion of any outcome that is due to a specified risk factor and that subsequently might be prevented if the effects of that risk factor were completely eliminated. Attributable risk is a function of two variables, the strength of the risk factor in increasing relative risk for the outcome, and the prevalence of the risk factor. The combination of prevalence (P) and relative risk (RR) are formalized as attributable risk in the epidemiology literature using the formula AR = P(RR − 1)/1 + P(RR − 1) (Kahn & Sempos, 1989). Reasonable estimates of the prevalence of children's exposure to stressors and the relative risk from such exposure allow us to estimate attributable risk for a number of mental health problems. Illustratively, parental divorce has a relatively modest impact on increasing children's conduct problems (RR = 1.7, for clinical levels of conduct problems) (Lindner, Hagan, & Brown, 1992) but is very prevalent (occurring to 40% of children) (Cherlin, 1992) and has an attributable risk of 21.9% for conduct problems. Similarly, poverty is a highly prevalent stressor (22% of children) that increases children's risk for mental health problems (RR = 2, for psychiatric diagnosis), yielding an attributable risk of 18% for psychiatric diagnosis. A stressor that is relatively rare may also have a considerable impact on the prevalence of a problem because of its strong effect. Parental death occurs in only 3.4% of the population. However, two studies indicate a very high relative risk for serious problems in childhood [RR = 7, for depression (Gersten, Beals, & Kallgren, 1991) and RR = 7, for overall clinical level of psychological disturbance (Worden & Silverman, 1996)]. Based on these figures, the attributable risk is 18.5% for depression and 16.9% for overall clinical level of disturbance. Clearly, stress creates a significant public health problem for children.

TRANSACTIONAL MODEL FOR ADAPTATION TO STRESSFUL SITUATIONS

Considerable research on the effects of stressful situations on children and adolescents has focused on identifying factors that contribute to resilience, defined as accomplishing positive developmental outcomes in the face of adversity. Progress has been made in identifying sources of resilience, including characteristics of the child, relationships with the primary caretakers, and support from extrafamilial community resources (Werner & Smith, 1982; Cowan, Cowan, & Schultz, 1996; Gore & Eckenrode, 1994; Cowen, Wyman, Work, & Parker, 19909). Research on resilience has progressed over the past decade from identifying static protective factors that are associated with better developmental outcomes under stress to a concern with mechanisms or the complex chain of events that lead to positive outcomes under conditions of stress (Rutter, 1994; Cowan et al., 1996). Illustratively, interparental quarrels may lead to more ineffective parenting, increased distress on the part of the parent, and feelings of emotional insecurity on the part of the child. Each of these, in turn, may lead to increased acting out behavior on the part of the child. However, children's response to interparental quarrels may be affected by what they are told about the conflict (Cummings & Davies, 1994), how they interpret and cope with the conflict (Grych & Fincham, 1993; Rossman & Rosenberg, 1992), and the family context within which the quarrels occur (O'Brien, Margolin, John, & Krueger, 1991).

Several authors have proposed that a broad stress and coping framework is useful in specifying a family of variables and research questions that concern adaptation to stress events (McGrath, 1970; Lazarus & Folkman, 1984; Dohrenwend & Dohrenwend, 1978). A stress framework refers to a process in which individuals encounter adverse events as they interact with their environment (*stressors*), interpret these events as threatening to their well-being (*appraisals*), and utilize *coping* strategies and *social resources* to manage their affect and/or attempt to change the situation (Lazarus & Folkman, 1984; McGrath, 1970). The process of adaptation occurs over time and results in changes in the individual's beliefs, affect, behavior, and approach to future stressful situations. The process also changes the environment to increase or decrease exposure to further stressors. Processes of person–environment transaction are emphasized rather than more stable structures of person (e.g., personality) or environment (e.g., household structure). Illustratively, from this perspective, research on children of divorce would study what stressors follow divorce, how children appraise them, what children do to respond, what assistance they receive from their social environment, and the developmental outcomes of these processes. We now consider each of three domains of constructs that are posited to be part of the process of children's adaptation to stress.

Environmental Stress

Early approaches to the assessment of stress in children (Coddington, 1972) attempted to assess the total amount of environmental change that recently occurred. These measures were based on a homeostatic model that posits change that disrupts the steady state and that the work of readjustment is stressful (Selye, 1956). An alternative theoretical model emphasized that stress derives from the negative quality of events (Lazarus & Folkman, 1984). Based on this model, stress was assessed as negative change, rather than as change per se. From a change perspective, positive as well as negative events are predicted to be stressful, while a desirability model predicts that only negative events are stressful. Numerous studies have been conducted to test these alternative predictions, with the consistent finding that undesirable but not desirable events relate to higher levels of psychological symptoms in children and adolescents (Rowlison & Felner, 1988; Sandler, Wolchik, Braver, & Fogas, 1991).

Undesirability is a very broad concept and several researchers have attempted to investigate more narrow-band properties of stressful events. For example, Seidman, Allen, Aber, Mitchell, & Feinman (1994) identified five dimensions of events for inner-city adolescents: school, neighborhood, family, peer, and resources. Guerra, Huesmann, Tolan, Van Acker, & Eron (1995) identified family stressors and neighborhood violence stressors for inner-city children. Sandler and Ramsey (1982) identified six dimensions of stressful events based on a factor analysis of expert ratings of their similarity. Thus, several studies have identified multiple negative characteristics of events rather than a single dimension of negativity.

From a transactional perspective, event stressfulness cannot be determined solely on the basis of the characteristics of the event, but also depends on the characteristics of the child, such as their goals, values, and self-system vulnerabilities (Lazarus, 1991). For example, events could be characterized in terms of the roles they affect. Events may impact on school functioning, friendship, family relationships, and so forth. The stressfulness of the event might be a function of the degree to which the event indicates the failure to obtain a desired goal in that domain and the importance of that domain to the child. Illustratively, Hammen and Goodman-Brown (1990) found that for children of depressed mothers, negative events that occurred in areas where they attached a particular meaning for their sense of self were associated with the onset or worsening of depression over a 6-month period.

From a motivational perspective, Skinner and Wellborn (1994; see also Chapter 14, this volume) conceptualize events as being stressful to the extent that they threaten basic needs for autonomy, competence, and relatedness. The stressfulness of events is a joint function of the event property (i.e., chaos, coercion, and neglect) and the vulnerability of the child's self-system in relation to that need which leads to a subjective appraisal of threat or challenge.

Research on the ecological properties of events has considered three major concepts: size of the event, chronicity, and the dynamic interrelatedness of events. Early research on children and stress largely focused on children exposed to single large events. Thus, a literature developed around specific major stressors such as parental divorce, poverty, bereavement, interparental conflict, child abuse, and parental mental illness. As presented in the chapters of this volume, each of these literatures has studied the impact of a major event and has investigated biological, individual difference, and social environmental factors that affect this impact.

Similar to the literature with adults, life stress event inventories subsequently were developed to assess the cumulative effects of all the major events that occurred during a specified time (Johnson & Bradlyn, 1988). Studies have consistently found that the scores reflecting the total number of major negative events are predictive of child and adolescent health and mental health problems in both cross-sectional and longitudinal analyses (Rowlison & Felner, 1988; DuBois, Felner, Brand, Adan, & Evans, 1992; Sandler, Tein, & West, 1994; Siegel & Brown, 1988). Over the past decade, research has shifted from a focus on the effects of major events that occur relatively infrequently to more minor events that constitute the stressors of everyday life. For children, these small events include problems in multiple domains of everyday life including school, friends, siblings, and parents. Research has consistently found that small events are correlated with major event scores, and correlate with child and adolescent problems over and above the effects of major events (Rowlison & Felner, 1988; DuBois et al., 1992; Wagner, Compas, & Howell, 1988).

Another important distinction between characteristics of environmental stress is between time-limited negative events and chronic stressful conditions. For example, poverty, having a chronic illness, or living with an alcoholic parent describe negative chronic conditions that can have pervasive effects over the child's environment. Such chronic stressful conditions can be differentiated from the acute major negative changes that occur in children's lives due to events such as parental death or divorce. Gersten, Langner, Eisenberg and Simcha-Fagan (1977) found that negative change events contributed little additional variance to the prediction of children's psychological problems after accounting for the effects of ongoing negative conditions.

Chronic conditions and negative changes are not mutually exclusive characteristics of children's social environment. Events are dynamically related in that major stressful events may be precipitated by chronic stressful conditions, and both may lead to increased occurrence of smaller stressors over time. This dynamic relation between stressors has important implications for the conceptualization and assessment of the effects of any major stressor. Although chronic (e.g., poverty) and acute major stressors (e.g., parental divorce or parental death) are sometimes considered to be single major events, they might be better conceptualized as ongoing processes involving the occurrence of multiple smaller stressors (Felner, Terre, & Rowlison, 1988). Illustratively, parental divorce may precipitate the occurrence of multiple stressors involving loss of time with the custodial or noncustodial parent, interparental quarrels, moving, increased parental distress, loss of family income, and so forth. There is considerable variability among divorces in the occurrence of these smaller stressors, and the stressfulness of the divorce can be assessed by variability in the occurrence of these divorce-related events. Illustratively, we have developed a measure of the small stressors that follow parental divorce and have found that divorce-related negative events predict the postdivorce adjustment of children in both cross-sectional and longitudinal studies (Sandler, Wolchik, Braver, & Fogas, 1986; Sandler, Wolchik, & Braver, 1988; Sandler et al., 1994). The assessment of smaller events has become an important tool in disaggregating the effects of a wide range of major stressors, such as parental alcoholism (Roosa, Sandler, Gehring, Beals, & Cappo, 1988), parental depression (Adrian & Hammen, 1993), poverty (Felner et al., 1995; Gonzales, Gunnoe, Jackson, & Samaniego, 1996), sexual abuse (Spacarelli, 1994), and transition to middle school (Seidman et al., 1994).

Several alternative models of the causal relations between stressful events and adjustment problems have been proposed (Dohrenwend & Dohrenwend, 1978). One model is that stressful events have a direct causal effect on increasing children's adjustment problems. Major and small events may have additive effects or small events may be caused by major events and mediate their effects, but in either case stressful events are conceptualized as causally related to increased adjustment problems. The strongest support for the causal relations between stressful events and mental health problems is derived from prospective longitudinal studies in which the effects of stressful events at time 1 are found to be significantly related to adjustment problems at time 2, controlling for the effects of initial adjustment problems (DuBois et al., 1992; Sandler et al., 1994; Seidman et al., 1994; Siegel & Brown, 1988; see, however, Swearingen & Cohen, 1985; Gersten et al., 1977; Roosa, Beals, Sandler, & Pillow, 1990, for failure to find prospective* effects for stress). It should be noted that these

---

*It is notable that relatively little is known about the appropriate time lag necessary to assess the effects of stress on mental health problems.

prospective longitudinal models are very conservative in that they assess the time-lagged effects of stress only, controlling for the effects of stress that are already present in the time 1 assessment.

An alternative model is one of bidirectional person–environment causality, with children's adjustment problems leading to increased environmental stressors as well as being caused by them. In support of this model, several prospective longitudinal studies have found that children's adjustment problems at time 1 predict the occurrence of stressors at time 2 (Roosa et al., 1990; Swearingen & Cohen, 1985; Compas, Wagner, Slavin, & Vannatta, 1986; DuBois et al., 1992; Sandler et al., 1994). Alternative models that have received some support, and will be considered later in this chapter, are that the effects of stressful events are mediated or moderated by characteristics of the child (e.g., coping) or social environment (e.g., social support).

Implications of Stressor Research for Intervention Design

The design of interventions to improve children's adaptation to stress can be informed in three important ways by research on stressful events (Fig. 1). First, the program might decrease the occurrence of the small events that are precipitated by the major events or chronic stressors by strategically working with influential social agents or institutions (path a). For example, reduction in children's exposure to the stressors of interparental conflict might be brought about by working with the custodial or noncustodial parent, or by institutional changes in the court system that attempt to minimize postdivorce conflict (e.g., mediation of disputes). Second, identifying the small events that are precipitated by the major stressor helps identify the social roles or motivational states that are negatively impacted by the stressors. For example, children of divorce need to deal with distressed parents who are fighting with each other, loss of time with parents, new relations with parental dating partners, and moving to a new neighborhood. Programs can be designed to help children develop coping strategies or marshal support to deal with the social roles that are disrupted by the stressors (path b) and negative motivational states (path c) that result from these events. For example, children of divorce might be helped to more effectively develop new role relations with their custodial parent, noncustodial parent, stepparent, or friends in a new school. Similarly, the program might help children cope in a way that maintains their self-esteem, sense of control, and sense of positive relatedness with their intimate social network.

Appraisal and Coping Variables

Appraisal

According to cognitive models, the critical process that leads to a stress response is the individual's appraisal that an event has negative implications for one's well-being. Appraisals have been studied both as styles of evaluating stressful events in general and as they occur in specific situations. One approach to assessing appraisal style involves systematic positive or negative distortions in the appraisal of negative events (Leitenberg, Yost, & Carroll-Wilson, 1986; Nolen-Hoeksema, Girgus, & Seligman, 1986). Mazur, Wolchik,

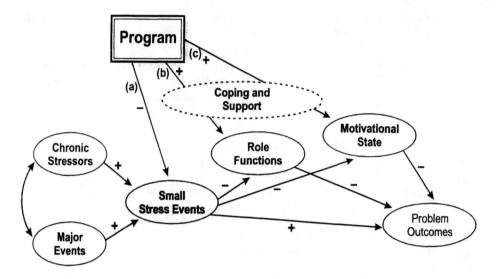

Figure 1. Program effects on stressors, role function, and motivational state. Note: Proximal mediators are shown in shaded ovals.

and Sandler (1992), for example, assessed children's negative cognitive errors (overgeneralization, personalization, catastrophizing) and positive illusions (high self-regard, control, and optimism) for hypothetical divorce-related stressors. They found that, after controlling for negative events and gender, total negative cognitive errors predicted mothers' reports of children's behavior problems and positive illusions predicted children's reports of anxiety.

Lazarus (1991) identified three components of appraising the implications of specific events, which correspond to three questions: (1) goal relevance (should I care?), (2) goal congruence (is this positive or negative?), and (3) type of ego-involvement (in what way am I or my goals and commitments involved?). Children's appraisals of the relevance and positivity or negativity of events that occurred to them have been assessed using ratings of whether an event is good or bad and of the degree of impact of the event (Johnson & Bradlyn, 1988). Several recent studies have also assessed type of ego involvement (Gamble, 1994; Grych, Seid, & Fincham, 1992; Sheets, Sandler, & West, 1996). Illustratively, Sheets et al. (1996) developed a measure of children's appraisals of divorce-related negative events. Based on open-ended interviews with children of divorce, they developed a self-report checklist of negative appraisals. Confirmatory factor analysis found developmental differences in the dimensional structure of appraisals. For children ages 8–10, a one-dimensional model provided an adequate fit for the data, whereas for children ages 11–12, a one-dimensional model was not adequate and a three-dimensional model provided an adequate fit, with the dimensions labeled threat to self, threat to others, and material loss. Negative appraisals were significant predictors of children's psychological problems in both cross-sectional and prospective longitudinal models. However, there was also evidence for bidirectional causality in that higher anxiety was also a significant prospective longitudinal predictor of children's negative appraisals.

Coping

Although the construct of appraisal is pivotal, it has received considerably less research attention than the construct of coping that focuses on how children respond once they have made a threatening appraisal for a stressful situation. Definitions of coping have varied in accord with different theoretical perspectives, such as psychoanalytic, transactional, and motivational. From the psychoanalytic perspective, coping typically has referred to the most mature ego processes, involving realistic and flexible thoughts and acts that contribute to more adaptive functioning (e.g., Haan, 1977, 1982). A problem with this approach is that it eliminates many thoughts and behaviors that individuals utilize to "cope" with the problems but which are not necessarily successful. As Stone, Helder, and Schneider (1988) argue, to understand which particular coping efforts are efficacious in any given situation, researchers first need to adopt a "neutral stance" regarding effectiveness.

Currently, the most prominent definition of coping is offered by Lazarus and Folkman (1984), who define coping as "constantly changing cognitive and behavioral efforts to manage specific external and/or internal demands that are appraised as taxing or exceeding the resources of the person" (p. 141). This transactional definition is relational in its focus and emphasizes that coping should be viewed as all cognitive and behavioral efforts, regardless of their outcomes, that are used to respond to specific external and internal demands. The definition highlights the importance of the characteristics of the situation and individual's appraisal of the stressful event. From Folkman and Lazarus's perspective, coping is intentional (rather than reflexive), and the functions of coping efforts are to manage the affective arousal in threatening situations and/or to change the situation.

From a motivational perspective, Skinner and Wellborn (1994) conceptualize coping as "an organizational construct that describes how people regulate their own behavior, emotion and motivational orientation under conditions of psychological distress" (p. 112). In this model, stress results from some environmental assault on basic psychological needs of relatedness, autonomy, and competence. Coping is energized by people's commitments to these needs and "encompasses peoples' struggles to maintain, restore, replenish, and repair the fulfillment of these needs" (p. 112). The immediate outcome of coping is to manage the individuals' engagement with versus disaffection from the stressful situation, and the longer-term outcome is to impact social, cognitive, and personality development. This conceptualization ties coping closely with developmental theory on regulation of emotion, behavior, and motivation and closely relates the specific coping behaviors with the nature of the stressful experience.

Similar to Menaghan (1993), we distinguish three broad categories of individual difference coping variables: coping resources, coping styles, and coping efforts or strategies. Coping resources refers to relatively stable characteristics of the individual that influence how children cope in specific situations. Coping resources include children's temperamental or personality characteristics, their generalized beliefs about themselves and their world (e.g., self-esteem, locus of control, optimism), and their skills (e.g., knowledge of problem-solving techniques). Coping styles refer to "generalized coping strategies defined as typical, habitual preferences for ways of approaching problems" (Menaghan, 1983, p. 159). Examples of constructs that assess coping style are repression–sensitization (Krohne & Rogner, 1982) and monitoring–blunting (e.g., Miller, Brody, & Summerton, 1988). Coping styles might also be assessed as strategies that people generally use to cope across a wide range of stressors (Carver, Scheier, & Weintraub, 1989). Lazarus and Folkman (1984) conceptualize coping efforts or strategies as cognitive and behavioral actions in a specific stressful situation which are intended to manage affective arousal or improve the problematic situation. Coping efforts continue over time and may change in response to the changing demands of the situation. Examples of such efforts or strategies include asking for help, thinking about alternative courses of action, refusing to think about the problem, and so forth.

The few empirical studies on the relations between resources, styles, and efforts indicate that these relations are complex and not always intuitively obvious (Ebata & Moos, 1994; Kliewer, 1991). Coping resources may directly influence children's use of coping strategies or they may make children more effective in carrying out specific strategies (Lengua & Sandler, 1996). Ebata and Moos (1994) found that adolescents with a more active temperament use more approach coping, while those with a temperament of higher negative emotionality used more avoidant strategies. Ayers, Sandler, West, and Roosa (in press) found moderate correlations between children's self-reported coping styles and the coping strategies they reported using in specific stressful situations (median r of .57 across 10 different coping categories). It is interesting to note that the relations between self-reported coping styles and situation-specific coping are higher for children than those found for adults (Carver et al., 1989), perhaps reflecting children's greater tendency to be less responsive to the specific demands and opportunities across stressful situations. Lengua and Sandler (1996) found that temperament moderated the relations between coping and children's psychological symptoms. Illustratively, for children with a more flexible and approach-oriented temperament, active coping was directly related to lower symptoms, while active coping was unrelated to symptoms for children who were less flexible and approach oriented.

Development of a categorization system is a fundamental step in studying the relations between coping and mental health problems. Theoretically, Lazarus and Folkman (1984) identified two broadband dimensions based on the intended functions of coping. Problem-focused strategies are aimed at changing the problematic situation, while emotion-focused strategies are aimed at managing or reducing the emotional distress. An alternative theoretical framework was based on the focus of coping, either toward or away from the stressful situation (Ebata & Moos, 1991). Approach coping involves cognition (e.g., positive reappraisal) or behaviors (e.g., direct action, support seeking) that focus on the stressful situation. Avoidant strategies involve cognitive or behavioral efforts to either not think about the stressor or to avoid encountering the stressful situation.

Broadband dimensions, however, are not very useful in studying the effects of coping efforts. For example, it may be that some efforts to manage emotional arousal are much more effective than others, a distinction that would be missed by studying only the broadband coping dimensions. Recently, several researchers have empirically identified narrow-band dimensions of coping using factor analytic approaches. Several studies using exploratory factor analysis have derived different dimensional structures (Causey & Dubow, 1992; Brodzinsky et al., 1992; Glyshaw, Cohen, & Towbes, 1989). Using confirmatory factor analysis, Ayers et al. (1996) empirically tested the adequacy of alternative theoretically derived dimensions of coping. They found that a four-dimensional model consisting of active coping, avoidance, distraction, and support seeking provided a better fit to the data than either an approach versus avoidance model or a problem-focused versus emotion-focused model. In this model, active coping includes both emotion-focused strategies (positive thinking) and problem-focused strategies (e.g., cognitive decision making and direct action). Distraction strategies such as listening to music or physical activity are distinguished from cognitive efforts to suppress thoughts about the situation (avoidance).

An issue with important implications for the design of preventive interventions involves the relation between specific coping strategies and mental health or substance use outcomes. We focus our discussion on identifying dimensions of coping that are consistently related to lower or higher levels of problems and also point out those dimensions where the findings have been inconsistent. Because of interpretation difficulties, we do not discuss findings on dimensions of coping such as internalizing or externalizing problems or substance use (Causey & Dubow, 1992) that are contaminated with the maladaptive outcomes they are predicting.

There is consistent evidence that dimensions of active coping that include problem solving and positive cognitions about a stressful situation are related to lower mental health and substance use problems. For example, both cross-sectional and longitudinal studies found that active coping strategies are related to lower emotional and behavioral problems and substance use (Ayers et al., 1996; Compas, Malcarne, & Fondacaro, 1988; Ebata & Moos, 1991; Glyshaw et al., 1988; Sandler et al., 1994; Wills, 1985, 1988). Other researchers have reported that problem focused coping significantly related to several positive developmental outcomes such as self-efficacy, self-esteem, and perceived competence in multiple domains (Brodzinsky et al., 1992; Causey & Dubow, 1992; Wills, 1985, 1988). Theoretically, the positive relations between problem-focused and positive-thinking strategies and better child adjustment may be due to their improving the stressful situation or leading to more benign interpretation of the stressor (e.g., that it will not threaten relatedness, autonomy, control, or esteem).

There is relatively consistent evidence that use of avoidance coping strategies (e.g., trying to not think about or avoiding dealing with a stressful event) is related to higher mental health problems in children and adolescents (Brodzinsky et al., 1992; Ebata & Moos, 1991; Causey & Dubow, 1992; Sandler et al., 1994; Ayers et al., 1996). Illustratively, based on cross-sectional analyses Wills (1986, 1988) reported that cognitive avoidance* was positively related to substance use and negatively related to self-efficacy. Sandler et al. (1994),

---

*In Wills' discussion of these analyses, he uses the label "distraction" coping. However, his items for both the intention-based measure (i.e., try to put the problem out of your mind) and the behavior-based measure (i.e., I daydream, and I put the problem out of my mind) more closely resemble what we refer to as cognitive avoidance. Our studies of the dimensional structure of coping distinguishes avoidant coping from distraction (Ayers et al., 1996; Sandler et al., 1994).

however, in their prospective analysis found that anxiety predicted higher avoidance coping, while avoidance coping did not prospectively predict anxiety. This finding is consistent with an interpretation that anxiety leads to a higher use of avoidance coping rather than the reverse causal direction. At a theoretical level the effects of avoidance coping strategies might be expected to differ as a function of the characteristics of the situation or of the individual. For example, in extremely high-stress situations, in uncontrollable stressful situations, or in acute stressful situations, avoidance may be adaptive in lowering the level of negative arousal, perhaps allowing the person time to mobilize for more active problem solving or positive cognitive reappraisal (Roth & Cohen, 1986; Suls & Fletcher, 1985). Individual differences in temperament or personality may also influence the degree to which use of avoidant coping leads to increased adjustment problems (Lengua & Sandler, 1996; Miller & Green, 1985). Thus, although the empirical evidence consistently indicates a positive relation between avoidant coping and mental health problems, the causal processes involved and the condition under which this relation occurs are not well understood.

Empirical evidence on the relations between distraction strategies and problem outcomes has been inconsistent. For example, in some studies distraction strategies such as social entertainment were positively related to substance use and higher mental health problems; however, they did not predict self-esteem or self-efficacy (Glyshaw et al., 1989; Wills, 1985, 1988). It may also be that types of distraction strategies affect outcomes differently. For example, physical exercise has been shown to relate to decreased subjective stress and negative life events over time (Wills, 1988) and higher concurrent levels of self-esteem (Glyshaw et al., 1989). Although Ayers (1991) and Sandler et al. (1994) did not find a significant cross-sectional relation between distraction coping and mental health problems, Sandler et al. (1994) reported significant inverse prospective paths between initial use of distraction and anxiety and depression 5½ months later.

Coping measures usually assess support as the act of seeking support and sometimes differentiate whether support is sought from parents or peers. Evidence is mixed concerning the relations of support-seeking coping with problem outcomes. Causey and Dubow (1992) found few significant relations between support seeking and children's adjustment. Wills (Wills, 1989; Wills & Vaughn, 1989) found that in a sample of adolescents seeking support from adults was positively related to self-esteem and negatively related to substance use, while peer support was positive related to substance use.* Glyshaw and colleagues (1989) found significant negative relations between parental support seeking and self-reports of depression in her cross-sectional analyses, but failed to find significant prospective effects. Ayers (1991) and Sandler et al. (1994) did not find any significant relations between support-seeking coping and child adjustment in cross-sectional analyses, although Sandler et al. (1994) reported a prospective positive relation between support coping and higher depression, controlling for initial levels of depression.

---

*It is important to note that the direction of causality between peer support and substance use cannot be inferred from these findings.

Implications of Coping and Appraisal Research for Intervention Programs

The design of interventions to improve children's adaptation to stressful situations can be informed by research on theoretical issues of coping and appraisal: (1) distinctions between coping resources, styles, and strategies; (2) the transactional values of coping; and (3) dimensions of coping. Figure 2 provides a schematic overview of alternative program approaches to enhance coping.

Two distinguishable approaches to intervention to enhance adaptive coping are building stable coping resources and styles and assisting in coping with the tasks of specific stressful situations. Coping resources (e.g., affect regulation skills, problem-solving competencies, and belief systems) and cross-situational styles of coping are relatively stable characteristics of the individual that develop as a function of constitutional factors (e.g., temperament) and life experience (e.g., relations with parents, prior encounters with stress). Theoretically, planned interventions that teach general skills (paths a and b) occur in the years prior to the occurrence of major stressors and will improve children's ability to cope effectively when they encounter specific stressful events. Considerable research has focused on building coping resources and styles (Greenberg, Kusche, Cook, & Quamma, 1995; Weissberg & Greenberg, in press). Illustratively, Greenberg et al. (1995) focused on "increasing children's ability to discuss emotions, utilize a larger emotional vocabulary, and understand meta-cognitive aspects of emotions" (p. 120). Currently, there is a large literature that demonstrates that problem-solving and affect awareness skill training programs have positive effects to strengthen these skills and to reduce a wide range of child mental health problems (Cowen et al., 1990; Durlak & Wells, in press; Elias & Weissberg, 1990). With a few exceptions (Dubow, Schmidt, McBride, Edwards, & Merk, 1993; Short et al., 1995), however, most of these programs have not specifically studied their effects on coping strategies with specific stressors. One program that studied the link between skills training and coping found that teaching fifth grade children social problem-solving skills resulted in increased feelings of effectiveness in coping with the stressors they encountered during the transition to middle school the following year (Elias, Gara, Schuyler, Branden-Muller, & Sayette, 1986).

One limitation of the experimental evaluations of programs to improve coping styles or resources is that they have generally not been successful in identifying the mediational paths between improvements in such competencies and improvements in children's mental health. Thus, we know little about how improvements in coping styles and resources lead to better mental health and/or improved coping strategies. One encouraging exception is a recent study that demonstrated that change in children's explanatory style mediated the effects of a cognitive training program to decrease depressive symptoms over a 2-year period (Gillham, Reivish, Jaycox, & Seligman, 1995).

The transactional definition of coping strategies focuses on what children think and do to handle the demands of specific situations that threaten their well-being. Interventions (path c) have been developed to assist children in coping with a specific stressful situation (Compas et al., 1989). Typically, such programs provide accurate information about the stressor; counteract patholog-

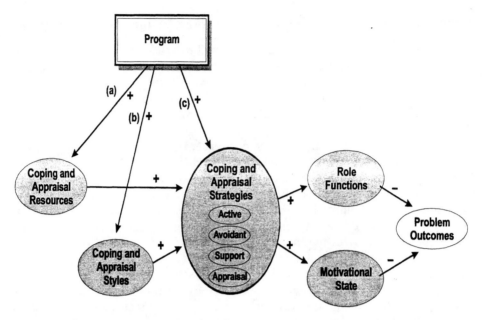

Figure 2. Program effects on coping and appraisal. Note: Proximal program mediators are shown in shaded ovals.

ical appraisals; teach problem-solving strategies, affect awareness, and affect regulation skills; provide social support from children confronting a similar stressor; and provide guided practice in applying the coping skills. Illustratively, several programs have been developed to help children cope with parental divorce, and experimental tests of these programs have shown positive effects to reduce children's psychological problems and improve their school adjustment (e.g., Pedro-Carroll & Cowen, 1987; Stolberg & Mahler, 1994). However, these evaluations have not systematically investigated the mediators that account for the positive effects of these programs, so we know little about how they achieve their positive effects. As described below, understanding of mediating mechanisms has important implications for strengthening and effectively disseminating such programs and contributing to our theoretical understanding of the coping process.

There is relatively consistent evidence that the dimension of active or approach-oriented coping strategies relate to fewer mental health problems. There is little empirical evidence, however, about how such strategies might work to meet the demands of specific stressful situations, particularly ones such as parental divorce, parental alcoholism, or living in poverty, that are beyond a child's control. Nolen-Hoeksema (1992) proposed that by positively reconstruing events, developing and achieving proximal goals, and using positive imagery that children could learn to adapt effectively in highly stressful situations where there is little apparent opportunity for control. Theoretically such processes help children maintain important role function (e.g., student, athlete) and positive motivational states (e.g., control, esteem) under adverse conditions. Studies are needed to investigate such processes and the effects of teaching specific strategies in these situations need to be carefully evaluated.

Social Support

In this section, we examine children's social support, one of several social resources that may protect children from the deleterious effects of stressful life events. We restrict our focus to social support rather than including other potential protective social resources, such as neighborhood context and support networks of parents, because of space limitations and because the empirical and theoretical literatures on social support are more extensive than those in other areas.

Researchers typically view social support as a complex, multidimensional construct including social relationships and supportive transactions (see Pierce, Sarason, Sarason, Joseph, & Henderson, 1996). Barrera (1986) makes the distinction between three aspects of social support: social embeddedness (connections or linkages between an individual and others in the environment), enacted support (frequency of supportive transactions), and perceived social support (subjective evaluation of the quality of support, availability of support, or relationships with supporters). Most inventories assess children's perceptions of the availability or quality of the following types of support: emotional, informational, instrumental, and social companionship (Cauce, Reid, Landesman, & Gonzales, 1990; Wills, Blechman, & McNamara, 1996), and most measures discriminate support from peers and parents/family members. In this chapter, we review only studies on support from parents/family and peers because of the predominance of research on these two types of support providers.

Research with adults has clearly indicated that measures of perceived social support are more strongly and consistently related to less adjustment problems than are measures of embeddedness or enacted support (Barrera, 1986; Cohen & Wills, 1985). Although the majority of researchers have used measures of perceived support in their work with children, the few studies that have assessed multiple aspects of support echo the finding in the adult literature that measures of perceived support show the most consistent evidence of negative relations with psychological problems (e.g., Barrera, 1981; Benson & Deeter, 1992; Greenberg, Seigel, & Leitch, 1983).

Two models of the beneficial effects of support have been tested: a direct effects model, which assumes that support is beneficial regardless of a child's current level of stress, and a stress-buffer model (e.g., Cogg, 1976; Cohen & Wills, 1985; Thoits, 1986), in which the negative effects of life events on adjustment problems are reduced under high support. A large body of cross-sectional research shows consistent, significant associations between family/parental support and a variety of positive outcomes, such as fewer internalizing and externalizing problems, fewer suicide behaviors, less drug and alcohol use, higher self-esteem, and better academic performance (e.g., Barrera & Garrison-Jones, 1992; Barrera, Chassin, & Rogosch, 1993; Licitra-Kleckler & Waas, 1993; Maton, 1990; Reifman & Windle, 1995; Rowlison & Felner, 1988; Stice, Barrera, & Chassin, 1993; Taylor, Casten, & Flickinger, 1993; Wills & Vaughan, 1989).

Although the results of longitudinal studies are not entirely consistent, a growing body of studies indicates that family/parental support is inversely related to later behavior problems and drug and alcohol use (e.g., DuBois et al., 1992; Slavin & Rainer, 1990; Windle, 1992).

In contrast, the findings on the direct effects of peer support are mixed. Some cross-sectional studies show nonsignificant relations or positive relations between peer support and adjustment problems (e.g., Cauce, Felner, Primavera, & Ginter, 1982; Cauce, Hannan, & Sargeant, 1992; Chassin, Presson, Sherman, Montello, & McGrew, 1986; Hirsch & Reischl, 1985; Windle, 1992; Wills & Vaughan, 1989; Wills, Mariani, & Filer, 1996; Wolchik, Ruehlman, Braver, & Sandler, 1989). However, other researchers have documented that peer support and adjustment problems are inversely related (Burke & Weir, 1978; DuBois & Ullman, 1989; Greenberg et al., 1983; Hirsch & DuBois, 1992; Rowlison & Felner, 1988). Findings from the few prospective studies are also mixed (e.g., DuBois et al., 1992; Dubow, Tisak, Causey, Hryshko, & Reid, 1991; Hirsch & DuBois, 1992; Windle, 1992). On the basis of 20 studies that included both peer and family support, Barrera and Li (1996) concluded that family support was more strongly and consistently related to psychological distress and behavior problems than was peer support.

Studies on whether social support buffers the negative effects of stress on children's adjustment have fairly consistently indicated a protective role for parental/family support but not for peer support (e.g., Greenberg et al., 1983; Quamma & Greenberg, 1994; Wills, 1986; Wills, Vaccaro, & McNamara, 1992; Wolchik et al., 1989). In sum, whereas the research on the beneficial effects of peer support is equivocal, there is consistent empirical support for both the direct and stress-buffer effects of family/parental support.

Although few researchers have studied the interrelations between parental and peer support, recent studies underscore the importance of examining how the parent–child relationship influences adolescents' reliance on peer support or the relation between peer support and developmental outcomes. For example, Fuligni and Eccles (1993) reported that early adolescents who viewed their parents as providing few opportunities for decision making were higher in peer advice seeking. Several studies find that in the absence of parental or adult support, peer support may have negative rather than positive effects. Wills (1990) found that teens with low adult support and high peer support were disproportionately at risk for substance abuse. Similarly, Barrera and Garrison-Jones (1992) reported that the effects of peer and family support interacted in the prediction of adolescent adjustment, such that peer support was inversely related to depression when family support was low.

How does social support achieve its protective effects? Several researchers have speculated that support mitigates the debilitating effects of stress through its impact on self-esteem, perceptions of control, social integration, or coping (Kliewer, Sandler, & Wolchik, 1994; Sandler, Miller, Short, & Wolchik, 1989; Skinner & Wellborn, 1994; Wills et al., 1996). These researchers assume a set of causal linkages between the stressors, social support, the intervening process, and mental health outcomes. For example, stress might decrease self-esteem, while social support counteracts that effect by increasing self-esteem; self-esteem in turn affects mental health problems and mediates the effects of stress and support on mental health problems. In this model, supportive transactions allow positive social comparisons or provide or reinforce esteem-enhancing messages. Although there is a reasonable amount of research supporting portions of the stress/self-esteem/outcome model (see DuBois, Felner, Meares, & Krier, 1994, for a discussion of this research), to date only one study has tested a mediational model. The findings of this prospective study provide support for self-esteem mediating the relation between social support and internalizing but not externalizing problems (DuBois et al., 1994).

Social support may influence children's coping processes in four ways: (1) directly instructing or reinforcing specific coping efforts and threat appraisals; (2) modeling coping and adaptive appraisals for dealing with stress; (3) providing a family context that supports effective coping and appraisals of stressors; or (4) facilitating access to helpful resources (Kliewer et al., 1994; Skinner & Wellborn, 1994; Wills et al., 1996). Recently, Hoffman and Levy-Shiff (1994) reported a significant association between adolescents' and mothers' coping profiles, evidence that is consistent with a modeling mechanism. Also, Wills et al. (1996) found that parental support was related to increased adaptive coping, decreased nonadaptive coping, and decreased substance use over time.

Another mechanism through which support may mitigate the effects of stress involves children's perceptions of control (Sandler et al., 1989; Skinner & Wellborn, 1994). Supportive relationships may reduce children's exposure to control-threatening events by maintaining a predictable social environment for them as well as encouraging realistic interpretation of the ability to control the stressful experiences (Sandler et al., 1989). It is also plausible that support affects the adjustment of children under stress by impacting their sense of security of social relationships (Sandler et al., 1989; Skinner & Wellborn, 1994). Supportive exchanges may help children maintain a belief that they are part of a continuing and caring social unit or provide predictable experiences that promote a sense of social integration.

It is important to note that these mechanisms of action are not independent and that supportive exchanges are likely to affect multiple intervening processes. For example, supportive actions that enhance perceptions of control are likely to positively impact self-esteem; supportive exchanges that affect self-esteem may enhance one's sense of belonging and social integration. These likely relations highlight the need for researchers to investigate multiple mechanisms simultaneously. Although there are extensive data for some of the linkages included in this model (see Sandler et al., 1989; Skinner & Wellborn, 1994), to date, the full model has not been empirically examined.

This discussion of mediating mechanism has focused on how supportive actions mitigate the effects of stressors once they have occurred. However, supportive exchanges that occur outside of the context of stressors also affect children's ability to deal with them. Analogous to our earlier discussion of coping resources, one can conceptualize supportive resources that facilitate children receiving and effectively using support for stressful situations. As noted by Wills et al. (1996) and Wellborn and Skinner (1994), consistent supportive exchanges can promote the development of positive internal working models of relationships that facilitate children's ability to seek the support and assistance they need to master small and large stressors. Successive mastery experiences can lead to a wide range of positive outcomes, such as academic and social competencies, which have direct as well as stress-buffer effects on adjustment problems (e.g., Kliewer & Sandler, 1992; Wills & Cleary, 1996; Wills et al., 1996). Supporters may also regulate children's exposure to stressors by taking actions themselves or encouraging children to take actions to prevent the occurrence of stressors and by shielding them from stressors that do occur (Skinner & Wellborn, 1994). Illustratively, a recent study found that parental support at the initial assessment was significantly related to lower levels of negative events a year later (Wills et al., 1996).

Implications of Support Research for the Development of Interventions

What are the implications of the research on children's social support for programs to bring about more positive developmental outcomes and prevent the negative effects of stress on mental health? The consistent evidence that children who perceive high levels of support from their parents are better adjusted and that support from parents reduces the negative effects of stressors on children's mental health outcomes strongly suggests that a focus on parental support in prevention programs would be productive. As shown in Fig. 3, program-induced enhancement of perceptions of parental support may affect children's mental health outcomes by increasing their self-esteem, sense of social integration, perceptions of control, and/or the effectiveness of their coping efforts. Although the specific parental behaviors that lead to enhanced perceptions of parental support have not been studied, examination of the most commonly used measures of perceived support suggests that programs designed to enhance parents' basic listening skills, empathy skills, and skills in helping children think through problems might increase children's perceptions that their parents are supportive.

Although evidence is equivocal as to whether support from peers has general beneficial effect on children's mental health outcomes, an important direction for future research involves identifying settings and personality variables that may moderate the impact of peer support. It may be that when adolescents are disaffected from adult supporters, they reinforce each other for counternormative ways of coping. It may be that programs might be effective if they can induce peer groups that have shared a common stress experience to reinforce each other for adaptive coping (Felner & Adan, 1988; Pedro-Carroll & Cowen, 1987; Silver, Coupey, Bauman, Doctors, & Boeck, 1992).

Furthermore, many child-focused programs that teach skills to deal with stressful situations include a component in which key social network members (e.g., parents, teachers, peers) are utilized to promote effective use of these skills (Weissberg, Caplan, & Spivo, 1989). The potential positive impact of such programs has been demonstrated (e.g., Elias et al., 1986), although other programs have had less success in enhancing coping by marshaling key social resources (Stolberg & Mahler, 1994).

This section has presented a brief overview of three major constructs used in transactional models of adaptation to stress, stressful events, coping and appraisal, and social support. Advances have been made in conceptualizing and assessing these constructs and beginning to study their relations to the

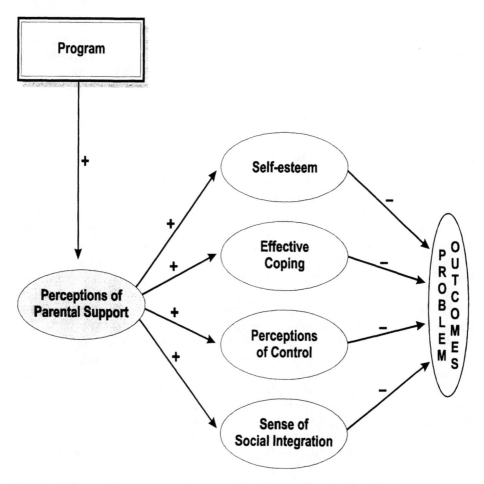

Figure 3. Program effects on parental support. Note: Proximal program mediators are shown in shaded ovals.

health, mental health, and substance use problems that often result from poor adaptation in stressful situation. The next section shifts the focus of the chapter to the design and evaluation of theoretically derived interventions to promote more adaptive outcomes.

DESIGN AND EVALUATION OF THEORETICALLY GUIDED INTERVENTIONS FOR CHILDREN IN STRESS

Theoretical models of adaptation to stress provide a guiding framework for the development and evaluation of interventions for the prevention of a wide range of mental and physical health problems and for the promotion of positive developmental outcomes for children in stressful situations. We propose that clearly articulated and empirically supported theory provides the foundation for strategic decisions concerning program development, evaluation, and dissemination (Lorion, Price, & Eaton, 1989; Lipsey, 1990). This section discusses four steps in the development and evaluation of theory guided interventions: (1) selection of the proximal processes to change (mediators) to bring about desired outcomes; (2) development of an experimental design to assess program effects on mediators and desired outcomes; (3) analysis and interpretation of the results of the experimental trial; and (4) redesign of the intervention to strengthen effects or disseminate the program.

Developing the Theory of the Intervention: Selection of Proximal Mediators to Improve Children's Adaptation

Children's adaptation to stressful situations is affected by multiple interrelated variables. For example, there is evidence that children's adaptation to divorce is affected by the occurrence of smaller divorce-related stressors, ongoing conflict between the parents, psychological distress of the custodial parent, parenting on the part of the custodial and noncustodial parent, children's locus of control, and children's coping (Grych & Fincham, 1993; Emery & Forehand, 1994). In addition, there may be complex causal chains between these variables. Interparental conflict may increase parental distress, which may in turn affect the quality of parenting. If these variables are causally connected to children's postdivorce adjustment, they are potential mediators of the effects of a planned intervention; changing them should improve adjustment.

How do researchers make their way through the overwhelming assortment of possible potential mediators to design an intervention? Two issues must be confronted in making these strategic decisions: (1) Is it plausible that the potential mediators are causally related to the outcomes? (2) Is it plausible that the mediators are modifiable by an intervention that can be effectively delivered to the population experiencing the stressful situation?

Empirical evidence of the relations between the potential mediator and the outcome variables is critical for identifying plausible causes of the outcomes. Optimally, such evidence comes from a test of a prospective longitudinal model that includes latent constructs of the major plausible causal constructs. Support for a given causal model is particularly compelling when alternative theoretical models have also been tested and rejected as inconsistent with the data. While tests of such models do not justify conclusions about the causal nature of these relations, they do justify continuing to consider them plausible causes (Games, 1988). Plausible causes of the outcomes are selected as the immediate (proximal) targets of the intervention (Fig. 4a), and the theory of the intervention is that change in these variables (paths a, b, c) leads to change in the more distal outcomes. Stronger paths from a variable to the outcome make a variable potentially a more powerful mediator of program effects. However, because variables are typically moderately correlated, even weak paths may indicate useful mediators that share meaningful effects with other variables.

More complicated models that test chains of causal connections between variables leading to an outcome may provide useful hypotheses about points of maximal influence on the outcomes. For example, for children of divorce, distress of the custodial parent may be a common cause of poor parenting and increased bad-mouthing of the ex-spouse, which in turn fully mediate the effects of parental distress on child mental health outcomes (Fig. 4b). An effi-

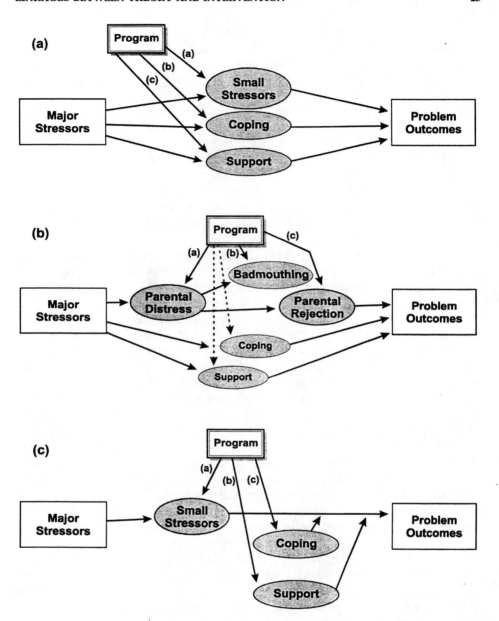

Figure 4. Developing theory of the intervention. Note: Proximal program mediators are shown in shaded ovals. Dotted arrows in b indicate potential intervention paths that are not discussed in text.

cient intervention in this case may be directed at changing the most distal variable in the causal chain (parental distress), expecting that this change will lead to improved parenting and decreased bad-mouthing and improved outcomes for the child. Alternatively, one might design a strategy to change each of the more proximal variables directly. Choice of whether to target more distal or proximal mediators depends on the researchers beliefs about which ones can be most effectively and efficiently changed.

A moderating pathway in which a variable weakens the effect of a second variable on mental health outcomes is particularly significant for stress based models. For example (Fig. 4c), there is evidence that social support from parents (path b) and active coping (path c) by children of divorce reduces the effects of stressful events on children's depressive symptoms (Sandler et al., 1994; Wolchik et al., 1989). A moderating variable might be a reasonable intervention under one of two conditions: (1) the variable that is being moderated has a relatively strong effect on the outcome but is relatively difficult to change directly (path a), or (2) the participants who come into the intervention disproportionately include those who have high scores on the variable whose effects are being moderated. For example, if families who self-select into a program for children of divorce experience higher levels of divorce-related stressors, then variables that are most strongly related to symptoms at high levels of stress are reasonable intervention targets.

A second consideration in the choice of proximal variables to target is their potential modifiability by a program that can be delivered to the population. Variables that might be important in a general etiologic theory of problem development (e.g., personality variables of agreeableness or negative affectivity) are less changeable than specific communication or self-talk skills that can influence outcomes in a stressful situation. Confidence that a variable is modifiable is maximized where the efficacy of existing technology to change a specific mediator has been demonstrated in previous experimental trials. Often such trials have been done in other contexts so that program developers need to adapt the existing technology to the current problem. For example, there is convincing evidence from the treatment literature for the efficacy of techniques to improve parenting (Graziano & Diament, 1992; Patterson, 1975). Since there is strong evidence that parenting is an important mediator of the effects of divorce on children's outcomes, the issue becomes whether these techniques can be adapted to fit the context of a short program for divorced parents. Illustratively, Fig. 5 shows an experimental intervention for custodial parents following divorce that is designed to use the parent as a change agent to improve four potentially modifiable mediators of children's adjustment: quality of mother–child relationship, effective discipline, father–child contact, and interparental conflict (Wolchik, Sandler, West, and Anderson, 1997). In this model, four intervention elements are designed to change the quality of the mother–child relationship, three elements are used to improve discipline, and two elements are used to improve father–child contact and to reduce interparental conflict.

Modifiability of a mediator may also depend on the conceptualization of the problem and the reality-based constraints placed on program design. If the problem is conceptualized as assisting coping with the transition that occurs around some change in family structure (e.g., parental divorce) (Felner et al., 1988), intervention design may call for a relatively short-term intervention. Programs would work with the change agents who provide maximal leverage to change the putative mediators. The custodial mother might be targeted to learn parenting skills, reduce children's exposure to stress, and support the child's coping. The child may be targeted to improve coping with the stressors of the

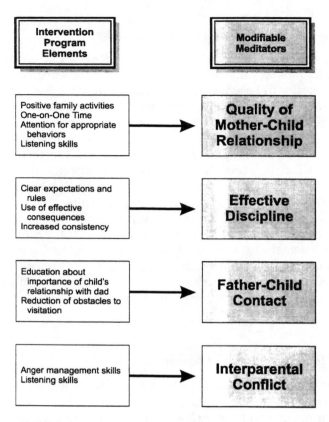

Figure 5. Links between program elements and modifiable mediators in program for custodial parents following divorce.

postdivorce environment. The noncustodial parent might be targeted to improve parenting skills or reduce children's exposure to interparental conflict. If a program focuses on chronic stressors such as poverty, a chronic physical illness, or disability, then interventions might target more stable characteristics of the child or the social environment. For example, deaf children might benefit from education programs that teach more effective cognitive affective development (Greenberg, Lengua, & Calderon, Chapter 11, this volume), or by social policies that create settings that ensure adequate educational and vocational opportunities. Children in poverty might benefit from programs that build competencies that serve as coping resources by providing adequate health care and early educational experiences and by supporting effective parenting in the early stages of life. More contemporaneously, a neighborhood or family-based program might help shield children from the environmental dangers in the inner city or might build settings that support the accomplishments of proximal goals to counteract feelings of loss of control or low self-worth (Nolen-Hoeksema, 1992; Tolan, Guerra, & Montaini-Klovdahl, Chapter 16, this volume).

Experimental Design for Evaluating the Effects of the Program on the Proximal Mediators and Mental Health Outcomes

The primary objective of using theory for program development is to design maximally effective and efficient programs. Theoretically, maximal program effectiveness will be achieved by changing all of the processes that mediate adaptation to stress. Thus, programs might be designed to simultaneously reduce the occurrence of stressful events, increase social support, and increase adaptive coping. However, the objective of changing all plausible mediators must be balanced by considerations of efficiency and practicality of program delivery, as well as by strategic decisions as to the critical questions to be addressed in an experimental trial (Sandler, Braver, Wolchik, Pillow, & Gersten, 1991). Two strategies will be discussed concerning the development and testing of experimental change programs, testing of alternative combinations of intervention components that are designed to change different mediators, and use of mediation analysis (see West & Aiken, in press; MacKinnon, 1994, for a fuller discussion of design and analysis issues in such studies). Our examples are drawn from research with children of divorce because of the extensive theoretical research and recent program development work focusing on this stressor.

Testing Multiple Intervention Components

Potential mediating variables are often clustered according to potential agents of influence. For example, following divorce the custodial parent has a great deal of influence over providing appropriate warmth and discipline in the home, the level of children's exposure to family stressors such as bad-mouthing and interparental quarrels, and perhaps some influence over the child's coping. Children have primary control over their choice of coping strategies, how they appraise divorce stressors, and how they communicate with parents. Noncustodial parents have influence over children's exposure to interparental conflict, the quality and quantity of their relationships with their children, and economic stressors on the custodial parent. Program components can be designed to work with specific change agents to change those processes over which they have most influence, and experimental designs can be developed to change the single and additive effects of these components (West & Aiken, in press).

Results of the experimental studies testing multiple component interventions with children of divorce have been surprising. Stolberg and Garrison (1985) used a 2 × 2 factorial design to test the effects of a parenting support group, a child support group, a combined condition (parenting support group and child support group), and a no-treatment control condition. Results indicated that children in the child-support-only group showed more improvement than children in the combined condition in self-concept at immediate posttest and social skills at 5-month follow-up. Similarly, parental adjustment improved more for the parent support group as compared to the combined condition on the measure of parental divorce adjustment. These results indicate subtractive rather than additive effects on child mental health for the combined condition. In the second trial, Stolberg and Mahler (1994) again found that adding multiple components did not have the expected effects, but instead improved the outcome on one variable, delayed gains on a second variable, and reduced gains on a third variable. These two studies indicate that the addition of components may as easily weaken as strengthen program effects. Unfortunately, because the evaluation design did not test the mediating mechanisms, it is difficult to understand the underlying theoretical processes that account for them.

Analysis of Mediating Mechanisms

Mediational analysis is a family of techniques to empirically test the mechanism by which an intervention affects a designed outcome. The general model is that the program changes a mediator, which in turn affects an outcome, and the significance of the mediated effect can be tested using techniques outlined in the next section. The mediational hypotheses are derived from theory concerning the causal relations between the intervention and the stress, support and coping variables, and between these variables and problematic outcomes. Four aspects of research design that are critical for mediation analysis are randomization, measurement, sample size, and sampling of participants.

If randomization to conditions is done correctly, any observed program effects can be attributed to the intervention and not to some other unmeasured variable. The randomization of units to conditions is particularly important for mediation analysis because the relation between the mediator and the outcome variable is correlated, not experimental, and is subject to multiple alternative explanations. If units are not assigned randomly to the program conditions, then the relations between the program and the mediator may also be due to multiple factors, greatly increasing the number of alternative explanations of the mediated effect.

Unreliability in the measures is more serious in mediation analysis than in analysis of direct program effects on outcomes, because error in both the mediator and the outcome measures attenuates estimates of mediated effects. One strategy to deal with the problem of unreliability is to use measurement models for the mediators and outcomes targeted using covariance structure modeling. The mediation effect is then calculated using structural coefficients among true or latent measures. A limitation to the use of these methods is that the constructs are latent or unobserved, leading to some ambiguity in the interpretation of results (Freedman, 1987).

Although detailed studies of the statistical power of tests of mediated effects are only now being completed, it is clear that a larger sample is needed to detect mediated effects than direct program effects. The methods used to create confidence intervals for mediated effects are based on asymptotic statistical theory, but they appear to be quite accurate starting at a sample size of 50 for a one-mediator model and normally distributed measures (MacKinnon, Warsi, & Dwyer, 1995).

Although random sampling ensures generalizability of the effects of the population, not all subjects might be optimally changed by the program. Research has often found that programs to facilitate adaptive outcomes in stressful situations are more effective for participants who are experiencing more problems initially than with participants who are adapting well (Sandler et al., 1992; Wolchik et al., 1993). Thus, studies that oversample participants who are experiencing problems on the outcomes and the mediators will have increased power to detect program effects (Pillow, Sandler, Braver, Wolchik, & Gersten, 1991). Theoretically, if the identified mediators account for differences in adaptation and are the mechanisms by which the program affects change, then only participants who are low on the mediators will benefit from the program.

Analysis and Interpretation of the Test of Mediation of Intervention Effects

An overview of the steps to test mediation of the effects of a program to improve adaptation to stress is described (see MacKinnon & Dwyer, 1993, for details on the statistical analyses). We describe a hypothetical mediation analysis for a program designed to reduce stressful events, improve coping, and improve social support, and each of these variables is assessed as a latent variable. As shown in Fig. 6, the theory of the intervention is that program-induced change in these three proximal mediators will lead to a reduction in the distal outcome. We assume that the program has been delivered to approximately half the participants who have been randomly assigned to conditions. The four questions in testing mediation are briefly reviewed below.

1. Is there a program effect on symptoms? The statistical significance of the program effect on the outcome measure is the primary focus of all prevention studies. If there is a statistically significant program effect, then mediation analysis may suggest the processes through which it worked. Mediation analysis is also important when there is not a statistically significant program effect because some mediators may reduce the problem behavior and others increase it (a suppressor effect), leading to a nonsignificant overall program effect on outcomes when mediation actually exists. The surprising finding of a subtractive effect of a multicomponent program for children of divorce (Stolberg & Garrison, 1985) described above may be because the multicomponent program affected different mediators in opposite directions.

2. Is there a program effect on the mediators? The test of the program's effect on the mediators (paths a1 through a3) serves as a manipulation check for the technology of the program. It is critical that the measures of these mediators are reliable and consistent with the theory of the intervention. For example, if it is hypothesized that the program affects outcomes by changing perceived support, then a measure of social embeddedness or enacted support would provide an inappropriate test of program effects on the theoretical mediator.

3. Is the effect of the mediator statistically significant when both program exposure and the mediators are included as predictors of the outcome variable? For there to be mediation, the mediator must be significantly related to the outcome variable when both the mediator and the program exposure variable are included in the model (paths b1 through b3). If the program effect is zero when adjusted for the mediator (path b4), then there is evidence for mediation.

4. Is the mediated effect statistically significant? The mediated effect is calculated as the multiplication of the parameter coding the program effect on the mediator times the parameter coding the mediator effect on the outcome

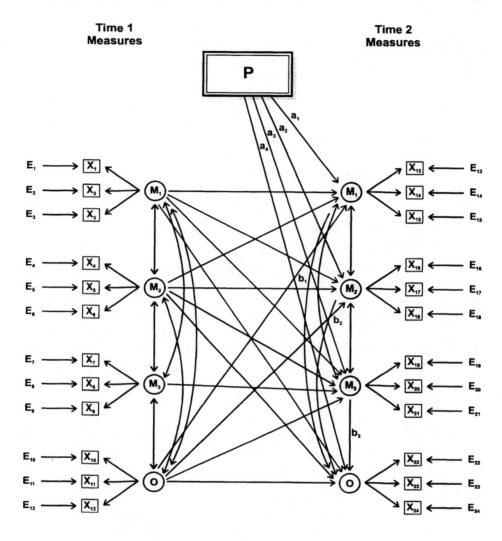

Note: **M1** - Small Stressors
        M2 - Active Coping
        M3 - Perceived Support
        P - Program
        O - Outcome

Figure 6. Model for the evaluation of mediators of the effects of an experimental program.

(a1b1, a2b2, a3b3). The standard error of the mediated effect was derived by Sobel (1982) and Folmer (1981) using the multivariate delta method. Confidence limits for the mediated effect are then used to determine if the size of the effect is large enough to conclude that the mediated effect is statistically significant. A significant mediated effect provides strong support that the program effect is due to changes in the mediator and is supportive of the theory of the intervention.

Because adaptation to stress is determined by multiple variables and interventions often target multiple potential mediators, it is unlikely that a single mediator would completely explain program effects on distal outcomes (Baron & Kenny, 1986). Measures of the percent of the program effect that is mediated and the ratio of the mediated to the nonmediated effect help in interpretation of results. Calculation of the percent of program effect that is mediated (mediated effect divided by the total program effect) allows the researcher to state, for example, that 43% of the program effect was due to changes in the perceived support variable. Simulation studies (MacKinnon et al., 1995) suggest that sample sizes of 500 are needed for accurate estimates of the proportion of the program effect that was mediated.*

Implications of Mediational Analysis for Program Redesign and Dissemination

When the program has not had the desired effects on mental health outcomes, mediational analysis can provide important information for program redesign. Two alternative explanations need to be considered: failure of technology and failure of theory. Failure of technology occurs when the program did not lead to significant changes in the targeted mediators. Several possible explanations for the absence of change in the mediator should be considered:

1. Was there sufficient power to detect effects on the mediating variables? Power at a given level of alpha is a function of sample size and size of the effect to be detected and is affected by reliability of measurement of the mediators and outcomes.
2. Was the program designed in a way to optimize behavior change? The program may not be sufficiently engaging, may not be credible, may not provide sufficient opportunities for practice or feedback of program skills, or it may not lead participants to believe that they can effectively apply the program skills. Some of these program concerns can be assessed by reviewing program manuals, observing tapes of the sessions, or interviewing participants about their perceptions of the program.
3. Were the program components delivered with sufficient strength and integrity? Process evaluation can identify problems in program delivery such as inadequate training of the program delivery agents, lack of attendance, or failure to complete specific program elements.
4. Are program effects assessed at the appropriate time? Program effects on some mediating variables may require extensive use of program skills and may not be apparent immediately after program completion. Illustratively, children may need repeated experience of receiving helpful support to change their perception that helpful support is available when they need it.
5. Are other program components detracting from program effects on one of the mediators? Illustratively, the success of one component in pre-

---

*It should be noted that the accuracy of the measure of the proportion of effect that was mediated depends on the size of the nonmediated effect (MacKinnon et al., 1995).

venting the occurrence of stressful events reduces the opportunity to engage in activities taught in other program components (e.g., use of coping strategies or obtaining social support).

Failure of theory occurs when the program has successfully changed a putative coping, support, or stress mediator, but change in that putative mediator does not lead to a corresponding change in a mental health outcome. In such cases it may be useful to reexamine how the construct is being measured. For example, coping has been assessed as resources (e.g., knowledge of appropriate coping strategies) and as use of those strategies in specific stressful situations to accomplish some functions (e.g., maintain self-esteem, sense of control or efficacy, etc.). While many programs teach knowledge of specific strategies, there is little theoretical reason to expect that such knowledge, without corresponding effective use, leads to better mental health outcomes.

When experimental trials with a high degree of internal validity have provided evidence of program efficacy, the next step involves replication and dissemination studies in which the program is delivered on a larger scale and in multiple contexts. Information derived from analysis of mediators can be very useful to guide decisions concerning how to deliver an effective program under these conditions. The objective in disseminating interventions is to maintain their effectiveness when the program is delivered in different sites, within different organizational contexts, and to different populations. A dilemma is created in that effectiveness is believed to be a function of two apparently contradictory principles (Mayer & Davidson, in press; Price & Lorion, 1989). The first principle is that effectiveness is a function of fidelity of implementation of the program that has demonstrated effects. Alterations of the original program detracts from fidelity, and thus reduces confidence that program effects will replicate. On the other hand, it has been argued that differences in local conditions require that the program be changed. For example, programs may need to adapt to organizational constraints, limited resources, and different populations. Modifying the original program may also be critical for an organization to feel a sense of ownership and commitment to the program. Research has provided support for both sides of the fidelity versus adaptation argument. For example, Blakely et al. (1987) found that fidelity of implementation was positively related to program effectiveness in a study of the dissemination of educational and criminal justice programs. However, modifications that involved additions to the program also contributed to effectiveness over and above fidelity of implementation.

Price and Lorion (1989) propose that the program developers identify core elements of their programs that are essential and must be implemented with a high degree of fidelity and adaptive elements that can be modified to meet local conditions. If we conceptualize program components as being primarily responsible for change in different potential mediators, assessment of the mechanisms by which programs have their effects is an important step in making decisions about core and adaptive program components. Program components that involve changing variables that are found to be partial or complete mediators of program effects should be considered core program components. Disseminated versions of the program should implement these components with high fidelity and evaluate whether the mediating effects are replicated under the new conditions. The identification of program components that are not linked to mediating variables should be done conservatively, being aware of the multiple reasons why a true mediating variable might not be significant. Even if they are not themselves mediators, some components might be essential parts of the program because they have other facilitative effects. They may promote the nonspecific elements of credibility, commitment, or support that enhance program effects but are not assessed in the mediational analysis. They might facilitate change on other mediating mechanisms. For example, completion of activities that improve the mother–child relationship might be a prerequisite for teaching effective joint problem-solving skills or discipline skills. Thus, while failure to demonstrate mediation for a variable should not rule out its potential importance, affirmative evidence of mediation by a variable should support the conclusion that all components linked to that variable are core elements to be implemented with a high degree of fidelity in dissemination efforts.

CONCLUDING SUMMARY

The objective of this chapter is to strengthen the linkages between theoretical research on resilience and the design and evaluation of interventions to promote resilience. The linking theoretical constructs have derived from transactional models of stress and coping. Research and theory have begun to better define and measure the key constructs of stressful events, coping, and support and to provide evidence about how they contribute to better adaptation to adverse conditions. Interventions can be designed to modify variables that are empirically supported as leading to better adaptation. Methodologically it was proposed that experimental tests of the interventions be designed to assess mediating mechanisms by which the program effects on the theoretical mediators account for effects of the program on the desired outcomes. Such tests provide an experimental assessment of the causal relations between the theoretical mediators and the desired outcomes and can lead to the development of stronger and more disseminatable interventions to promote more adaptive outcomes for children in stressful situations.

ACKNOWLEDGMENTS
Support for writing this chapter was provided by NIMH Grant #P50-MH39246 to support a Preventive Intervention Research Center at Arizona State University, which is gratefully acknowledged. Many of the ideas in this chapter are the result of ongoing dialogue with our colleagues at the center, particularly Sanford Braver and Stephen West. We thank them for their stimulating ideas. We thank the students at the center who work with us on our shared action research agenda and we thank Mindy Herman-Stahl, who contributed some very interesting ideas in the early stages of the project. Special thanks are due to Kathy Wilcox for her diligent work in developing the references and to Earnest Fairchild for his creative graphics.

REFERENCES

Adrian, C., & Hammen, C. (1993). Stress exposure and stress generation in children of depressed mothers. *Journal of Consulting and Clinical Psychology, 61,* 354–359.

Ayers, T. S. (1991). *A dispositional and situational assessment of children's coping: Testing alternative theoretical models.* Unpublished doctoral dissertation, Arizona State University, Tempe.

Ayers, T. S., Sandler, I. N., West, S. G., & Roosa, M. W. (1996). A dispositional and situational assessment of children's coping: Testing alternative models of coping. *Journal of Personality, 64,* 923–958.

Baron, R. M., & Kenny, D. A. (1986). The moderator–mediator variable distinction in social psychological research: Conceptual, strategic, and statistical considerations. *Journal of Personality and Social Psychology, 51,* 1173–1182.

Barrera, M., Jr. (1981). Social support in the adjustment of pregnant adolescents: Assessment issues. In B. Gottlieb (Ed.), *Social networks and social support* (pp. 69–96). Beverly Hills, CA: Sage.

Barrera, M., Jr. (1986). Distinctions between social support concepts, measures and models. *American Journal of Community Psychology, 14,* 413–441.

Barrera, M., Jr., & Garrison-Jones, C. (1992). Family and peer social support as specific correlates of adolescent depressive symptoms. *Journal of Abnormal Child Psychology, 20,* 1–16.

Barrera, M., Jr., Chassin, L., & Rogosch, F. (1993). Effects of social support and conflict on adolescent children of alcoholic and nonalcoholic fathers. *Journal of Personality and Social Psychology, 64,* 602–612.

Barrera, M., Jr., & Li, S. (1996). The relation of family support to adolescents' psychological distress and behavior problems. In G. R. Pierce, B. S. Sarason, & I. G. Sarason (Eds.), *Handbook of social support and the family* (pp. 313–343). New York: Plenum Press.

Benson, L. T., & Deeter, T. E. (1992). Moderators of the relation between stress and depression in adolescents. *The School Counselor, 39,* 189–194.

Blakely, C., Mayer, J., Gottschalk, R., Schmitt, N., Davidson, W., Roitman, D., & Emshoff, J. (1987). The fidelity-adaptation debate: Implications for the implementation of public sector social programs. *American Journal of Community Psychology, 15,* 253–268.

Bloom, B. L. (1990). Stressful life events and the prevention of psychopathology. In NIMH (Ed.), *Conceptual research models for preventing mental disorders* (pp. 63–90). DHHS Publication No. (ADM) 90-1713, Washington, DC.

Brodzinsky, D. M., Elias, M. J., Steiger, C., Simon, J., Gill, M., & Hitt, J. C. (1992). Coping scale for children and youth: Scale development and validation. *Journal of Applied Developmental Psychology, 13,* 195–214.

Burke, R. J., & Weir, T. (1978). Benefits of adolescents of informal helping relationships with their parents and peers. *Psychological Reports, 42,* 1175–1184.

Caplan, R. D., Vinokur, A. D., Price, R. H., & van Ryn, M. (1989). Job seeking, reemployment, and mental health: A randomized field experiment in coping with job loss. *Journal of Applied Psychology, 74,* 759–769.

Carver, C. S., Scheier, M. F., & Weintraub, J. K. (1989). Assessing coping strategies. *Journal of Personality and Social Psychology, 56,* 267–283.

Cauce, A. M., Felner, R. D., Primavera, J., & Ginter, M. A. (1982). Social support in high risk adolescents: Structural components and adaptive impact. *American Journal of Community Psychology, 10,* 417–428.

Cauce, A. M., Hannan, K., & Sargeant, M. (1992). Life stress, social support, and locus of control during early adolescence: Interactive effects. *American Journal of Community Psychology, 20,* 787–798.

Cauce, A. M., Reid, M., Landesman, S., & Gonzales, N. (1990). Social support in young children: Measurement, structure, and behavioral impact. In B. Sarason, I. Sarason, & G. Pierce (Eds.), *Social support: An interactional view* (pp. 64–94). New York: Wiley.

Causey, D. L., & Dubow, E. F. (1992). Development of a self-report coping measure for elementary school children. *Journal of Clinical Child Psychology, 21,* 47–59.

Chassin, L., Presson, C., Sherman, S. J., Montello, D., & McGrew, J. (1986). Changes in peer and parent influence during adolescence: Longitudinal versus cross-sectional perspectives on smoking initiation. *Developmental Psychology, 22,* 327–334.

Cherlin, A. (1992). *Marriage, divorce and remarriage*. Cambridge, MA: Harvard University Press.

Cobb, S. (1976). Social support as a moderator of life stress. *Psychosomatic Medicine, 38,* 300–314.

Coddington, R. D. (1972). The significance of life events as etiologic factors in the diseases of children: A study of a normal population. *Journal of Psychosomatic Research, 16,* 205–213.

Cohen, S., & Wills, T. A. (1985). Stress, social support, and the buffering hypothesis. *Psychological Bulletin, 98,* 310–317.

Coie, J. D., Watt, N., West, S. G., Hawkins, D., Asarnow, J., Markman, H., Ramsey, S., Shure, M., & Long, B. (1993). The science of prevention: A conceptual framework for and some directions for a national research program. *American Psychologist, 48*(10), 1013–1022.

Compas, B. E., Malcarne, V., & Fondacaro, K. (1988). Coping with stressful events in older children and young adolescents. *Journal of Consulting and Clinical Psychology, 56,* 405–411.

Compas, B. E., Phares, V., & Ledoux, N. (1989). Stress and coping preventive interventions for children and adolescents. In L. A. Bond & B. E. Compas (Eds.), *Primary prevention and promotion in the schools* (pp. 319–340). Newbury Park, CA: Sage.

Compas, B. E., Wagner, B. M., Slavin, S. L., & Vannatta, K. (1986). A prospective study of life events, social support, and psychological symptomatology during the transition from high school to college. *American Journal of Community Psychology, 14,* 241–258.

Cowan, P. A., Cowan, C. P., & Schulz, M. S. (1996). Thinking about risk and resilience in families. In E. M. Hetherington & E. A. Blechman (Eds.), *Stress, coping and resiliency in children and families* (pp. 10–38). Mahwah, NJ: Erlbaum.

Cowen, E. L. (1980). The wooing of primary prevention. *American Journal of Community Psychology, 8,* 258–284.

Cowen, E. L. (1985). Person centered approaches to primary prevention in mental health: Situation-focused and competence enhancement. *American Journal of Community Psychology, 13,* 31–48.

Cowen, E. L., Wyman, P. A., Work, W. C., & Parker, G. R. (1990). The Rochester Child Resilience Project (RCRP): Overview and summary of first year findings. *Development and Psychopathology, 2,* 193–212.

Cummings, E. M., & Davies, P. (1994). *Children and marital conflict: The impact of family dispute and resolution*. New York: Guileford Press.

Dohrenwend, B. S., & Dohrenwend, B. P. (1978). Some issues in research on stressful life events. *Journal of Nervous and Mental Disease, 166,* 7–15.

DuBois, D. L., Felner, R. D., Brand, S., Adan, A., & Evans, E. G. (1992). A prospective study of life stress, social support, and adaptation in early adolescence. *Child Development, 63,* 542–557.

DuBois, D. F., Felner, R. D., Meares, H., & Krier, M. (1994). Prospective investigation of the effects of socioeconomic disadvantage, life stress, and social support on early adolescent adjustment. *Journal of Abnormal Psychology, 103,* 511–522.

DuBois, E. R., & Ullman, D. G. (1989). Assessing social support in elementary school children: The survey of children's social support. *Journal of Clinical Child Psychology, 18,* 52–64.

Dubow, E. F., Schmidt, D., McBride, J., Edwards, S., & Merk, F. L. (1993). Teaching children to cope with stressful experiences: Initial implementation and evaluation of a primary prevention program. *Journal of Clinical Child Psychology, 22,* 428–440.

Dubow, E. F., Tisak, J., Causey, D., Hryshko, A., & Reid, G. (1991). A two-year longitudinal study of stressful life events, social support, and social problem-solving skills: Contributions to children's behavioral and academic adjustment. *Child Development, 62,* 583–599.

Durlak, J., & Wells, A. (in press). Primary prevention mental health programs for children and adolescents: A meta-analytic review. *American Journal of Community Psychology,*

Ebata, A. T., & Moos, R. H. (1991). Coping and adjustment in distressed and healthy adolescents. *Journal of Applied and Developmental Psychology, 12,* 33–54.

Ebata, A., & Moos, R. (1994). Personal, situational, and contextual correlates of coping in adolescence. *Journal of research on adolescence, 4,* 99–125.

Elias, M., Gara, M., Schuyler, T., Branden-Muller, L., & Sayette, M. (1986). The promotion of social competence: Longitudinal study of a preventive school-based program. *American Journal of Orthopsychiatry, 61,* 409–417.

Elias, M., Gara, M., Ubriaco, M., Rothbaum, P., Clabby, J., & Schuyler, T. (1986). The impact of a preventive social problem-solving intervention on children's coping with middle-school stressors. *American Journal of Community Psychology, 14,* 259–275.

Elias, M., & Weissberg, R. (1990). School-based social competence promotion as a primary prevention strategy: A tale of two projects. In R. P. Lorion (Ed.), *Protecting the children: Strategies for optimizing emotional and behavioral development* (pp. 177–200). New York: Haworth Press.

Emery, R., & Forehand, R. (1994). Parental divorce and children's well-being: A focus on resilience. In R. Haggerty, L. Sherrod, N. Garmezy, & M. Rutter (Eds.), *Stress, risk, and resilience in children and adolescents: Processes, mechanisms, and interventions* (pp. 64–100). New York: Cambridge University Press.

Felner, R. D., & Adan, A. (1988). The school transitional environment project: An ecological intervention and evaluation. In R. H. Price, E. L. Cowen, R. P. Lorion, & J. Ramos-McKay (Eds.), *Fourteen ounces of prevention: A casebook for practitioners* (pp. 111–123). Washington, DC: American Psychological Association.

Felner, R. D., Brand, S., DuBois, D. L., Adan, A., Mulhall, P. F., & Evans, E. G. (1995). Socioeconomic disadvantage, proximal environmental experiences, and socioemotional and academic adjustment in early adolescence: Investigation of a mediated effects model. *Child Development, 66,* 774–792.

Felner, R. D., Terre, L., & Rowlison, R. (1988). A life transition framework for understanding marital dissolution and family reorganization. In S. Wolchik & P. Karoly (Eds.), *Children of divorce: Empirical perspective on adjustment* (pp. 35–66). New York: Gardner Press.

Folkman, S. (1984). Personal control and stress and coping processes: A theoretical analysis. *Journal of Personality and Social Psychology, 46,* 839–852.

Folmer, H. (1981). Measurement of the effects of regional policy instruments by means of linear structural equation models and panel data. *Environmental and Planning A, 13,* 1435–1448.

Freedman, D. A. (1987). As other see us: A case study in path analysis. *Journal of Educational Statistics, 12,* 101–128.

Fuligni, A. J., & Eccles, J. S. (1993). Perceived parent–child relationship and early adolescents' orientation toward peers. *Developmental Psychology, 29,* 622–632.

Gamble, W. (1994). Perceptions of controllability and other stressor event characteristics as determinants of coping among young adolescents and young adults. *Journal of Youth and Adolescence, 23,* 65–84.

Games, P. (1988). Correlation and causation: An alternative view. *The Score,* 9–10.

Gersten, J. C., Beals, J., & Kallgren, C. A. (1991). Epidemiology and preventive interventions: Parental death in childhood as a case example. *American Journal of Community Psychology, 19,* 481–500.

Gersten, J. C., Langner, T. S., Eisenberg, J. G., & Simcha-Fagan, O. R. (1977). An evaluation of the etiological role of stressful life changes in psychological disorders. *Journal of Health and Social Behavior, 18,* 228–244.

Gillham, J., Reivish, K., Jaycox, L., & Seligman, M. (1995). Prevention of depressive symptoms in schoolchildren: Two-year follow-up. *Psychological Science, 6,* 343–351.

Glyshaw, K., Cohen, L. H., & Towbes, L. C. (1989). Coping strategies and psychological distress: Prospective analyses of early and middle adolescents. *American Journal of Community Psychology, 17,* 607–623.

Gonzalez, N., Gunnoe, M., Jackson, K., & Samaniego, R. (1996). *Validation of a multicultural events scale for urban adolescents: Preliminary strategies for enhancing cross-ethnic and cross-language equivalence.* Manuscript submitted for publication.

Gore, S., & Eckenrode, J. (1994). Context and process in research on risk and resilience. In R. Haggerty, L. Sherrod, N. Garmezy, & M. Rutter (Eds.), *Stress, risk, and resilience in children and adolescents: Processes, mechanisms, and interventions* (pp. 19–63). New York: Cambridge University Press.

Graziano, A. M., & Diament, D. M. (1992). Parent behavioral training: An examination of the paradigm. *Behavior Modification, 16,* 3–38.

Greenberg, M. T., Seigel, J. M., & Leitch, C. J. (1983). The nature and importance of attachment relationships to parents and peers during adolescence. *Journal of Youth and Adolescence, 12,* 373–386.

Greenberg, M., Kusche, C., Cook, E., & Quamma, J. (1995). Promoting emotional competence in school-aged deaf children. The effects of the PATHS curriculum. *Developmental Psychopathology, 5,* 191–213.

Grych, J., & Fincham, F. (1993). Children's appraisals of marital conflict: Initial investigations of the cognitive–contextual framework. *Child Development, 64,* 215–230.

Grych, J., Seid, M., & Fincham, F. (1992). Assessing marital conflict from the child's perspective: The children's perception of interparental conflict scale. *Child Development, 63,* 558–572.

Guerra, H. G., Huesmann, L. R., Tolan, P. H., Van Acker, R., & Eron, L. (1995). Stressful events and individual beliefs as correlates of economic disadvantage and aggression among urban children. *Journal of Consulting and Clinical Psychology, 63,* 518–528.

Haan, N. (1977). *Coping and defending, processes of self-environment organization.* New York: Academic Press.

Haan, N. (1982). The assessment of coping, defense, and stress. In L. Goldberg & S. Brezwitz (Eds.), *Handbook of stress: Theoretical and clinical aspects* (pp. 254–269). New York: Free Press.

Haggerty, R., Sherrod, L., Garmezy, N., & Rutter, M. (1994). *Stress, risk, and resilience in children and adolescents: Processes, mechanisms, and interventions.* New York: Cambridge University Press.

Hammen, C., & Goodman-Brown, T. (1990). Self-schemas and vulnerability to specific life stress in children at risk for depression. *Cognitive Therapy and Research, 14,* 215–227.

Hetherington, E. M., & Blechman, E. A. (1996). *Stress, coping and resiliency in children and families.* Mahwah, NJ: Erlbaum.

Hirsch, B. J., & DuBois, E. F. (1992). The relation of peer social support and psychological symptomatology during the transition to junior high school: A two-year longitudinal analysis. *American Journal of Community Psychology, 20,* 333–347.

Hirsch, B. J., & Reischl, T. (1985). Social networks and developmental psychopathology: A comparison of adolescent children of depressed, arthritic, or normal parent. *Journal of Abnormal Psychology, 94,* 272–281.

Hoffman, M. A., & Levy-Shiff, R. (1994). Coping and locus of control: Cross-situational transmission between mothers and adolescents. *Journal of Early Adolescence, 14,* 391–405.

Johnson, J., & Bradlyn, A. (1988). Life events and adjustment in childhood and adolescence: Methodological and conceptual issues. In L. Cohen (Ed.), *Life events and psychological functioning: Theoretical and methodological issues* (pp. 64–95). Newbury Park, CA: Sage.

Kahn, H. A., & Sempos, C. T. (1989). *Statistical methods in epidemiology.* New York: Oxford.

Kliewer, W. (1991). Coping in middle childhood: Relations to competence, type A behavior, monitoring, blunting, and locus of control. *Developmental Psychology, 27,* 689–697.

Kliewer, W., & Sandler, I. (1992). Locus of control and self-esteem as moderators of stressor–symptom relations in children and adolescents. *Journal of Abnormal Child Psychology, 20,* 393–413.

Kliewer, W., Sandler, I. N., & Wolchik, S. A. (1994). Family socialization of threat appraisal and coping: Coaching, modeling and family context. In K. Hurrelman & F. Nestmann (Eds.), *Social networks and social support in childhood and adolescence* (pp. 271–291). Berlin: Walter de Gruyter.

Knitzer, J., & Aber, J. (1995). Young children and poverty: Facing the facts. *American Journal of Orthopsychiatry, 65,* 174–176.

Krohne, H. W., & Rogner, J. (1982). Repression–sensitization as a central construct in coping research. In H. W. Krohne & L. Laux (Eds.), *Achievement, stress, and anxiety* (pp. 167–193). Washington, DC: Hemisphere.

Lazarus, R. S., & Folkman, S. (1984). *Stress, appraisal and coping.* New York: Springer.

Lazarus, R. S. (1991). *Emotion and adaptation.* New York: Oxford University Press.

Leitenberg, H., Yost, L. W., & Carroll-Wilson, M. (1986). Negative cognitive errors in children: Questionnaire development, normative data, and comparisons between children with and without self-reported symptoms of depression, low self-esteem, and evaluation anxiety. *Journal of Consulting and Clinical Psychology, 54,* 528–536.

Lengua, L. J., & Sandler, I. N. (1996). Self-regulation as a moderator of the relation between coping and symptomatology in children of divorce. *Journal of Abnormal Child Psychology, 24,* 681–701.

Licitra-Kleckler, D. M., & Waas, G. A. (1993). Perceived social support among high-stress adolescents: The role of peers and family. *Journal of Adolescent Research, 8,* 381–402.

Lindner, M. S., Hagan, M. S., & Brown, J. C. (1992). The adjustment of children in nondivorced, divorced single-mother, and remarried families. In E. M. Hetherington & W. G. Clingempeel (Eds.), *Coping with marital transitions: Monographs of the Society for Research in Child Development, 57* (No. 2-3), 35–72.

Lipsey, M. (1990). Theory as method: Small theories of treatments. In L. Sechrest, E. Perrin, & J. Bunker (Eds.), *Research methodology: Strengthening causal interpretations of nonexperimental data* (pp. 33–53). Washington, DC: US Department of Health and Human Services.

Lorion, R., Price, R., & Eaton, W. (1989). The prevention of child and adolescent disorders: From theory to research. In D. Schaffer, I. Philips, & N. Enzer (Eds.), *Prevention of mental disorders, alcohol and other drug use in children and adolescents* (pp. 55–97). Washington, DC: Office of Substance Abuse Prevention Monograph-2 (DHHS Publication No. ADM 90-1646).

MacKinnon, D. (1994). Analysis of mediating variables in prevention and intervention research. *National Institute on Drug Abuse Research Monograph Series, 139,* 127–153.

MacKinnon, D., & Dwyer, J. (1993). Estimating mediated effects in prevention studies. *Evaluation Research, 17,* 144–158.

MacKinnon, D., Warsi, G., & Dwyer, J. (1995). A simulation study of mediated effects measures. *Multivariate Behavioral Research, 30,* 41–62.

Mayer, J., & Davidson, W. (in press). Dissemination of innovations. In J. Rappaport & E. Seidman (Eds.), *The handbook of community psychology.* New York: Plenum Press.

Maton, K. (1990). Meaningful involvement in instrumental activity and well-being: Studies of older adolescents and at risk urban teen-agers. *American Journal of Community Psychology, 18,* 297–320.

Mazur, E., Wolchik, S. A., & Sandler, I. N. (1992). Negative cognitive errors and positive illusions for negative divorce events: Predictors of children's psychological adjustment. *Journal of Abnormal Child Psychology, 20,* 523–542.

McGrath, J. E. (1970). A conceptual formulation for research on stress. In J. E. McGrath (Ed.), *Social and psychological factors in stress* (pp. 10–21). New York: Holt, Rinehart, and Winston.

Menaghan, E. G. (1983). Individual coping efforts: Moderators of the relationship between life stress and mental health outcomes. In H. B. Kaplan (Ed.), *Psychosocial stress: Trends in theory and research* (pp. 157–191). New York: Academic Press.

Miller, S. M., Brody, D. S., & Summerton, J. (1988). Styles of coping with threat: Implications for health. *Journal of Personality and Social Psychology, 54,* 142–148.

Miller, S., & Green, M. (1985). Coping with stress and frustration: Origins, nature, and development. In M. Lewis & C. Saarni (Eds.), *The socialization of emotions* (pp. 263–313). New York: Plenum Press.

Mrazek, P. J., & Haggerty, R. (Eds.). (1994). *Reducing risks for mental disorders: Frontiers for preventive intervention research.* Washington, DC: National Academy Press.

National Institute of Mental Health. (1995). *A plan for prevention research for the national institute of mental health: A report to the national advisory mental health council.* NIH Publication 96-4093. Rockville, Maryland.

Nolen-Hoeksema, S. (1992). Children coping with uncontrollable stressors. *Applied and Preventive Psychology, 1,* 183–189.

Nolen-Hoeksema, S., Girgus, J. S., & Seligman, M. E. P. (1986). Learned helplessness in children: A longitudinal study of depression, achievement, and explanatory style. *Journal of Personality and Social Psychology, 51,* 435–442.

Nowachek, P. A., & Stoddard, J. J. (1994). Prevalence and impact of multiple childhood chronic illnesses. *Journal of Pediatrics, 124,* 40–48.

O'Brien, M., Margolin, G., John, R., & Krueger, L. (1991). Mother's and son's cognitive and emotional reactions to simulated marital family conflict. *Journal of Consulting and Clinical Psychology, 59,* 692–703.

Patterson, G. R. (1975). *Families: Application of social learning to family life.* Champaign, IL: Research Press.

Pedro-Carroll, J., & Cowen, E. (1987). Preventive interventions for children of divorce. In J. P. Vincent (Ed.), *Advances in family intervention, assessment and theory,* Vol. 4 (pp. 281–307). Greenwich, CT: JAI Press.

Pierce, G., Sarason, B., Sarason, I., Joseph, H., & Henderson, C. (1996). Conceptualizing and assessing social support in the context of the family. In G. Pierce, B. Sarason, & I. Sarason (Eds.), *Handbook of social support and the family* (pp. 3–23). New York: Plenum Press.

Pillow, D. R., Sandler, I. N., Braver, S., Wolchik, S., & Gersten, J. (1991). Theory-based screening for prevention: Focusing on mediating processes in children of divorce. *American Journal of Community Psychology, 19*, 809–837.

Price, R. (1983). The education of a prevention psychologist. In R. Felner, L. Jason, J. Moritsugu, & S. Farber (Eds.), *Preventive psychology: Theory, research and practice* (pp. 290–296). Elmsford, NY: Pergamon.

Price, R. H., Cowen, E. L., Lorion, R. P., & Ramos-McKay, J. (Eds.). (1988). *14 ounces of prevention: A casebook for practitioners.* Washington, DC: American Psychological Association.

Price, R., & Lorion, R. (1989). Prevention programming as organizational reinvention: From research to implementation. In OSAP Prevention Monograph-2, *Prevention of mental disorders, alcohol and other drug use in children and adolescents* (pp. 97–123). DHHS Publication No. (ADM)90-1646. Washington, DC.

Quamma, J. P., & Greenberg, M. T. (1994). Children's experience of life stress: The role of family social support and social problem-solving skills as protective factors. *Journal of Clinical Child Psychology, 23*, 295–305.

Reifman, A., & Windle, M. (1995). Adolescent suicidal behaviors as a function of depression, hopelessness, alcohol use, and social support: A longitudinal investigation. *American Journal of Community Psychology, 23*, 329–354.

Rolf, J., Masten, A. S., Cicchetti, D., Nuechterlein, K. H., & Weintraub, S. (Eds.). (1990). *Risk and protective factors in the development of psychopathology.* Cambridge, England: Cambridge University Press.

Roosa, M., Beals, J., Sandler, I., & Pillow, D. (1990). The role of risk and protective factors in predicting symptomatology in adolescent self-identified children of alcoholic parents. *American Journal of Community Psychology, 18*, 725–741.

Roosa, M. W., Sandler, I. N., Gehring, M., Beals, J., & Cappo, L. (1988). The Children of Alcoholics Life Events Schedule: A stress scale for children of alcohol abusing parents. *Journal of Studies on Alcohol, 49*, 422–429.

Rossman, B., & Rosenberg, M. (1992). Family stress and functioning in children: The moderating effects of children's beliefs about their control over parental conflict. *Journal of Child Psychology and Psychiatry, 33*, 699–715.

Roth, S., & Cohen, L. (1986). Approach, avoidance, and coping with stress. *American Psychologist, 41*, 813–819.

Rowlison, R. T., & Felner, R. D. (1988). Major life events, hassles, and adaptation in adolescence: Confounding in the conceptualization and measurement of life stress and adjustment revisited. *Journal of Personality and Social Psychology, 55*, 432–444.

Russell, M., Henderson, C., & Blume, S. (1985). *Children of alcoholics: A review of the literature.* New York: Children of Alcoholics Foundation.

Rutter, M. (1994). Stress research: Accomplishments and tasks ahead. In R. Haggerty, L. Sherrod, N. Garmezy, & M. Rutter (Eds.), *Stress, risk, and resilience in children and adolescents: Processes, mechanisms, and interventions* (pp. 354–385). Cambridge, England: Cambridge University Press.

Sameroff, A., & Seifer, R. (1990). Early contributors to developmental risk. In J. Rolf, A. Masten, D. Cicchetti, K. Neuchterlein, & S. Weintraub (Eds.), *Risk and protective factors in the development of psychopathology* (pp. 52–67). New York: Cambridge University Press.

Sandler, I., Braver, S., Wolchik, S., Pillow, D., & Gersten, J. (1991). Small theory and the strategic choices of prevention research. *American Journal of Community Psychology, 19*, 873–880.

Sandler, I. N., Miller, P., Short, J., & Wolchik, S. A. (1989). Social support as a protective factor for children in stress. In D. Belle (Ed.), *Children's social networks and social supports* (pp. 277–307). New York: Wiley.

Sandler, I., & Ramsey, T. B. (1982). Dimensional analysis of children's stressful life events. *American Journal of Community Psychology, 8*, 285–302.

Sandler, I., Tein, J., & West, S. (1994). Coping, stress, and the psychological symptoms of children of divorce: A cross-sectional and longitudinal study. *Child Development, 65*, 1744–1763.

Sandler, I., Wolchik, S., & Braver, S. (1988). The stressors of children's postdivorce environments. In S. A. Wolchik & P. Karoly (Eds.), *Children of divorce: Empirical perspective on adjustment* (pp. 111–143). New York: Gardner Press.

Sandler, I., Wolchik, S., Braver, S., & Fogas, B. (1986). Significant events of children of divorce: Toward the assessment of risky situations. In S. M. Auerbach & A. Stolberg (Eds.), *Crisis intervention with children and families* (pp. 65–83). New York: Hemisphere.

Sandler, I., Wolchik, S., Braver, S., & Fogas, B. (1991). Stability and quality of life events and psychological symptomatology of children of divorce. *American Journal of Community Psychology, 19,* 501–520.

Sandler, I. N., West, S. G., Baca, L., Pillow, D. R., Gersten, J., Rogosch, F., Virdin, L., Beals, J., Reynolds, K., Kallgren, C., Tein, J., Kriege, G., Cole, E., & Ramirez, R. (1992). Linking empirically based theory and evaluation: The family bereavement program. *American Journal of Community Psychology, 20,* 491–521.

Seidman, E., Allen, L., Aber, J., Mitchell, C., & Feinman, J. (1994). The impact of school transitions in early adolescence on the self-system and perceived social context of poor urban youth. *Child Development, 65,* 507–522.

Selye, H. (1956). *The stress of life.* New York: McGraw-Hill.

Sheets, V., Sandler, I., & West, S. (1996). Appraisals of negative events by preadolescent children of divorce. *Child Development, 67,* 2166–2182.

Short, J., Roosa, M., Sandler, I., Ayers, T., Gensheimer, L., Braver, S., & Tein, J. (1995). Evaluation of a preventive intervention for a self-selected subpopulation of children. *American Journal of Community Psychology, 23,* 223–248.

Siegel, J. M., & Brown, J. D. (1988). A prospective study of stressful circumstances, illness symptoms, and depressed mood among adolescents. *Developmental Psychology, 24,* 715–721.

Silver, E. J., Coupey, S. M., Bauman, L. J., Doctors, S. R., & Boeck, M. A. (1992). Effects of peer counseling training intervention on psychological functioning of adolescents. *Journal of Adolescent Research, 7,* 110–128.

Skinner, E. A., & Wellborn, J. G. (1994). Coping during childhood and adolescence: A motivational perspective. In R. Lerner, D. Featherman, & M. Perlmuter (Eds.), *Life-span development and behavior,* Vol. 12 (pp. 91–123). Hillsdale, NJ: Erlbaum.

Slavin, L. A., & Rainer, K. L. (1990). Gender differences in emotional support and depressive symptoms: A prospective analysis. *American Journal of Community Psychology, 18,* 407–421.

Sobel, M. E. (1982). Some new results on indirect effects and their standard errors in structural equation models. In N. Tuma (Ed.), *Sociological methodology 1986* (pp. 159–186). San Francisco: Jossey Bass.

Spacarelli, S. (1994). Stress, appraisal, and coping in child sexual abuse: A theoretical and empirical review. *Psychological Bulletin, 116,* 340–362.

Stice, E., Barrera, M., Jr., & Chassin, L. (1993). Relation of parental support and control to adolescents' externalizing symptomatology and substance use: A longitudinal examination of curvilinear effects. *Journal of Abnormal Child Psychology, 21,* 609–629.

Stolberg, A. L., & Garrison, K. M. (1985). Evaluating a primary prevention program for children of divorce. *American Journal of Community Psychology, 13,* 111–124.

Stolberg, A. C., & Mahler, J. (1994). Enhancing treatment gains in a school based intervention for children of divorce through skill training, parental involvement, and transfer procedures. *Journal of Consulting and Clinical Psychology, 62,* 147–156.

Stone, A. A., Helder, L., & Schneider, M. S. (1988). Coping with stressful events: Coping, dimensions and issues. In L. H. Cohen (Ed.), *Life events and psychological functioning: Theoretical and methodological issues* (pp. 182–210). Newbury Park, CA: Sage.

Suls, J., & Fletcher, B. (1985). The relative efficacy of avoidant and nonavoidant coping strategies: A meta-analysis. *Health Psychology, 4,* 249–288.

Swearingen, E., & Cohen, L. (1985). Life events and psychological distress: A prospective study of young adolescents. *Developmental Psychology, 21,* 1045–1054.

Taylor, R. D., Casten, R., & Flickinger, S. M. (1993). Influence of kinship social support on the parenting experiences and psychosocial adjustment of African-American adolescents. *Developmental Psychology, 29,* 382–388.

Thoits, P. A. (1986). Social support as coping assistance. *Journal of Consulting and Clinical Psychology, 54,* 416–423.

Trickett, E., Dahiyal, C., & Selby, P. (1994). *Primary prevention in mental health: An annotated bibliography 1983–1991*. NIH Publication No. 94-3767. Rockville, MD: NIMH.

US Bureau of the Census, Current Population Reports. (1994). *Marital status and living arrangements: March, 1994* Washington, DC: US Government Printing Office.

Wagner, B. M., Compas, B. E., & Howell, D. C. (1988). Daily and major life events: A test of an integrative model for psychosocial stress. *American Journal of Community Psychology, 16,* 189–207.

Weissberg, R. P., Caplan, M., & Spivo, P. J. (1989). A new conceptual framework for establishing school-based social competence promotion programs. In L. A. Bond & B. E. Compas (Eds.), *Primary prevention and promotion in the schools* (pp. 255–296). Newbury Park, CA: Sage.

Weissberg, R., & Greenberg, M. (in press). School and community competence-enhancement and prevention programs. In W. Damon, I. Sigel, & K. Renninger (Eds.), *Handbook of child psychology: Vol. 5, Child psychology in practice* (5th ed.). New York: Wiley.

Werner, E., & Smith, R. (1982). *Vulnerable but invincible: A longitudinal study of resilient children and youth.* New York: McGraw Hill.

West, S., & Aiken, L. (in press). Towards understanding individual effects in multiple component prevention programs: Design and analysis strategies. In K. Bryant, M. Windle, & S. West (Eds.), *New methodological approaches to prevention research.* Washington, DC: American Psychological Association.

Wills, T. A. (1985). Stress, coping and tobacco and alcohol use in early adolescence. In S. Shiffman & T. A. Wills (Eds.), *Coping and substance use* (pp. 67–94). New York: Academic Press.

Wills, T. A. (1986). Stress and coping in early adolescence: Relationships to substance use in urban school samples. *Health Psychology, 5,* 503–529.

Wills, T. A. (1988). Coping and self-efficacy: Prospective analyses for adolescents in urban school samples. Submitted for publication.

Wills, T. A. (1989). *Coping processes and self-efficacy: Prospective analyses in cohorts of urban adolescents.* Unpublished manuscript, Ferkauf Graduate School of Psychology and Albert Einstein Medical School, Bronx, NY.

Wills, T. A. (1990). Social support and the family. In E. Blechman (Ed.), *Emotions and the family* (pp. 75–98). Hillsdale, NJ: Erlbaum.

Wills, T. A., Blechman, E. A., & McNamara, G. (1996). Family support, coping and competence. In E. M. Hetherington & E. A. Blechman (Eds.), *Stress, coping and resiliency in children and the family* (pp. 107–133). Hillsdale, NJ: Erlbaum.

Wills, T. A., & Cleary, S. D. (1996). How are social support effects mediated: A test with parental support and adolescent substance use. Manuscript submitted for publication.

Wills, T. A., Mariani, J., & Filer, M. (1996). The role of family and peer relationship in adolescent substance use. In G. R. Pierce, B. R. Sarason, & I. G. Sarason (Eds.), *Handbook of social support and the family* (pp. 521–549). New York: Plenum Press.

Wills, T. A., Vaccaro, D., & McNamara, G. (1992). The role of life events, family support, and competence in adolescent substance use: A test of vulnerability and protective factors. *American Journal of Community Psychology, 20,* 349–374.

Wills, T. A., & Vaughn, R. (1989). Social support and substance use in early adolescence. *Journal of Behavioral Medicine, 12,* 321–339.

Windle, M. (1992). A longitudinal study of stress buffering for adolescent problem behaviors. *Developmental Psychology, 28,* 522–530.

Wolchik, S. A., Ruehlman, L. S., Braver, S. L., & Sandler, I. N. (1989). Social support of children of divorce: Direct and stress buffering effects. *American Journal of Community Psychology, 17,* 485–501.

Wolchik, S. A., West, S. G., Westover, S., Sandler, I., Martin, A., Lustig, J., Tein, J., & Fisher, J. (1993). The children of divorce parenting intervention: Outcome evaluation of an empirically based program. *American Journal of Community Psychology, 21*(3), 293–331.

Wolchik, S., Sandler, I., West, S., & Anderson, E. (1997). *Children of divorce: 6-year follow-up of preventive efforts.* Unpublished manuscript. Arizona State University.

Worden, J. W., & Silverman, P. R. (1996). Parental death and the adjustment of school-age children. *Omega Journal of Death and Dying, 33,* 91–102.

2

Coping with Stress
The Roles of Regulation and Development

NANCY EISENBERG, RICHARD A. FABES, and IVANNA K. GUTHRIE

Our goals for this chapter are threefold. Our first goal is to consider coping within the larger framework of regulation, thereby broadening our perspective to include work on aspects of regulation that are relevant to an understanding of coping but frequently have not been considered by coping theorists. A second related goal is to present a preliminary heuristic model in which the roles of various modes of regulation in the coping process are considered. Finally, we use our heuristic model as a framework for briefly reviewing the developmental literature concerning factors related to coping and regulation.

COPING AS REGULATION

Although there is a tradition of defining coping in terms of defense mechanisms (e.g., Haan, 1977; Vaillant, 1977), for the study of normal children we find Lazarus and Folkman's (1984) conceptual framework more useful. Lazarus and Folkman have defined coping as "the process of managing demands (external or internal) that are appraised as taxing or exceeding the resources of the person" (p. 283). In their view, coping includes "not just approach–avoidance behavior or defensive processes to cope with the complex demands and constraints of a given stressful encounter, but a wide range of cognitive and behav-

NANCY EISENBERG and IVANNA K. GUTHRIE • Department of Psychology, Arizona State University, Tempe, Arizona 85287-1104.   RICHARD A. FABES • Department of Family Resources and Human Development, Arizona State University, Tempe, Arizona 85287-1108.
Handbook of Children's Coping: Linking Theory and Intervention, edited by Wolchik and Sandler. Plenum Press, New York, 1997.

ioral strategies that have both problem-solving and *emotion-regulation* functions" (Folkman & Lazarus, 1988, p. 466; italics are ours). In research on coping,
mechanisms of interest typically are specific categories of behavior (e.g., confrontative coping, seeking social support, escape–avoidance, planful problem
solving; see Folkman & Lazarus, 1988) that are viewed as modifying the source
of the problem (i.e., problem-focused coping) or the emotional distress (emotion-focused coping).

Based on this definition, the emerging literature on emotion regulation
would appear to be highly relevant to an understanding of coping. The term
emotion regulation has been defined in a variety of ways, but a current and
representative example is that of Kopp (1989): "Emotion regulation (ER) is a
term used to characterize the processes and characteristics involved in coping
with heightened levels of positive and negative emotions including joy, plea-
sure, distress, anger, fear, and other emotions" (p. 343). Like most other researchers and theorists, Kopp has focused primarily on the regulation of, or
coping with, negative emotions, including distress and stress reactions.

In our view, coping and emotion regulation are instances of the more
general category of regulation. Self-regulation has been defined as

> those processes, internal and/or transactional, that enable an individual to
> guide his/her goal-directed activities over time and across changing circum-
> stances (contexts). Regulation implies modulation of thought, affect, behav-
> ior, or attention via deliberate or automated use of specific mechanisms and
> supportive metaskills. (Karoly, 1993, p. 25)

We view coping as involving regulatory processes in a subset of contexts—
those involving stress.

In contrast to Karoly's (1993) inclusion of automated responses in his
definition of self-regulation, Lazarus and Folkman (1984), as well as others
(e.g., Compas, 1987), have argued that coping does not involve automated
regulatory mechanisms; it is effortful and under the individual's volitional
control. However, as was suggested by Skinner and Wellborn (1994), a focus on
purpose and effort excludes phenomena of relevance to coping in children
such as learned helplessness and limits consideration of early coping responses. Further, it is debatable whether processes such as shifting one's attention away from a distressing stimulus are always purposeful. Indeed, Masters
(1991) argued that attempts to regulate emotional arousal may be deliberate or
automatic, although automatic strategies may be less flexible and more vulnerable to dysregulation. Thus, although we would agree that coping and emotion
regulation generally involve effort, in our view coping may not always be
intentional and conscious. By broadening the focus from traditional coping
responses to include the literature on emotion regulation, we greatly expand
the theoretical and research base of relevance to the discussion of coping and
regulation. For example, there is considerable work on infants' and toddlers'
developing abilities to regulate emotion as a consequence of developmental
changes in reflex adaptations, early cognitive abilities (e.g., making discrimina-
tions and associations, memory, development of intentionality, representational thinking), and social interactive skills (Kopp, 1982, 1989; Thompson, 1994).

Although work on infant emotion regulation generally is not emphasized in this chapter (due to space constraints), this work is relevant to a developmental perspective on the origins of coping skills.

Another body of research on emotion regulation that is very useful for a regulation approach to coping is embedded in the work on temperament. In some recent conceptualizations of temperament, aspects of temperament are viewed as reflecting individual differences in both reactivity (including emotionality) and regulation (e.g., Rothbart & Derryberry, 1981; Fox, 1989). For example, Rothbart and Derryberry (Rothbart & Derryberry, 1981; Derryberry & Rothbart, 1988) view temperament as involving the regulation of impinging stimuli and internal states. Behavioral mechanisms used for temperamentally based regulation include shifting attention away from an arousing or unpleasant stimulus to modulate distress (attentional shifting), sustaining attention (attentional focusing), voluntarily initiating or continuing action (activation control), and inhibiting action (inhibition control). Clearly, there are similarities or links between these modes of regulation and emotion- and problem-focused coping. Consequently, information on these mechanisms is relevant to an understanding of how people cope with stressful situations and individual differences in the ability to do so successfully.

Researchers such as Compas (1987) previously have noted the possible relevance of temperament for understanding coping. However, he considered temperament as a stable, nonvolitional factor, whereas he viewed coping as an effortful response. In addition, Compas, like Lazarus and Folkman (1984), focused primarily on coping as a response in a specific context, rather than individual differences in coping style (although Lazarus and Folkman acknowledge the existence of preferred modes of coping).

Nonetheless, many coping researchers have noted the existence (or possible existence) of coping styles that are somewhat consistent across time and contexts, and measures of coping styles have proved productive for predicting situational behavior and socially relevant outcomes (e.g., Carver, Scheier, & Weintraub, 1989; Eisenberg, Fabes, Carlo, & Karbon, 1992; Eisenberg, Fabes, Nyman, Bernzweig, & Pinuelas, 1994). Although modes of coping and emotion regulation change with age (an issue to which we return) and vary across situations, there appear to be individual differences that are somewhat stable over the years in preferred mode of coping in certain types of stressful contexts (e.g., peer conflicts; Eisenberg, Fabes, Murphy et al., 1995). Indeed, individuals probably vary in both their tendencies to select relatively constructive (e.g., planful problem solving) versus nonconstructive (e.g., confrontative) methods of dealing with stress (e.g., Eisenberg, Fabes, Murphy et al., 1995) and in the flexibility and appropriateness of their coping reactions. Thus, individual differences in regulation capabilities such as those reflected in temperament are relevant to an understanding of coping.

Modes of Coping-Relevant Regulation

Even in the coping literature, operationalizations of coping vary considerably. However, most systems for coding coping responses include categories reflective of both problem-focused and emotion-focused coping; some also include categories pertaining to the regulation of emotionally driven behavior (see Chapter 1, this volume).

The most common problem-focused coping categories include active coping, direct problem solving, and planning (e.g., Carver et al., 1989; Eisenberg et al., 1992; Folkman & Lazarus, 1988; Sandler, Tein, & West, 1994); sometimes, but not always, categories such as cognitive decision making and seeking information (Sandler et al., 1994) or instrumental social support (Carver et al., 1989) are grouped within problem-focused modes of coping. In general, however, one can talk about modes of coping that are used to change the environment in a manner that makes it less stressful.

In contrast, emotion-focusing coping typically includes accepting responsibility, positive reappraisals, acceptance, denial, and/or cognitive or behavioral avoidance or distraction (e.g., Carver et al., 1989; Eisenberg et al., 1992; Folkman & Lazarus, 1988; Kliewer, 1991; Sandler et al., 1994). In the emotion regulation literature, behaviors such as attention shifting and attention focusing can be used to regulate emotional arousal; for example, shifting attention from a negative stimulus appears to diminish arousal or frustration (see Derryberry & Rothbart, 1988; Fabes, Eisenberg, & Eisenbud, 1993; Miller & Green, 1985; Mischel & Mischel, 1983; Rothbart, Ziaie, & O'Boyle, 1992; Tronick, 1989). Further, inhibition of behavior can be useful at times in avoiding contact with a stressful stimulus. Thus, categories of response used in both the coping and temperament literatures can be viewed as useful for managing emotional arousal per se (and not the behavioral outcomes of emotion).

A third category of regulatory responses relevant to an understanding of coping is the regulation of emotionally driven behavior. In this category, we include the regulation of behavior that is driven by emotion and that is not specifically directed at changing aspects of the situation causing the problem. Behavioral regulation becomes relevant primarily when emotion regulation is not adequate in a stressful context and the individual is still experiencing negative emotion. For example, people sometimes deal with stress by enacting behaviors such as venting of emotion (e.g., crying or yelling) (Eisenberg et al., 1992; Rossman, 1992), aggression, hostility, or confrontation (Carver et al., 1989; Cummings & Cummings, 1988; Eisenberg et al., 1992; Eisenberg, Fabes, Nymen et al., 1994; McCrae, 1984), or the inhibition of such overt behavioral expression (a construct that is central to many measures of both temperamental regulation and self-control) (Derryberry & Rothbart, 1988; Kendall & Wilcox, 1979). Often these behaviors simply reflect the absence of sufficient regulation and are not either attempts to master the situation or aimed at making oneself feel better.

The same behavior, for example, the venting of negative emotion, could in different situations, reflect attempts to regulate the situation, emotion, or behavior. Moreover, a given response may serve more than one function in a single situation. However, on a conceptual level, it is useful to differentiate among these three functions of regulation.

Measures tapping the regulation of emotionally driven behavior most often are used in studies of children rather than adults. This is probably because children are more likely than adults to act out in stressful situations and because behavioral (e.g., observational) measures of coping are obtained more often with children (e.g., Fabes & Eisenberg, 1992). In addition, children's behavioral reactions to the experience of negative emotion are topics of considerable importance to investigators studying aggression, social competence, externalizing behaviors, behavioral inhibition, and a number of other contemporary topics.

The Blocks' (Block & Block, 1980) work on ego control is an example of developmental work focused primarily on behavioral regulation. They defined ego control as the threshold or operating characteristic of an individual with regard to the expression or containment of impulses, feelings, and desires. *Overcontrol* is characterized by "the containment of impulse, delay of gratification, inhibition of action, and insulation from environmental distractors" (Block & Block, 1980, p. 43). Thus, the ego overcontroller has a high modal threshold for response and is high in behavioral regulation; indeed, the overcontroller often is unduly constrained and inhibited. The other end of the continuum, *undercontrol,* is defined as "insufficient modulation of impulse, the inability to delay gratification, immediate and direct expression of motivations and affects, and vulnerability to environmental distractors" (p. 43). Thus, the undercontroller translates needs and impulses relatively directly into behavior and is low in behavioral regulation (and probably also emotional regulation). Therefore, the dimension of ego control reflects the range of behavioral regulation.

In brief, we are suggesting that there are at least three broad categories of coping/regulation that are relevant to dealing with stress: attempts to directly regulate emotion (e.g., emotion-focused coping; henceforth labeled emotion regulation), attempts to regulate the situation (e.g., problem-focused coping, including thinking about how to do so), and attempts to regulate emotionally driven behavior (i.e., behavioral regulation). By conceptualizing coping reactions in this manner, we include the broad array of behaviors in the literature on emotional and behavioral regulation, as well as responses typically discussed in research on coping. We are not implying that researchers should use only these three broader categories of coping/regulation or that measures of each of the three types necessarily be grouped in analyses; categorizing various modes of regulating stress in the aforementioned manner is useful primarily for conceptual analyses. We turn to discussion of these three modes of regulation within a broader conceptual model shortly.

Optimal Coping

As frequently has been noted (Compas, 1987; Lazarus & Folkman, 1984), what is effective (in terms of reaching one's goal) or constructive coping (in terms of social outcomes) in one context may be ineffective or inappropriate in another. For example, as noted previously, problem-focused coping seems to be associated with better outcomes in settings in which the individual has some control over the situation, whereas emotion-focused coping may be more effective (and less frustrating) in uncontrollable contexts (e.g., Altshuler & Ruble, 1989; see Compas, Banez, Malcarne, & Worsham, 1991). Based on findings of this sort, Compas (1987) has argued that effective coping is "likely characterized by flexibility and change" (p. 399), because no single coping strategy is effective for all types of stress. This is not a new idea; the notion of flexibility is central to Block and Block's (1980) important work concerning the regulation of emotion and emotionally driven behavior.

In addition to ego control, the Blocks (Block & Block, 1980) described an aspect of personality they labeled *ego resiliency*. Ego resiliency refers to the dynamic capacity of individuals to modify their modal level of ego control as a function of the demands of the environment. At one extreme of the dimension, ego resiliency is defined as resourceful adaptation to changing circumstances and contingencies, a fit between situational demands and behavioral possibilities, and the flexible use of the available repertoire of problem-solving strategies (broadly defined to include social and personal as well as cognitive strategies). The other end of the continuum, called ego brittleness, implies little adaptive flexibility, an inability to respond to changing demands, a tendency to perseverate or become disorganized when confronted with changes in circumstances or when stressed, and difficulty in recovering from traumatic experiences.

The Blocks differentiated the construct of ego resiliency from that of coping because contemporaneous researchers often defined coping in ways that were not independent of the outcome, that is, of whether or not the behavior "works." However, their notion of ego resiliency is quite similar to Lazarus and Folkman's (1984) definition of coping.

In an impressive longitudinal study, the Blocks (1980) obtained considerable support for their construct of ego resiliency (as well as ego control). Among other findings, ego-resilient children, in comparison to ego-brittle children, were viewed by teachers as better able to cope with stress. Findings at age 7 were similar, albeit weaker (perhaps due to the method of measurement). Further, Eisenberg, Fabes, Guthrie et al. (1996) have found that resiliency is related to low levels of problem behavior.

The Blocks found no statistical relation between measures of ego resiliency and ego control, and they argued that the two constructs are independent. However, they noted that "extreme placement at either end of the ego-control continuum implies a constancy in mode of behavior that, given a varying world, can be expected to be adaptively dysfunctional" (p. 44). This statement seems to reflect the belief that moderate ego control is adaptive and entails more flexibility than ego over- or undercontrol. Indeed, children who are not over- or undercontrolled are likely to possess many of the positive qualities associated with ego resiliency. Thus, Eisenberg and Fabes (1992) suggested that there is a relation between ego control and ego resiliency, but this relation is nonlinear. Specifically, they hypothesized that ego resiliency is negatively related to both ego overcontrol and undercontrol, but positively related to moderate ego control. Such a relation was hypothesized, although moderate ego control may not always be associated with the flexibility and ability to adapt (the hallmark of the construct of ego resiliency). Consistent with Eisenberg and Fabes' arguments, Arend, Gove, and Sroufe (1979) found that securely attached children were both high on resiliency and between the avoidant infants (who were overcontrolled) and the anxious/resistant infants (who were undercontrolled).

Although no one mode of coping is optimal in all situations and flexibility may be essential for optimal adaptation, it appears that some types of coping often are more effective at reducing stress and more constructive than are others. For example, problem-focused coping seems to be associated with positive outcomes in many settings, albeit not in uncontrollable contexts (e.g., Compas, Malcarne, & Fondacaro, 1988; Folkman & Lazarus, 1988). Further, the ability to shift or refocus attention has been associated with lower levels of distress, frustration, and other negative emotions (e.g., Bridges & Grolnick, 1995; Derryberry & Rothbart, 1988; Miller & Green, 1985; Rothbart et al., 1992). Thus, planful problem solving and the use of attentional strategies seem in general, if not always, to be effective ways of coping with stress. In contrast, aggressive, hostile responses to stress, although they sometimes may reduce the stress experienced by the actor in the immediate context, in general are likely to be ineffective in reducing stress (and may exacerbate it), particularly in the long term (e.g., Fabes & Eisenberg, 1992; Folkman & Lazarus, 1988; Folkman, Lazarus, Dunkel-Schetter, Delongis, & Gruen, 1986). For example, aggressive coping is likely to lead to peer rejection (Coie, Dodge, & Kupersmidt, 1990), which is likely to generate stress on an ongoing basis.

Based on the Block's work and on empirical data pertaining to the effectiveness of various modes of regulation and coping, we have proposed three general styles of regulation (Eisenberg & Fabes, 1992): optimal regulation, underregulation, and highly inhibited regulation. *Optimal regulation* involves the flexible use of regulatory mechanisms, relatively high use of constructive modes of regulation such as activational control, attentional control (e.g., attention shifting and focusing), planning and problem solving, and moderately high use of inhibitory control. *Underregulation* is less flexible and involves relatively low use of generally constructive modes of regulation such as attentional control, inhibition control, activational control (the ability to initiate and maintain behavior, particularly behaviors that are not pleasurable) (Derryberry & Rothbart, 1988), planning and direct problem solving, and other modes of emotion regulation such as positive cognitive restructuring. Due to the lack of regulation of both emotion and emotionally driven behavior, impulsive, acting-out responses are likely to occur (see Pulkkinen, 1986). *Highly inhibited regulation,* although similar to underregulation in terms of lack of flexibility and relative underutilization of adaptive modes of regulation, is characterized by high levels of inhibition control. Block and Block's (1980) overcontrolled children and Kagan's (e.g., Kagan, 1989) behaviorally inhibited children are examples of people characterized by a highly inhibited regulation style (see also Cummings & Cummings, 1988). Although inhibition and avoidance sometimes may be effective coping strategies (Eisenberg et al., 1992; Kliewer, 1991; Roth & Cohen, 1986), stable high use of inhibition and avoidance in dealing with stress may be associated with fearfulness and difficulty in dealing with stress and novelty (see Rubin, LeMare, & Lollis, 1990), as well as psychological symptoms when dealing with an ongoing stressor such as divorce (Sandler et al., 1994).

These three general types of coping clearly do not capture all the variation in either coping in specific settings or in coping styles. Nonetheless, they are useful in considering the correlates and outcomes (short- and long-term) of individual differences in general styles of coping (see Eisenberg & Fabes, 1992).

From a developmental perspective, it is important to explore whether style of coping is associated with social, psychological, and even health-related outcomes (see Skinner & Wellborn, 1994); a focus merely on adaptation in specific situations is not highly informative in regard to developmental outcomes.

A MODEL OF COPING

From the extant literature, it is clear that developmental changes in children's competencies and behaviors have significance for understanding their choices among, and execution of, various coping and regulatory strategies. For example, the resources (internal, external, and/or social) that children can bring to bear in stressful contexts change with development. Additionally, children's susceptibility to stress (i.e., threats to oneself) and the situations that produce stress change over the course of development (Thompson, 1990). Events that induce stress in young children often appear innocuous to older children and adults, whereas cognitively induced stressors are likely to occur more often for older children and adults than for younger children. Thus, from a developmental point of view, it is unlikely that there is any simple linear increase or decrease in children's overall likelihood of experiencing stress (Maccoby, 1983), and the limited research supports this notion (i.e., Silverman, La Greca, & Wasserstein, 1995; Yamamoto, Soliman, Parsons, & Davies, 1987).

What factors influence the development of coping and regulatory responses? Additionally, what factors contribute to changes in the contexts that produce stress? To address these questions, we now turn to a discussion (albeit limited) of processes that may influence children's stress-related responses (e.g., appraisals, coping, regulation).

To facilitate our thinking and discussion about both the coping process and variables influencing and resulting from that process, we have constructed a heuristic model (presented in Fig. 1). Our goals in presenting this model are twofold: (1) to illustrate how the distinction among various modes of regulation is useful in considering the process of coping, and (2) to stimulate thinking about individual, socialization/environmental, and contextual characteristics that influence the coping process, as well as about the role of coping in important developmental outcomes. Space does not allow full discussion of this model; thus, we primarily focus our attention on the far left side of the figure (Characteristics of Child, Socialization and Environment of the Child, and Context of the Stressful Event) after brief consideration of the middle components of the model (other authors in this volume cover more of the processes identified in five middle-level boxes of Fig. 1; e.g., Chapter 1, this volume).

The Role of Regulation in the Coping Process

Before we begin our discussion of the boxes on the left side of Fig. 1, we believe it is important to differentiate among the various types of coping/regulation that may function somewhat differently in the coping process. In our view, attempts to directly regulate the experience of emotion often occur quite early in the coping process, prior to or while the first physiological and

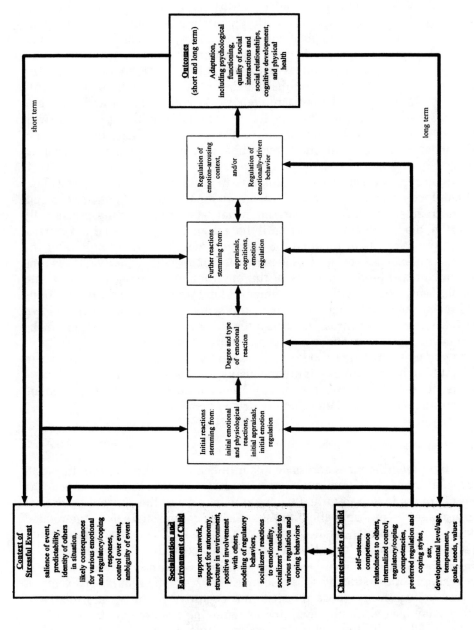

Figure 1. Heuristic model of the influences on regulation, the regulation process, and its outcomes. Shaded areas are discussed in the text.

emotional responses to a stressor are occurring. As soon as a situation is appraised as stressful, the individual may employ emotion regulation strategies
such as shifting attention or physically inhibiting approach behavior and further contact with the stressful stimulus in order to limit the escalation of
negative affect (see Rothbart & Derryberry, 1981). Further, once the individual
has clearly experienced negative affect, additional attempts at emotion regulation are likely. Thus, attempts at emotion regulation probably occur both prior
to full elicitation of physiological and emotional responses and again when an
emotional response (such as distress) has occurred (see Fig. 1). Further, as a
consequence of coping or changes in the situation, a new emotional response
may occur and additional emotional regulation strategies may be called into
play. The aforementioned ideas are consistent with Folkman and Lazarus's
(1988) assertion that coping may mediate emotional reactions, as well as with
the basic assumptions that emotional reactions to stress elicit efforts to cope,
and that coping occurs continually over time with feedback loops (see Lazarus,
1991).

In contrast, we suggest that attempts to regulate both the context (e.g.,
problem-focused coping) and one's own emotionally driven behavior (i.e., behavioral regulation) usually occur somewhat later in the coping process. By
definition, the latter cannot occur until there is an emotional reaction to stress.
In addition, attempts to regulate the situation would be likely only after the
stressful context has been appraised in at least some depth; usually it takes time
and thought to pinpoint aspects of the environment causing the stress and
possible ways to modify the environment. Many times, particularly for young
children, by the time such cognitive processing has occurred, a full-blown
emotional reaction to stress may be present, although identification of the
cause of the stress sometimes may evoke initial distress.

In summary, different types of regulation may occur at different points in
time (although sometimes simultaneously) in the coping process. Consequently, it is useful to conceptually distinguish among attempts to regulate
emotion, the context, and emotionally driven behavior.

Characteristics of the Child

Individual differences across people influence their choice of coping strategies. Children's developmental level is a factor that doubtlessly affects the
types of coping in an individual's repertoire, as well as the appropriateness of
their use and the probable effectiveness of some coping strategies. Age-related
changes in motor skills, memory, cognitive processing, language, understanding of others' and one's own internal states, metacognitive skills, and capacity
for planning have obvious relevance for children's abilities to choose and execute various coping strategies (see Compas, 1987; Kopp, 1989). For example,
the very young child, whose physical and cognitive resources are relatively
limited, may have difficulty avoiding or removing a source of stress without
assistance. Older children, whose motor, cognitive, and material resources are
more diverse and mature, often can leave a stressful situation, physically master the stressor (i.e., remove a barrier or turn off a noisy toy), or muster the
necessary cognitive and communication resources (i.e., recognition, memory)

for coping with stressful situations (e.g., Kopp, 1992). A review of the literature pertaining to all person variables relevant to developmental or individual differences in children's coping would be quite large, especially if one includes the work on emotion and behavioral regulation. Consequently, we do not attempt to review all of the relevant literature. Rather, we merely highlight some examples that are of particular interest from a developmental perspective.

Developmental Change and Coping

How children perceive and appraise events and people in potentially stressful situations is related to their behavioral responses, and these perceptions and appraisals vary considerably across development (see Shantz, 1983). Relatedly, children's tendency and/or ability to use various modes of coping involving mental images or control of attention seems to vary with children's development, as do their coping-relevant self-perceptions and notions of control.

Type of Coping. Researchers have found that children's use of emotion-focused coping strategies (attempts to manage emotional distress) generally increases with age (Band & Weisz, 1988; Compas et al., 1988). In contrast, although problem-focused strategies (attempts to deal with the stressor) are more fully developed in older children and adults than in younger children, some types of problem-focused strategies decrease with age (Band & Weisz, 1988). For example, Harris and Lipian (1989) found that 6-year-olds suggested concrete strategies to make themselves feel better when they felt sad, whereas 10-year-olds discussed more mentalistic strategies than instrumental strategies. Similarly, Masters (1991) reported that young children's (5-year-olds) strategies for regulating their own negative affect relied more on physical interaction and other physical and material interventions, whereas older children (8-year-olds) offered more cognitive interventions. Moreover, older children, in comparison to young children, are likely to utilize a greater number and variety of coping responses and focus on positive factors associated with the stressor (Brown, O'Keefe, Sanders, & Baker, 1986). These developmental differences probably are due, in part, to age-related changes in children's abilities to employ (as well as verbalize) cognitions designed to regulate emotions and stressful conditions.

Older and younger children may differ in their tendencies to use avoidant physical and cognitive coping responses. Bernzweig, Eisenberg, and Fabes (1993) found that second-grade children reported using more cognitive avoidance when coping with their own distress (and somewhat less support-seeking) than did kindergarten children. Altshuler and Ruble (1989) reported that younger children used complete avoidance (leaving or going away from the stressor) in stressful situations they could not control, whereas older children were more likely than younger children to use cognitive avoidance or distraction in these situations. Altshuler, Genevro, Ruble, and Bornstein (1995) obtained similar results in terms of knowledge of coping strategies; however, they also found that problem-solving ability moderated the effects of age, with older children who also were high in problem solving having the greatest knowledge of behavioral and cognitive distraction.

Mischel and Mischel (1983) found developmental differences in children's

knowledge of self-control strategies, including mentalistic strategies. Specifically, Mischel and Mischel found that by the end of their fifth year, children
begin to understand two basic rules for effective delay of gratification: to cover
rather than expose the reward and to engage in task-oriented rather than consummatory ideation while waiting. By grade 6, children realized that abstract
ideation would foster delay more than would consummatory ideation. Moreover, Mischel and Mischel reported that children under age 5 create self-defeating dilemmas for themselves by choosing tempting environments without adequately anticipating that they will be unable to execute strategies to overcome
the temptation. For example, young children expect that exposure to rewards
will help them delay gratification more than covering the rewards up. Young
children's preoperational thought may result in greater reliance on wish-fulfill-
ing strategies rather than on objectively effective strategies.

Age-related changes in children's attentional processes likely play an important role in coping. In comparison to older children and adults, young
children have limited attentional capacities. Young children have difficulty in
responding simultaneously to multiple inputs that require attention. Thus,
with development, children become increasingly able to cope with a potentially distressing event even if there is a great deal of change occurring in other
aspects of their environment (Maccoby, 1983). Moreover, young children's attention appears to be easily drawn to arousing rather than abstract properties of
a stimulus, thereby making self-control exceedingly difficult (Mischel, Shoda,
& Rodriguez, 1989). In contrast, older children recognize the problem of directing attention to the arousing attributes of the stimulus and try to distract their
attention away from the tempting stimulus.

Self-Perceptions and Perceptions of Control. Children's self-perceptions
regarding the degree to which they can successfully manage and control stressful events appear to influence whether an event is experienced as stressful. For
example, Compas and Phares (1991) noted that children who were vulnerable
to interpersonal stress reported lower self-perceptions of social competence
than did children resistant to social stress. Perceptions of control probably
influence children's responses to stressful situations in several ways (Skinner &
Wellborn, 1994). First, they protect the child from interpreting potential
stressors as threatening. Second, they support the development of new coping
strategies. For example, perceptions of control seem to influence the ability to
process information in stressful situations; Bugental, Cortez, and Blue (1992)
found that preschoolers and second graders who were high in perceived control acquired more accurate information in a fear-inducing situation than did
children with low self-perceived control. Moreover, adolescents high in perceived internal control used practice (e.g., problem-focused) coping (Hoffman
& Levy-Shiff, 1994), which is often a constructive reaction in controllable contexts.

Children's perceptions of their own competencies likely change as they
develop a more comprehensive, coherent, and integrated self-concept. Younger
children's self-referent beliefs focus predominantly on physical or behavioral
characteristics, whereas older children's beliefs reflect predominantly dispositional and personalistic beliefs (see Harter, 1983; Ruble & Dweck, 1995; Shantz,

1983). Moreover, younger children tend to be less accurate than older children in their assessments of their abilities; they tend to overestimate their abilities, remaining optimistic and confident, even in the face of negative feedback (Stipek, Recchia, & McClinic, 1992). One reason for young children's optimistic view of their competencies is that they believe that ability is a changing attribute that can be improved through practice or effort. In contrast, older children make a greater distinction between ability and effort, and regard competence as a relatively enduring trait that promotes or limits success (Benenson & Dweck, 1986). Thus, if older children have experiences that induce them to feel incapable of coping with specific stressors, they are unlikely to persist at coping efforts.

As children age, their ability to differentiate between situations where they can exert some control over a stressful situation and those where they cannot appears to increase (Band & Weisz, 1988; Harris, 1989). This ability is important for effective coping because, as noted previously, emotion-focused coping strategies seem to be the most effective means of coping in uncontrollable contexts (Blount, Landolf-Fritsche, Powers, & Sturges, 1991; Compas, Malcarne, & Banez, 1992). In contrast, events that are perceived as controllable tend to elicit more strategies for directly coping with the problem, and such strategies are believed to be related to positive outcomes (Band & Weisz, 1988; Compas et al., 1988, 1992). Children who use problem-focused coping in stressful situations perceived to be controllable and emotion-focused coping when the situation is perceived as uncontrollable evidence fewer behavior problems than do other children (Compas et al., 1988; Rossman & Rosenberg, 1992).

Developmental changes in sociocognitive capacities not only may provide children with new tools and skills for mastering their environment, but also may contribute to the likelihood of children experiencing stress. Because older children can more effectively alter their emotional arousal via mentally strategic means (e.g., distraction, altering goals, etc.), they are less likely than younger children to become overwhelmed in stressful situations. However, because older children are likely to internalize negative experiences and information and may be more realistic in their self-perceptions, their self-concepts may be more easily threatened than is the case for younger children (Thompson, 1990).

Attributions regarding Intentionality. Children's understanding of others' intentions is another important factor in children's stress-related responses and coping. Maccoby (1983) noted that the understanding of others' intentions is important for learning how to elicit cooperation and persuade others to help, for the development of a plan of action, and for successfully interacting with others. Consistent with Maccoby's observations, Dodge and his colleagues (e.g., Dodge & Coie, 1987) have shown that deficits in this domain of social cognition are related to ineffective coping. Specifically, they have found that aggressive children tend to perceive conflict situations that are ambiguous in regard to intent as intentionally caused. Children who were rated by their teachers and peers as neglected and rejected attributed hostile intent to prosocial and accidental actions, which in turn increased the likelihood of responding aggressively (Dodge, Murphy, & Buchsbaum, 1984). Popular children and average children's ability to make correct attributions about others' intents increased from kindergarten to fourth grade (Dodge et al., 1984); thus, these children might be expected to cope with certain interpersonal stressors more effectively with age.

In addition, perceptions of intent affect the experience of emotions (Dodge, 1991). Graham, Hudley, and Williams (1992) found that aggressive young adolescents who perceived an ambiguous action as intentionally caused reacted with higher feelings of anger. Moreover, this anger was linked to prescriptions of aggressive responding. Dodge (1991) hypothesized that aggressive children may be "emotionally vulnerable," and in arousing conditions are not able to process information effectively. In addition, under conditions of arousal, children may rely on both their dominant response pattern and cognitive heuristics when coping rather than on more reflective cognitive processing (see Bugental, Cortez, & Blue, 1992).

In brief, children's ability to make accurate inferences about themselves and others increases from childhood through adolescence (Shantz, 1983), and these inferences influence children's social coping strategies (Compas, 1987). The more mature the social inference, the more likely children will have the ability to select an effective coping strategy in the given context. As such, older children are more likely to be more effective at coping than younger children.

Temperamental and Dispositional Differences in Coping

Temperament and related individual differences in personality are person variables that likely influence coping and regulation. For example, temperamental factors such as reactivity and inhibition control (which probably become part of personality) (Caspi, in press) are likely to affect how children and adults respond to stress and the ways in which they attempt to regulate their emotional response to stress. Eisenberg and Fabes (1992) hypothesized that children who are high in emotionally reactivity are relatively likely to become overaroused in stressful contexts, particularly if they are low in dispositional regulation, and consequently are likely to choose and execute inappropriate coping strategies (see also Eisenberg, Fabes, Nyman et al., 1994). In contrast, children who are relatively high in temperamental emotional and behavioral regulation (see Derryberry & Rothbart, 1988) are believed to be relatively likely to react in a measured, socially competent rather than unregulated manner (Eisenberg, Fabes, Murphy et al., 1995).

There is evidence that individual differences in stress and coping responses are observable from a very early age. For example, Davis and Emory (1995) found that boys exhibited greater physiological and behavioral reactivity to some forms of stress at birth than did newborn girls. Because of the age of the children in her study (20–58 hours of age), these differences in stress-related reactivity existed before extensive socialization had occurred.

Positive Emotion, Sociability, and Activity Level. Positive emotionality, sociability, and activity level all have been linked to competence in dealing with stress and social conflict. For example, Werner and Smith (1982) found that infants who were active and socially responsive were likely to be resistant

to stress in childhood and adulthood. Similarly, children with positive socio-emotional characteristics (e.g., positive mood, sociability, low intensity of reaction) cope better with high levels of stress than do other children (Carson & Bittner, 1994; Garmezy, 1985). Temperamental attributes such as positive mood and sociability may contribute to stress resistance and coping because they enhance the goodness of fit between the individual and his or her physical and social environment (Lerner & East, 1984). Further, children high in positive emotionality likely have secure and positive relationships with others (although the causal relation between temperament and quality of relationships doubtlessly is bidirectional), and feelings of relatedness with others are believed to enhance the quality of coping (Skinner & Wellborn, 1994).

It also is likely that more active and persistent children, in comparison to children who are less active and persistent, are relatively effective at problem-focused coping in controllable situations because they expend greater effort and try more solutions than do other children when coping (Karraker & Lake, 1991; see also Carson & Bittner, 1994). However, we might expect active and persistent children to be less effective in situations that are uncontrollable and in which problem-focused strategies are likely to lead to frustration (Altshuler & Ruble, 1989).

Negative Emotional Intensity. As noted previously, children's negative emotional intensity may be particularly relevant to coping. For example, high dispositional negative emotional intensity and/or general emotional intensity has been negatively related to constructiveness of children's coping with anger (Eisenberg, Fabes, Nyman et al., 1994), low levels of socially appropriate behavior and social/prosocial behavior, and relatively high levels of problem behavior, particularly for boys (Eisenberg, Fabes, Murphy et al, 1995). Children who are high in temperamental reactivity and low in regulation are particularly likely to score low on measures of social functioning (e.g., socially appropriate behavior and peer status) (Eisenberg et al., 1993, 1995; Eisenberg, Fabes, Minore, et al., 1994). In addition, children with a low threshold of reactivity are likely to be more easily stressed by low evocative stress-related stimuli than are those children who have higher thresholds (see Kagan, 1989).

Inhibitory Control. The ability to inhibit behavior appears to be especially linked to quality of coping. As noted by Maccoby (1983), there is reason to believe that the maturation of the nervous system during early childhood contributes to children's increasing ability to inhibit disorganizing responses to stressful situations. Thus, with age, children become increasingly competent at maintaining behavioral and physiological organization in the face of stressful and arousing events (also see Kopp, 1982).

Of course, there are individual differences in people's abilities to inhibit inappropriate behavioral responses in response to stress. Recall our earlier discussion of Block and Block's (1980) findings that undercontrolled children were less behaviorally regulated than overcontrolled children. Further, antisocial behavior has been associated with dysregulation when stressed (e.g., Zahn-Waxler et al., 1994). In a sample of normal children, individual differences in regulation (including the ability to inhibit behavior) were associated with children's socially appropriate behavior and problem behavior (Eisenberg et al., 1995).

Pierce, Tout, and de Haan (1993) found that inhibitory control was inversely related to salivary cortisol production (which is produced when stressed). Moreover, children who were sociable and socially skilled evidenced less cortisol reactivity than other children. These results suggest that there is a relation between inhibitory regulatory mechanisms, as well as sociability (another aspect of temperament), and stress-sensitive physiological systems.

Other evidence of the relation between inhibition control and coping comes from a recent study with adults (Fabes & Eisenberg, in press). In this study, measures of adults' temperamental inhibitory control (as well as emotion regulation) were inversely related to reports of daily stress and intense emotional reactions in these stressful situations. Indices of regulation were related to adults' reported daily coping strategies; individuals who reported more inhibitory and emotional control were less likely to vent their emotions or to use drugs when stressed. However, the relation of regulatory control (as assessed with vagal tone) to coping was moderated by the level of stress experienced by the individual. Individuals who had greater regulatory control were more likely to utilize positive coping responses (e.g., seek support from others, thinking about or trying out solutions to problems) than were those low or moderate in regulatory control, but only under conditions of high stress. Thus, the relation between temperamental regulation and coping depended on situational factors. Whether similar relations hold for children and how the association between inhibition control and adaptive coping changes with development are important questions for the future.

Although moderately high levels of inhibition appear to be associated with effective coping, very high levels may undermine effective coping, at least in some contexts. Behaviorally inhibited children tend to display distress and anxiety in response to stressful psychosocial stimuli, whereas behaviorally uninhibited children are often spontaneous and sociable with strangers and explore unfamiliar environments (Kagan, 1989; Kagan, Reznick, and Snidman, 1986). As such, behaviorally inhibited children evidence a lowered response threshold to psychosocial stressors, resulting in exaggerated responses to these stressors.

Longitudinal evidence suggests that behavioral inhibition is moderately stable; three fourths of the children classified as either behaviorally inhibited or uninhibited at 21 months retained their classifications at 7½ years (Kagan, 1989). Similarly, Block (1987) found considerable continuity in impulse control from age 4 to age 18. Thus, inhibitory control appears to be a relatively stable aspect of individuals' functioning and would be expected to relate to coping throughout childhood.

Attentional Control. Another temperamental mechanism relevant to coping with stress is attentional control. Individuals can direct their attention toward or away from a source of stimulation to reduce stressful reactivity. Fabes et al. (1993) found that children who were physiologically aroused (as measured by skin conductance reactivity) were more likely to visually disengage the visually distressing stimulus (an evocative film). In that study, boys who evidenced more attentional disengagement reported feeling relatively less distress than did those boys who did not visually disengage the stressful film. Thus, it appears that boys were successful in their attempts to reduce their aversive arousal by visually disengaging the visual stimulus (see, however, Cortez & Bugental, 1994, for different findings). Moreover, Rothbart and colleagues found that both infants (Rothbart et al., 1992) and adults (Derryberry & Rothbart, 1988) who were able to shift their attentional focus were less susceptible to discomfort, fear, and frustration. Consistent with these findings, attentional control has been negatively correlated with 4- to 6-year-olds' negative affect and the intensity of negative emotions and positively related to socially appropriate behavior, popularity, and constructive reactions when angered (Eisenberg et al., 1993; Eisenberg, Fabes, Nyman et al., 1994). Thus, attentional mechanisms can be considered to be an important means of emotional regulation.

Summary. No doubt there are other temperamental characteristics that contribute to children's abilities to cope with stress (e.g., irritability, soothability). Because temperamental factors underlie children's affective, cognitive, and social functioning, it is likely that they are intimately involved in children's susceptibility and reactions to stress. However, it is important to keep in mind that temperamental characteristics and their expression are modified by development and experience (Lerner & East, 1984; Rende & Plomin, 1992). Consideration of the complex relations among temperament, the stressful context, situational emotional responses, and emotionally driven behavior is necessary for a more complete understanding of coping.

Socialization and Environment of the Child

Numerous aspects of the child's socialization history and his or her antecedent and ongoing environment would be expected to influence the degree to which a child is a flexible and effective coper in stressful situations. Again, space permits consideration of only a few examples.

Structure and Autonomy

Skinner and Wellborn (1994) suggested two aspects of the ongoing social context that buffer the effects of stress and promote effective coping: structure (i.e., the provision of clear expectations, consistent contingencies, and help) and support for autonomy (including the provision of choice, minimal coercion, and rationales for disciplinary rules). In their view, individuals construct self-system processes based on the quality of their interactions with the environment. An involved social context promotes children's perceptions of relatedness to others; structured environments foster success experiences and self-perceived competence. Further, structured social contexts are viewed as fostering active attempts at problem solving in some contexts. In an analogous manner, contexts that allow children to experience themselves as self-determining promote self-perceptions of autonomy (and, one suspects, actual autonomy); the more supportive of autonomy the social context, the more flexible and self-determined the child's coping is likely to be.

There is evidence supporting Skinner and Wellborn's assertions. Parents who provide consistent structure and contingencies allow the child to develop a sense of control over their environment, and these perceptions of control have been found to be related to how efficacious children feel (Baumrind, 1989; Grolnick & Ryan, 1989; cf. Hardy, Power, & Jaedicke, 1993). For example, parents' use of consistent contingencies for children's behavior has been found to be positively related to self-regulation (Kopp, 1982). Additionally, Bryant (1987) found that parental use of principled discipline and parental consistency of expectations were positively related to coping with social stressors in middle childhood. In adolescence, parental monitoring and firmness have been linked to low emotion-focused coping (e.g., angry reactions and avoidance of stressors through drugs and denial); it also was linked to low levels of coping through prayer and talking with various professionals (Dusek & Danko, 1994).

In contrast, children who are not provided with structure and contingent responses tend to experience feelings of helplessness and incompetence, which in turn lower their feelings of effectiveness in coping with their world (Baumrind, 1989). Indulgent and uninvolved parents, by providing few rules and making few demands for mature behavior, are relatively unlikely to foster the development of regulation. Children reared in a permissive family environment lack impulse control as preschoolers and are relatively low in social and cognitive competence as elementary school children (Baumrind, 1989).

Parental Socialization of Children's Emotional Responses

Parents' reactions to children's emotions have been linked with children's abilities to regulate emotions (e.g., emotion-focused coping/regulation). Through social interactions with caregivers, the infant and young child learn to control the degree of excitation they experience (Kopp, 1989). For example, parents manage and guide children's emotional experiences by directly relieving distress, fear, frustration, and other negative emotions and helping children to modulate emotional arousal. Furthermore, parents influence development of emotion regulation through modeling, selective reinforcement of emotional expressions, social referencing, verbal instruction about emotions, induction of emotion, and controlled opportunities for emotional arousal (Eisenberg et al., 1992; Thompson, 1994).

Because children generally experience negative emotions in stressful situations, it is likely that socializers' emotion-related socialization practices affect the ways in which children deal with stress. Within the family, parents may foster constructive coping by directly instructing children on how to appraise stressful events, suggesting various courses of action to deal with problems and reinforcing appraisals and coping behavior. Moreover, parents model coping behaviors and shape the family environment within which coping is learned (Kliewer, Sandler, & Wolchik, 1994; see also Hoffman & Levy-Shiff, 1994).

As one example, Eisenberg et al. (1991) found that boys whose parents encouraged them to engage in direct problem-solving when anxious or sad seemed to manage their vicariously induced distress in a relatively optimal manner compared to others boys (i.e., they were more likely to experience sympathy rather than a distressed reaction when exposed to an empathy-inducing stimulus). Similarly, parental emphasis on either solving the problem or on comforting their child when the child experiences negative emotion has been correlated with lower levels of children's seeking revenge when dealing with anger, as well as with high peer status (Eisenberg et al., 1992). Consistent with these findings, Roberts and Strayer (1987) found that parental problem-solving responses when their children were upset were related to children's social competence; children likely model the problem-solving behaviors of their parents. In contrast, parental punitive responses to children's displays of negative emotion have been associated with children coping with anger by seeking revenge or avoiding the conflict situation (Eisenberg et al., 1992). Thus, it is likely that parents and other socializers play a relatively direct role in shaping children's preferred coping responses (Miller, Kliewer, Hepworth, & Sandler, 1994), although genetic factors also may partially account for relations between parental behaviors and children's coping reactions.

Quality of Social Relationships

The ongoing quality of the children's relationships with others would be expected to relate to children's ability to cope with stress (e.g., Skinner & Wellborn, 1994). For example, research on the quality of children's attachments provides evidence of the importance of the early relationship between parent and child for children's coping competence. Children's attachments to their caregivers impact their resilience to stress (Garmezy, 1985) and are likely related to children's perceptions of themselves and their effectiveness, as well as children's emotional regulation in relationships (Bridges & Grolnick, 1995; Sroufe, 1988). Further, the support and effectuality provided by secure attachments are thought to foster effective coping skills and intellectual and social competence. For example, Sroufe (1988) found that children who were classified as securely attached evidenced more positive affect, persistence, and compliance as toddlers than did insecurely attached children. In the preschool years, children classified as securely attached were rated by teachers as being competent in coping with peers and in establishing friendships. In contrast, anxious and avoidant children were more likely to be have problematic interactions with peers (i.e., to be victimized) and were found to be noncompliant with teachers.

Consistent with the attachment-related data, Herman and McHale (1993) found that parental warmth and intimacy were associated with higher rates of children's talking to parents and problem-solving strategies for coping with parental negativity. Further, Hardy et al. (1993) noted that children from families with high maternal support and relatively low family structure (i.e., consistency and organization of household) used the greatest variety of coping strategies. Maternal support also was associated with children's use of avoidant strategies in uncontrollable situations (viewed as an appropriate strategy), whereas family structure was correlated with low levels of children's aggressive coping. Moreover, in another study, adolescent boys' (but not girls') perceptions of their parents as warm and supportive were related to practical coping (e.g., problem-focused and support-seeking) (Dusek & Danko, 1994).

Sibling and peer relationships provide different contexts than parent–

child relationships for the development of coping strategies. These relationships are based more on reciprocity and relative equality than is interaction with parents (Skinner & Wellborn, 1994; Sroufe, 1988; Youniss, 1980). Thus, peer and sibling interactions may provide an optimal setting for children's learning to cope with stress in relationships with equals.

In addition, Bryant and Litman (1987) argued that siblings can provide a buffer for children when parents are unavailable. For example, when mothers are distant or absent, older siblings in particular tend to comfort their younger sibling. This behavior alleviates younger siblings' distress and may facilitate active exploration, learning about the environment, and feelings of competence and control. Comforting, helping, praising, and cooperating with siblings also may enhance children's coping by increasing their feelings of self-efficacy. In addition, siblings facilitate children's learning to cope with aggressive behaviors. Through sibling conflict interactions, children learn how to discriminate when aggressive behaviors are appropriate and when they are not (Bryant & Litman, 1987). Thus, children's experiences with their siblings likely influence the development of coping abilities.

Peers, like siblings, likely provide a context for learning coping skills. For example, peers serve as models for coping with stressful contexts (Schunk & Hanson, 1989). Klingman, Melamed, Cuthbert, and Hermecz (1984) found that children exposed to peers who modeled the use of controlled breathing and imagery under stressful conditions enacted more problem-focused and emotion-focused coping when coping with stress (i.e., going to the dentist) than did those children who were not exposed to peer models. Moreover, if a peer treats a potentially stressful situation as nonthreatening, children may learn from the peer's example, and hence experience less distress. Thus, it is likely that children's stress-related appraisals, as well as behavioral and emotional responses, are influenced by observing peers (Compas et al., 1992; Thompson, 1994).

Another important role played by peers is that of meeting children's needs for social and emotional support. Contacts with peers, especially with friends, represent important sources of companionship and recreation, with peers serving as trusted confidants, allies, and sources of advice and assistance in times of stress (Asher, 1990). As discussed previously, children with adequate social support may cope better with stress. Given the increasing number of working mothers and single-parent families, peers may play an even more important role in social support and coping today than they did in years past.

The importance of peer relationships for children's effective coping is highlighted by substantial evidence that poor peer relations predict certain negative outcomes for children (Newcomb, Bukowski, & Pattee, 1993; Parker & Asher, 1987). For example, social rejection and isolation in childhood are predictors of early school withdrawal, delinquency and adult criminality, and mental health problems (Kupersmidt, Cole, & Dodge, 1990). Thus, one would expect the quality of children's peer relationships to be related to their coping skills, although it is likely that the causal influence in this relation is bidirectional.

Developmentally, peers probably represent increasingly important sources of influence on children's coping as frequency of contact with family members declines (Compas et al., 1992; Feiring & Lewis, 1991). Children become increasingly dependent on peers, not only for companionship but also for self-validation and support (Nelson-LeGall & Gumerman, 1984). Moreover, the basis for peer relations changes with age; young children stress the importance of activities and common interests, whereas older children and adolescents stress the importance of emotional support and loyalty (Rotenberg & Mann, 1986). Older children expect and demand more from their friends, and the quality of older children's friendships are more intense and intimate than is the case of younger children. With increased age, children increasingly regard peer relationships as a forum for self-disclosure, advice, and support when stressed (Greene & Larson, 1991). Thus, with age, positive relationships with peers, particularly in the context of friendships, may play an increasing role in children's ability to cope with stress.

Quality of Social Support

One factor that is part of an individual's ongoing everyday life and frequently has been linked with the coping process is the individual's social support resources. Supportive relationships with peers (Cauce, Felner, & Primavera, 1982) and one's family (Holahan & Moos, 1987) appear to foster effective coping (see Compas, 1987). For children in nonsupportive, disturbed families, a relationship with an adult outside the family seems to enhance the child's resilience to stress (Garmezy, 1983). Skinner and Wellborn (1994) argued that a social context in which adults are involved with the child (i.e., express affection and dedicate time and resources) both buffers the effects of stress and allows the child to turn to others for help and comfort when necessary.

Context of the Stressful Event

The role of the stressful context in the coping process has been discussed in some detail by coping theorists (e.g., Lazarus & Folkman, 1984; Krohne, 1988). Thus, due to our focus on children and development, we discuss primarily the ways in which stressful contexts may differ for children of different ages.

Age-related changes in children and their social environments may affect which specific situations elicit children's stress. Children's early interactions with their environment initially revolve around their caregivers. Thus, it is not surprising that separation from infants' caregivers is a common stressful context; by the end of the first year, even brief periods of separation from the caregiver are believed to be stressful to infants (Bowlby, 1969). Children's separation from their caregiver produces a set of physiological responses (i.e., increased heart rate, increased salivary cortisol production) that is indicative of stress (see Gunnar & Brodersen, 1992). Even in the first years of life, children exhibit individual differences in the ability to cope with their distress when separated from mother (Connell & Thompson, 1986; see Bridges & Grolnick, 1995). Moreover, as children get older, stress increasingly is likely to be induced as a result of caregivers' efforts to control and elicit compliance from their children (see Kopp, 1982).

With age, children also increasingly come into contact with stressors that do not involve their caregivers. For example, as children come into contact with other children, stress associated with anger and conflict is a common occurrence. Parke and Slaby (1983) noted that approximately half of the interactions among infants 12 to 18 months of age are disruptive or conflictual. Although the proportion of such stressful conflicted interactions decreases with age, even among older preschoolers, stressful conflict occurs in a sizable proportion of their interactions (20% of all interactions) (Parke & Slaby, 1983).

Moreover, the situations that elicit these stressful conflicts with peers change over age. During the preschool years, children's conflicts primarily revolve around material objects and space issues. Hay and Ross (1982) found that 72% of conflicts among 21-month-old children involved conflicts over objects or possession struggles. Using an older sample of preschoolers (mean age was about 55 months), Fabes and Eisenberg (1992) found that about 50% of the conflicts between these older preschoolers involved material or possession conflicts. Additionally, Fabes and Eisenberg reported that older children (especially girls) were more likely to be involved in stressful conflicts due to social rejection (i.e., being ignored or not allowed to play with others) than were younger children.

Entrance into elementary school also brings about changes in stress-related situations. Researchers have found that children manifest behavioral problems related to school entry and that these behaviors typically dissipate after a short adjustment period (see Rutter, 1983). The increased focus on intellectual skills, evaluation, and achievement in the school context produces stress in the form of homework, tests, and increased social comparisons (Higgins & Parsons, 1983). Entry into school also is associated with increased concerns and stress related to peer acceptance and increased exposure to a variety of personality styles to which children must accommodate (see Minuchin & Shapiro, 1983). Many of these changes are likely to disrupt a child's equilibrium and consequently elicit the need for coping reactions.

The adolescent period often has been characterized as a period that is wrought with stress and tension (Blos, 1979). Although contemporary researchers often have failed to find much evidence for universal or dramatic stress and disorganization during adolescence (e.g., Brooks-Gunn, 1989; Offer, 1987), the social and environmental (and physiological) changes (i.e., dating, sexuality, entry into new school settings, etc.) experienced by young adolescents provide numerous opportunities for stressful events (Brooks-Gunn, 1992). Depending on the mix of events, their timing and sequencing, and the circumstances in which they occur, adolescents are likely to experience stress-related situations that differ from those of younger children.

Finally, it is important to note that there is an interaction of individual differences in coping-relevant person characteristics with features of the particular context. For example, as noted by Skinner and Wellborn (1994), individual differences in relatedness (i.e., the feeling of being securely connected to others, worthy, and capable of love) would be expected to be particularly relevant in coping with stressors that involve interpersonal loss or separation, such as divorce, adjustment to the birth of a sibling, or adjustment to child care or school. If a child has a secure internal working model of relationships and if individuals with whom the child has a close attachment are available, the child likely will experience such situations as less stressful and would be expected to react in constructive ways (e.g., by trying to establish new relationships). Similarly, individual differences in perceived control would be expected to be intimately related to reactions to events involving failure, noncontingency, and unpredictability, whereas individual differences in perceived autonomy would be expected to predict flexibility and independent coping in situations in which the child's autonomy is threatened (and perhaps in a wider range of situations in which autonomous responding is an option).

Outcomes

Coping with stress is likely to have both short-term and long-term consequences. In the short term, how the individual copes/regulates may alter interactions in the immediate context. For example, if an individual reacts in a socially appropriate and constructive manner, the stressful situation is likely to be resolved (e.g., Sackin & Thelen, 1984). In contrast, reactions that are hostile or confrontative may perpetuate and escalate the stressful context (Carver et al., 1989).

Because of their interest in optimal development, developmentalists and child clinicians are particularly likely to be concerned with the long-term implications of coping/regulation reactions, particularly in regard to social adaptation and psychological symptoms (e.g., Block, Gjerde, & Block, 1991; Cummings & Cummings, 1988; Eisenberg et al., 1993; Sandler et al., 1994). From a developmental perspective, coping reactions tend to elicit social and environmental consequences and evaluations (e.g., they influence how adults and peers perceive the child and his or her acceptance), which are then reflected back and alter the child's self-perceptions and style of reaction and regulation in future stressful situations.

Skinner and Wellborn (1994) emphasized the long-term consequences of coping for social development (i.e., the capacity to love and be loved), cognitive development (i.e., the ability to discover and understand how to produce desired outcomes and the capacities to execute those strategies), and personality development (i.e., the construction of a coherent self that integrates one's unique talents and proclivities with the demands internalized from society). They noted the importance of (1) coping responses that do not inhibit development in one area of functioning in the service of gain (often short term) in another, and (2) the ability to reengage in the face of obstacles for cognitive, social, and personality development. Engagement in stressful contexts is viewed as an opportunity to exercise and develop skills.

Initial work indicates that there are indeed correlational associations between children's regulatory behaviors in stressful contexts and important long-term outcomes such as the development of socially appropriate behavior, popularity, problem behavior, and psychological symptoms (Block & Block, 1980; Block et al., 1991; Eisenberg et al., 1993; Eisenberg, Fabes, Murphy et al., 1995; Kliewer, 1991; Pulkkinen, 1988; Sandler et al., 1994). However, work of this sort is limited in quantity, and there is little relevant longitudinal work.

Clearly, work on the long-term consequences of quality of coping is a research priority.

CONCLUSIONS

In this chapter we have explored the construct of coping from a developmental perspective. This was done in several ways. First, the construct of coping was embedded in the larger developmental literature on regulation, including the work on emotion and behavioral regulation. A heuristic model of the coping process was proposed, one that emphasizes developmental antecedents and outcomes of coping, as well as the multiple roles of regulation in the coping process. Then the developmental literature relevant to changes in children's stress-related vulnerability and their coping and regulation was reviewed.

One of our goals was to bring more of the developmental literature into theory and research on coping. Although the coping literature generally is treated as a separate body of research—one more relevant to clinical and personality psychology than to developmental psychology—there is much in the developmental literature of relevance to an understanding of coping. Further, given the consistency across time of temperamental emotionality and its regulation and the role of socialization and relationships in the development of regulation, developmental research and theory are essential for an understanding of individual differences in coping styles, even in adulthood. Analogously, work on coping is relevant to developmentalists interested in regulation, especially emotion regulation. Thus, more exchange is needed between developmental researchers and investigators studying coping from other perspectives.

ACKNOWLEDGMENTS

The writing of this chapter was partially supported by a grant from the National Science Foundation (DBS9208375) to the first two authors and a Research Scientist Development Award from the National Institute of Mental Health (K02 MH 00903) to Nancy Eisenberg.

REFERENCES

Altshuler, J. L., & Ruble, D. N. (1989). Developmental changes in children's awareness of strategies for coping with uncontrollable stress. *Child Development, 60*, 1337–1349.

Altshuler, J. L., Genevro, J. L., Ruble, D. N., & Bornstein, M. H. (1995). Children's knowledge and use of coping strategies during hospitalization for elective surgery. *Journal of Applied Developmental Psychology, 16*, 53–76.

Arend, R., Gove, F. L., & Sroufe, L. A. (1979). Continuity of individual adaptation from infancy to kindergarten: A predictive study of ego-resiliency and curiosity in preschoolers. *Child Development, 50*, 950–959.

Asher, S. R. (1990). Recent advances in the study of peer rejection. In S. R. Asher & J. D. Coie (Eds.), *Peer rejection in childhood* (pp. 3–16). Cambridge, England: Cambridge University Press.

Band, E. B., & Weisz, J. R. (1988). How to feel better when it feels bad: Children's perspectives on coping with everyday stress. *Developmental Psychology, 24*, 247–253.

Baumrind, D. (1989). The permanence of change and the impermanence of stability. *Human Development, 32*, 187–195.

Benenson, J. F., & Dweck, C. S. (1986). The development of trait explanations and self evaluations in the academic and social domains. *Child Development, 57,* 1179–1187.

Bernzweig, J., Eisenberg, N., & Fabes, R. A. (1993). Children's coping in self- and other-relevant contexts. *Journal of Experimental Child Psychology, 55,* 208–226.

Block, J. H. (1987, April). *Longitudinal antecedents of ego-control and ego-resiliency in adolescence.* Paper presented at the biennial meeting of the Society for Research in Child Development, Baltimore.

Block, J. H., & Block, J. (1980). The role of ego-control and ego-resiliency in the organization of behavior. In W. Andrew Collins (Ed.), *Development of cognition, affect, and social relations. The Minnesota Symposia on Child Psychology* (Vol. 13, pp. 39–101). Hillsdale, NJ: Erlbaum.

Block, J., Gjerde, P. F., & Block, J. H. (1991). Personality antecedents of depressive tendencies in 18-year-olds: A prospective study. *Journal of Personality and Social Psychology, 60,* 726–738.

Blos, P. (1979). *The adolescent passage.* New York: International Press.

Blount, R. L., Landolf-Fritsche, B., Powers, S. W., & Sturges, J. W. (1991). Differences between high and low coping children and between parent and staff behaviors during painful medical procedures. *Journal of Pediatric Psychology, 16,* 795–809.

Bowlby, J. (1969). *Attachment and loss: Attachment* (Vol. 1). New York: Basic Books.

Bridges, L. J., & Grolnick, W. S. (1995). The development of emotional self-regulation in infancy and early childhood. In N. Eisenberg (Ed.), *Review of personality and psychology* (pp. 185–211).

Brooks-Gunn, J. (1989). Adolescents as children and as parents: A developmental perspective. In I. E. Sigel & G. H. Brody (Eds.), *Methods of family research: Biographies of research projects, Vol. I: Normal families* (pp. 213–248). Hillsdale, NJ: Erlbaum.

Brooks-Gunn, J. (1992). Growing up female: Stressful events and the transition to adolescence. In T. M. Field, P. M. McCabe, & N. Schneiderman (Eds.), *Stress and coping in infancy and childhood* (pp. 119–148). Hillsdale, NJ: Erlbaum.

Brown, J. M., O'Keefe, J., Sanders, S. H., & Baker, B. (1986). Developmental changes in children's cognition to stressful and painful situations. *Journal of Pediatric Psychology, 11,* 343–357.

Bryant, B. K. (1987). Mental health, temperament, family, and friends: Perspectives on children's empathy and social perspective taking. In N. Eisenberg & J. Strayer (Eds.), *Empathy and its development* (pp. 245–270). Cambridge, England: Cambridge University Press.

Bryant, B. K., & Litman, C. (1987). Siblings as teachers and therapists. *Journal of Children in Contemporary Society, 19,* 185–205.

Bugental, D. B., Cortez, V., & Blue, J. (1992). Children's affective responses to the expressive cues of others. In N. Eisenberg & R. A. Fabes (Eds.), *New directions in child development* (pp. 75–89). San Francisco: Jossey-Bass.

Carson, D. K., & Bittner, M. T. (1994). Temperament and school-aged children's coping abilities and responses to stress. *Journal of Genetic Psychology, 155,* 289–302.

Carver, C. S., Scheier, M. F., & Weintraub, J. K. (1989). Assessing coping strategies: A theoretically based approach. *Journal of Personality and Social Psychology, 56,* 267–283.

Caspi, A. (in press). Personality development. In W. Damon (Ed.), *Handbook of child psychology (Vol. 3, N. Eisenberg, ed., Social and personality development).* New York: Wiley.

Cauce, A. M., Felner, R. D., & Primavera, J. (1982). Social support in high-risk adolescents: Structural components and adaptive impact. *American Journal of Community Psychology, 10,* 417–428.

Coie, J. D., Dodge, K. A., & Kupersmidt, J. B. (1990). Peer group behavior and social status. In S. R. Asher & J. D. Coie (Eds.), *Peer rejection in childhood* (pp. 17–59). Cambridge, England: Cambridge University Press.

Compas, B. E. (1987). Coping with stress during childhood and adolescence. *Psychological Bulletin, 101,* 393–403.

Compas, B. E., Banez, G. A., Malcarne, V., & Worsham, N. (1991). Perceived control and coping with stress: A developmental perspective. *Journal of Social Issues, 47,* 23–34.

Compas, B. E., Malcarne, V. L., & Banez, G. A. (1992). Coping with psychological stress: A developmental perspective. In B. N. Carpenter (Ed.), *Personal coping: Theory, research, and application* (pp. 47–64). Westport, CT: Praeger.

Compas, B. E., Malcarne, V. L., Fondacaro, K. M. (1988). Coping with stressful events in older children and young adolescents. *Journal of Consulting and Clinical Psychology, 56,* 405–411.

Compas, B. E., & Phares, V. (1991). Stress during childhood and adolescence: Sources of risk and vulnerability. In E. M. Cummings, A. L. Greene, & K. H. Karraker (Eds.), *Life-span developmental psychology: Perspectives on stress and coping* (pp. 111–130). Hillsdale, NJ: Erlbaum.

Connell, J. P., & Thompson, R. A. (1986). Emotion and social interaction in the Strange Situation: Consistencies and asymmetric influences in the second year. *Child Development, 57,* 733–745.

Cortez, V. L., & Bugental, D. B. (1994). Children's visual avoidance of threat: A strategy associated with low social control. *Merrill-Palmer Quarterly, 40,* 82–97.

Cummings, E. M., & Cummings, J. L. (1988). A process-oriented approach to children's coping with adults' angry behavior. *Developmental Review, 8,* 296–321.

Davis, M., & Emory, E. (1995). Sex differences in neonatal stress reactivity. *Child Development, 66,* 14–27.

Derryberry, D., & Rothbart, M. K. (1988). Arousal, affect, and attention as components of temperament. *Journal of Personality and Social Psychology, 55,* 958–966.

Dodge, K. A. (1991). Emotion and social information processing. In J. Garber & K. A. Dodge (Eds.), *The development of emotion: Regulation and dysregulation* (pp. 159–181). Cambridge, England: Cambridge University Press.

Dodge, K. A., & Coie, J. D. (1987). Social-information-processing factors in reactive and proactive aggression in children's peer groups. *Journal of Personality and Social Psychology, 53,* 1146–1158.

Dodge, K. A., Murphy, R. R., & Buchsbaum, K. (1984). The assessment of intention-cue detection skills in children: Implications for development of psychopathology. *Child Development, 55,* 163–173.

Dusek, J. B., & Danko, M. (1994). Adolescent coping styles and perceptions of parental child rearing. *Journal of Adolescent Research, 9,* 412–426.

Eisenberg, N., & Fabes, R. A. (1992). Emotion, regulation, the development of social competence. In M. S. Clark (Ed.), *Review of personality and social psychology: Vol. 14. Emotion and social behavior* (pp. 119–150). Newbury Park, CA: Sage.

Eisenberg, N., Fabes, R. A., Bernzweig, J., Karbon, M., Poulin, R., & Hanish, L. (1993). The relations of emotionality and regulation to preschoolers' social skills and sociometric status. *Child Development, 64,* 1418–1438.

Eisenberg, N., Fabes, R. A., Carlo, G., & Karbon, M. (1992). Emotional responsivity to others: Behavioral correlates and socialization antecedents. N. Eisenberg & R. A. Fabes (Eds.), *New Directions in Child Development, 55,* 57–73.

Eisenberg, N., Fabes, R. A., Guthrie, I. K., Murphy, B. C., Maszk, P., Holmgren, R., & Suh, K. (1995). The relations of regulation and emotionality to problem behavior in elementary school children. *Development and Psychopathology, 8,* 141–162.

Eisenberg, N., Fabes, R. A., Minore, D., Mathy, R., Hanish, L., & Brown, T. (1994). Children's enacted interpersonal strategies: Their relations to social behavior and negative emotionality. *Merrill-Palmer Quarterly, 40,* 212–232.

Eisenberg, N., Fabes, R. A., Murphy, M., Maszk, P., Smith, M., & Karbon, M. (1995). The role of emotionality and regulation in children's social functioning: A longitudinal study. *Child Development, 66,* 1239–1261.

Eisenberg, N., Fabes, R. A., Nyman, M., Bernzweig, J., & Pinuelas, A. (1994). The relations of emotionality and regulation to young children's anger-related reactions. *Child Development, 65,* 109–128.

Fabes, R. A., & Eisenberg, N. (1992). Young children's coping with interpersonal anger. *Child Development, 63,* 116–128.

Fabes, R. A., & Eisenberg, N. (in press). Regulatory control and adults' stress and coping responses to daily life events. *Journal of Personality and Social Psychology.*

Fabes, R. A., Eisenberg, N., & Eisenbud, L. (1993). Physiological and behavior correlates of Children's reactions to others in distress. *Developmental Psychology, 29,* 655–663.

Fabes, R. A., Eisenberg, N., Nyman, M., & Michelieu, Q. (1991). Children appraisals of others' spontaneous emotional reactions. *Developmental Psychology, 27,* 858–866.

Feiring, C., & Lewis, M. (1991). The development of social networks from early to middle childhood: Gender differences and the relation to school competence. *Sex Roles, 25,* 237–253.

Folkman, S. (1991). Coping across the life span: Theoretical issues. In E. M. Cummings, A. L.

Greene, & K. H. Karraker (Eds.), *Life-span developmental psychology: Perspectives on stress and coping* (pp. 3–18). Hillsdale, NJ: Erlbaum.

Folkman, S., & Lazarus, R. A. (1988). Coping as a mediator of emotion. *Journal of Personality and Social Psychology, 54,* 466–475.

Folkman, S., Lazarus, R. S., Dunkel-Schetter, C., DeLongis, N., & Gruen, R. (1986). Dynamics of a stressful encounter: Cognitive appraisal, coping, and encounter outcomes. *Journal of Personality and Social Psychology, 50,* 992–1003.

Fox, N. A. (1989). Psychophysiological correlates of emotional reactivity during the first year of life. *Developmental Psychology, 25,* 364–372.

Garmezy, N. (1983). Stressors of childhood. In N. Garmezy & M. Rutter (Eds.), *Stress, coping and development in children* (pp. 43–84). New York: McGraw-Hill.

Garmezy, N. (1985). Stress-resistant children. The search for protective factors. In J. E. Stevenson (Ed.), *Recent research in developmental psychopathology* (pp. 213–233). Oxford: Pergamon.

Gibson, E. J. (1994). Has psychology a future? *Psychological Science, 5,* 69–76.

Graham, S., Hudley, C., & Williams, E. (1992). Attributional and emotional determinants of aggression among African-American and Latino young adolescents. *Developmental Psychology, 28,* 731–740.

Greene, A. L., & Larson, R. W. (1991). Variation in stress reactivity during adolescence. In E. M. Cummings, A. L. Greene, & K. H. Karraker (Eds.), *Life-span developmental psychology: Perspectives on stress and coping* (pp. 151–176). Hillsdale, NJ: Erlbaum.

Grolnick, W. S., & Ryan, R. M. (1989). Parent styles associated with children's self-regulation and competence in school. *Journal of Educational Psychology, 81,* 143–154.

Gunnar, M. R., & Brodersen, L. (1992). Infant stress reactions to brief maternal separations in human and nonhuman primates. In T. M. Field, P. M. McCabe, & N. Schneiderman (Eds.), *Stress and coping in infancy and childhood* (pp. 1–18). Hillsdale, NJ: Erlbaum.

Haan, N. (1977). *Coping and defending.* New York: Academic.

Hardy, D. F., Power, T. G., & Jaedicke, S. (1993). Examining the relation of parenting to children's coping with everyday stress. *Child Development, 64,* 1829–1841.

Harris, P. (1989). *Children and emotion.* Cambridge, MA: Basil Blackwell.

Harris, P. L., & Lipian, M. (1989). Understanding emotion and experiencing emotion. In C. Saarni & P. L. Harris (Eds.), *Children's understanding of emotion* (pp. 241–258). New York: Cambridge University Press.

Harter, S. (1983). Developmental perspectives on the self-system. In P. H. Mussen (Ed.), *Handbook of child psychology: Vol. IV. Socialization, personality, and social development* (ed. E. M. Hetherington) (pp. 275–385). New York: Wiley.

Hay, D. F., & Ross, H. S. (1982). The social nature of early conflict. *Child Development, 53,* 105–113.

Herman, M. A., & McHale, S. M. (1993). Coping with parental negativity: Links with parental warmth and child adjustment. *Journal of Applied Developmental Psychology, 14,* 131–136.

Higgins, E. T., & Parsons, J. E. (1983). Social cognition and the social life of the child: Stages as subcultures. In E. T. Higgins, D. N. Ruble, & W. W. Hartup (Eds.), *Social cognition and social development* (pp. 15–62). Cambridge, England: Cambridge University Press.

Hoffman, M. A., & Levy-Shiff, R. (1994). Coping and locus of control: A cross-generational transmission between mothers and adolescents. *Journal of Early Adolescence, 14,* 391–405.

Holahan, C. J., & Moos, R. H. (1987). Personal and contextual determinants of coping strategies. *Journal of Personality and Social Psychology, 52,* 946–955.

Kagan, J. (1989). The concept of behavioral inhibition to the unfamiliar. In J. S. Reznick (Ed.), *Perspectives on behavioral inhibition* (pp. 1–23). Chicago: Chicago University Press.

Kagan, J., Reznick, J. S., & Snidman, N. (1986). Temperamental inhibition in early childhood. In R. Plomin & J. Dunn (Eds.), *The study of temperament: Changes, continuities, and challenges* (pp. 53–65). Hillsdale, NJ: Erlbaum.

Karoly, P. (1993). Mechanisms of self-regulation: A systems view. *Annual Review of Psychology, 44,* 23–52.

Karraker, K. H., & Lake, M. (1991). Normative stress and coping processes in infancy. In E. M. Cummings, A. L. Greene, & K. H. Karraker (Eds.), *Life-span developmental psychology: Perspectives on stress and coping* (pp. 85–110). Hillsdale, NJ: Erlbaum.

Kendall, P. C., & Wilcox, L. E. (1979). Self-control in children: The development of a rating scale. *Journal of Consulting and Clinical Psychology, 47,* 1020–1030.

Kliewer, W. (1991). Coping in middle childhood: Relations to competence, type A behavior, monitoring, blunting, and locus of control. *Developmental Psychology, 27,* 689–697.

Kliewer, W., Sandler, I., & Wolchik, S. (1994). Family socialization of threat appraisal and coping: Coaching, modeling and family context. In F. Nestmann & K. Hurrelmann (Eds.), *Social networks and social support in childhood and adolescence* (pp. 271–293). New York: Walter de Gruyter.

Klingman, A., Melamed, B. G., Cuthbert, M. I., & Hermecz, D. A. (1984). Effects of participant modeling on information acquisition and skill utilization. *Journal of Consulting and Clinical Psychology, 52,* 414–422.

Kopp, C. B. (1982). Antecedents of self-regulation: A developmental perspective. *Developmental Psychology, 18,* 199–214.

Kopp, C. B. (1989). Regulation of distress and negative emotions: A developmental view. *Developmental Psychology, 25,* 343–354.

Kopp, C. (1992). Emotional distress and control in young children. In N. Eisenberg & R. A. Fabes (Eds.), *Emotion and its regulation in early development. New Directions in Child Development, 55,* 41–56.

Krohne, H. W. (1988). Coping research: Current theoretical and methodological developments. *The German Journal of Psychology, 12,* 10–30.

Kupersmidt, J. T., Coie, J. D., & Dodge, K. A. (1990). The role of poor peer relations in the development of disorder. In S. R. Asher & J. D. Coie (Eds.), *Peer rejection in childhood* (pp. 274–308). Cambridge, England: Cambridge University Press.

Lazarus, R. S. (1991). *Emotion and adaptation.* New York: Oxford University Press.

Lazarus, R. S., & Folkman, S. (1984). Coping and adaptation. In W. D. Gentry (Ed.), *The handbook of behavioral medicine* (pp. 282–325). New York: Guilford.

Lerner, R. M., & East, P. L. (1984). The role of temperament in stress, coping, and socioemotional functioning in early development. *Infant Mental Health Journal, 5,* 148–159.

Maccoby, E. E. (1983). Social–emotional development and response to stressors. In N. Garmezy and M. Rutter (Eds.), *Stress, coping, and development in children* (pp. 217–234). New York: McGraw-Hill.

Masters, J. C. (1991). Strategies and mechanisms for the personal and social control of emotion. In J. Garber & K. A. Dodge (Eds.), *The development of emotion: Regulation and dysregulation* (pp. 182–207). Cambridge, England: Cambridge University Press.

McCrae, R. R. (1984). Situational determinants of coping responses: Loss, threat, and challenge. *Journal of Personality and Social Psychology, 46,* 919–928.

Miller, P. M., Kliewer, W., Hepworth, J. T., & Sandler, I. N. (1994). Maternal socialization of children's postdivorce coping: Development of a measurement model. *Journal of Applied Developmental Psychology, 15,* 457–487.

Miller, S. M., & Green, M. L. (1985). Coping with stress and frustration: Origins, nature and development. In M. Lewis & C. Saarni (Eds.), *The socialization of emotions* (pp. 263–314). New York: Plenum Press.

Minuchin, P. P., & Shapiro, E. K. (1983). The school as a context for social development. In P. Mussen (Ed.), *Handbook of child psychology* (Vol. IV, pp. 197–274). New York: Wiley.

Mischel, H. N., & Mischel, W. (1983). The development of children's knowledge of self-control strategies. *Child Development, 54,* 603–619.

Mischel, W., Shoda, Y., & Rodriguez, M. L. (1989). Delay of gratification in children. *Science, 244,* 933–938.

Nelson-LeGall, S. A., & Gumerman, R. A. (1984). Children's perceptions of helpers and helper motivation. *Journal of Applied Developmental Psychology, 5,* 1–12.

Newcomb, A. F., Bukowski, W. M., & Pattee, L. (1993). Children's peer relations: A meta-analysis review of popular, rejected, neglected, controversial, and average sociometric status. *Psychological Bulletin, 113,* 99–128.

Offer, D. (1987). In defense of adolescence. *Journal of the American Medical Association, 257,* 3407–3408.

Parke, R. D., & Slaby, R. G. (1983). The development of aggression. In P. Mussen (Ed.), *Handbook of child psychology* (Vol. IV, pp. 547–641). New York: Wiley.

Parker, J. G., & Asher, S. R. (1987). Peer relations and later personal adjustment: Are low-accepted children at risk? *Psychological Bulletin, 102,* 357–389.

Pierce, S. L., Tout, K., & de Haan, M. (1993, March). *Individual differences in neuroendocrine activity in preschoolers: Relations with temperament characteristics.* Paper presented at the biennial meeting of the Society for Research in Child Development, New Orleans, LA.

Pulkkinen, L. (1986). The role of impulse control in the development of antisocial and prosocial behavior. In D. Olweus, J. Block, & M. Radke-Yarrow (Eds.), *Development of antisocial and prosocial behavior: Research, theories, and issues* (pp. 149–206). Orlando, FL: Academic Press.

Pulkkinen, L. (1988). A two-dimensional model as a framework for interindividual differences in social behavior. In D. H. Saklofske & S. B. G. Eysenck (Eds.), *Individual differences in children and adolescents* (pp. 27–37). London: Hodder & Stoughton.

Rende, R. D., & Plomin, R. (1992). Relations between first grade stress, temperament, and behavior problems. *Journal of Applied Developmental Psychology, 13,* 435–446.

Roberts, W., & Strayer, J. (1987). Parents' responses to the emotional distress of their children: Relations with children's competence. *Developmental Psychology, 23,* 415–432.

Rossman, B. B. R. (1992). School-age children's perceptions of coping with distress: Strategies for emotion regulation and the moderation of adjustment. *Journal of Child Psychology and Psychiatry, 33,* 1373–1397.

Rossman, B. B. R., & Rosenberg, M. S. (1992). Family stress and functioning in children: The moderating effects of children's beliefs about their control over parental conflict. *Journal of Child Psychology and Psychiatry, 33,* 699–715.

Rotenberg, K. J., & Mann, L. (1986). The development of the norm of reciprocity of self-disclosure and its function in children's attraction to peers. *Child Development, 57,* 1349–1357.

Roth, S., & Cohen, L. J. (1986). Approach, avoidance, and coping with stress. *American Psychologist, 41,* 813–819.

Rothbart, M. K., & Derryberry, D. (1981). Development of individual differences in temperament. In M. E. Lamb & A. L. Brown (Eds.), *Advances in developmental psychology* (Vol. 1, pp. 37–86). Hillsdale, NJ: Erlbaum.

Rothbart, M. K., Ziaie, H., & O'Boyle, C. G. (1992). Self-regulation and emotion in infancy. In N. Eisenbergy & R. A. Fabes (Eds.), *New directions in child development: The development of self-regulation and emotion* (pp. 7–24). San Francisco: Jossey-Bass.

Rubin, K. H., LeMare, L. J., & Lollis, S. (1990). Social withdrawal in children: Developmental pathways to peer rejection. In S. R. Asher & J. D. Coie (Eds.), *Peer rejection in childhood* (pp. 217–249). Cambridge, England: Cambridge University Press.

Ruble, D. N., & Dweck, C. (1995). Self-conceptions, person conceptions and their development. In N. Eisenberg (Ed.), *Review of personality and social psychology,* Vol. 15, (pp. 109–139). Thousand Oaks, CA: Sage.

Rutter, M. (1983). Stress, coping, and development: Some issues and some questions. In N. Garmezy and M. Rutter (Eds.), *Stress, coping, and development in children* (pp. 1–42). New York: McGraw-Hill.

Sackin, S., & Thelen, E. (1984). An ethological study of peaceful associative outcomes to conflict in preschool children. *Child Development, 55,* 1098–1102.

Sandler, I. N., Tein, J., & West, S. G. (1994). Coping, stress and the psychological symptoms of children of divorce: A cross-sectional and longitudinal study. *Child Development, 65,* 1744–1763.

Schunk, D. H., & Hanson, A. R. (1989). Influence of peer-model attributes on children's beliefs and learning. *Journal of Educational Psychology, 81,* 431–434.

Shantz, C. U. (1983). Social cognition. In P. Mussen (Ed.), *Handbook of child psychology* (Vol. III, pp. 495–555). New York: Wiley.

Silverman, W. K., La Greca, A. M., & Wasserstein, S. (1995). What do children worry about? Worries and their relation to anxiety. *Child Development, 66,* 671–686.

Skinner, E. A., & Wellborn, J. G. (1994). Coping during childhood and adolescence: A motivational perspective. In R. Lerner, D. Featherman, & M. Perlmuter (Eds.), *Life-span development and behavior* (Vol. 12, pp. 91–123). Hillsdale, NJ: Erlbaum.

Sroufe, L. A. (1988). The role of infant–caregiver attachment in development. In J. Belsky & T. Nezworski (Eds.), *Clinical implications of attachment* (pp. 18–38). Hillsdale, NJ: Erlbaum.

Stipek, D. J., Recchia, S., & McClinic, S. (1992). Self-evaluation in young children. *Monographs of the Society for Research in Child Development, 57,* Serial No. 226, 1–79.

Thompson, R. A. (1990). Vulnerability in research: A developmental perspective on research risk. *Child Development, 61,* 1–16.

Thompson, R. A. (1994). Emotional regulation: A theme in search of definition. *Child Development Monographs, 59,* 25–52.

Tronick, E. Z. (1989). Emotions and emotional communication in infants. *American Psychologist, 44,* 112–119.

Vaillant, G. E. (1977). *Adaptation to life.* Boston: Little, Brown.

Werner, E. E., & Smith, R. S. (1982). *Vulnerable, but invincible: A study of resilient children.* New York: McGraw-Hill.

Yamamoto, K., Soliman, A., Parsons, J., & Davies, O. L. (1987). Voices in unison: Stressful events in the lives of children in six countries. *Journal of Child Psychology and Psychiatry, 28,* 855–864.

Youniss, J. (1980). *Parents and peers in social development: A Sullivan–Piaget perspective.* Chicago: University of Chicago Press.

Zahn-Waxler, C., Cole, P. M., Richardson, D., Friedman, R. J., Michel, M. K., & Belouad, F. (1994). Social problem solving in disruptive preschool children: Reactions to hypothetical situations of conflict and distress. *Merrill-Palmer Quarterly, 40,* 98–119.

II

Family Stressors

3

Children's Coping with Maltreatment

JEFFREY J. HAUGAARD, N. DICKON REPPUCCI, and MARGARET M. FEERICK

Millions of children in the United States, and millions more around the world, experience some form of maltreatment. These experiences appear to have little or no effect on some children and they significantly impair the development of others. Although several programs to prevent physical abuse, sexual abuse, and neglect have been implemented over the past 20 years, there is no evidence that the incidence of child maltreatment has been reduced meaningfully. A variety of efforts to help children overcome the consequences of their maltreatment have been instituted; as noted later in this chapter, however, the effectiveness of these efforts has not been demonstrated clearly. In this chapter we review some of the literature on child maltreatment. We begin by discussing the research regarding the prevalence of child maltreatment and the consequences of maltreatment on children. We then explore ways in which these consequences might be ameliorated.

EPIDEMIOLOGY OF CHILD MALTREATMENT

Defining Child Maltreatment

Prior to an assessment of the prevalence of any event, that event must be defined precisely. Without a precise definition, the way that one person counts the occurrences of an event will not match the way that another person counts

JEFFREY J. HAUGAARD and MARGARET M. FEERICK • Department of Human Development and Family Studies, Cornell University, Ithaca, New York 14853.   N. DICKON REPPUCCI • Department of Psychology, University of Virginia, Charlottesville, Virginia 22903.
Handbook of Children's Coping: Linking Theory and Intervention, edited by Wolchik and Sandler. Plenum Press, New York, 1997.

them, resulting in varying prevalence estimates. Since theorizing in the social-sciences about the causes of an event is often based on correlations between the prevalence of the event across different groups [e.g., physical abuse is more prevalent in families with very low incomes, so abuse may be partly caused by the stress of economic hardship (Pelton, 1994)], significant differences in theory may result from the use of varying definitions of an event.

The field of child maltreatment continues to function without consistent definitions. Several reasons have been suggested for this, including that the definitions must be useful in fields that often have conflicting goals (e.g., law enforcement, social work, mental health), and that the meaning of some potentially abusive acts will vary for children at different developmental stages and for children living in different sociocultural and socioeconomic contexts (Aber & Zigler, 1981; Haugaard & Reppucci, 1988; McGee & Wolfe, 1991).

Perhaps the biggest impediment to a common definition of child maltreatment is the lack of societal agreement about the harmful or beneficial nature of many behaviors toward children. For example, there appears to be broad-based agreement about the harmful nature of a parent having sexual intercourse with a 10-year-old or of locking a 10-year-old in a closet for days on end. However, there is less agreement about the potential harm of a parent bathing a 10-year-old or of the possible harm or benefit of spanking a child (Haugaard & Reppucci, 1988). Furthermore, when assessing the abusive nature of some behaviors, their frequency, intent, and context are considered. Since these factors can each vary independently, it is often difficult to classify the behaviors themselves as abusive or not.

Most legal definitions of child abuse and neglect are stated generally. This allows child protection and legal professionals to make judgments about particular incidents that take into consideration characteristics of the child, abusive act, parent, and parent's history with similar behavior. For example, Section 1012 of the New York Family Court Act defines abuse as

> inflicts or allows to be inflicted upon such child physical injury by other than accidental means which causes or creates a substantial risk of death . . . or protracted impairment of the physical or emotional health . . . creates or allows to be created a substantial risk of physical injury to such child . . . commits or allows to be committed a sex offense against such child . . . using a child in a sexual performance and promoting a sexual performance by a child.

Research definitions tend to be more objectively defined, with specific acts and ages forming the criteria. Researchers have not agreed about which acts should be considered abusive, however, which results in a variety of research definitions (Giovannoni, 1989).

For the purposes of this discussion, it is sufficient to note that care must be taken when viewing the results of epidemiology studies of child maltreatment. Attention must be paid to the definition used by each researcher. Abuse and neglect definitions that are inclusive may result in a large prevalence estimate, but also will result in a very heterogeneous group of victims. More circumscribed definitions will result in a more homogeneous group of victims and lower prevalence estimates.

Prevalence Estimates

There are three basic sources of prevalence estimates for child maltreatment: reports to various legal agencies, community or national surveys, and surveys of college students. There are limitations associated with each source. Consequently, the use of all three sources together is likely to provide more accurate information about child maltreatment. Although it is generally assumed that research underestimates the number of abuse and neglect cases, the number of cases is dramatically high. Child maltreatment is clearly a problem of great magnitude.

Reports to Legal Agencies

It is generally assumed that only a minority of cases of child maltreatment are reported to legal agencies (National Center on Child Abuse and Neglect (NCCAN), 1995). Furthermore, there is some research suggesting bias in reporting child maltreatment. Several studies have found a disproportionately large percentage of minority families among reported cases of physical abuse (e.g., Hampton, 1987; Lindholm & Willey, 1986). Other research has found a greater propensity to report minority and low-income families (Gelles, 1982; Hampton, 1987). Thus, reports to legal agencies are likely to underestimate the number of maltreated children and may not accurately represent the extent to which abuse and neglect is distributed across the population. In addition, agencies typically include only substantiated cases in their reports. There may be many actual cases of maltreatment for which there is not enough evidence for substantiation, further increasing the extent to which reports from legal agencies underestimate the prevalence of abuse and neglect.

Each state currently collects reports of child abuse and neglect, and these are compiled at the national level by NCCAN. The most recent report (NCCAN, 1995) concerned data gathered in 1993, when state agencies investigated nearly 2 million reports of child abuse and neglect involving approximately 2.3 million children. The rate of reported maltreatment in 1993 was 43 per 1000 children in the population. For the first time since the national government began collecting this information in 1976, the rate of reported maltreatment did not increase from the previous year. The cases for 1,019,000 children were substantiated (39% of all reports). Forty-nine percent of the victims experienced physical neglect, 24% experienced physical abuse, 14% experienced sexual abuse, 5% experienced emotional neglect, and 15% experienced some other type of maltreatment (some children experienced more than one type). Fifty-one percent of the victims were female and about 51% were 7 years of age or younger. Fifty-four percent of the children were white, 25% were black, 9% were Hispanic, 2% were Native American, and the remainder were of other ethnic groups (NCCAN, 1995). The US Advisory Board on Child Abuse and Neglect (1995) estimated that there are 142,000 serious injuries, 18,000 serious disabilities, and 2000 fatalities due to child abuse and neglect each year in the United States.

National and Community Samples

National and community samples have been used primarily to estimate the prevalence of physical and sexual abuse. Advantages of these samples are that they include a broad range of households and that the occurrence of abuse that has and has not been reported can be assessed. The rate of participation of potential subjects and the honesty of the subjects' responses present important concerns with these samples. Some research has suggested that troubled families are less likely to participate in survey research (Cox, Rutter, Yule, & Quinton, 1977), and it seems logical that many families would be reluctant to report maltreatment behavior honestly. Thus, these studies may underestimate maltreatment in general, and may particularly underestimate the most violent or intrusive types of maltreatment.

Straus, Gelles, and Steinmetz (1980) and Straus and Gelles (1986) completed two surveys of the prevalence of family violence. Violence was defined as any purposeful act that caused pain or injury to the child. The 1975 study involved 1146 households and the 1985 study involved 1428 households that included a parental couple and at least one child between the ages of 3 and 17. All households were from a national probability sample. A substantial majority of the households had experienced some type of minor violence (e.g., spanking a child). More severe forms of violence occurred less frequently: The 1975 and 1985 data showed (respectively) the percent of households reporting at least one incident in the past year of (1) kicked, bit, hit with fist: 3.2% and 1.3%; (2) hit, tried to hit with an object: 13.4% and 9.7%; (3) beat up: 1.3% and 0.6%; and (4) threatened use of or use of a knife or gun: 0.2% and 0.4%.

Studies of the prevalence of child sexual abuse have included women from probability-sampled households in San Francisco (Russell, 1983) and Los Angeles (Wyatt, 1985). Russell and Wyatt interviewed women about sexual encounters involving physical contact and noncontact (such as an encounter with an exhibitionist) prior to the age of 18. Russell counted as sexual abuse all intrafamilial sexual contact and only extrafamilial contact that was unwanted. Wyatt counted all sexual contact with girls under the age of 13 and unwanted contact with older girls.

Thirty-eight percent of the women in Russell's sample had experienced some type of unwanted physical sexual encounter prior to the age of 18. Most had been abused by a friend or acquaintance. Five percent had been abused by a father or father figure, 2% by a brother, and less than 1% by a mother or sister. Approximately one third of those abused by a father or father figure had experienced vaginal, oral, or anal intercourse, one third had experienced genital fondling, and one third had experienced other sexual behavior. In Wyatt's sample, 59% reported an unwanted physical or nonphysical sexual encounter before age 18. One percent had been abused by their father, 7% by a stepfather, foster father, or mother's boyfriend, and 4% by a brother. Approximately 50% of the women responding to both surveys had experienced one unwanted sexual encounter.

College Student Samples

The primary strength of these studies is the availability of college undergraduates, allowing for relatively easy testing of various hypotheses. However, college students generally are not representative of either the general population or others their age. To the extent that maltreatment is harmful to the emotional or intellectual development of a child, college students are likely to underrepresent children who have been subjected to repeated or severe mal-treatment.

Berger, Knutson, Mehm, and Perkins (1988) surveyed 4695 undergraduates about "punitive childhood experiences." Percentages of students who reported that the following experiences occurred at least once in their home were: spanked, 80%; hit other than spanking, 20%; hit with an object, 35%; punched, 6%; kicked, 5%; choked, 3%; and severely beaten, 2%. Twelve percent had been injured as the result of punishment. Most of the injuries involved bruises or cuts; however, 7% were broken bones, 8% were burns, 5% were dental injuries, and 11% were head injuries.

Finkelhor (1979) and Haugaard and Emery (1989) were among researchers who investigated the prevalence of child sexual abuse in college samples. Both included abuse occurring before a child's 17th birthday. Finkelhor included noncontact abuse experiences and experiences that were both wanted and unwanted. Haugaard and Emery included only unwanted experiences that involved physical contact. Haugaard and Emery found that 12% of women and 5% of men reported a sexual abuse experience. Finkelhor found a prevalence of 19% for women and 9% for men.

Summary

Community and college surveys show that many children experience some form of sexual abuse. Although approximately half of these children have only one encounter, typically with a friend or member of their extended family, thousands of children experience long-term, intrusive abuse. Physical abuse or family violence is present at least occasionally in most homes with young children. The extent to which many of these incidents would be considered appropriate punishment or inappropriate abuse is not clear. However, even if the category of abuse is shrunk to include only violence resulting in injury, college surveys suggest that abuse occurs in 10% of homes. Most striking from the reports to legal agencies is that neglect comprises half of all reports. Despite the number of cases of neglect, research regarding the causes and consequences of neglect is rare.

CONSEQUENCES OF CHILD MALTREATMENT

Several extensive reviews of the impact of child maltreatment have been completed in the past few years (e.g., Beitchman, Zucker, Hood, daCosta, & Akman, 1991; Beitchman et al., 1992; Kendall-Tackett, Williams, & Finkelhor, 1993; Malinosky-Rummell & Hansen, 1993; O'Beirne & Reppucci, in press; Trickett & McBride-Chang, 1995; Widom, 1989). The focus of these reviews is the short- and long-term impact of child maltreatment at different developmental periods, especially physical and sexual abuse and neglect. Studies of short-term or acute consequences typically employ cross-sectional designs and use samples of children and adolescents after maltreatment has been officially identified or disclosed. Studies of long-term effects commonly use retrospective designs with adults who have identified themselves as having been maltreated. Few longitudinal studies exist, and Trickett and McBride-Chang (1995) found none that followed maltreated children for longer than 2 years. Moreover, most studies suffer from basic methodological problems such as small sample sizes and no comparison groups, they do not consider age or developmental period as a variable even when the subjects range from 7 to 17 years of age, and they seldom try to disentangle such issues as frequency and duration of the abuse. Nonetheless, some general conclusions regarding consequences are possible, based on findings common to many studies.

Maltreatment has been shown to have a pervasive negative influence on the development of infants, children, and adolescents. Maltreatment affects individual functioning through an apparent influence on the development of a number of problematic behaviors and by interfering with cognitive development. Maltreatment is associated with deficits in social functioning throughout childhood and adolescence and also is associated with problematic and abusive marital and other social relationships in adulthood.

The mechanisms through which maltreatment influences development are diverse. This can complicate the assessment of the consequences of maltreatment. For example, some maltreated children are depressed and withdraw from social contact. Other maltreated children are aggressive and are rejected by peers and adults. Both types of maltreated children are likely to have deficits in social development, but the pathways to these deficits are different. In addition, it is important to note that the specific role of the maltreatment on development, as opposed to living in an environment where maltreatment occurs, has not been isolated. Maltreating families are likely to be different from nonmaltreating families in ways other than simply their maltreatment. For example, there may be less overall concern about the children's welfare or substantial substance abuse problems. This is an important issue when designing treatment programs. If the maltreatment itself is the cause of the negative consequences seen in the children, then efforts to end the maltreatment may be sufficient. If, however, the maltreatment has a relatively small role compared to other family characteristics, then simply stopping the maltreatment will have minimal influence on a child's development.

Some maltreated children show few or no apparent negative influences of their experiences. For example, several studies of child sexual abuse found that between 21% (Conte & Schuerman, 1987) and 49% (Caffaro-Rouget, Lang, & van Santen, 1989) of children were symptom free. It is not clear whether symptoms would appear at other points in these children's lives or whether they were less affected by their maltreatment. No work seems to have been done to isolate which children are more likely to show no symptoms of maltreatment.

Physically abused and sexually abused children are consistently found to be higher on both internalizing and externalizing disorders (Trickett & McBride-Chang, 1995). Aggression appears to be particularly common in physically abused children and adolescents (Malinosky-Rummell & Hansen, 1993) and sexual aggression or promiscuity is reported for victims of child sexual abuse (e.g., Friedrich, Beilke, & Urquiza, 1987). Children who are the victims of repeated or violent sexual abuse are reported to experience higher levels of dissociative experiences and disorders (Putnam, Helmers, & Trickett, 1993). Sexually abused adolescents are reported to have higher rates of self-injurious and suicidal behaviors than nonmaltreated children, and these behaviors have not been reported to be as high in physically abused or neglected children (Fromuth & Burkhart, 1989).

Peer and other social problems are reported for physically abused and neglected children from early childhood on (Erickson & Egeland, 1987; Oates, Peacock, & Forrest, 1984). Physically abused male adolescents are more likely to engage in both aggressive and sexually aggressive behaviors with peers and children (Malinosky-Rummell & Hansen, 1993).

Findings in the cognitive/academic domain are generally consistent for physically abused and neglected children and adolescents. From the earliest ages with socioeconomic status controlled, they demonstrate poorer cognitive development and poorer school performance than comparison groups, with neglected children showing the worst delays and the lowest performance (e.g., Eckenrode, Laird, & Doris, 1993; Wodarski, Kurtz, Gaudin, & Howing, 1990). There is less consistent evidence regarding the academic performance of sexually abused children (Eckenrode et al., 1993). One long-term outcome of maltreatment may be lower educational attainment and consequently lower occupational attainment. If this is the case, university samples may be undesirable for assessing the long-term impact of maltreatment because of an overselection of adults who suffered less severe impact of the abuse.

Differences in consequences to boys and girls have been examined in relatively few instances, and no clear consistencies have resulted. For example, while Dodge, Bates, and Pettit (1990) found that physically abused boys and girls exhibited no differences in externalizing problems (as rated by teachers and observers in kindergarten), they reported that girls did show more internalizing problems than boys. In contrast, Trickett (1993) found that parents reported physically abused, school-aged girls and boys to have high internalizing and externalizing behaviors, while observers rated girls as wary and withdrawn and boys as demanding and negativistic. White, Halpin, Strom, and Santilli (1988) reported that young sexually abused girls showed greater developmental delays than boys, but the boys exhibited more internalizing problems than girls.

THEORETICAL EXPLANATIONS FOR THE CONSEQUENCES OF CHILD MALTREATMENT

Several theories have been used to explain the negative emotional and behavioral consequences observed in maltreated children. Some of these theories are discussed briefly in this section.

Biological Explanations

Physically abused children may have experienced some sort of neurological damage during their abuse, particularly if they were abused during infancy. Research has implicated physical abuse as the cause of brain damage (Buchannan & Oliver, 1977), cerebral palsy (Diamond & Jaudes, 1983), and pinpoint hemorrhages in brain tissue (Caffey, 1972). Severe neglect also may impair a child's biological development. These biological consequences may have a significant influence on a maltreated child's emotional, cognitive, or behavioral development. For example, a variety of neurological abnormalities have been associated with human aggression (Carlson, 1991).

Recent work has shown an association between child sexual abuse and elevated levels of urinary catecholamines and dysregulation of the hypothalamic–pituitary–adrenal axis (DeBellis, Lefter, Trickett, & Putnam, 1994). These findings suggest that sexually abused girls' stress-related systems may function at elevated levels. Many abused children show symptoms of anxiety-related psychological disorders or stress-related biological disorders and these may be related to the children's biological response to abuse (Trickett & McBride-Chang, 1995).

Psychoanalytic Theory

Psychoanalytic theory focuses on the disruptive influence of maltreatment on the child's developing ego (Sugarman, 1994). The pain of the abuse and neglect and the child's strong ambivalent feelings toward the abuser (particularly if the abuser is a parent) can result in psychological trauma and emotional helplessness. These feelings can be heightened by the child's sense of guilt for the maltreatment. This guilt is caused by the self-centeredness of the child, and can be heightened by statements from the abuser and by pleasurable physical sensations that often accompany sexual abuse (Kramer, 1994). Psychoanalytic theory suggests that children abused at younger ages will experience more negative consequences. The younger child's ego must use the most primitive defense mechanisms to cope with the trauma. These mechanisms can influence negatively the child's ongoing psychic development (Tyson, 1986). Empirical research, however, is equivocal on this issue (Kendall-Tackett et al., 1993).

Operant Learning Theory Explanations

Operant learning theory suggests that a maltreated child's behaviors will be shaped by the environmental responses to these behaviors. The child will engage in various behaviors in response to the maltreatment, and the extent to which these behaviors are reinforced or punished will influence the likelihood of them occurring in future abusive or neglectful situations. The reinforced behaviors may generalize so that they are employed, for example, in all situations involving an authority figure. Thus, these learned behavioral patterns can form the foundation for a lifetime pattern of behaviors.

Learning theory helps to explain children's diverse responses to abuse and neglect. For example, in one situation a child whose initial resistance to sexual abuse results in increased violence from an adult and whose subsequent submissive behavior results in a cessation of this violence will have a withdrawn, submissive behavioral style negatively reinforced. Another abused child may learn that abuse is reduced or stopped when the child acts aggressively toward the abuser. The cessation of the abuse would be a strong negative reinforcer for the child's aggressive behavior.

Attachment Perspective Explanations

Bowlby (1969) described attachment as a biologically based bond with a caregiver. Through the early attachment experiences, the child develops an internal working model of relationships that influences the child's future relationships (Alexander, 1992; Crittenden & Ainsworth, 1989). Main and Solomon (1986) found several patterns of attachment in research with maltreated infants that did not fit the initial three categories described by Ainsworth, Blehar, Waters, and Wall (1978), and labeled these disorganized/disoriented. Many of the commonly reported behaviors of maltreated children can be accounted for by this perspective. For example, the fear activated by the potential of abuse will conflict with the abused child's natural attachment tendencies toward that parent. This can result in behaviors that appear paradoxical: excessive anger at a parent accompanied by closeness to the parent that often makes the child unwilling to implicate the parent in the abuse. In addition, in order to deny their anger, maltreated children may compulsively care for an abusive parent. This pattern may be repeated in subsequent relationships, resulting in a pattern of caregiving and victimization.

Cognitive Explanations

Cognitive therapy is based on the theory that how a person thinks has a significant influence on how that person feels and behaves (Beck, 1979, 1985). All people process information from the environment, since doing so is essential for survival. Some people develop biases in the way they process information. These biases predispose them to interpret environmental information in dysfunctional ways, and these interpretations can result in consistent patterns of behavior. Cognitive theory effectively explains the development of the anxiety and depression that is commonly associated with child abuse and neglect. Children who are abused or neglected during their early years are likely to develop schema based, in some part, on their abuse experiences (e.g., people who love you hurt you, I am a fundamentally bad person, there is no escape from pain). These schema will influence their interactions with others, and their interpretations of these interactions will reinforce their schema. Because of their experiences, maltreated children may interpret social cues as more hostile than nonabused children do. They are less able cognitively to take into account relevant social cues and to generate appropriate behavioral actions. As a result, maltreated children may be regularly misinterpreting social situations and responding in a hostile way, resulting in hostility and rejection from peers.

CHILDREN'S ADAPTATION TO MALTREATMENT

Research using clinical samples of children, adolescents, and adults typically suggests that child maltreatment can influence the development of both acute and chronic physical and psychological problems. However, as noted above, research with nonclinical samples of maltreated children or adolescents often shows a wide range of effects, from severe impairment to no apparent impairment at all. An important question for researchers and practitioners, then, centers on whether there are identifiable factors that influence the consequences to a child of maltreatment experiences. Identification of these factors may suggest which family or individual interventions are more likely to facilitate a child's recovery from maltreatment. They also may show what types of preventive efforts could enhance a child's ability to cope with maltreatment.

Theoretically, the consequences of maltreatment can be influenced by a variety of factors. Unfortunately, only minimal work has been done in the area of understanding the influences of these factors on a child's response to maltreatment. Research relating to these factors is described in this section. The research has been divided into four categories: child characteristics, home and social characteristics, abuse characteristics, and postabuse experiences.

Child Characteristics

Several studies have assessed the association between a child's personality characteristics and his or her adaptation to maltreatment. Farber and Egeland (1987) studied 44 maltreated children raised by a sample of 267 women who were recruited before their children's birth and who were considered to be at high risk for child maltreatment. Assessments of children's and mothers' behaviors and of mother–child interactions were done several times over the children's lives prior to entering elementary school. Some individual characteristics of the maltreated children as newborns and infants predicted their level of competence as toddlers and preschoolers. Maltreated children who were rated as more competent on problem-solving tasks with their mothers at 24 months of age had been higher on orientation, alertness, and physiological response to stress as newborns. At 42 months, the maltreated children who were rated as more competent had been rated as more alert and attentive as newborns. Although no maltreated child was rated as competent during all of the assessments, there was a clear pattern of children who were incompetent during early assessments remaining incompetent throughout the assessments.

Cicchetti, Rogosch, Lynch, and Holt (1993) examined factors that predicted adaptive functioning in 127 disadvantaged, school-age, maltreated children. Three child characteristics predicted adaptive functioning among maltreated children: higher ego resiliency and ego control as measured by the California Child Q-Sort and higher self-esteem as measured by the Coopersmith Self-Esteem Inventory. Ego control referred to the children's ability to control their impulses and feelings and ego resiliency referred to children's ability to modify their level of ego control depending on environmental demands. Among maltreated children, those who could successfully modulate their level of ego control across several environments showed more adaptive functioning than those maltreated children who could not do this. In addition, ego overcontrol, characterized by a reserved, controlled, and rational way of interacting and relating, was associated with adaptive functioning among maltreated children. This suggested that an organized, problem-solving coping style was important for maltreated children, who often are forced to restrict their emotions and behavior in order to protect themselves in their home environments. Ego overcontrol was not associated with adaptive functioning for 70 nonmaltreated comparison children, suggesting that ego overcontrol may be an important coping mechanism specific to maltreatment environments.

Hazzard, Celano, Gould, Lawry, and Webb (1995) studied 56 sexually abused 8- to 13-year-old girls and their primary female caretakers. The girls' behavior was assessed through the Child Behavior Checklist (CBCL) completed by the caretaker, and overall child functioning was assessed by a psychologist using the Global Assessment Scale (GAS). No child characteristics were related to CBCL scores. However, a lower sense of self-blame and a lower sense of powerlessness were related to better scores on the GAS.

Valentine and Feinauer (1993) interviewed 22 women, recruited through newspaper advertising in Utah, who had been sexually abused as children. Many women described "believing in myself and believing I was worth something" (p. 220) as having been an important influence on their ability to lead competent lives. Being able to recognize that their abuse was not their fault and being able to say to themselves, during the time of the abuse, that they would be able to get away from it someday also were related to being able to cope effectively with their experiences. A lack of comparison between women coping successfully with child abuse and those coping unsuccessfully with it, however, makes it impossible to know whether the beliefs of those coping successfully with abuse were also held by those who coped unsuccessfully with their abuse.

In summary, these studies suggest that some characteristics and/or beliefs of a maltreated child may assist the child in coping with his or her maltreatment. Being able to interact relatively effectively with adults and others in a maltreating environment may provide a child with some relief from maltreatment and may promote more positive parent–child interactions at other times. Being able to externalize blame for the maltreatment, which may be related to a child being able to preserve a more positive sense of self, also may increase the child's ability to adapt to maltreatment. In addition, having more effective ways of dealing with social situations and having a better sense of self may enable a child to be successful in several settings other than the one in which the maltreatment occurs, which may allow for more successful overall development.

Home and Social Characteristics

Some research has suggested that characteristics of a child's home and relationships with parents may have a substantial impact on the long-term adjustment of maltreated children. Farber and Egeland (1987) found that at each developmental stage a child's history of attachment to his or her caretaker was the best predictor of child competence. In addition, the presence of a male partner in the home and the mother's emotional support of the child predicted competence. Mothers of competent abused children at age 42 months were more likely to have been more cooperative in their feeding and play behaviors when the child was 6 months old. In addition, mothers of competent children at age 42 months used more positive and effective teaching techniques during the 42-month assessment. Although most children showed decreasing competence over time, for those who showed improvement, positive change was associated with the availability of a caring adult and intensive family intervention. A structured school environment, caring teacher, and enrollment in high-quality day care also were associated with higher likelihood of later competence. Aber, Allen, Carlson, and Cicchetti (1991) found that higher levels of parents' enjoyment of their children and access to community resources were associated with lower levels of symptomatology in maltreated children, while parent's encouragement of maltreated children's autonomy was positively associated with children's cognitive maturity. Such research supports findings from studies of high-risk, nonmaltreated children that indicate that under substantial stress children may benefit from the availability of supportive relationships with other adults, which may make them less vulnerable to maladaptive outcomes (Werner, 1990).

Several studies of sexually abused children also found that the child's perception of her relationship with her mother was related to higher levels of competence and lower levels of behavioral disturbance. Lovett (1995) gave a measure of perceived maternal warmth/rejection to 60 sexually abused 7- to 12-year-old girls and the CBCL to their mothers. She found that lower levels of perceived maternal rejection were associated with higher levels of competency and lower levels of behavioral disturbance on the CBCL, even after the influence of several abuse-related characteristics were considered. Hazzard et al. (1995) found that the strength of the parent–child relationship was the only variable that was significantly related to lower internalizing and externalizing scores on the CBCL. Child characteristics and abuse characteristics were not significantly associated with CBCL scores. Spaccarelli and Kim (1995) studied 43 10- to 17-year-old sexually abused girls and their nonoffending parents. They found that the child's perception of parental support was the only significant predictor of social competence measured on the CBCL. Abuse-related characteristics and the children's coping styles were not related to social competence. Level of behavioral symptoms was related to both parent support and abuse stress. Waterman and Kelly (1993) studied a group of 88 preschoolers who had been involved in ritualistic sexual abuse. Family factors were associated with the most variance in CBCL scores for the children taken 5 years after the abuse was discovered. Children from families that experienced significant internal stress and whose mothers engaged in frequent yelling and chastising had more behavior problems than did children from families with less stress. Romans, Martin, Anderson, O'Shea, and Mullen (1995) interviewed 138 women who had been sexually abused as children. They found that girls who had poor relationships with their mothers and fathers were at increased risk for psychopathology as adults. Girls who enjoyed high school, reported a good social life in high school, or who were good at sports were at decreased risk for adult psychopathology. Finally, Valentine and Feinhauer's (1993) interviews suggested that having a supportive parent or adult outside the family was seen as being of primary importance to women's recovery from sexual abuse experiences.

In summary, parent or caretaker support consistently has been found to be related to child adaptation to maltreatment. Research that has considered family, child, and abuse characteristics have tended to find that family characteristics are the strongest predictor of competence and lack of behavioral problems.

The correlational nature of this body of research presents the problem of not being able to assess whether family characteristics influence a child's adaptation, or whether other characteristics (e.g., child temperament) may influence both the family environment and the child's adaptation to maltreatment. Additional longitudinal research in this area should begin to address these questions.

Abuse Characteristics

There have been many efforts to establish whether certain maltreatment characteristics are associated with better or poorer adaptation to child maltreatment. A few studies have examined whether the type of maltreatment (physical abuse, sexual abuse, or neglect) is associated with adaptation. Manly, Cicchetti, and Barnett (1994) examined whether maltreatment type was associated with social competence or behavior problems, as measured by the CBCL, for 145 5- to 11-year-old maltreated children participating in a summer camp for low-income children. They found that the group of children who had been sexually abused were more socially competent than children in the other maltreatment groups and that their competence was similar to children in the nonmaltreated comparison group. The physically abused group showed higher behavior problems than the nonmaltreated comparison group, with the sexually abused and physically neglected groups in between the physically abused and nonmaltreated groups and not statistically significantly different from either.

Eckenrode et al. (1993) analyzed the school performance of 420 maltreated children and 420 matched controls. Although there were slightly different patterns of results across the various dependent measures of school grades, achievement test scores, and school discipline problems, the general pattern was for children who had a combination of physical or sexual abuse and neglect, physical abuse by itself, and neglect by itself to have lower academic performance and more school behavior problems than the nonmaltreated children. Children who experienced sexual abuse by itself were generally no different from the nonmaltreated comparison group and showed fewer problems than children with other types of maltreatment.

Kendall-Tackett et al. (1993) recently completed an analysis of research focused on the consequences of child sexual abuse. They found only a few generally consistent results when examining research that attempted to determine whether abuse characteristics were associated with poorer outcome. Even when the same results were found frequently, they were not found consistently. Abuse characteristics that frequently were associated with increased symptoms in child victims were: having a perpetrator who was in a close relationship with the child, duration of the abuse, the abuse including acts of vaginal, anal, or oral intercourse, and the use of physical force. Abuse characteristics such as age at time of abuse, sex of the child, and the time elapsed between abuse and reporting of abuse were not related to number of symptoms. It is unclear from this research, however, whether each of these characteristics had a unique influence on increased symptoms. This is because each of these characteristics can be confounded with the others (Haugaard & Reppucci, 1988).

Typically, perpetrators in close relationships with a child have the opportunity to engage in more long-term abuse than those who are strangers or only acquaintances to the child. This is partly due to the person with a close relationship typically having more influence over the actions of a child and increased accessibility to the child for long periods of time. In many cases, abuse of long duration proceeds from less intrusive forms such as nongenital fondling to more intrusive forms such as intercourse. Since this pattern can occur with some frequency, it is not clear whether any one of the characteristics would be associated with more symptoms by itself (e.g., would longer duration be associated with more symptoms after the influence of the identity of the perpetrator was accounted for).

Postabuse Experiences

Two postabuse experiences have received the most research attention: the reaction of a nonoffending parent (usually the mother) to the discovery of the abuse and the involvement of an abused child in court proceedings. Both of these issues have been addressed with victims of sexual abuse only. Another postabuse experience, involvement in psychotherapy, is covered later in this chapter.

The Tufts (1984) study of sexually abused children found that mothers' negative reactions following disclosure of abuse were associated with more behavioral disturbances among children. Interestingly, however, they did not find that a supportive reaction resulted in fewer behavioral disturbances than a more neutral reaction. This result was similar to that found by Everson, Hunter, Runyon, Edelsohn, and Coulter (1989). Everson et al. examined 88 6- to 17-year-old female victims of sexual abuse and classified the supportiveness of their mother's response to disclosure as none/low, ambivalent, or high. Clinicians' ratings of children's behaviors on the Child Assessment Schedule showed that children whose mothers provided little support had significantly more behavioral and emotional problems than those whose mothers were ambivalent or highly supportive. There were no differences between the ambivalent and high-support groups in child problems. However, there was no relation between maternal support and child behavior problems as rated by the children's mothers on the CBCL.

In an examination of the effects of court testimony, Goodman, Taub, Jones, et al. (1992) followed a group of sexually abused children recruited through the Denver, Colorado's District Attorney's Office. Fifty-five of these children testified in criminal court. Their behaviors, as rated by the parent and teacher versions of the CBCL, were compared to a group of 75 sexually abused children who did not have to testify. Comparisons were made at 3 months and 7 months after the children testified and at the time the testifying children's cases were closed. Compared to behaviors at the time the child began involvement with the legal system, both the testifying and nontestifying groups had improved behavior at the 3-month comparison and there were no behavioral differences between the testifying and nontestifying groups. At 7 months, behavior ratings for the testifying group were more problematic than the nontestifying group. By the time the cases had closed, the problematic behaviors of both groups had decreased. Children who had to testify multiple times, who did not have maternal support, and for whom there was no corroborating testimony had higher levels of behavioral disturbance.

Runyan, Everson, Edelsohn, Hunter, and Coulter (1988) studied 100 incest victims who had some involvement with the legal system. Five months after their first legal contact, the children who had already testified had a greater reduction in behavioral problems than the children who would never have to testify, with the children who had not yet testified showing the poorest behavioral improvement.

These two studies suggest that, although court testimony may be stressful to maltreated children, it does not necessarily have long-term negative consequences. Some children may find that the experience of being able to participate in legal proceedings against their abuser is empowering. The research does suggest, however, that children who receive little support and must testify repeatedly do experience more symptoms of problematic behaviors.

Summary and Critique

There are several limitations to much of this research. Many studies involved specific subsets of maltreated children. For example, Farber and Egeland (1987), Cicchetti et al. (1993), and Aber et al. (1991) involved only families determined to be at high risk for the development of maltreatment. The range of functioning of the children from these homes may have been constrained, and a sample with a higher range of infant and child functioning may have identified other child or environmental characteristics associated with competence in maltreated children. Similarly, the studies of sexual abuse victims included only those children whose abuse became known to child protective or mental health agencies. Since only a minority of sexual abuse cases are ever reported, these cases may not be representative of all sexual abuse cases.

Another problem common to many of these studies is that the dependent measure was parental reports on the CBCL. Spaccarelli and Kim (1995) compared results from parental reports on the CBCL and children's reports of their own behavioral symptoms on measures such as the Children's Depression Inventory. They found that of 19 youths classified as resilient based on measures they completed, 9 were viewed by their parents as anxious or depressed. Of 20 youth classified as anxious or depressed by their parents, 10 were classified as resilient based on their self-reports. Without additional assessments it is impossible to know whether the youths or their parents were more accurate. The contradictory results do raise questions about using parental report as the only measure of children's competence and indicate the importance of including some type of third-party assessment in maltreatment research.

Farber and Egeland's (1987) finding that competent maltreated children were more likely to have mothers who were capable of providing appropriate parenting was similar to the finding of Aber et al. (1991) that appropriate parenting of maltreated children was associated with lower behavioral symptomatology and higher cognitive maturity. These studies suggest that the parenting of maltreating parents is not monolithically bad. Although the consequences of maltreatment clearly indicate that it should be considered inappropriate parenting, research shows that there is a range of overall parenting skills among maltreating parents. This suggests that increasing the ability of a mother to engage in some effective parenting, even in the face of the inability to eliminate her maltreating behavior, may provide her child with a better chance to develop competence.

The most consistent result in this research is that support from parents and other adults is associated with better adaptation in maltreated children. This is seen in research assessing supportive caretaking directly and also in the research on postabuse experiences that shows that overall parental support and support during court testimony is associated with fewer behavioral problems. Even some of the research on child characteristics can be seen as supporting the importance of supportive environments. It may be that many of the child characteristics associated with better outcomes are due to those characteristics evoking more developmentally appropriate parenting. Children who are more adept at engaging their parents or other adults and children whose behaviors are less troublesome to parents and other adults may receive better overall caretaking. Given the apparent strength of the relationship between supportive caretaking and adaptation to maltreatment, any child behaviors that encourage more parental support are likely to have an indirect influence on the child's adaptation.

The findings also indicate that positive social or academic experiences postabuse are related to better functioning. Again, because of the correlational nature of this research, it is impossible to know what mechanism was responsible for this finding (e.g., was it the actual success in the activity or a personality characteristic that resulted in both the successful experience and better adaptation to maltreatment). However, the results suggest the possibility that increasing the chance of maltreated children to succeed in some aspect of their lives that is important to them may enhance their ability to adapt to their maltreatment.

These findings have important implications for interventions with maltreated children. They suggest that interventions with the child's parents or other caretakers is of great importance. The possibility that the child will adapt successfully to maltreatment may be influenced by the extent to which a positive relationship can be restored or developed between a parent and the child. What is unclear at this point is the extent to which a supportive relationship between a maltreating parent and the child who is the target of the maltreatment is beneficial to the child, or whether it is primarily the supportive nature of relationships with nonmaltreating adults that is of benefit to the child. The research also suggests that efforts to promote social competence in maltreated children may help to reduce any maltreatment they experience and may help them to be successful in school or social settings, providing the children with positive developmental experiences that may help to offset the negative influence of the maltreatment. Helping the children to assess the blame for their abuse accurately also may reduce the negative influence of the maltreatment.

RESEARCH ON TREATMENT WITH MALTREATED CHILDREN

Over the past 20 years, a variety of treatment programs have been established to address the needs of maltreated children. The number of these programs grew dramatically in the late 1970s and early 1980s (Cohen & Daro, 1987). Despite this upward trend in the numbers of children receiving services and in the variety of treatments that have been established, limited empirical information exists to evaluate the effectiveness of the treatments that are available. Most studies focused on the effectiveness of such programs have provided only descriptive reports. Few studies have used adequate control or comparison groups or have conducted extended follow-ups, which makes interpretation of the results difficult. Further, in programs with multiple components, it is often difficult to isolate the effectiveness of particular aspects of the treatment (for reviews, see Becker, Alpert, BigFoot, Bonner, et al., 1995; Wolfe, 1994). Consequently, the results of the research must be viewed with caution.

A review of articles, chapters, and books on psychotherapy concerned with child maltreatment shows the general trend of focusing much more of the therapy on the child victim in cases of sexual abuse than is done in cases of physical abuse or neglect, where the focus is often on the parents (see Wolfe, 1994). To the extent that there is any emphasis on treatment of physically abused and neglected children, it tends to be on very young children (e.g., see Culp, Little, Letts, & Lawrence, 1991). The literature provides little information about therapeutic programs for physically abused and neglected school-age and older children. This is in contrast to the many therapeutic programs for child, adolescent, and adult victims of child sexual abuse.

While preparing to write this chapter, a search was done of the American Psychological Association's computerized version of Psychological Abstracts for journal articles in the past 10 years. The results were instructive. In response to a search using the descriptors *psychotherapy, child abuse,* and *sexual abuse,* over 90 articles were found. In response to *psychotherapy, child abuse,* and *physical abuse,* about 10 articles were found. In response to *psychotherapy* and *child neglect,* only 3 articles were found. Based on research showing that physical abuse and neglect can be just as damaging, if not more damaging, than sexual abuse, it is unclear why there is such little emphasis on therapy with physically abused and neglected children.

Physical Abuse

The majority of treatment programs developed for physically abused children have involved the use of therapeutic day care or day treatment programs. Such programs are usually offered to preschoolers as one component of a family preservation program that includes services to parents as well as individual therapy and group activities for children. Although therapeutic day care programs differ in the specific activities children engage in, most involve peer interaction and individual activities that aim to facilitate cognitive, language, and motor development (Becker et al., 1995; Melton & Barry, 1994). Residential infant programs focus on improving the cognitive and developmental skills of infants with severe impairments and who have been removed from abusive homes (Oates & Bross, 1995). Day hospital programs typically serve school-age children and adolescents who present with severe emotional and behavioral disturbances. A range of treatment components are provided which include psychodynamically oriented therapies aimed at improving children's self-expression and services to parents designed to remove threats in the home environment (R. Shindledecker, personal communication, July 9, 1996). Interventions to improve academic functioning and social skills with peers and adults also are typically included.

A variety of individual outpatient therapies have been developed for physically abused children, including cognitive control therapy, modeling, cognitive–behavioral approaches, and social skills training. Such programs typically address the social and behavioral needs of abused children, using a variety of techniques to improve deficits in social or cognitive functioning (Becker et al., 1995; Oates & Bross, 1995).

Efficacy of Programs for Physically Abused Children

Although a variety of programs have been developed to address the needs of physically abused children, there is limited empirical research on the effectiveness of different forms of treatment. Overall, however, the research has suggested that treatment is effective, particularly when programs focus on improving the developmental and cognitive abilities of children (Oates & Bross, 1995). In their review of federal demonstration programs, for example, Cohn and Daro (1987) reported that of the 70 children who received direct services in the early 1970s, 50% demonstrated improvement in the developmental and emotional areas that presented problems when treatment began. Similarly, of the 1600 children receiving direct services in the 1982 study, over 70% demonstrated developmental gains across all functional domains during treatment. The direct services in these studies included individual therapy, group counseling, therapeutic day care, speech and physical therapy, and medical care. The measures employed, however, varied between the evaluations, and mostly consisted of clinical judgments. Thus, although there is some evidence for treatment efficacy, the reliance on clinical judgments may have resulted in biases in outcome reporting. In addition, with few studies having no-treatment comparison groups, it is impossible to know whether a similar positive response would have occurred if the abuse had been stopped and no treatment for the children offered.

Treatment success also has been reported for therapeutic day care programs (for review, see Wolfe & Wekerle, 1993). For example, Culp, Heide, and Richardson (1987) compared 35 physically abused and neglected children participating in a therapeutic day treatment program with 35 abused and neglected children not participating in the program, who were matched on demographic and abuse variables. The program involved group and individual treatment as well as services to parents. Compared to the comparison children, those enrolled in the therapeutic day treatment program showed greater improvements in social–emotional, cognitive, motor, and language development as measured by the Michigan Developmental Profile. In a later study, Culp et al. (1991) compared 17 maltreated preschoolers in their day treatment program to 17 maltreated preschoolers who could not be admitted to the program because of space limitations. After 9 months of treatment, the children's developmental profile as measured by the staff and their self-reported self-esteem was measured. The children in treatment had significantly higher levels of self-esteem and had superior developmental profiles than those not in treatment.

Elmer (1986) evaluated a residential treatment program for physically abused infants. Infants stayed an average of 3 months and were visited by their mothers once a week. When compared to a group of infants from families at risk for maltreatment, there were no differences on mental or motor development at time of intake, discharge, or at the infants' first birthdays. Differences in interaction patterns between the abused and comparison infants and their mothers appeared at the time of discharge. Although three categories of interactions between mothers and infants improved more in the treatment than the comparison group, the mothers in the comparison group showed more improvement than the treatment mothers in four categories of mother behavior. Disappointingly, improvements in interactions in the treatment group generally disappeared by the first birthday of the child.

The home treatment program (Wood, Barton, & Schroeder, 1988), which involved family therapy and practical support, reported rates of 74% of treatment children remaining in the home compared with 45% of a comparison group.

Sexual Abuse

Individual psychotherapy is the most common form of treatment for child sexual abuse and a variety of treatment techniques have been described for use with sexually abused children, including play therapy, therapeutic storytelling, drama therapy, role plays, sex education, body integrity/prevention, self-esteem exercises, cognitive–behavioral techniques, and behavioral techniques (for review, see Becker et al., 1995). The philosophies underlying such treatments tend to be substantially different, resulting in a wide range of therapeutic aims and techniques (Beutler, Williams, & Zetzer, 1994).

Family therapy appears to be the second most common treatment for sexual abuse, frequently used for cases of father–daughter incest. According to Silovsky and Hembree-Kigin (1994), the goals for treatment for dysfunctional family relationships are similar across different models of family therapy and include preventing future abuse occurrences, having the perpetrator acknowledge and accept responsibility for the abuse, and reestablishing an appropriate hierarchy in the family. Typically, family therapy involves a variety of components including court intervention, individual therapy for the child, offender, nonoffending parent and siblings, family therapy, group therapy, and dyadic therapy.

Group therapy interventions also have been established to address the feelings and needs of sexually abused children. Issues addressed in group therapy typically involve feelings related to the abuse, depression, self-esteem, sexual behavior, social skills, dissociation, and problems related to separation and abandonment (Silovsky & Hembree-Kigin, 1994). Group therapy also allows abused children to understand that others have had experiences similar to them. Abused children often report that knowing this has been beneficial, since it makes them feel less responsible for their abuse (Haugaard & Reppucci,

1988). Group therapy sessions typically involve discussions of abuse-related themes and coping strategies, as well as structured activities such as role-playing and trust-building exercises. With specialized groups of children, such as sexually abused boys with problems with aggression, behavior management techniques also may be used (Silovsky & Hembree-Kigin, 1994).

Efficacy of Treatment for Sexually Abused Children

Although specialized treatments for sexually abused children have become increasingly common in the literature, the diversity of approaches used within each type of treatment, as well as a number of methodological problems (including different definitions of abuse and lack of standardized outcome measures), makes it difficult to determine the relative effectiveness of different types of treatments (Becker et al., 1995; Beutler et al., 1994). However, some evidence suggests that each type of treatment may be effective with some children. In reviewing several studies of individual psychotherapy, for example, Becker et al. (1995) concluded that psychological treatment can have an impact on many of the short-term effects of sexual abuse, although they caution that methodological limitations make it difficult to interpret and generalize results. Similarly, Beutler et al. (1994), in evaluating naturalistic studies of individual therapy that focus on the child's thoughts about the abuse, relationships in the child's life, or the child's behavior, conclude that while such studies have demonstrated some benefits, the size of such benefits is small.

Studies of family treatment programs have found low recidivism rates following treatment (Silovsky & Hembree-Kigin, 1994). For example, Giaretto (1982) found in an study of 250 families who completed individual, dyadic, group, and family therapy that there was no recidivism reported, although no follow-up period was specified. Similar results using family therapy were reported by Trepper and Traicoff (1983) in a study of 50 families. Neither study had a no-treatment control group, however, so the value of therapeutic intervention, rather than simply the legal intervention that accompanies being identified as an incestuous family, is unknown.

Studies of group therapy seldom have no-treatment control conditions. In one study that did, Verleur, Hughes, and De Rios (1986) conducted group therapy in a residential setting with 30 female incest victims, ranging in age from 13 to 17. After 6 months of treatment, the girls in treatment had higher levels of self-esteem, as measured by the Coopersmith Self-Esteem Inventory, than did 30 incestuously abused residents who had not participated in the group treatment. Friedrich, Luecke, Bielke, and Place (1992) and Hiebert-Murphy, De Luca, and Runtz (1992) reported behavior improvements in sexually abused children in their group treatment programs but did not have a comparison group of abused children who received no group treatment.

Neglect

Although neglect is the most frequently reported type of abuse, comprising nearly 50% of all cases of child maltreatment (NCCAN, 1995), there is very little empirical information available on specialized treatments for neglected children. Most of the treatments described for neglected children are the same as those for physically abused children, which typically involve some form of therapeutic day care for preschool age children (Becker et al., 1995).

Efficacy of Programs for Neglected Children

Because programs for neglected children typically treat both physically abused and neglected children, most of the outcome research on neglected children has already been reviewed in the section on physical abuse. As indicated earlier, this research suggests that treatment programs may be effective, particularly when they focus on improving the developmental and cognitive abilities of children (Oates & Bross, 1995). However, as with the research on physically abused children, there is little information available on long-term treatment gains and virtually no research has addressed interventions for older children or adolescents (Becker et al., 1995; Wolfe, 1994).

Fantuzzo et al. (1988) conducted a social skills training intervention with 18 neglected children, 9 physically abused children, and 12 children from high-risk families. Children were randomly assigned to one of three groups: peer initiation, adult initiation, and control. In each group, children participated in eight play sessions. In the peer initiation condition, a child modeled prosocial behavior for two treatment children. In the adult initiation condition, an adult modeled prosocial behavior for two treatment children. In the control condition, the additional peer or adult responded but did not model any behavior. Results demonstrated significant increases in positive, prosocial responses for children in the peer-initiation group, with no differences found between the adult initiation and control groups. Other research by Fantuzzo and his associates (Fantuzzo, Stovall, Schachtel, Goins, & Hall, 1987; Davis & Fantuzzo, 1989) has suggested that social skills training may be effective for increasing prosocial behavior among maltreated children, although there is some evidence that maltreated children who tend to be aggressive show an increase in negative social behaviors in response to social initiations (Davis & Fantuzzo, 1989).

Summary

Despite an upward trend in the number and variety of programs available for maltreated children, there is limited empirical information about the efficacy of such treatments. Although some research suggests that treatment may be effective, there are few methodologically sound studies available on which to base conclusions. A few studies of the effectiveness of treatment for young physically abused and neglected children have shown some short-term improvement. The work by Elmer (1986), however, raises significant concerns about the long-term effectiveness of treatment that does not focus substantially on parenting behaviors.

Treatment involving parents is rare in the child sexual abuse literature, which seems to go against all of the research showing that a supportive and developmentally appropriate family life is one of the strongest predictors of a child's ability to cope successfully with child sexual abuse. There is almost no empirical evidence suggesting that psychotherapy with victims of child sexual abuse is effective at meeting the goals of therapy.

FUTURE EFFORTS TO ESTABLISH THE EFFICACY OF TREATMENT FOR CHILD MALTREATMENT

There are several obstacles to the development of treatment outcome research in child maltreatment. Some of these obstacles could be overcome without too much difficulty, while others will be more problematic to overcome.

One way that outcome research could be done is by individual agencies, or consortiums of agencies, implementing treatment outcome research with their clients. There are several obstacles to this approach. A primary ethical obstacle is that outcome research typically involves a comparison group of possible clients who do not receive services or who do not receive them for a certain period of time. It is unethical to withhold treatment from someone who needs it simply to create a methodologically sound study. Withholding treatment from child victims of maltreatment may be seen as especially unprincipled. Some researchers have overcome this obstacle, however. As noted above, Culp et al. (1987, 1991) made use of the great demand for their treatment program by forming a comparison group from children who could not be admitted to it because of space limitations. Agencies with waiting lists for services might use those on the waiting list as a comparison group, although this would limit the length of their study to the time that the children remained on the waiting list. Another strategy was used by Nicole et al. (1988), who provided different types of treatment to maltreating families and compared the effectiveness of the two types. Using another strategy, Verleur et al. (1986) added a group treatment component to the regular inpatient treatment received by one group of sexually abused girls and compared their outcome to girls who received regular inpatient treatment without group therapy.

Each of these strategies requires that data be gathered from children and their families receiving treatment and, in some cases, by families not receiving treatment. This can be an expensive and time-consuming effort, and one that most agencies cannot afford to do. In addition, many agencies focused on treatment do not have research experts on staff. Money is required to solve this problem—to hire additional staff and gather and analyze data. Unfortunately, federal and state agencies focused on child maltreatment have provided little money for methodologically sound research on treatment outcome (Melton, 1994).

A second strategy for outcome research would be to gather a large number of maltreated children and give them specific forms of treatment. Such research is typically done in conjunction with a university or other research agency. Meaningful work on attention deficit hyperactivity disorder (Hinshaw, 1994) and conduct disorder (Kazdin, 1993), to mention two examples, has been done in this manner. There is, however, a significant obstacle to this type of research, which also constrains the type of agency-based research described in the previous paragraph. Most treatment-outcome research has focused on specific psychological disorders. This allows researchers to (1) determine whether or not a potential research participant meets the requirements for a disorder, (2) use valid instruments to measure periodically the level of the disorder, and (3) employ treatments that have been linked theoretically or empirically to the mechanisms believed to be causing the disorder. However, child maltreatment is not a disorder. Child maltreatment is an experience that has been linked to a variety of disorders. As noted above, some maltreated children are anxious, others are depressed or have conduct problems, and still others show no apparent disorder. Thus, it is not maltreatment that is being treated; rather, treatment is aimed at preventing or mollifying the variety of disorders and other problems that have been associated with child maltreatment.

Therapists have identified many characteristics of therapy that they believe are valuable when working with maltreated children. For example, providing a maltreated child with the knowledge that other children have had the same experience, allowing children to express their range of feelings about the abuser and other family members, and helping children to learn socially appropriate physical contact with others (see Haugaard & Reppucci, 1988, for review). Given that there is a growing body of research on the effectiveness of therapy with children exhibiting a variety of psychological disorders (Weisz & Weisz, 1993), it might be more beneficial to assess the effectiveness of therapy aimed at a particular psychological disorder of maltreated children, with and without the addition of the characteristics that some therapists have argued are important for therapy with maltreated children. The focus would then shift from treatment of child maltreatment to, for example, treatment of depressed children who have been maltreated. The usefulness of the inclusion of specific therapeutic interventions aimed at maltreated children (e.g., inclusion in a group where other children describe their experiences) could then be assessed relatively easily, just as the inclusion of some interventions with depressed children are now done (e.g., the addition of social skills training to a program of cognitive therapy).

SUMMARY AND CONCLUSIONS

Child maltreatment is a significant public health problem in the United States. For individual children, its consequences can be severe and enduring. Case reports from individual, group, and family therapy show that maltreated children and their families can recover from their experiences, although the process by which they recover, and those who are more likely to recover than others, remains unclear. Research in this area needs to focus on the process of recovery, rather than simply examining the end result of therapy or other interventions. For example, is the functioning of maltreated children improved because (1) they learn that others have had the same experiences, (2) they are able to express anger at the perpetrator and family members, or (3) their family begins to function more effectively. Several of these changes (as well as others) may be useful to some children, and a different set of changes may be beneficial to some children and not others. However, until we can begin to identify more clearly what it is about an intervention that makes it beneficial, the interventions will be less effective than they could be.

Research shows that a substantial number of maltreated children show no symptoms of emotional or behavioral disturbance after their maltreatment is discovered. Because of a lack of longitudinal research, however, it is unclear whether emotional or behavioral problems are more likely to develop in these children during subsequent developmental periods than in nonmaltreated children. Such information is important for policy makers and clinicians who must decide whether asymptomatic maltreated children should receive some intervention to prevent the onset of future problems (thus spreading the resources available to maltreated children thinner), or whether such children do not need professional intervention (thus making more resources available to symptomatic maltreated children).

There is a surprisingly small amount of research regarding factors, other than professional intervention, that aid children in their adaptation to maltreatment. Research in this area is of great importance. The prevalence of child maltreatment makes it impossible for community mental health agencies and private practitioners to provide services to all maltreated children. Knowing which factors are associated with better adaptation to maltreatment could assist agencies in deciding which children are in the most need of individual, group, or family therapy. In addition, agencies could use information about these factors to develop interventions other than, or in addition to, direct therapy for children. For example, research showing the importance of parental support in promoting adaptation to maltreatment could indicate that groups or classes designed to increase the capacity of parents to provide constructive support could promote recovery from maltreatment even more effectively than time-consuming individual child therapy in many cases. Finally, research on these factors could inform therapeutic strategies. For example, if having supportive friends was shown to be related to adaptation to maltreatment, then an important goal of therapy might be to help a child develop the social skills necessary to develop a group of supportive friends.

The high prevalence of maltreatment and the wide heterogeneity of the experiences of maltreated children require that a range of formal and informal interventions be available to them. By working to discover which children need more intense interventions and which can adapt to their experiences through less formal interventions by school personnel, caseworkers, community volunteers, parents, and others, we will be able to provide needed services to many more maltreated children than we are currently reaching.

REFERENCES

Aber, J. L., Allen, J. P., Carlson, V., & Cicchetti, D. (1991). The effects of maltreatment on development during early childhood: Recent studies and their theoretical, clinical, and policy implications. In D. Cicchetti & V. Carlson (Eds.), *Child maltreatment: Theory and research on the causes and consequences of child abuse and neglect* (pp. 280–301). Cambridge, MA: Cambridge University Press.

Aber, J. L., & Zigler, E. (1981). Developmental considerations in the definition of child maltreatment. In R. Rizly & D. Cicchetti (Eds.), *Developmental perspectives on child maltreatment* (pp. 1–29). San Francisco: Jossey-Bass.

Ainsworth, M. D. S., Blehar, M. C., Waters, E., & Wall, S. (1978). *Patterns of attachment: A psychological study of the Strange Situation.* Hillsdale, NJ: Erlbaum.

Alexander, P. C. (1992). Application of attachment theory to the study of sexual abuse. *Journal of Consulting and Clinical Psychology, 60*, 185–195.

Beck, A. T. (1979). *Cognitive therapy of depression*. New York: Guilford.

Beck, A. T. (1985). *Anxiety disorders and phobias: A cognitive perspective.* New York: Basic Books.

Becker, J. V., Alpert, J. L., BigFoot, D. S., Bonner, B. L., Geddie, L. F., Henggeler, S. W., Kaufman, K. L., & Walker, C. E. (1995). Empirical research on child abuse treatment: Report by the child abuse and neglect treatment working group, American Psychological Association. *Journal of Clinical Child Psychology, 24*, 23–46.

Beitchman, J. H., Zucker, K. J., Hood, J. E., daCosta, G. A., & Akman, D. (1991). A review of the short-term effects of child sexual abuse. *Child Abuse & Neglect, 15*, 537–556.

Beitchman, J. H., Zucker, K. J., Hood, J. E., da Costa, G. A., Akman, D., & Cassavia, E. (1992). A review of long-term effects of child sexual abuse. *Child Abuse & Neglect, 16*, 101–118.

Berger, A. M., Knutson, J. F., Mehm, J. G., & Perkins, K. A. (1988). The self-report of punitive experience of young adults and adolescents. *Child Abuse & Neglect, 12*, 251–262.

Beutler, L. E., Williams, R. A., & Zetzer, H. A. (1994). Efficacy of treatment for victims of child sexual abuse. *The Future of Children, 4*, 156–175.

Bowlby, J. (1969). *Attachment and loss. Vol. I: Attachment.* New York: Basic Books.

Buchannan, A., & Oliver, J. E. (1977). Abuse and neglect as a cause of mental retardation. *British Journal of Psychiatry, 131*, 458–467.

Caffaro-Rouget, A., Lang, R. A., & van Santen, V. (1989). The impact of child sexual abuse. *Annals of Sex Research, 2*, 29–47.

Caffey, J. (1972). On the theory and practice of shaking infants. *American Journal of Diseases of Children, 124*, 161–169.

Carlson, N. R. (1991). *Physiology of behavior* (4th ed.). Boston: Allyn & Bacon.

Cicchetti, D., Rogosch, F. A., Lynch, M., & Holt, K. (1993). Resilience in maltreated children: Processes leading to adaptive outcome. *Development and Psychopathology, 5*, 629–647.

Cohn, A. H., & Daro, D. (1987). Is treatment too late: What ten years of evaluative research tell us. *Child Abuse & Neglect, 11*, 433–442.

Conte, J. R., & Schuerman, J. R. (1987). Factors associated with an increased impact of child sexual abuse. *Child Abuse & Neglect, 11*, 201–211.

Cox, A., Rutter, M., Yule, B., & Quinton, D. (1977). Bias resulting from missing information: Some epidemiological findings. *British Journal of Preventive and Social Medicine, 31*, 131–136.

Crittenden, P. M., & Ainsworth, M. D. S. (1989). Child maltreatment and attachment theory. In D. Cicchetti & V. Carlson (Eds.), *Child maltreatment: Theory and research on the causes and consequences of child abuse and neglect* (pp. 432–463). Cambridge, MA: Cambridge University Press.

Culp, R. E., Heide, J., & Richardson, M. T. (1987). Maltreated children's developmental scores: Treatment versus nontreatment. *Child Abuse & Neglect, 11*, 29–34.

Culp, R. E., Little, V., Letts, D., & Lawrence, H. (1991). Maltreated children's self-concept: Effects of a comprehensive treatment program. *American Journal of Orthopsychiatry, 61*, 114–121.

Davis, S. P., & Fantuzzo, J. W. (1989). The effects of adult and peer social initiations on the social behavior of withdrawn and aggressive maltreated preschool children. *Journal of Family Violence, 4*, 227–248.

DeBellis, M. D., Lefter, L., Trickett, P. K., & Putnam, F. W. (1994). Urinary catecholamine excretion in sexually abused girls. *Journal of the American Academy of Child and Adolescent Psychiatry, 33*, 320–327.

Deblinger, E., McLeer, S. V., Atkins, M. S., Ralphe, D., & Foa, E. (1989). Post-traumatic stress in sexually abused, physically abused, and nonabused children. *Child Abuse & Neglect, 13*, 403–408.

Diamond, L. J., & Jaudes, P. K. (1983). Child abuse in a cerebral-palsied population. *Developmental Medicine and Child Neurology, 25*, 169–174.

Dodge, K. A., Bates, J. E., & Pettit, G. S. (1990). Mechanisms in the cycle of violence. *Science, 250*, 1678–1683.

Eckenrode, J., Laird, M., & Doris, J. (1993). School performance and disciplinary problems among abused and neglected children. *Developmental Psychology, 29*, 53–62.

Elmer, E. (1986). Outcome of residential treatment for abused and high risk infants. *Child Abuse & Neglect, 10*, 351–360.

Erickson, M. F., & Egeland, B. (1987). A developmental view of the psychological consequences of maltreatment. *School Psychology Review, 16,* 156–168.

Everson, M. D., Hunter, W. M., Runyon, D. K., Edelsohn, G. A., & Coulter, M. L. (1989). Maternal support following disclosure of incest. *American Journal of Orthopsychiatry, 59,* 197–207.

Fantuzzo, J. W., Stovall, A., Schachtel, D., Goins, C., & Hall, R. (1987). The effects of peer social initiations on the social behavior of withdrawn, maltreated preschool children. *Journal of Behavior Therapy and Experimental Psychiatry, 4,* 357–363.

Fantuzzo, J. W., Jurecic, L., Stovall, A., Hightower, A. D., Goins, C., & Schachtel, D. (1988). Effects of adult and peer social initiations on the social behavior of withdrawn, maltreated preschool children. *Journal of Consulting and Clinical Psychology, 56,* 34–39.

Farber, E. A., & Egeland, B. (1987). Invulnerability among abused and neglected children. In E. J. Anthony & B. Cohler (Eds.), *The invulnerable child* (pp. 253–288). New York: Guilford Press.

Finkelhor, D. (1979). *Sexually victimized children.* New York: Free Press.

Friedrich, W. N., Beilke, R. L., & Urquiza, A. (1987). Children from sexually abusive families: A behavioral comparison. *Journal of Interpersonal Violence, 2,* 391–402.

Freidrich, W. N., Luecke, W. J., Bielke, R. L., & Place, U. (1992). Psychotherapy outcome of sexually abused boys: An agency study. *Journal of Interpersonal Violence, 7,* 396–409.

Fromuth, M. E., & Burkhart, B. R. (1989). Long-term psychological correlates of childhood sexual abuse in two samples of college men. *Child Abuse & Neglect, 10,* 5–15.

Gelles, R. J. (1982). Child abuse and family violence: Implications for medical professionals. In E. Newberger (Ed.), *Child abuse* (pp. 25–41). Boston: Little, Brown and Company.

Giaretto, H. (1982). Humanistic treatment of father–daughter incest. In National Institute of Mental Health, *Sexual abuse of children* (pp. 39–46). (DHHS Publication No. 78-30161). Washington, DC: United States Department of Health and Human Services.

Giovannoni, J. (1989). Definitional issues in child maltreatment. In D. Cicchetti & V. Carlson (Eds.), *Child maltreatment: Theory and research on the causes and consequences of child abuse and neglect* (pp. 3–37). New York: Cambridge University Press.

Goodman, G., Taub, E., Jones, D., England, P., Port, L., Rudy, L., & Prado, L. (1992). Testifying in criminal court. *Monographs of the Society for Research in Child Development, 57,* 1–160.

Hampton, R. L. (1987). Race, class and child maltreatment. *Journal of Comparative Family Studies, 18,* 113–126.

Haugaard, J. J., & Emery, R. E. (1989). Methodological issues in child sexual abuse research. *Child Abuse & Neglect, 13,* 89–100.

Haugaard, J. J., & Reppucci, N. D. (1988). *The sexual abuse of children.* San Francisco: Jossey-Bass.

Haugaard, J. J., & Samwel, C. (1992). Legal and therapeutic interventions with incestuous families. *International Journal of Medicine and Law, 11,* 469–484.

Hazzard, A., Celano, M., Gould, J., Lawry, S., & Webb, M. (1995). Predicting symptomatology and self-blame among child sex abuse victims. *Child Abuse & Neglect, 19,* 707–714.

Hiebert-Murphy, D., De Luca, R., & Runtz, M. (1992). Group treatment for sexually abused girls: Evaluating outcome. *Families in Society, 73,* 205–213.

Hinshaw, S. (1994). *Attention deficits and hyperactivity in children.* Thousand Oaks, CA: Sage.

Kazdin, A. (1993). Treatment of conduct disorder. *Development and Psychopathology, 5,* 277–310.

Kendall-Tackett, K., Williams, L. M., & Finkelhor, D. (1993). Impact of sexual abuse on children: A review and synthesis of recent empirical studies. *Psychological Bulletin, 113,* 164–180.

Kramer, S. (1994). Further considerations on somatic and cognitive residues of incest. In A. Sugarman (Ed.), *Victims of abuse* (pp. 69–95). Madison, CT: International Universities Press.

Lindholm, K. J., & Willey, R. (1986). Ethnic differences in child abuse and sexual abuse. *Hispanic Journal of Behavioral Sciences, 8,* 111–125.

Lovett, B. (1995). Child sexual abuse: The female victim's relationship with her nonoffending mother. *Child Abuse & Neglect, 19,* 729–738.

Lynch, M., & Cicchetti, D. (1991). Patterns of relatedness in maltreated and nonmaltreated children: Connections among multiple representational models. *Development and Psychopathology 3,* 207–226.

Main, M., & Solomon, J. (1986). Discovery of a disorganized disoriented attachment pattern. In T. B. Brazelton & M. W. Yogman (Eds.), *Affective development in infancy* (pp. 95–124). Norwood, NJ: Ablex.

Malinosky-Rummell, R., & Hansen, D. (1993). Long-term consequences of childhood physical abuse. *Psychological Bulletin, 114,* 68–79.

Manley, J., Cicchetti, D., & Barnett, D. (1994). The impact of subtype, frequency, chronicity, and severity of child maltreatment on social competence and behavior problems. *Development and Psychopathology, 6,* 121–143.

McGee, R. A., & Wolfe, D. A. (1991). Psychological maltreatment: Toward an operational definition. *Development and Psychopathology, 3,* 3–18.

Melton, G. B. (1994). Research policy and child maltreatment. *Child Abuse & Neglect, 18* (Suppl. 1), 1–28.

Melton, G. B., & Barry, F. D. (1994). *Protecting children from abuse and neglect.* New York: Guilford.

National Center on Child Abuse and Neglect. (1995). *Child maltreatment in 1993: Reports from the states to the National Center on Child Abuse and Neglect.* Washington, DC: Department of Health and Human Services.

Nicole, A. R., Smith, J., Kay, B., Hall, D., Barlow, J., & Williams, B. (1988). A focused casework approach to the treatment of child abuse: A controlled comparison. *Journal of Child Psychology and Psychiatry, 29,* 703–711.

Oates, R. K., & Bross, D. C. (1995). What have we learned about treating child physical abuse: A literature review of the last decade. *Child Abuse & Neglect, 19,* 463–473.

Oates, R. K., Peacock, A., & Forrest, D. (1984). The development of abused children. *Developmental Medicine and Child Neurology, 26,* 649–656.

O'Beirne, H., & Reppucci, N. D. (in press). The sequelae of childhood sexual abuse: Implications of empirical research for clinical, legal and public policy domains. In D. Cicchetti & S. Toth (Eds.), *New directions in child psychopathology.*

Pelton, L. H. (1994). The role of material factors in child abuse and neglect. In G. B. Melton & F. D. Barry (Eds.), *Protecting children from abuse and neglect* (pp. 131–181). New York: Guilford.

Putnam, F., Helmers, K., & Trickett, P. (1993). Development, reliability, and validation of a child dissociation scale. *Child Abuse & Neglect, 17,* 731–740.

Romans, S., Martin, J., Anderson, J., O'Shea, M., & Mullen, P. (1995). Factors that mediate between child sexual abuse and adult psychological outcome. *Psychological Medicine, 25,* 127–142.

Runyan, D. K., Everson, M. D., Edelsohn, G. A., Hunter, W. M., & Coulter, M. L. (1988). Impact of legal intervention on sexually abused children. *Journal of Pediatrics, 113,* 647–653.

Russell, D. (1983). The incidence and prevalence of intrafamilial and extrafamilial sexual abuse of female children. *Child Abuse & Neglect, 7,* 133–146.

Sales, B. (1994). In a dim light: Admissibility of child sexual abuse memories. *Applied Cognitive Psychology, 8,* 399–406.

Silovsky, J. F., & Hembree-Kigin, T. L. (1994). Family and group treatment for sexually abused children: A review. *Journal of Child Sexual Abuse, 3,* 1–20.

Spacarelli, S., & Kim, S. (1995). Resilience criteria and factors associated with resilience in sexually abused girls. *Child Abuse & Neglect, 19,* 1171–1182.

Straus, M. A., & Gelles, R. J. (1986). Societal change and change in family violence from 1975–1985. *Journal of Marriage and the Family, 48,* 465–479.

Straus, M. A., Gelles, R. J., & Steinmetz, S. K. (1980). *Behind closed doors: Violence in the American family.* Garden City, NY: Anchor.

Sugarman, A. (Ed.). (1994). *Victims of abuse.* Madison, CT: International Universities Press.

Trepper, T. S., & Traicoff, M. E. (1985). Treatment of intrafamily sexuality: Issues in therapy and research. *Journal of Sex Education and Therapy, 4,* 14–18.

Trickett, P. K. (1993). Maladaptive development of school-aged, physically abused children: Relations with the child rearing context. *Journal of Family Psychology, 7,* 134–147.

Trickett, P. K., & McBride-Chang, C. (1995). The developmental impact of different forms of child abuse and neglect. *Developmental Review, 15,* 311–337.

Trickett, P. K., McBride-Chang, C., & Putnam, F. W. (1994). The classroom performance and behavior of sexually abused females. *Development and Psychopathology, 6,* 183–194.

Tufts New England Medical Center, Division of Child Psychiatry. (1984). *Sexually exploited children: Service and research project.* Washington, DC: US Department of Justice.

Tyson, R. L. (1986). The roots of psychopathology and our theories of development. *Journal of the American Academy of Child Psychiatry, 25,* 12–22.

US Advisory Board on Child Abuse and Neglect. (1995). *A nation's shame: Fatal child abuse and neglect in the United States.* Washington, DC: Department of Health and Human Services.

Valentine, L., & Feinauer, L. (1993). Resilience factors associated with female survivors of childhood sexual abuse. *American Journal of Family Therapy, 21,* 216–224.

Verleur, D., Hughes, R. E., & De Rios, M. D. (1986). Enhancement of self-esteem among female adolescent incest victims: A controlled comparison. *Adolescence, 21,* 843–854.

Waterman, J., & Kelly, R. (1993). Mediators of effects on children. In J. Waterman, R. Kelly, M. K. Oliveri, & J. McCord (Eds.), *Behind the playground walls: Sexual abuse in preschools* (pp. 168–192). New York: Guilford.

Weisz, J., & Weiss, B. (1993). Effects of psychotherapy with children and adolescents. Newbury Park, CA: Sage.

Werner, E. M. (1990). Protective factors and individual resilience. In S. J. Meisels & J. P. Shonkoff (Eds.), *Handbook of early childhood intervention* (pp. 97–116). Cambridge, England: Cambridge University Press.

White, S., Halpin, B. M., Strom, G. A., & Santilli, G. (1988). Behavioral comparisons of young sexually abused, neglected, and nonreferred children. *Journal of Clinical Child Psychology, 17,*53–61.

Widom, C. S. (1989). The cycle of violence. *Science, 244,* 160–166.

Wodarski, J., Kurtz, P. D., Gaudin, J., & Howing, P. (1990). Maltreatment and the school-age child: Major academic, socioemotional, and adaptive outcomes. *Social Work, 35,* 506–513.

Wolfe, D. A. (1994). The role of intervention and treatment services in the prevention of child abuse and neglect. In G. B. Melton & F. D. Barry (Eds.), *Protecting children from abuse and neglect* (pp. 224–304). New York: Guilford.

Wolfe, D. A., & Wekerle, C. (1993). Treatment strategies for child physical abuse and neglect: A critical progress report. *Clinical Psychology Review, 13,* 473–500.

Wood, S., Barton, K., & Schroeder, C. (1988). In-home treatment of abusive families: Cost and placement at one year. Special Issue: Psychotherapy and the new health care systems. *Psychotherapy, 25,* 409–414.

Wyatt, G. E. (1985). The sexual abuse of Afro-American and White-American women in childhood. *Child Abuse & Neglect, 10,* 231–240.

4

Parental Alcoholism as a Risk Factor

LAURIE CHASSIN, MANUEL BARRERA, Jr., and HEATHER MONTGOMERY

Parental alcoholism is a risk factor of great public health significance because it has the potential to affect a large number of children and adolescents. Although prevalence estimates for alcoholism vary with the operational definition of the disorder, recent data suggest that approximately 25% of adult males and 4–5% of adult females in the US population meet lifetime criteria for alcohol abuse or dependence (Robins et al., 1984). Based on these epidemiological data, Russell, Henderson, and Blume (1985) estimated that there were approximately 6.6 million children of alcoholic parents (COAs) under 18 years of age and approximately 22 million "adult" children of alcoholic parents (i.e., age 18 or over). Thus, a large segment of the population is exposed to parental alcoholism. The potential importance of parental alcoholism as a risk factor has produced great clinical interest in children of alcoholics as targets for intervention, including the recent popularity of self-help groups for adult children of alcoholics, and the codependence movement (see Sher & Mothershead, 1991, for a review of this literature).

Parental alcoholism has also received substantial empirical attention, particularly among researchers who are interested in the etiology of alcohol abuse and dependence. Because COAs are known to be at elevated risk for the development of adult alcoholism, there has been a great deal of study devoted to identifying factors characteristic of COAs that might be of etiologic significance for the development of adult alcoholism. This literature has included studies of personality characteristics, psychopathology, neuropsychological functioning, psychophysiological responsiveness, responses to alcohol consumption, and,

LAURIE CHASSIN, MANUEL BARRERA, Jr., and HEATHER MONTGOMERY • Department of Psychology, Arizona State University, Tempe, Arizona 85287-1104.

Handbook of Children's Coping: Linking Theory and Intervention, edited by Wolchik and Sandler. Plenum Press, New York, 1997.

to a lesser extent, studies of the psychosocial environments to which COAs are exposed. This rather large literature on characteristics of COAs has been the subject of several recent excellent, comprehensive reviews (Searles & Windle, 1988; Sher, 1991; West & Prinz, 1987), which cannot be duplicated in this chapter. Instead, we will selectively emphasize studies of childhood and adolescence, studies that have appeared since recent reviews, studies that illustrate larger conceptual or methodological issues, and studies that have implications for preventive interventions. First, we will review literature on the impact of parent alcoholism on child and adolescent outcomes, considering methodological problems that limit our conclusions. Second, we will consider component features of parental alcoholism as a stressor and will describe some potential mediating mechanisms underlying parental alcoholism effects, as well as possible moderators of parental alcoholism effects. Third, we will describe some efforts at preventive intervention and discuss dilemmas faced in constructing preventive interventions for COAs.

METHODOLOGICAL ISSUES

Recent reviews have summarized the many methodological limitations that have plagued this area of research (Sher, 1991; West & Prinz, 1987). Sampling has been a major problem, with studies often having only small samples with little power to detect parental alcoholism effects. In addition to using small samples, few studies have attempted to access representative samples of community-dwelling alcoholics. Instead, studies have relied on samples of convenience, which can potentially overrepresent pathology (e.g., samples of alcoholic parents in treatment) or underrepresent pathology (e.g., samples of college student COAs). This variation in sampling has produced frequently conflicting findings concerning parental alcoholism effects.

Measurement issues have also been a major limiting factor in COA research. As West and Prinz (1987) noted, studies have often relied on a single reporter providing data on both parental alcoholism and offspring psychopathology, so that reporter bias potentially overestimates parental alcoholism effects. Studies have often failed to directly ascertain parental alcoholism, relying instead on offspring report. Although some methods of offspring report have demonstrated adequate reliability (Crews & Sher, 1992), offspring reports show weak sensitivity, and studies relying on offspring report typically fail to determine important sources of heterogeneity within parental alcoholism. For example, these studies rarely obtain information about co-occurring parental pathology (e.g., antisocial personality, depression, anxiety disorders), age of onset of parental alcoholism, gender of the alcoholic parent, severity, or recency of parental alcoholism. Studies of adult alcoholism have convincingly demonstrated that alcoholism is not a unitary disorder; different subtypes of alcoholism appear to have different patterns of intergenerational transmission, and thus are likely to differentially affect children (Cloninger, 1987). However, few studies have been able to consider this important heterogeneity within parental alcoholism.

Finally, studies have been limited by a failure to consider variables that co-occur with parental alcoholism that have potentially important impacts on offspring. Because alcoholism often co-occurs with a variety of other disorders (e.g., depression, antisocial personality) as well as a variety of environmental disruptions (e.g., divorce, lowered socioeconomic status, family conflict), the extent to which obtained effects are specific to parental alcoholism has not been clear. These factors that co-occur with parental alcoholism are important to assess because they can constitute "third" variables (which create spurious relations between parental alcoholism and child outcomes) or they may represent important mediators of the effects of parental alcoholism on child outcomes. These mediators are potentially important targets for preventive interventions.

In short, COA research has been limited by severe methodological problems including the use of small samples, reliance on treated samples or college student samples, failure to obtain data from multiple sources, failure to directly ascertain parental alcoholism, failure to consider important sources of heterogeneity in parental alcoholism, and failure to consider the effects of important factors that co-occur with parental alcoholism.

PARENTAL ALCOHOLISM AND OFFSPRING OUTCOMES

Alcohol and Drug Use Outcomes

Parental alcoholism is a well-established risk factor for the development of adult alcoholism. Russell (1990) reviewed adoptee studies and reported consistent elevations in the prevalence of alcoholism among adults COAs who were raised in adoptive, nonalcoholic homes. However, there was considerable variation in the magnitude of the risk ratios. The highest risk (risk ratios of 9) was associated with sons of severely alcoholic fathers with early-onset serious criminality, and the lowest risk (risk ratios of 1.5–3) was found among sons of mildly alcoholic parents and adopted daughters of alcoholic biological mothers. Similar variability in the magnitude of risk by gender was noted by McGue (1994), who suggests that genetic factors exert a moderate influence on male risk for alcoholism and a modest influence on female risk for alcoholism. However, two recent studies found stronger associations between parental alcoholism and female alcohol use outcomes than between parental alcoholism and male alcohol use outcomes (Russell, Cooper, & Frone, 1990; Sher, Walitzer, Wood, & Brent, 1991). Because these were not adoptee studies, this elevated risk for female COAs may reflect mechanisms of transmission other than genetic influences. Moreover, this greater parental alcoholism effect for females than for males was limited to non-Hispanic Caucasian subjects (Russell et al., 1990).

Evidence also suggests that COAs show elevations in alcohol and drug use in the adolescent years, although these findings have been somewhat less consistent (Herjanic, Herjanic, Penick, Tomelleri, & Armbruster, 1977; Merikangas, Weissman, Prusoff, Pauls, & Leckman, 1985). Pandina and Johnson (1989) found significant differences between high- and low-risk subjects only at the oldest age groups (18–21). However, their high-risk group included those with a family history of alcoholism in second-degree relatives, who have sometimes been considered to be at "moderate" rather than high risk (Alterman, Searles, & Hall, 1989).

Our own data (Chassin, Rogosch, & Barrera, 1991), using a community sample, found that early- to middle-adolescent COAs showed elevated levels of alcohol and drug use. The magnitude of their risk varied with the recency of parental alcoholism, with the strongest risk ratios found for those with "current" alcoholic parents and more moderate risk for those with "recovered" alcoholic parents. Moreover, this elevated risk was unique to parental alcoholism, and could not be explained by co-occurring parental antisociality, depression, or environmental disruption. Finally, we found that paternal alcoholism was associated with steeper escalation of substance use involvement over a 3-year period during adolescence (Chassin, Pillow, Curran, Molina, & Barrera, 1993; Chassin, Curran, Hussong, & Colder, 1996). This increasing involvement with substance use could not be fully explained by co-occurring parental pathology, by environmental stress and negative affect, by temperamental emotionality or sociability, or by disruptions in parental monitoring and affiliation with substance-using peers. Thus, other mediators (unmeasured in our study) must be invoked to explain the effect of paternal alcoholism on adolescent substance use. Some data (see Newlin & Thomson, 1990, for a review) suggest that male offspring of alcoholic fathers may experience more positive effects from alcohol and less negative impact of alcohol consumption than do non-COA males. Such individual differences in the reinforcement value obtained from substance use could explain the more rapid escalation of substance use involvement that we found in our adolescents who had alcoholic fathers.

In summary, research has demonstrated that COAs are at increased risk for alcohol and drug use and abuse outcomes in adolescence and adulthood, that this risk is specific to parental alcoholism (above and beyond comorbidities), and that the magnitude of the risk varies with aspects of parental alcoholism and with gender of the COA and gender of the alcoholic parent. These findings suggest that COAs are an important target audience for substance use preventive interventions. However, the magnitudes of effect also show substantial overlap between COA and non-COA groups (suggesting either differential exposure to the risk mediators or protective factors that buffer risk). Little is known about the mediators of parental alcoholism risk for substance use outcomes, although possible mechanisms have included high-risk temperament, impaired parental socialization, increased environmental stress and negative affect, and differential reinforcement value obtained from the pharmacological effects of alcohol and drugs (see Sher, 1991, for a description of these theoretical mechanisms). From the point of view of developing preventive interventions, further information on the mechanisms underlying COA risk for substance use is of great importance.

Externalizing Symptomatology

Most studies suggest that COAs are at risk for higher levels of externalizing symptomatology, including aggression, oppositional behavior, and delinquent or antisocial behavior. West and Prinz's (1987) review noted that five of six studies supported an association between parental alcoholism and childhood conduct problems. However, researchers have pointed out that the majority of COAs do not show clinically elevated levels of externalizing symptoms (Jacob & Leonard, 1986). Moreover, exceptions to these findings have also been noted. For example, Jacob and Leonard (1986) failed to find elevations in externalizing symptomatology among COAs in comparison to children with a depressed parent. This suggests that the effect may not be specific to parental alcoholism. However, that study had small sample sizes and a COA group that might be less likely to be impaired (because of the selection of mothers without significant psychopathology and alcoholic fathers with no significant comorbidities). Other studies have also challenged the specificity of the link between parent alcoholism and externalizing symptoms. Our data (Chassin et al., 1991) found that adolescents' externalizing symptomatology was more clearly linked to parental antisocial personality disorders than unique to parental alcoholism.

From the point of view of preventive intervention, it is also important that children's conduct problems have been linked to the familial disruption that goes along with parental alcoholism (West & Prinz, 1987). For example, Roosa, Dumka, Tein, and Tweed (1992) found that the effects of parental problem drinking on children's conduct problems were mediated by family strengths (adaptability and cohesion). Pollack et al. (1990), using retrospective data from young adults, found that a history of physical abuse rather than parental alcoholism significantly predicted antisocial behavior. To the extent that ongoing family disruption mediates the effects of parental alcoholism on childhood conduct problems, interventions focused on preserving familial adaptability and cohesion may help to prevent conduct problems among COAs.

It has also been suggested that parental alcoholism can raise risk for attention deficit hyperactivity disorder (ADHD) in childhood (Cantwell, 1975; Morrison & Stewart, 1971). Pihl, Peterson, and Finn (1990) asserted that there are common biological links among disorders of disinhibition such as alcoholism, conduct problems, and ADHD. They focus on a subgroup of COAs who are male, have alcoholic fathers, and have a high density of alcoholic relatives (i.e., sons of male, multigenerational alcoholics, referred to as SOMMAs). Pihl et al. (1990) suggest that SOMMAs show a pattern of hypoactive responding in situations where there is a need for effortful, sustained attention. Such an attentional dysfunction would be consistent with attentional problems of children diagnosed with ADHD.

There have been empirical links between parental alcoholism and other individual symptoms of ADHD (such as high activity level and impulsivity). For example, Tarter, Kabene, Escallier, Laird, and Jacob (1990) and Moss, Blackson, Martin, and Tarter (1992) found that COAs had elevated levels of behavioral activity. Fitzgerald et al. (1993) found a relation between paternal alcoholism and impulsivity (assessed by a delay of gratification task) in a sample of preschoolers with alcoholic parents recruited from driving under the influence (DUI) records. This study is noteworthy because of the young age of the subjects and the use of a nonclinical sample of alcoholic parents. Links between parental alcoholism, hyperactivity, and attentional deficits have also been noted as a result of fetal alcohol syndrome (Streissguth, Landesman-Dwyer, Martin, & Smith, 1980; Streissguth, Sampson, & Olson, 1994). Although links have been shown between parental alcoholism and symptoms of inattention, impulsivity, and activity level, this is not the equivalent of diagnosed ADHD. Studies that have attempted to link diagnosed ADHD to parental alcoholism starting with clinically diagnosed ADHD children as the probands have not consistently supported a relation (West & Prinz, 1987). Finally, studies attempting to link parental alcoholism and ADHD have often failed to control for the child's co-occurring conduct problems, which could account for any correlation with parental alcoholism. Thus, although there have been studies to link parental alcoholism with symptoms of ADHD, the evidence has not been entirely consistent.

Finally, given the covariation among symptoms of aggression, inattention, impulsivity, and overactivity, some researchers have suggested that there is a common deficit in self-regulation among COAs (e.g., Martin et al., 1994) and some have described COAs as "behaviorally undercontrolled" (Sher et al., 1991; Windle, 1990). Martin et al. (1994) compared preadolescent boys with and without paternal substance abuse (including but not limited to alcoholism) on a profile of mother report, teacher report, child report, and laboratory measures of these dimensions. In addition to providing support for covariation among these dimensions, Martin et al. (1994) found that boys with substance-abusing fathers scored higher in aggression, inattention, and impulsivity (but not in hyperactivity). Thus, although links between clinical diagnoses of ADHD and parental alcoholism are not firmly established, evidence exists that links parental alcoholism with a temperamental constellation of behavioral undercontrol or dysregulation that includes aggression, impulsivity, and inattention.

Internalizing Symptomatology

Parental alcoholism has also been linked to internalizing disorders in offspring. Adult children of alcoholics have been reported to have higher levels of anxiety and depression (Domenico & Windle, 1993; Tweed & Ryff, 1991) and higher rates of panic disorders with agoraphobia and social phobia, and these relations have been maintained even when considering parents' comorbid anxiety disorders (see Sher, 1991, for a review). Adult children of alcoholics also show elevated rates of depressive disorder (Sher et al., 1991), although some evidence has suggested that these elevations are due to co-occurring parental depression or are environmentally mediated (Goodwin, Schulsinger, Knop, Mednick, & Guza, 1977; Russell et al., 1985).

Parental alcoholism has also been associated with elevations in internalizing symptomatology in childhood and adolescence, with West and Prinz (1987) noting these elevations in 10 of 11 published studies. There may be differential impact on anxiety and depression, in that Roosa, Sandler, Beals, and Short (1988) found elevations in depressive symptoms and lowered self-esteem but no increases in anxiety among children of problem-drinking parents. Moreover, as with the adult literature, the specificity of the relation between parental alcoholism and childhood internalizing symptomatology has been questioned. Jacob and Leonard (1986) found that COAs showed elevations in internalizing symptomatology in comparison to offspring of normal controls but not in comparison to children of depressed parents. Our own data (Chassin et al., 1991) found some unique effects of maternal alcoholism on adolescents' internalizing symptomatology, but this effect was not robust across reporters.

As with the adult data, it has been suggested that the relation between parental alcoholism and children's internalizing symptomatology may be environmentally mediated. Moos and Billings (1982) reported that children of actively alcoholic parents had significantly higher levels of anxiety and depression than did normal controls. However, children of "recovered" alcoholic parents did not significantly differ from children of normal controls. These data suggest that, with environmental "recovery" after parental alcoholism has been successfully controlled, COAs may return to normal levels with regard to internalizing symptomatology. However, the findings may also reflect differences in subtype or severity of parental alcoholism, with the most severe alcoholism both persisting over time and being associated with childhood symptomatology.

In short, parental alcoholism has been associated with increases in anxiety and depression in both adulthood and childhood. The relation between parental alcoholism and anxiety has been documented more clearly in adulthood than in childhood, and the relation between parental alcoholism and depression may be due to comorbid parental depression and/or may be environmentally mediated.

School Achievement and Cognitive Functioning

Studies have suggested that COAs are at risk for poor school achievement, with lower grade point averages, higher likelihood of repeating grades, and less likelihood of pursuing higher education. West and Prinz's (1987) review noted that five of six studies found significant decrements in academic achievement among COAs, including a study that had other high-risk control groups (children of depressed parents and children of divorced parents) (Schuckit & Chiles, 1978). The mechanism for this lowered school achievement is not clear, however. Some studies have reported that COAs have lower IQ scores (6 of 9 studies in the West & Prinz, 1987, review) and cognitive deficits could be responsible for lowered academic achievements. Cognitive deficits and lowered intellectual abilities have been demonstrated as a result of fetal alcohol effects. Aside from the fetal alcohol mechanism, however, the reasons behind lowered academic achievement for COAs have not been clear, and either conduct problems, cognitive deficits, environmental disruptions (or all three) could result in lowered achievement. Cognitive deficits among COAs would be an important mechanism, because these deficits could have broader implications for COAs' abilities to succeed in school, to develop coping strategies, and to assess the risks and benefits of different behaviors (including "risky" behaviors such as substance use). Thus, if COAs do have cognitive deficits, these deficits could, in turn, raise risk for a broad array of social and interpersonal problems.

Because of these important implications, a large literature has been directed at neuropsychological assessment of COAs, with the goal of identifying cognitive deficits that may underlie lowered academic achievement (and that may be related to later alcohol abuse). A complete review of this literature is beyond the scope of this chapter, but recent reviews can be found in Sher (1991), Tarter, Laird, and Moss (1990), Pihl et al. (1990), and Pollack and Earleywine (1994). In general, results have been quite inconsistent and have varied widely across laboratories that use different neuropsychological measures and different sampling strategies (e.g., smaller effects in college student samples). The most consistent evidence points to lowered verbal reasoning and abstract reasoning abilities, with less consistent findings of differences in visual–spatial abilities and learning and memory. Effect sizes also have been small, with COA groups scoring within normal ranges on these measures. Moreover, because neuropsychological tests of complex functions are multidimensional in their requirements, lowered scores on these measures cannot uniquely identify specific deficits. Lowered scores may be due to motivational factors, attentional deficits, memory deficits, or more complex planning abilities (as well as verbal skills). Thus, it is difficult to pinpoint any particular functional deficit among COAs.

The small effect sizes may also suggest that only a subgroup of COAs show cognitive deficits. In an important study, Begleiter, Porjesz, Bihari, and Kissin (1984) reported that sons of alcoholic fathers showed a pattern of attenuated P300 waves after a complex visual stimulus, suggesting difficulties in the voluntary allocation of attention. Because these male COAs were preadolescents with little drinking exposure, the deficit could not be explained as an effect of their alcohol use. Other researchers have also suggested that cognitive deficits are most likely to occur in male offspring of male alcoholics, particularly those with a high density of alcoholism in the family history. Whipple, Parker, and Noble (1988) found that subjects with both an alcoholic father and a second-degree alcoholic relative had lower performance IQ scores, digit spans, verbal learning and memory abilities, and deficits in spatial organization. Pihl et al. (1990) suggest that sons of male, multigenerational alcoholics are characterized by hyperactivity, poor academic performance, deficits in verbal and abstract reasoning, and poor academic performance, and that they are hyperreactive to stimuli with inherent motivational properties but hyporeactive to stimuli requiring the voluntary allocation and maintenance of attention (see also Peterson, Finn, & Pihl, 1992). Thus, cognitive deficits may be present in only a subgroup of COAs.

Even among SOMMAs, however, the effect sizes for findings of cognitive deficits are not always large. Moreover, the mechanism underlying these effects is not clear. For example, Tarter et al. (1990) reported that cognitive deficits in SOMMAs were related to the severity of disruption in the home environment, and that differences between COAs and non-COAs were eliminated when environmental disruption was considered in prediction. Similarly, Noll, Zucker, Fitzgerald, and Curtis (1992) found that preschool sons of male alcoholics had lower developmental quotients than their non-COA peers. However, both groups were within age norms, and the differences between the groups were attenuated when the degree of stimulation in the home environment was considered in the prediction.

In short, literature suggests that COAs show lowered academic achievement, and researchers have suggested that cognitive deficits may underlie this outcome. Some evidence exists for deficits in complex verbal abilities and in abstract reasoning. However, results have not been robust across laboratories, and effect sizes have generally been small. These effects may be concentrated within one subgroup of COAs (SOMMAs), and the home environment may play a role in accounting for these deficits.

Social Competencies: Coping, Problem Solving, Interpersonal Relationships

In contrast to the large empirical literature on alcohol and drug use, psychopathology, and neuropsychological functioning, little is known about the development of social competence among COAs. The clinical literature suggests that adult COAs have difficulty with intimate relationships, are overly dependent on approval from others, are overly loyal even when loyalty is undeserved, assume responsibility for others, and feel different from other people (cf. Sher & Mothershead, 1991). However, there is little systematic empirical research to conclude that these problems are characteristic of COAs. For example, Tweed and Ryff (1991) found that adult COAs were indistinguishable from controls in terms of a sense of well-being, capacity for intimacy, and identity. Moreover, some researchers have criticized descriptions of COAs' social and interpersonal problems as being so general that the majority of college students endorsed these descriptors as applying to themselves, consistent with a "Barnum" effect (Logue, Sher, & French, 1992).

Consistent with the notion that COAs have interpersonal difficulties, data from the Piedmont Health Survey (Greenfield, Swartz, Landerman, & George, 1993) showed that parental problem drinking was associated with divorce (above and beyond reported histories of physical abuse, economic deprivation, and parental divorce). Similarly, Domenico and Windle (1993) reported that (in a sample of middle-class, middle-aged women) COAs had lower levels of marital satisfaction and higher levels of marital conflict. However, the effect sizes were relatively small, and COAs were not "clinically" maladaptive on these measures. Moreover, the mechanisms underlying parental alcoholism effects on marital functioning are unclear.

Even less is known about social and developmental competencies among COAs in childhood and adolescence. Shell and Roosa (1991) found that COAs used more problem-focused and avoidant coping than did controls, but few other studies have attempted to examine the development of coping strategies as a function of parental alcoholism. Moreover, as noted by Windle (1990), there has been a general absence of a developmental perspective in the empirical literature, such that little is known about the development of attachment, autonomy, identity, capacity for intimacy, or other important developmental phenomena. In one exception, Tweed and Ryff (1991) found that adult COAs were indistinguishable from controls on measures of identity development. By and large, however, the lack of developmental studies remains a significant gap in the literature. Finally, although authors have discussed the possibility of "resilient" COAs (Werner, 1986), there has been little systematic research concerning unusual levels of social competencies.

Summary of Offspring Outcomes

In summary, parental alcoholism has been demonstrated to raise risk for alcohol and drug use and abuse, externalizing symptomatology and "behavioral undercontrol," internalizing symptomatology, and lowered academic achievement. There is also some evidence to suggest that COAs have deficits in verbal ability and abstract reasoning. These outcomes have been shown in both childhood and adulthood, raising the possibility that parental alcoholism has long-lasting effects on offspring. However, the specificity of the link between parental alcoholism and these outcomes has been challenged, and many of these outcomes may be linked to co-occurring parental psychopathology (such as antisocial personality and depression) or to the environmental and family disruption that is associated with parental alcoholism. Moreover, the magnitude of parental alcoholism effects varies significantly with the samples that are studied, and in all cases, there is substantial overlap in outcomes between COA and non-COA samples (Clair & Genest, 1987; Heller, Sher, & Benson, 1982). Furthermore, there is significant heterogeneity within parental alcoholism, and some research suggests that SOMMAs are at particular risk for cognitive deficits, behavioral undercontrol, and alcohol and drug use. Little is known about the associations between parental alcoholism and social competencies. Because of the general absence of a developmental perspective, little is known about how COAs resolve important developmental tasks.

PARENT ALCOHOLISM AS A STRESSOR: COMPONENTS, MEDIATORS, AND MODERATORS OF PARENT ALCOHOLISM RISK

The determination that COAs do, in fact, show higher rates of psychological disorders and substance use than children of nonalcoholic parents is a critical first step in a larger research effort to understand the processes that contribute to this risk. How does parental alcoholism cause the variety of negative outcomes that are experienced by COAs? What are the mechanisms that might explain why some COAs are adversely influenced by parental alcoholism while others appear to be relatively unaffected? These questions are the familiar challenges that lead researchers to consider the mediators and moderators of parental alcoholism's effects on children.

Considering parental alcoholism as a stressor, however, is a complex enterprise, because it is not a single circumscribed "event" but a more chronic condition that affects outcomes by multiple pathways. An important mechanism for parental alcoholism effects is, of course, teratogenic effects of alcohol on the developing fetus. However, a review of fetal alcohol syndrome is beyond the scope of this chapter (see Steinhausen & Spohr, 1986, for a review). Considering parental alcoholism as a "stressor" is also made more complex by the fact that alcoholism is rarely a steady state, but one that alternates between periods of sobriety and intoxication and between abstinence and relapse (Jacob & Krahn, 1988; Jacob, Ritchey, Cvitkovic, & Blane, 1981; Moos & Billings, 1982). Family research has shown that family environments, marital satisfaction, and parenting behaviors vary between sober and intoxicated states, and even that the context of the drinking (in the home vs. out of the home) can change the nature of the effect (Dunn, Jacob, Hummon, & Seilhamer, 1987; Steinglass, Bennett, Wolin, & Reiss, 1987). This variation in the environment from sober to intoxicated parental states suggests that instability and unpredictability may be components of the stress of parental alcoholism. Indeed, items tapping such instability appear on life stress scales designed for COA populations and are endorsed more frequently by COAs than non-COAs (Roosa, 1988). COAs are more likely to endorse items suggesting disruptions in family routines and organization, unreliability of parental role performance, and inconsistency in parental social support (Li, Barrera, & Chassin, 1994; Roosa, 1988).

Given the complexity of parental alcoholism as a stressor, a large number of factors have been hypothesized to be mediators or moderators of parental alcoholism effects. These factors include potentially heritable characteristics such as temperament or individual differences in the body's reactions to alcohol, macro-level variables such as socioeconomic status, and a host of socioenvironmental features such as stress, parenting, coping, family disorganization, and peer affiliations. Sher (1991) provided a comprehensive heuristic model of the many processes by which parental alcoholism could lead to pathological alcohol involvement in offspring, and this model incorporated many of these factors. Embedded within this large model were three interrelated submodels that Sher labeled (1) the enhanced reinforcement model, (2) the deviance-proneness model, and (3) the negative affect model. Although the first submodel is specific to substance use outcomes, the deviance-proneness model and the negative affect model provide useful structures for considering mechanisms underlying parental alcoholism effects on a broad range of negative outcomes.

The enhanced reinforcement model emphasizes COAs' relatively high sensitivity to the effects of alcohol, as well as alcohol expectancies that contribute to COAs' pathological alcohol use. Some data suggest that COAs derive greater reinforcement value from alcohol consumption and/or suffer fewer negative effects (Newlin & Thomson, 1990), and these effects may be particularly prominent among COAs who are also high in behavioral undercontrol (Sher & Levenson, 1982). An increased pharmacological benefit of alcohol consumption may be one pathway that accounts for greater alcohol use and abuse among COAs. Moreover, COAs may receive different socialization about the use of alcohol and drugs than do their non-COA peers. Alcoholic parents present models of maladaptive consumption of alcohol and drugs, of the use of substances to cope with life stressors, and of an inability to regulate intake. Both enhanced reinforcement from alcohol and this differential modeling and socialization about alcohol may influence COAs' beliefs and expectancies about alcohol effects. Research has shown that, as early as the preschool years, COAs show greater knowledge about alcohol than their non-COA peers (Noll, Zucker, & Greenberg, 1990). Adolescent COAs have been shown to have more positive beliefs about alcohol effects than do their non-COA peers (Sher et al., 1991; Mann, Chassin, & Sher, 1987; Brown, Creamer, & Stetson, 1987). Formal tests of mediation have produced mixed results, with one cross-sectional study of college students finding such mediation (Sher et al., 1991) and one longitudinal study of adolescents failing to support expectancies as a mediator of parental alcoholism effects on escalating substance use over time (Colder, Chassin, & Curran, 1995). Despite mixed evidence concerning mediation, COAs' beliefs and expectancies about alcohol and drug use remain potentially important targets for intervention in substance use prevention programs.

In Sher's deviance-proneness model, ineffective parenting is hypothesized to interact with COAs' difficult temperamental characteristics and cognitive dysfunctions to set off a process of school failure and association with deviant peers. This process increases the likelihood of antisocial outcomes, including substance use and delinquency. Sher's (1991) model did not detail the aspects of parenting that moderate these relationships, but both control aspects of parenting as well as nurturance have been included in other models of parental alcoholism and parenting (e.g., Jacob & Leonard, 1994; Seilhamer & Jacob, 1990). In the deviance-proneness model, parenting is a moderator of the relation between difficult temperament and deviant peer affiliations and between school failure and deviant peer affiliations. These hypothesized relations are founded on the belief that good parenting can intervene to decrease the effects of difficult temperament and school failure on children's associations with deviant peers.

In the negative affect model, parental alcoholism is depicted as increasing children's exposure to stressful life events that produce emotional distress. This distress can lead to pathological involvement with alcohol or drugs as a means of regulating negative affect. Moreover, environmental stress can produce internalizing symptomatology (anxiety and depression) and can increase risk for externalizing symptomatology as distressed children turn to a deviant peer group to relieve their negative affect (Kaplan, 1980). In the negative affect model, COAs' ability to cope with stressful life events plays a critical role in determining their outcomes. An important feature of this model is a hypothetical pathway that suggests that parent alcoholism can also impair children's coping capacities. Coping is proposed as a moderator of the relation between life stress and emotional distress and as a moderator of the relation between emotional distress and externalizing outcomes. Thus, parental alcoholism was hypothesized to influence the stress–distress–alcohol use process by both increasing children's exposure to stress and by decreasing their capacity to cope effectively with stress and its emotional distress sequelae.

To summarize, stressful life events, coping, ineffective parenting, school failure, associations with deviant peers, and alcohol expectancies were the primary socioenvironmental factors that were identified by Sher in his heuristic model as mediators and (in the case of coping and parenting) moderators of parental alcoholism's effect on children's alcohol involvement. There have been few formal tests of these models, but some evidence is accumulating about the association between parent alcoholism and these hypothesized mediators.

EVIDENCE IN SUPPORT OF MEDIATION

In the absence of formal tests of mediation, potential mediators of parental alcoholism's effect on children's outcomes can be identified through the framework outlined by Baron and Kenny (1986). Assuming that an overall relation between parental alcoholism and a child's outcome has been established, a mediator of parental alcoholism must (1) show a clear statistical relation to both parental alcoholism and child outcomes (criteria), and (2) account for parental alcoholism's relation to the child outcomes. Although this last point can only be determined in formal tests of mediation, we can examine the literature for evidence that the potential mediator is related to parental alcoholism and to child outcomes. In addition to genetic transmission of biological vulnerabilities to alcohol effects and personality traits, many of the socioenvironmental factors captured by Sher's (1991) models have been explored as mediators of parental alcoholism: (1) life stress, (2) family disruptions, (3) parenting, (4) coping, and (5) peer affiliations. Following a review of studies that investigated the possible link between parental alcoholism and these factors, the few formal model tests that integrated several of these constructs will be described.

Life Stress

Not only can the immediate alcohol-induced impairment of a parental caregiver create adversity for a child, but a parent's extensive and protracted alcohol abuse can set into motion a series of stressful events. Studies of young children (Roosa, Tein, Groppenbacher, Michaels, & Dumka, 1993), adolescents (Chassin et al., 1993), high school students (Roosa, Sandler, Gehring, Beals, and Cappo, 1988; Roosa, Beals, Sandler, & Pillow, 1990), and adults (Velleman & Orford, 1990) show that COAs experience more stressful events than do their peers. For example, Velleman and Orford (1990) reported that compared to controls, offspring of problem-drinking parents reported more neglect ("being on own a lot," 47.3% vs. 25%), unreliability ("arrangements going wrong," 50.3% vs. 25%), exposure to conflict ("forced to participate in parents' rows," 44.8% vs. 8.8%), and burdensome caregiving ("having to take care of parent," 27.3% vs. 7.5%). These events illustrate how the concept of life stress can easily spill over into other constructs such as parenting, family adversity, and even elements of social support. Part of the strength of associations between measures of life stress and other constructs in research on COAs might be attributed to the range of domains that are contained within the stress construct.

Life stress appeared as a construct in several mediational models that have been reported (Chassin et al., 1993; Roosa et al., 1990, 1993). For example, Roosa et al. (1990) estimated a simple mediational model in which positive and negative life events were proposed as mediators of parental alcoholism's effect on late adolescents' depression and anxiety symptoms. This study included two assessment periods that were separated by 3 months, thus allowing for the evaluation of cross-sectional as well as prospective effects. Subjects were 43 high school students who were self-identified as being children of alcoholics and 102 peers who did not report having alcoholic parents. The cross-sectional results were consistent with the hypothesized model in which positive and negative events mediated the effects of parental alcoholism on symptomatology; however, none of the predicted prospective effects was obtained. Despite the lack of prospective effects, the results of this and our own cross-sectional analysis that will be described more fully below (Chassin et al., 1993) suggest the value of continuing to pursue an understanding of life stress as a mediator of parental alcoholism's effects.

Adversity within the Family

Although it overlaps with the concept of life stress, special attention has been drawn to parental alcoholism's impact on family organization and functioning (Seilhamer & Jacob, 1990; Velleman, 1992). One of the three mediational models included in a review by Velleman (1992) described a general environmental mechanism involving disruption and upheaval within alcoholic families. He cited the following mediators: (1) parental violence, (2) marital conflict, (3) marital separation, and (4) inconsistency in parenting. This model was similar to the one proposed by Seilhamer and Jacob (1990). Others have also noted the greater prevalence of separation, divorce, and other parental absences in families with an alcoholic parent (e.g., Schulsinger, Knop, Goodwin, Teasdale, & Mikkelson, 1986).

Conflict is a form of adversity that commonly distinguishes COA families and non-COA comparison families (Barry & Fleming, 1990; Benson & Heller, 1987; Clair & Genest, 1987; Moos & Billings, 1982). In our data, adolescent COAs reported more overall family conflict than did controls (Barrera, Li, & Chassin, 1995), as well as more specific parent–adolescent conflict with both their mothers and fathers (Barrera, Rogosch, & Chassin, 1993; Barrera, Stice, & Chassin, 1994).

In contrast to the numerous studies that have found an association between parental alcoholism and family conflict, there are few formal tests of family conflict as a mediator of parental alcoholism's relation to child outcomes. However, at least two studies have provided some relevant data. In our research, regression models that included parental alcoholism, ethnicity, life stress, and their interactions were estimated with and without the inclusion of a measure of family conflict (Barrera et al., 1995). Parental reports of adolescents' internalizing and externalizing symptoms were the criteria. The pattern of findings showed that family conflict mediated the effects of life stress on adolescents' internalizing and externalizing symptoms, but conflict did not mediate the effects of parental alcoholism on these outcomes. That is, the inclusion of family conflict in these regression models eliminated the previously significant effects of life stress but not those of parental alcoholism, which continued to show significant relations to all of the criteria. Although parental alcoholism was related to family conflict (and family conflict was correlated with adolescents' distress and problem behavior), family conflict did not adequately explain parental alcoholism's relation to adolescents' internalizing and externalizing symptoms.

The causal model estimated by Roosa et al. (1990) that we described previously also provided some evidence concerning family conflict's role as a mediator. Their measure of negative life events included a cluster of eight items that were identified by judges as indicators of family conflict. When this subset of eight family conflict events was used in place of their original 42-item measure of negative events, it produced a model that closely resembled the original. At least cross-sectionally, family conflict appeared to mediate the relation between high school students' reports of their parents' alcoholism and these students' reports of their own anxiety and depression.

Taken together, these findings produce a somewhat mixed picture for the role of family conflict as a mediator. There are rather consistent findings that show a relation between parental alcoholism and conflict within the family, but it is not clear that family conflict can account for parental alcoholism effects on children's outcomes. Adversity within the family is a meta-construct that embraces more distinct concepts such as marital strife, expressions of violence between family members, child–parent conflict, and parental loss through divorce, separation, or other absences. Intuitively, each of these could have specific relations to parental alcoholism and to child outcomes. Moreover, family conflict effects may be moderated by characteristics of an individual (e.g., personal competencies) or a family (e.g., supportive relations between family member). Models that do not include moderating factors might miss opportunities to understand how adversity within alcoholic families functions.

Parenting

Seilhamer and Jacob (1990) identified "disrupted parenting" as a central mediator in their model, which emphasized family characteristics as influences on COAs' adjustment. Three elements of disrupted parenting were highlighted: poor socialization, poor nurturance, and inconsistency (Rollins & Thomas, 1979). Poor socialization corresponds roughly with the control aspects of parenting, which would include discipline, rule enforcement, and monitoring of children's activities and interactions with peers. Poor nurturance captures the supportive dimensions of parenting that involve expressions of warmth, affection, understanding, and engagement in positive activities. Finally, inconsistency refers to the style parents use in providing control and support. Unpredictability in the administration of discipline or unreliability in the provision of support could contribute to the poor development of regulation and psychological distress in children (Li et al., 1994; Velleman, 1992).

Poor parental control has been associated with adolescent substance use and other forms of externalizing behavior problems, but these studies have not evaluated this form of parenting as a mediator of parental alcoholism (Brook, Whiteman, & Gordon, 1983; Jessor & Jessor, 1977; Stice & Barrera, 1995; Vuchinich, Bank, & Patterson, 1992). However, on a closely related topic, Dishion, Patterson, and Reid (1988) studied linkages between parental drug use, parental socialization, and adolescents' drug use. Consistent with Sher's deviance-proneness model, parental drug use impaired parents' monitoring, which in turn was related to involvement with deviant peers. Involvement with deviant peers was the proximal link to adolescents' substance use.

In the general literature, social support is often conceptualized as a moderator of life stress, but some studies have examined its role as a possible mediator of parental alcoholism effects. A relation has been found between parental alcoholism and social support, particularly social support from parents and other family members (Benson & Heller, 1987; Clair & Genest, 1987; Holden, Brown, & Mott, 1988; Li et al, 1994; Moos & Billings, 1982). Despite the many studies that found an association between parental alcoholism and family support, we did not find that adolescent COAs self-reported less parental social support than non-COAs (Barrera, Rogosch, & Chassin, 1993). In an analysis of data from this same sample that were collected 2 years later, adolescent COAs and non-COAs still did not differ in their self-reports of social support received from their fathers (Li et al., 1994). These two groups did differ, however, on fathers' reports of the consistency of their provision of social support to their adolescent children.

There is also a suggestion in the literature that support is impaired during the active phases of alcoholism and might not be a general characteristic of alcoholic parents (Moos & Billings, 1982). Alcoholic patients were classified as recovered or relapsed based on a number of criteria (such as rehospitalization, problems with drinking, quantity–frequency of alcohol consumption) that were assessed at 6-month and 2-year intervals. A group of control families that did not contain alcoholic parents were matched to the families of these alcoholics on sociodemographic factors, family size, ethnicity, and other features. Two subscales from the Family Environment Scale—Cohesion and Expressiveness—that are often used as measures of family support were rated by fathers and mothers, scores were averaged, and then used as criteria in between-group analyses. Results showed that the ratings by parents in the control and recovered alcoholic subsamples were remarkably similar. Only families of relapsed alcoholics significantly differed from the control families. Thus, social support from parents and other family members might be primarily affected by active alcohol abuse by one or more of the parents. Furthermore, parental alcohol abuse might affect the consistency with which parents provide social support more than the overall amount of support parents can provide to their children.

Coping

Coping was included in the heuristic model described by Sher (1991), but he acknowledged that there are few data that support its role as a mediator of parental alcoholism. This is surprising because coping appears to be a personal resource that might be effective in preventing or reducing individuals' experience of psychological distress and substance use (Wills & Shiffman, 1985).

One of the few studies to assess the coping of COAs was conducted by Clair and Genest (1987). They studied a sample of mostly college students that included 30 COAs (28 women) and 40 controls (34 women). Results showed that COAs were more likely to view problems in their families as unchangeable or as requiring acceptance. Furthermore, parental alcoholism was associated with the types of coping that these students reported. COAs were more likely to use emotion-focused coping than problem-focused coping; controls did not differ in their use of emotion-focused versus problem-focused coping. COAs also were more likely to use avoidant strategies (e.g., sleeping, drinking, smoking, eating) than were control subjects. Simple correlations calculated for the COA group showed that problem-focused coping was negatively correlated with depression and positively correlated with self-esteem. Emotion-focused coping was not significantly correlated with either criterion. Neither coping category was significantly correlated with the criteria for the control groups. Unfortunately, the data were not analyzed in a way that would help us determine if problem-focused coping was a viable mediator or moderator of parental alcoholism. The unique composition of the sample also limited the generalizability of these findings.

A person's ability to cope effectively with adversity is typically viewed as a positive personal resource. In the case of COAs, some have voiced concern that their coping efforts portend future pathology. As Seilhamer and Jacob (1990) wrote,

Descriptions of nonsymptomatic children of alcoholics, many of whom exhibit extraordinary coping skills, have earned them the label of "invulnerables" or "superkids." However, other writers claim that the exaggerated coping styles of many of these children lead to dysfunction in adulthood. (p. 169)

This is a provocative hypothesis that has not been substantiated as of yet. In general, coping is an appealing construct that has received very little systematic research with COA samples.

Formal Tests of Mediation

In planning our own research, we recognized the value of simultaneously testing three interrelated submodels that included several of the proposed mediators of parental alcoholism (Chassin et al., 1993). This model estimation followed initial analyses that demonstrated that adolescent COAs showed more externalizing and internalizing symptoms and substance use than did controls (Chassin et al., 1991). This work was then extended to identify possible mediational pathways leading from parental alcoholism to adolescents' substance use. Cross-sectional data from the first assessment of a longitudinal study of 454 adolescents were used in these analysis. Somewhat over half the sample (54.2%) were COAs and the remaining adolescents were from families in which neither parent was alcoholic. Extensive interviews were conducted with both parents and adolescents that allowed us to form several multiple-reporter constructs that were used in model estimations. A temperament submodel posited that parental alcoholism would increase the likelihood of elevated levels of temperamental emotionality and sociability. These characteristics in turn were thought to lead to negative affect and associations with drug-using peers, respectively, two factors that are linked more proximally to adolescents' drug and alcohol use.

Another submodel emphasized the mediational role of parenting. In this submodel, parental alcoholism was depicted as impairing parents' ability to monitor the behavior of their adolescent children. We proposed that this aspect of parents' ineffective control practices would lead to adolescents' involvement with peers who use substances, which would provide a key link to the initiation of substance use.

A third and final submodel was concerned with stress and negative affect. Parental alcoholism's initial influence was hypothesized to be on increasing their children's exposure to stressful life experiences. This stress was thought to give rise to negative affect, which was further associated with affiliations with drug-using peers. These affiliations could have the immediate effect of elevating self-esteem (Kaplan, 1980) and alleviating negative affect, but ultimately these affiliations increase the likelihood of early initiation of substance use.

The model estimates were consistent with the parenting and stress-negative affect submodels and partially consistent with the temperament submodel. Compared to controls, COAs were more likely to experience stressful events, less likely to have parents who monitored their behavior, and more likely to show a temperament characterized by emotionality. The model also pointed to the importance of adolescents' associations with drug-using peers. As predicted, this construct mediated the influence of both parental monitoring and the stress-negative affect pathways. However, although these mediational pathways were able to explain parent alcoholism effects on adolescent substance use in a cross-sectional design, longitudinal data suggested somewhat different conclusions (Chassin, Curran, Hussong, & Colder, 1996). Longitudinal latent growth curve analysis showed that COAs had steeper growth over time in substance use than did their non-COA peers. Moreover, parental monitoring, environmental stress, and negative affect predicted associations with drug-using peers, which significantly predicted the slope of this growth. However, the significant effect of parent alcoholism on substance use growth was largely unchanged when the mediators were included in the model, suggesting that they could not completely account for the effect of parental alcoholism on adolescents' growth in substance use over time.

Roosa et al. (1993) tested a model that hypothesized a series of pathways from parental problem drinking to stressful life events, parenting behaviors (parental support and inconsistent discipline), and ultimately to child conduct disorder and depression. Their sample of 303 families included 214 non-Hispanic (African American, Anglo, Native American, and other) and 70 Hispanic children in 4th to 6th grade. Parents were categorized as problem drinkers through their reports on the Diagnostic Interview Schedule (DIS) or Short-Michigan Alcoholism Screening Test (SMAST); children reported on their parents' parenting and their own conduct disorder and depression symptoms. Because there was evidence that the data matrices for Hispanics and non-Hispanics should not be combined, separate models were estimated for each group. In both models, parental problem drinking was positively related to children's negative life events. However, in neither model was parental problem drinking related to supportive parenting or inconsistent discipline. The findings for the two groups differed somewhat, but there was some suggestion that parenting at least partially mediated the effects of stressful life events on child conduct disorder and depression symptoms.

Overall there is a rather modest collection of findings that identify modifiable mediators, and only a few of these demonstrations have included formal tests of mediation. The available data suggest that stressful life events, parenting, associations with deviant peers, and, perhaps, family conflict are potentially important mediators. Research that clarifies the mediational pathways that lie between parental alcoholism and children's psychological adjustment contributes to theory and provides the empirical foundation for intervention efforts. As the basic links between parental alcoholism and child outcomes become more firmly established, there is a growing need to understand the mediational pathways. Because of the prominent role that peer associations play in the initiation of alcohol and substance use, there is a special need to explore the ways that parental alcoholism might influence factors that affect children's affiliation with deviant peers.

EVIDENCE IN SUPPORT OF MODERATION

Little is known about the mediators of parent alcoholism effects, but even less is known about moderators. Sher's (1991) review identified the following as possible moderators of parental alcoholism's effects on child outcomes:

social class, preservation of family rituals, mother's esteem for the alcoholic father, amount of attention from primary caregivers, family conflict during infancy, birth of another sibling within the first 2 years of life, social support, personality (self-awareness), cognitive–intellectual functioning, and coping. Seilhamer and Jacob (1990) presented a model in which parental alcohol abuse led to family stress (marital conflict, financial strain, ritual disruption, etc.), which in turn led to disrupted parenting (inconsistency, poor socialization, poor nurturance) and ultimately to child adjustment problems. They proposed, however, several possible constitutional factors (sex, age, intellectual level, temperament, and genetic propensities) and environmental factors (sex of non-alcoholic parent, exposure to drinking, treatment experience, peer influences, supportive social institutions, and informal social resources) that could moderate the relation between disrupted parenting and child outcomes. Unfortunately, there are not extensive data to support these factors as moderators of parental alcoholism effects.

Moderation implies an interaction between two predictor variables such that the relation of one predictor (e.g., parental alcoholism) to a criterion (i.e., offspring outcomes) is dependent on levels of a second predictor (e.g., some protective factor). Curiously, the most commonly cited examples of moderation effects in the COA literature did not actually test interactions between parental alcoholism and proposed moderating conditions (Bennett, Wolin, Reiss, & Teitelbaum, 1987; Werner, 1986; Wolin, Bennett, Noonan, & Teitelbaum, 1980).

Werner (1986) studied 49 children of alcoholics on the island of Kauai, Hawaii, in an attempt to discover why some children of alcoholics develop serious problems in childhood and adolescence while others do not. She followed these children from the time that they were 1 year of age to 18 years of age. She found that children of alcoholics who failed to develop serious problems by age 18 (i.e. "resilient" children) differed from the COAs who did develop problems by age 18 in several ways. COAs who adjusted successfully were more likely to have experienced fewer stressful events during the early part of their lives, to be viewed as having a "cuddly and affectionate" temperament during the first year of life, to have an internal locus of control, to have a more positive self-concept, and to have competent communication skills than COAs who developed problems by age 18. These are impressive findings that identified predictors of adjustment for COAs, but the lack of a comparison group limits the interpretation of these findings as evidence of moderation effects. We do not know, for example, how well these factors predict adjustment in non-COA samples or how the well-adjusted children would compare to a control sample.

Wolin and Bennett's studies on the maintenance of family rituals is another well-known research program on moderators of parental alcoholism. Wolin et al. (1980) examined the relationship between consistency of family rituals and risk of developing alcohol problems in COAs in a sample of 25 families in which at least one parent was an alcoholic. Family rituals include regular patterns of behavior associated with events such as dinner time, vacations, and holidays. Based on the degree to which changes in family rituals were tied to changes in the alcoholic parent's frequency and intensity of drinking, Wolin et al. characterized the families as either "subsumptive" (meaning that changes in family rituals were closely linked to changes in the alcoholic parent's drinking), "intermediate" (meaning that some rituals were affected by the alcoholic parent's drinking while others were not), or "distinctive" (meaning that family rituals remained relatively stable despite changes in the alcoholic parent's drinking). Wolin et al. found that children from distinctive families were significantly less likely to develop alcohol problems than children from subsumptive families. Thus, substantial change in family rituals was associated with increased risk for transmission of alcohol problems to COAs.

In a related study, Bennett et al. (1987) found that adult COAs who demonstrated a high degree of deliberateness and planning in choosing and establishing family rituals in their own marriages were at decreased risk for developing alcohol problems themselves. This study also replicated their earlier finding that children of alcoholics from "distinctive" families are at decreased risk for developing alcohol problems. As in their previous work, Bennett et al. did not include a group that could have indicated how the distinctive families compared to nonalcoholic families. Longitudinal studies would also add to our understanding of the nature of the relationship between family rituals and risk for alcoholism in that the characteristics of family rituals could be documented prior to the onset of alcohol problems. Furthermore, these findings warrant replication in a larger sample of families.

Research by Clair and Genest (1987) included groups of young adult children of alcoholic and nonalcoholic parents, but their data analyses did not include direct tests of moderation effects. As the authors noted, the samples were samples of convenience that consisted of 30 offspring of alcoholic fathers (28 females and 2 males) who were recruited through advertisements and contacts with Alcoholics Anonymous and Al-Anon and 40 control group subjects (34 females and 6 males) who were obtained through a university subject pool. Clair and Genest (1987) reported correlations between hypothesized "moderators" and criteria separately for COAs and controls. They found that cohesion, expressiveness, and emotional support were correlated with depression-proneness and self-esteem for both COAs and controls. This pattern of correlations would in fact argue against interpreting these variables as moderators. In contrast, they found that problem-focused coping was significantly related to both depression-proneness and self-esteem for COAs, but not for controls. These results could suggest interaction effects, but it is dangerous to interpret the presence of statistical significance in one group and the absence of significance in another as evidence of moderation, particularly when the group sizes are small ($n = 30$ and 40).

Tests of True Moderation Effects

Just a few studies of COAs have provided true tests of moderation. Illustrative research from two projects examined socioenvironmental factors (social support and conflict) as potential moderators. Ohannessian and Hesselbrock (1993) administered perceived social support scales (ISEL and PSS-Family and PSS-Friends) to 85 adult COAs and 68 controls. COAs were the adult children of inpatients who were being treated for alcoholism; the controls were adult children of dental patients. Interesting interactions between parental alcoholism and social support were observed. The pattern of means suggested that COAs with low friend support and low overall support had higher Michigan Alcoholism Screening Test (MAST) scores, drank more, and expressed more concern about their drinking than did other subjects. For the most part, COAs with high friend social support closely resembled the controls. Family support did not show moderation effects. The authors pointed out how their findings demonstrated the importance of drawing distinctions between support provided by family members and friends, not only during adolescence but also during adulthood.

We have found evidence of moderation effects in our own research on adolescent COAs. A compelling basic finding was that COAs were more vulnerable to the effects of stress than were children without alcoholic parents (Barrera, Li, & Chassin, 1993, 1995). This effect was found in cross-sectional analyses of two annual assessments and in prospective analyses of adolescents' internalizing and externalizing symptomatology.

There was some additional but limited evidence that ethnicity and family conflict moderated the effects of parental alcoholism (Barrera, Li, & Chassin, 1993, 1995). Compared to Caucasians, Hispanics were more resilient to the effects of parental alcoholism during the first annual assessment, but this effect was not replicated in subsequent assessments. Also, family conflict (Barrera et al., 1995) and parent–adolescent conflict and parental social support (Barrera et al., 1994) moderated the influences of parental alcoholism. In all of these cases, COAs who had parental support or who lacked conflict resembled our control subjects. On the other hand, COAs who lacked parental support or who reported conflict in family relations showed elevated levels of psychological distress.

We also examined the possibility that the quality of parenting provided by mothers could buffer the impact of paternal alcoholism on adolescent COAs. However, results showed that maternal parenting behaviors significantly predicted adolescents' outcomes but did not interact with paternal alcoholism (Curran & Chassin, 1996). Thus, mothers' parenting functioned as an independent determinant of adolescents' outcomes rather than exerting specific protective effects for COAs. Finally, our longitudinal data suggested that high levels of perceived control and self-esteem served as protective factors to reduce the risk that adolescent COAs would initiate substance use (Hussong & Chassin, 1997; McGrath & Chassin, 1995).

The evidence in support of moderators suggested by Ohannessian and Hesselbrock (1993) and by our own data needs to be tempered by the reality that these interactions tend to be small in magnitude, inconsistently observed across criteria, and rarely observed in prospective analyses. Other than social support, few of the potential moderators identified by reviewers (e.g., coping) have been tested as moderators. Furthermore, constructs commonly recognized as moderators that emerged from the pioneering research by Werner, Bennett, and Wolin have not appeared in true tests of moderation effects. Thus, as with tests of mediational models, the study of moderators of parent alcoholism effects remains a significant gap in the empirical literature.

PREVENTIVE INTERVENTIONS FOR ADAPTATION TO PARENTAL ALCOHOLISM

An important goal for research on risk and protective factors among children of alcoholics is to serve as a generative database for the design of preventive interventions for this target audience. Before preventive interventions can be developed, however, there are two questions that should be answered from this database that we have just reviewed. First, are COAs a group at risk for negative outcomes, so that preventive intervention might be an appropriate goal? Second, have we identified potentially modifiable mediators and moderators of this risk that can be used to guide the content of prevention programs?

Our review of the existing empirical literature suggests that COAs are indeed at elevated risk for negative outcomes including alcohol and drug abuse, externalizing and internalizing symptomatology, and school failure. However, results suggest that only a subset of COAs will develop these negative outcomes. This conclusion from the empirical literature is an important contrast to a clinical literature that has often assumed that all COAs are by definition pathological and in need of treatment (cf. Sher, 1991). The reason for concern here is that there exists very real possibilities of stigma and negative labeling effects that can occur by overpathologizing COAs. In terms of preventive intervention, this means that young children or adolescent children of alcoholics may be reluctant to participate in preventive intervention. For example, DiCicco, Davis, Travis, and Ornstein (1984) reported that children were reluctant to join COA groups in a school-based preventive intervention. Moreover, there is also evidence that negative labeling effects occur. For example, Burk and Sher (1990) showed mental health professionals videotapes of children labeled as a COA or a non-COA and as a socially successful school leader or a child with behavior problems. Independent of the "social success" label, targets labeled as COAs were seen as more pathological. Because such negative expectations on the part of adults could produce harm to COAs, prevention programs must be sensitive to the risks of labeling effects.

With respect to potentially modifiable mediators and moderators of COA risk, our literature review again indicates that considerable caution is warranted in the development of preventive intervention. That is, there have been few longitudinal studies that formally test mediational models or that appropriately test moderator variables. Thus, there is a slim empirical foundation on which to build preventive interventions. However, some possible targets for modification that have been identified include adolescents' expectancies about alcohol and drug effects (Sher et al., 1991), conditions of the family environment (e.g., family conflict, family stability, and family routines), parenting (e.g., parental support, control, and consistency), and environmental stress (suggesting that interventions for coping with environmental stress might be useful). Moreover, because some studies have demonstrated associations between parental recovery from alcoholism and improved outcomes for COAs (Moos & Billings, 1982), alcoholism treatment itself may function as a preventive intervention for children of alcoholics. Thus, although the empirical literature is quite limited, it suggests that prevention programs might attempt to change adolescents' expectancies about alcohol and drugs, to decrease family conflict, increase family stability and protect family rituals, improve parental support and consistency of discipline, and teach strategies for coping with environmental stress. Further research is warranted on preventive interventions targeted at these factors.

Given that little is known about the mediators and moderators of COA risk, it is perhaps not surprising that there have been very few studies to empirically evaluate preventive interventions for COAs. The Cambridge-Somerville Program for Alcoholism Rehabilitation (CASPAR) provides curriculum materials for school-based interventions (DiCicco, Davis, Hogan, MacLean, & Ornstein, 1984). DiCicco et al. (1984) evaluated a 10-session program in which students learned about alcoholism and the effects of consuming alcohol. Although the program was not restricted to COAs, there were deliberate attempts to recruit them. A pretest–posttest uncontrolled study showed that participants reported increased knowledge about alcohol and decreased drinking.

Roosa and his colleagues (Short et al., 1995) evaluated a preventive intervention for 4th to 6th graders in 13 schools. The intervention was aimed at improving coping, increasing self-esteem, and changing alcohol expectancies. To foster generalization of program effects outside of a school setting, this intervention also evaluated the effects of a "personal trainer" component in which a college student volunteer met weekly with the child to reinforce the child's coping skills. Moreover, to avoid labeling effects, the study recruited children by showing a film about parental alcoholism and inviting students interested in discussing issues presented in the film to attend a group meeting. This method was important to avoid public labeling as a COA. However, because parental alcoholism was not assessed, the number of actual COAs in the intervention was unknown.

This study is unique in the literature because it implemented and rigorously evaluated a theory-based intervention aimed at mediators of COA risk that have received empirical support. However, results showed limited program effects. The program was effective in increasing knowledge of program content and increasing emotion-focused and social support coping. Moreover, for a subgroup of children who reported concern about parental drinking, the intervention also produced small effects on teacher reports of increased problem solving and social competence. However, the program was not successful in improving self-esteem or in changing distal psychological outcomes (internalizing and externalizing symptoms), and the personal trainer component did not produce significant additional benefit. Moreover, program impact on alcohol expectancies was in the opposite of the intended direction (i.e., intervention increased perceptions that alcohol produced tension reduction). The limited magnitude of the program effects led the researchers to call for more extensive programs, perhaps including parental involvement. Given that many of the hypothesized mediators of COA risk focus on parenting and family environment factors, school-based programs without parental involvement may not be sufficiently powerful to affect COA outcomes. Moreover, given the difficulties with labeling and identifying COAs, school-based preventive interventions for COAs might need to start with universal rather than targeted programs. Because most schools offer substance use prevention programs (at least in the middle school years), some interventions concerning alcohol and drug expectancies could be integrated into these programs without producing negative labeling effects.

One alternative to school-based programs is to implement preventive interventions for children within alcohol treatment facilities. This approach has the potential advantage of involving parents, and thus being able to target parenting and family environment mediators. Moreover, these interventions do not need to publicly label COAs to their peers in school. Unfortunately, however, preventive interventions in alcohol treatment settings will reach only a minority of COAs, because only a minority of alcoholics receive treatment. Moreover, although there have been some attempts to implement preventive interventions within alcohol treatment settings, there has been limited success. Programs either fail to report clear evaluation data (Anderson & Quast, 1983) or have found only weak effects (perhaps because of limited statistical power associated with small sample sizes) (Woodward, 1985). Finally, there have been some attempts to evaluate the impact of Alateen on COAs' mental health outcomes. For example, Hughes (1977) compared COAs who received no services with those who attended Alateen, and found some positive program effects on mood but not on antisocial behavior. This study is noteworthy in that a substantial number of COAs in the "no-intervention" group were just about to begin attending Alateen. This minimizes the extent to which selection factors could account for the between-group differences in mood. That is, it is unlikely that the program's effects on mood could be explained by the factors that led some COAs to seek out Alateen as an intervention. However, the extent to which Alateen can reach a large, representative sample of COAs is unknown.

In short, although the clinical literature reflects substantial concern with interventions for COAs, the empirical literature contains almost no studies of rigorously evaluated programs designed to modify empirically supported mediators and moderators of COA risk. Thus, little is known about the effectiveness of preventive interventions. Caution is warranted in pursuing interventions because of the rather slim generative database that exists and the danger of labeling effects. Because of these labeling effects, school-based efforts may need to focus on universal interventions, and to some extent these may be usefully incorporated into existing alcohol and drug prevention programs. More powerful effects may be obtained by adding a parental involvement component, perhaps through alcohol treatment settings. However, these interventions are likely to reach only a minority of COAs.

SUMMARY AND DIRECTIONS FOR FUTURE RESEARCH

The goal of this chapter was to review the literature on outcomes for children of alcoholics, as well as studies of potential mediators and moderators of parental alcoholism effects. These studies form the generative database on which to build preventive interventions. Our review suggests that COAs are indeed an important target audience for preventive interventions, because parental alcoholism is a relatively prevalent risk factor that is linked to a variety of negative outcomes (although most specifically linked to alcohol and drug abuse problems). However, the magnitude of the risk also pointed to caution about overpathologizing COAs and the real risks of negative labeling effects. Moreover, our review revealed that there have been few longitudinal studies that appropriately test mediators and moderators of parental alcoholism effects, further limiting the empirical foundation for the design of preventive interventions. Potentially important mediators and/or moderators that have been identified include temperamental characteristics, life stress, expectancies about alcohol and drug effects, family conflict, impaired parental control and support, coping, self-esteem, perceived control, and the preservation of family rituals. However, there have been few efforts to target these mediators and moderators in preventive intervention programs (even considering the slim empirical foundation that does exist). Moreover, there have been almost no rigorously evaluated trials of preventive intervention programs. School-based interventions must take care to avoid labeling effects, and some universal interventions may be usefully incorporated into existing substance use prevention curricula. More powerful prevention effects may be obtained by adding parental involvement components, but alcoholic families may be difficult to enlist outside of alcohol treatment settings, which reach only a minority of alcoholic families. Based on our review, important directions for future research include longitudinal studies that appropriately test mediators and moderators of parental alcoholism effects. Moreover, if careful attention is paid to preventing potential labeling effects, research is warranted that provides rigorous tests of preventive interventions that target the mediating and moderating factors that have already been identified.

ACKNOWLEDGMENTS

Preparation of this chapter was supported by Grant DA05227 from the National Institute on Drug Abuse to Laurie Chassin and Manuel Barrera, Jr.

REFERENCES

Alterman, A. I., Searles, J. S, & Hall, J. G. (1989). Failure to find differences in drinking behavior as a function of familial risk for alcoholism: A replication. *Journal of Abnormal Psychology, 98,* 50–53.

Anderson, E. E., & Quast, W. (1983). Young children in alcoholic families: A mental health needs-assessment and an intervention/prevention strategy. *Journal of Primary Prevention, 3,* 174–187.

Barrera, M., Jr., Li, S. A., & Chassin, L. (1993). Ethnic group differences in vulnerability to parental alcoholism and life stress: A study of Hispanic and non-Hispanic Caucasian adolescents. *American Journal of Community Psychology, 21,* 15–35.

Barrera, M., Jr., Li, S. A., & Chassin, L. (1995). Exploring the role of ethnicity and family conflict in adolescents' vulnerability to life stress and parental alcoholism. In H. I. McCubbin, E. A. Thompson, A. I. Thompson, & J. E. Fromer (Eds.), *Resiliency in ethnic minority families. Vol. 1: Native and immigrant American families* (pp. 295–324). Madison, WI: Center for Family Studies, University of Wisconsin System.

Barrera, M., Jr., Rogosch, F., & Chassin, L. (1993). Social support and conflict among adolescent children of alcoholics. *Journal of Personality and Social Psychology, 64,* 602–613.

Barrera, M., Jr., Stice, E., & Chassin, L. (1994, June). Parent–adolescent conflict in the context of parental support. Poster presented at the Family Research Consortium II First Annual Summer Institute, Sante Fe, NM.

Baron, R. M., & Kenny, D. A. (1986). The moderator–mediator variable distinction in social psychological research: Conceptual, strategic, and statistical considerations. *Journal of Personality and Social Psychology, 51,* 1173–1182.

Barry, K. L., & Fleming, M. F. (1990). Family cohesion, expressiveness and conflict in alcoholic families. *British Journal of Addiction, 85,* 81–87.

Begleiter, H., Porjesz, B., Bihari, B., & Kissin, B. (1984). Event-related brain potentials in boys at risk for alcoholism. *Science, 225,* 1493–1496.

Bennett, L. A., Wolin, S. J., Reiss, D., & Teitelbaum, M. (1987). Couples at risk for alcoholism recurrence: Protective influences. *Family Process, 26,* 111–129.

Benson, C. S., & Heller, K. (1987). Factors in the current adjustment of young adult daughters of alcoholic and problem drinking fathers. *Journal of Abnormal Psychology, 90,* 305–312.

Brook, J. S., Whiteman, M., & Gordon, A. S. (1983). Stages of drug use in adolescence: Personality, peer, and family correlates. *Developmental Psychology, 19,* 269–277.

Brown, S. A., Creamer, V. A., & Stetson, B. A. (1987). Adolescent alcohol expectancies in relation to personal and parental drinking patterns. *Journal of Abnormal Psychology, 96,* 117–121.

Burk, J. P., & Sher, K. F. (1990). Labeling the child of an alcoholic: Negative stereotyping by mental health professionals and peers. *Journal of Studies on Alcohol, 51,* 156–163.

Chassin, L., Curran, P., Hussong, A., & Colder, C. (1996). The relation of parent alcoholism to adolescent substance use: A longitudinal follow-up study. *Journal of Abnormal Psychology, 105,* 70–80.

Chassin, L., Pillow, D., Curran, P., Molina, B., & Barrera, M. (1993). The relation of parental alcoholism to early adolescent substance use: A test of three mediating mechanisms. *Journal of Abnormal Psychology, 102,* 3–19.

Chassin, L., Rogosch, F., & Barrera, M. (1991). Substance use and symptomatology among adolescent children of alcoholics. *Journal of Abnormal Psychology, 100,* 449–463.

Clair, D., & Genest, M. (1987). Variables associated with the adjustment of offspring of alcoholic fathers. *Journal of Studies on Alcohol, 48,* 345–355.

Cloninger, C. R. (1987). Neurogenetic adaptive mechanisms in alcoholism. *Science, 236,* 410–416.

Colder, C. R., Chassin, L., & Curran, P. (1995). Alcohol expectancies as potential mediators of parent alcoholism effects on adolescent substance use. (under editorial review).

Curran, P., & Chassin, L. (1996). A longitudinal study of parenting as a protective factor for children of alcoholic fathers. *Journal of Studies on Alcohol, 57,* 305–313.

Crews, T. M., & Sher, K. J. (1992). Using adapted short MASTs for assessing parental alcoholism: Reliability and validity. *Alcoholism: Clinical and Experimental Research, 16,* 576–585.

DiCicco, L., Davis, R., Travis, J., & Ornstein, A. (1984). Recruiting children from alcoholic families into a peer education program. *Alcohol Health and Research World, 8,* 28–34.

DiCicco, L., Davis, R., Hogan, J., MacLean, A., & Ornstein, A. (1984). Group experiences for children of alcoholics. *Alcohol Health and Research World, 8,* 20–24.

Dishion, T. J., Patterson, G. R., & Reid, J. R. (1988). Parent and peer factors associated with drug sampling in early adolescence: Implications for treatment. In E. R. Rahdert & J. Grabowski (Eds.), *NIDA Research Monograph 77, Adolescent drug abuse: Analyses of treatment research* (pp. 69–93). Rockville, MD: NIDA.

Domenico, D., & Windle, M. (1993). Intrapersonal and interpersonal functioning among middle-aged female adult children of alcoholics. *Journal of Consulting and Clinical Psychology, 61,* 659–666.

Dunn, N. J., Jacob, T., Hummon, N., & Seilhamer, R. A. (1987). Marital stability in alcoholic–spouse relationships as a function of drinking pattern and location. *Journal of Abnormal Psychology, 96,* 99–108.

Fitzgerald, H. E., Sullivan, L. A., Ham, H. P., Zucker, R. A., Bruckel, S., Schneider, A. M., & Noll, R. B. (1993). Predictors of behavior problems in three-year-old sons of alcoholics: Early evidence for the onset of risk. *Child Development, 64,* 110–123.

Goodwin, D. W., Schulsinger, F., Knop, J., Mednick, S., & Guze, S. B. (1977). Alcoholism and depression in adopted-out daughters of alcoholics. *Archives of General Psychiatry, 34,* 751–755.

Greenfield, S. F., Swartz, M. S., Landerman, L. R., & George, L. K. (1993). Long-term psychosocial effects of childhood exposure to parental problem drinking. *American Journal of Psychiatry, 150,* 808–613.

Heller, K., Sher, K. J., & Benson, C. S. (1982). Problems associated with risk overprediction in studies of offspring of alcoholics: Implications for prevention. *Clinical Psychology Review, 2,* 183–200.

Herjanic, B., Jerjanic, M., Penick, E., Tomelleri, C., & Armbruster, R. (1977). Children of alcoholics. In F. Seixas (Ed.), *Currents in alcoholism* (Vol. 2, pp. 445–455). New York: Grune and Stratton.

Holden, M. G., Brown, S. A., & Mott, M. A. (1988). Social support network of adolescents: Relation to family alcohol abuse. *American Journal of Drug and Alcohol Abuse, 14,* 487–498.

Hughes, J. (1977). Adolescent children of alcoholic parents and the relationship of Alateen to these children. *Journal of Consulting and Clinical Psychology, 45,* 946–947.

Hussong, A., & Chassin, L. (1997). Substance use initiation among adolescent children of alcoholics: Examining protective factors. *Journal of Studies on Alcohol, 58,* 272–279.

Jacob, T., & Krahn, G. (1988). Marital interaction of alcoholic couples: Comparison with depressed and non-distressed couples. *Journal of Consulting and Clinical Psychology, 56,* 73–79.

Jacob, T., & Leonard, K. E. (1986). Psychological functioning in children of alcoholic fathers, depressed fathers, and control fathers. *Journal of Studies on Alcohol, 47,* 373–380.

Jacob, T., & Leonard, K. E. (1994). Family and peer influences in the development of adolescent alcohol abuse. In R. Zucker, G. Boyd, & J. Howard (Eds.), *The development of alcohol problems: Exploring the biopsychosocial matrix of risk* (pp. 123–156). NIAAA Research Monograph No. 26, USDHHS, NIH Publication No. 94-3495. Rockville, MD: Public Health Service, National Institute of Health, National Institute of Alcohol Abuse and Alcoholism.

Jacob, T., Ritchey, D., Cvitkovic, J. F., & Blane, H. T. (1981). Communication styles of alcoholic and nonalcoholic families when drinking and not drinking. *Journal of Studies on Alcohol, 42,* 466–482.

Jessor, R., & Jessor, S. L. (1977). *Problem behavior and psychosocial development: A longitudinal study of youth.* New York: Academic Press.

Kaplan, H. B. (1980). *Deviant behavior in defense of self.* New York: Academic Press.

Li, S. A., Barrera, M., & Chassin, L. (1994, August). Paternal inconsistent support and adolescent mental health. Presented at the annual meeting of the American Psychological Association, Los Angeles.

Logue, M. B., Sher, K. J., & French, P. A. (1992). Purported characteristics of ACOAs: A possible "Barnum" effect. *Professional Practice: Research and Practice, 3,* 226–232.

Mann, L. M., Chassin, L., & Sher, K. J. (1987). Alcohol expectancies and risk for alcoholism. *Journal of Consulting and Clinical Psychology, 55,* 411–417.

Martin, C. S., Earleywine, M., Blackson, T. C., Vanyukov, M. M., Moss, H. B., & Tarter, R. E. (1994). Aggressivity, inattention, hyperactivity, and impulsivity in boys at high and low risk for substance abuse. *Journal of Abnormal Child Psychology, 22,* 177–203.

McGrath, C., & Chassin, L. (1995). Testing self-enhancement models of adolescent problem behavior: The role of self-esteem in adolescent substance use. Presented at the annual meeting of the Society for Prevention Research, Scottsdale, AZ.

McGue, M. (1994). Genes, environment, and the etiology of alcoholism. In R. Zucker, G. Boyd, & J. Howard (Eds.), *The development of alcohol problems: Exploring the biopsychosocial matrix of risk* (pp. 1–40). NIAAA Research Monograph No. 26, USDHHS, NIH Publication No. 94-3495, Rockville, MD: Public Health Service, National Institute of Health and National Institute of Alcohol Abuse and Alcoholism.

Merikangas, K., Weissman, M., Prusoff, B., Pauls, D., & Leckman, J. (1985). Depressives with secondary alcoholism: Psychiatric disorders in offspring. *Journal of Studies on Alcohol, 46,* 199–204.

Moos, R. H., & Billings, A. G. (1982). Children of alcoholics during the recovery process: Alcoholic and matched control families. *Addictive Behavior, 7,* 155–163.

Moss, H., Blackson, T., Martin, C., & Tarter, R. (1992). Heightened motor activity level in male offspring of substance abusing fathers. *Biological Psychiatry, 32,* 1135–1147.

Newlin, D. B., & Thomson, J. B. (1990). Alcohol challenge with sons of alcoholics: A critical review and analysis. *Psychological Bulletin, 108,* 383–402.

Noll, R. B., Zucker, R. A., Fitzgerald, H. E., & Curtis, J. W. (1992). Cognitive and motoric functioning of sons of alcoholic fathers and controls: The early childhood years. *Child Development, 28,* 665–675.

Noll, R. B., Zucker, R. A., & Greenberg, G. S. (1990). Identification of alcohol by smell among preschoolers: Evidence for early socialization about drugs occurring in the home. *Child Development, 61,* 1520–1527.

Ohannessian, C. M., & Hesselbrock, V. M. (1993). The influence of perceived social support on the relationship between family history of alcoholism and drinking behaviors. *Addiction, 88,* 1651–1658.

Pandina, R. J., & Johnson, V. (1989). Familial drinking history as a predictor of alcohol and drug consumption among adolescent children. *Journal of Studies on Alcohol, 50,* 245–254.

Peterson, J. B., Finn, P. R., & Pihl, R. O. (1992). Cognitive dysfunction and the inherited predisposition to alcoholism. *Journal of Studies on Alcohol, 53,* 154–160.

Pihl, R. O., Peterson, J. B., & Finn, P. R. (1990). The inherited predisposition to alcoholism: Characteristics of sons of male alcoholics. *Journal of Abnormal Psychology, 99,* 291–301.

Pollack, V. E., Briere, J., Schneider, L., Knop, J., Mednick, S. A., & Goodwin, D. W. (1990). Childhood antecedents of antisocial behavior: Parental alcoholism and physical abusiveness. *American Journal of Psychiatry, 147,* 1290–1293.

Pollack, V. E., & Earleywine, M. (1994). Neuropsychological characteristics of individuals at risk for alcoholism: A meta-analysis. Presented at the annual meeting of the Research Society on Alcoholism.

Robins, L. N., Helzer, J. E., Weissman, M. M., Orvaschel, H., Gruenberg, E., Burke, J. D., Jr., & Regier, D. A. (1984). Lifetime prevalence of specific psychiatric disorders in three sites. *Archives of General Psychiatry, 41,* 949–958.

Rollins, B. C., & Thomas, D. L. (1979). Parental support, power, and control techniques in the socialization of children. In W. R. Burr, R. Hill, F. I. Nye, & I. L. Reiss (Eds.), *Contemporary theories about the family.* Vol. 1: *Research-based theories* (pp. 417–364). New York: Wiley.

Roosa, M. W., Beals, J., Sandler, I. N., & Pillow, D. R. (1990). The role of risk and protective factors in predicting symptomatology in adolescent children of alcoholics. *American Journal of Community Psychology, 18,* 725–741.

Roosa, M. W., Dumka, L., Tein, J., & Tweed, S. (1992, November). Family influences on child mental health in alcoholic families. Presented at the annual meeting of the National Council on Family Relations, Orlando, Fl.

Roosa, M. W., Sandler, I. N., Beals, J., & Short, J. L. (1988). Risk status of adolescent children of problem drinking parents. *American Journal of Community Psychology, 16,* 225–239.

Roosa, M. W., Sandler, I. N., Gehring, M., Beals, J., & Cappo, L. (1988). The Children of Alcoholics Life Events Schedule: A stress scale for children of alcohol abusing parents. *Journal of Studies on Alcohol, 49,* 422–429.

Roosa, M. W., Tein, J., Groppenbacher, N., Michaels, M., & Dumka, L. (1993). Mothers' parenting behavior and child mental health in families with a problem drinking parent. *Journal of Marriage and the Family, 55,* 107–118.

Russell, M. (1990). Prevalence of alcoholism among children of alcoholics. In M. Windle & J. Searles (Eds.), *Children of alcoholics: Critical perspectives.* (pp. 9–38). New York: Guilford.

Russell, M., Cooper, L., & Frone, M. R. (1990). The influence of sociodemographic characteristics on familial alcohol problems: Data from a community sample. *Alcoholism: Clinical and Experimental Research, 14,* 221–226.

Russell, M., Henderson, C., & Blume, S. (1985). *Children of alcoholics: A review of the literature.* New York: Children of Alcoholics Foundation.

Schuckit, M., & Chiles, J. (1978). Family history as a diagnostic aid in two samples of adolescents. *Journal of Nervous and Mental Disease, 166,* 165–176.

Schulsinger, F., Knop, J., Goodwin, D. W., Teasdale, T. W., & Mikkelson, U. (1986). A prospective study of young men at high risk for alcoholism. *Archives of General Psychiatry, 43,* 755–760.

Seilhamer, R. A., & Jacob, T. (1990). Family factors and adjustment of children of alcoholics. In M. Windle & J. S. Searles (Eds.), *Children of alcoholics: Critical perspectives* (pp. 168–186). New York: Guilford Press.

Shell, R. M., & Roosa, M. W. (1991, November). Family influences on children's coping as a function of parent alcoholism status. Presented at the annual meeting of the National Council on Family Relations, Denver.

Sher, K. J. (1991). *Children of alcoholics: A critical appraisal of theory and research.* Chicago: University of Chicago Press.

Sher, K. J., & Levenson, R. W. (1982). Risk for alcoholism and individual differences in the stress-response-dampening effect of alcohol. *Journal of Abnormal Psychology, 91,* 350–368.

Sher, K. J., & Mothershead, P. (1991). The clinical literature. In K. J. Sher (Ed.), *Children of alcoholics: A critical appraisal of theory and research* (pp. 148–170). Chicago: University of Chicago Press.

Sher, K. J., Walitzer, K. S., Wood, P. K., & Brent, E. E. (1991). Characteristics of children of alcoholics: Putative risk factors, substance use and abuse, and psychopathology. *Journal of Abnormal Psychology, 100,* 427–228.

Short, J. L., Roosa, M. W., & Tein, J. (1995). Evaluation of a preventive intervention for a self-selected sub-population of children. *American Journal of Community Psychology, 23,* 223–231.

Steinglass, P., Bennett, L. A., Wolin, S. J., & Reiss, D. (1987). *The alcoholic family.* New York: Basic Books.

Steinhausen, H.-C., & Spohr, H.-L. (1986). Fetal alcohol syndrome. In B. B. Lahey & A. E. Kazdin (Eds.), *Advances in clinical child psychology* (Vol. 9, pp. 217–243). New York: Plenum Press.

Stice, E. M., & Barrera, M., Jr. (1995). A longitudinal examination of the reciprocal relations between perceived parenting and adolescents' substance use and externalizing behaviors. *Developmental Psychology, 31,* 322–334.

Streissguth, A. P., Landesman-Dwyer, S., Martin, J. C., & Smith, D. W. (1980). Teratogenic effects of alcohol in humans and laboratory animals. *Science, 209,* 353–354.

Streissguth, A. P., Sampson, P. D., & Olson, H. C. (1994). Maternal drinking during pregnancy: Attention and short-term memory in 14-year-old offspring: A longitudinal prospective study. *Alcoholism: Clinical and Experimental Research, 18,* 202–210.

Tarter, R. E., Kabene, M., Escallier, E. A., Laird, S. B., & Jacob, T. (1990). Temperamental deviation and risk for alcoholism. *alcoholism: Clinical and Experimental Research, 14,* 380–382.

Tarter, R. E., Laird, S. B., & Moss, H. B. (1990). Neuropsychological and neurophysiological characteristics of children of alcoholics. In M. Windle & J. Searles (Eds.), *Children of alcoholics: Critical perspectives* (pp. 73–98). New York: Guilford.

Tweed, S. H., & Ryff, C. D. (1991). Adult children of alcoholics: Profiles of wellness amidst distress. *Journal of Studies on Alcohol, 52,* 133–141.

Velleman, R. (1992). Intergenerational effects—A review of environmentally oriented studies concerning the relationship between parental alcohol problems and family disharmony in the genesis of alcohol and other problems. II: The intergenerational effects of family disharmony. *International Journal of the Addictions, 27,* 367–389.

Velleman, R., & Orford, J. (1990). Young adult offspring of parents with drinking problems: Recollections of parents' drinking and its immediate effects. *British Journal of Clinical Psychology, 29,* 297–317.

Vuchinich, S., Bank, L., & Patterson, G. R. (1992). Parenting, peers, and the stability of antisocial behavior in preadolescent boys. *Developmental Psychology, 28,* 510–521.

Werner, E. E. (1986). Resilient offspring of alcoholics: A longitudinal study from birth to age 18. *Journal of Studies on Alcohol, 47,* 34–40.

West, M. O., & Prinz, R. J. (1987). Parental alcoholism and childhood psychopathology. *Psychological Bulletin, 102,* 204–218.

Wills, T. A., & Shiffman, S. (1985). Coping and substance use: A conceptual framework. In S. Shiffman & T. A. Wills (Eds.), *Coping and substance use* (pp. 3–24). Orlando, FL: Academic Press.

Whipple, S. C., Parker, E. S., & Noble, E. P. (1988). An atypical neurocognitive profile in alcoholic fathers and their sons. *Journal of Studies on Alcohol, 49,* 240–244.

Windle, M. (1990). Temperament and personality attributes of children of alcoholics. In M. Windle & J. Searles (Eds.), *Children of alcoholics: Critical perspectives,* (pp. 129–167). New York: Guilford.

Wolin, S. J., BEnnett, L. A., Noonan, D. L., & Teitelbaum, M. A. (1980). Disrupted family rituals. *Journal of Studies on Alcohol, 41,* 199–214.

Woodward, B. (1985). An assessment of a prevention program for children of alcoholics. *Dissertation Abstracts International, 45,* 2324-B.

5

Children of Depressed Parents
The Stress Context

CONSTANCE HAMMEN

In recent years, we have come to recognize the enormous toll that depression takes on peoples' lives. In exploring the impact of this disorder, it has also become clear that depression affects the lives of others, and nowhere is this effect more apparent and dramatic than in families. Studies of children of depressed parents have grown in number and sophistication recently, and they all point to a common conclusion: Depression runs in families, and children of depressed parents are highly likely to experience depression and other forms of disorder and maladjustment. The extent of children's impairment is striking, apparently equaling or even exceeding that of seemingly more severe parental disorders such as schizophrenia or bipolar affective disorder. Although a genetic model often implicitly guided earlier studies of children's risk, alternative approaches suggest a role for psychosocial factors in a diathesis—stress model: That children in families with a depressed parent are enormously stressed by the constellation of circumstances associated with their parents' debilities, and many may lack the skills and resources that would be necessary to deal with such stress.

The goal of this chapter, therefore, will be to develop the case for such an approach to understanding children's risk for disorder. After describing the potential magnitude of the problem of parental depression, we explore the nature and extent of the children's problems, the meaning and characteristics of parental depression as it affects children, the stress context of depression, and the special challenges to children in coping with parental depression. In view of the enormous and apparently increasing incidence of depression, such issues present not only theoretical but also practical challenges.

CONSTANCE HAMMEN • Department of Psychology, University of California, Los Angeles, Los Angeles, California 90095.

Handbook of Children's Coping: Linking Theory and Intervention, edited by Wolchik and Sandler. Plenum Press, New York, 1997.

THE SCOPE OF PARENTAL DEPRESSION

There are several striking features of the distribution of depression that command attention in the context of family life. It is common, and apparently increasing in frequency. It is largely a disorder of young women, and hence a risk to those of childbearing ages. Even nonclinical levels of depressive symptoms may be debilitating and may even portend clinical conditions. And, depression tends to be recurrent and in a sizable subgroup of cases, it is chronic, as we discuss in a later section.

Incidence and Prevalence of Depression

Rates of diagnosable depression and subclinical symptoms are remarkably high. The most recent large-scale epidemiological survey of psychiatric disorders in people ages 15–54 found that 24% of women and 14.7% of men had experienced a diagnosable mood disorder in their lifetimes (Kessler et al., 1994). Major depression was reported to have occurred within the past 12 months by one in every eight women (13%). Current prevalence of depression (within the past month) is also notably high; major depressive episodes were diagnosed in 5.9% of women and 3.8% of men (Blazer, Kessler, McGonagle, & Swartz, 1994). Because elevated symptom levels may also mark impaired functioning, rates of subclinical depression are also informative. Defining subclinical as at least two depressive symptoms for at least 2 weeks, Horwath, Johnson, Klerman, and Weissman (1992) found that 24% of the population had such periods in their lifetimes; rates for women alone would doubtless be higher, but only the overall population average was reported. Not only are rates of diagnosable depression relatively high, but also evidence is accumulating that such rates are increasing, especially among young people, according to studies of an apparent birth cohort effect of those born in more recent decades (e.g., Cross-National Collaborative Group, 1992; Klerman et al., 1985).

Depression in Young Women

Of particular note, the greatest elevations in depressive symptoms and disorders are reported by young women. Virtually all surveys indicate higher rates of depression for women than men, by about 2:1 (e.g., Nolen-Hoeksema, 1990). For example, current (30-day) prevalence rates of major depression were highest for women between the ages of 15 and 24 (especially for white and Hispanic women) (Blazer et al., 1994). Not only are the highest rates of diagnosable depressions typically observed in young women, but also in both adolescent and adult samples, young women with prior depressive episodes are the most likely to have recurrent episodes (e.g., Lewinsohn, Hoberman, & Rosenbaum, 1988; Lewinsohn et al., 1994).

Impairment Associated with Depression

Another reason to take note of depression in the population is not just that it is a common disorder and increasingly afflicts young adults, but also that it exacts an enormous toll of impairment. Depressed people reported worse role functioning, poorer physical and social adjustment, and more days spent in bed compared with those suffering from one of several chronic medical ailments (such as respiratory problems, diabetes, arthritis, and others) (Wells et al., 1989). Impairment in those with chronic low-level depression (dysthymia) is striking: They had the worst outcomes in a 2-year follow-up, and even those with subclinical depressive symptoms showed significant impairment over the 2 years (Wells, Burnam, Rogers, Hays, & Camp, 1992). Similarly, those with elevated depressive symptoms but no diagnosis were found to account for significant use of emergency services, use of psychotropic medications, self-reported poor emotional health, days lost from work, and suicide attempts (Johnson, Weissman, & Klerman, 1992), to account for even more disability days than those with major depressive episode (Broadhead, Blazer, George, & Tse, 1990), and to be at significant risk for developing a major depressive episode over a follow-up period (Horwath et al., 1992; Wells et al., 1992).

These findings emphasize that probably even more than severity of depressive symptoms, chronicity or recurrence contribute to impaired functioning. It is noteworthy, therefore, that we understand that clinical depressions are commonly recurrent. It is estimated that between 50 and 85% of individuals who seek treatment for a major depressive episode will have at least one recurrence (Keller, 1985), and many individuals have multiple episodes. Moreover, it is also estimated that 20–25% of depressed individuals have chronic symptoms of depression, and sometimes have superimposed episodes of major depression (double depression) (e.g., Depue & Monroe, 1986; Keller, Lavori, Rice, Coryell, & Hirschfeld, 1986).

Conclusions and Implications

The epidemiological figures suggest that at any given moment, about 6% of all women (but more than 8% of young adult women) are depressed to the degree to warrant a diagnosis of major depression (Blazer et al., 1994); moreover, nearly one quarter of women report major depression at some point, most commonly in the teenage or early adult years. These figures do not even count the additional numbers who might be experiencing significant impairment and disruption due to milder depressive symptoms. Obviously, the frequency of significant depressive symptoms, plus its relative concentration among young women, suggests that the early adult years may be a period of risk. Since these are often childbearing years for many women, the patterns suggest that children's exposure to maternal depression is not a rare occurrence, and that a good many youngsters are exposed to maternal depressive episodes or symptoms. Moreover, since the great majority of people suffering from a major depressive episode do not seek treatment, their families and social milieu may be exposed to weeks or even months of debility. Additionally, young women who have had one episode are at increased risk for recurrences, potentially exposing families to repeated bouts of depression.

OUTCOMES OF CHILDREN OF DEPRESSED PARENTS

The vast majority of studies of offspring of depressed parents have actually focused on maternal depression. The reasons are partly theoretical—the pre-

sumably more influential role of mothers as primary caretakers—but are probably largely practical. The greater prevalence of depression in women makes
them more available as subjects for study. Also, depression is commonly associated with divorce and marital disruption, such that the pool of depressed
fathers is further reduced by the relatively low frequency of such men who live
with their children. Thus, in the sections to follow, the great majority of studies
concern children of depressed women.

One of the difficulties in organizing a review of children's outcomes concerns the heterogeneity of indicators that have been used (and corresponding
lack of comparability) and the wide ranges of ages studied, with few guidelines
concerning age-related patterns of maladjustment according to children's developmental status. Also, the methodological shortcomings of studies have
generally precluded the accumulation of a body of comparable findings and
have included a lack of multiple informants or diverse indicators of functioning, emphasis on short-term rather than long-term adjustment, and heterogeneous samples of depressed parents (some studies even included bipolar
with unipolar).

Studies of Infants and Preschoolers

A number of observational studies of nondepressed compared with depressed women interacting with their babies or young children have indicated
that depressed mothers are unresponsive or noncontingently responsive, or
negative and rejecting, while the babies themselves are wary or distressed.
Even mildly or transiently depressed mothers may elicit negative reactions in
their infants. Some of these studies are noted below in a discussion of quality of
parent–child relations. One of the most extensive studies of young children of
clinically depressed (both unipolar and bipolar) mothers has been conducted at
the National Institute of Mental Health (NIMH) Laboratory of Developmental
Psychology. Infants and toddlers of such mothers have problems regulating
emotional reactions, including aggression, and in cooperative interactions with
others (Zahn-Waxler, Cummings, Iannoti, & Radke-Yarrow, 1984; Zahn-Waxler, Cummings, McKnew, & Radke-Yarrow, 1984; Zahn-Waxler, McKnew,
Cummings, Davenport, & Radke-Yarrow, 1984). An English study of depressed
and nondepressed mothers of 2- to 3-year-olds reported that 44% of children of
depressed women had "substantive" problems based on observations and assessments of children's functioning; the rates were even higher (63%) among
women with personality disorders and/or extensive prior history of depression
in addition to current depression (Pound, Cox, Puckering, & Mills, 1985). The
children's problems included emotional and behavioral disturbances and delayed expressive language development (Cox, Puckering, Pound, & Mills,
1987). Further underscoring the significant negative impact of maternal depression, a study of infants of women with postpartum depression found that they
tested lower than control infants on cognitive development on the Bayley
Scales of Infant Development and displayed more negative emotional reactions
during testing (Whiffen & Gotlib, 1989).

One of the strongest and most widely replicated findings concerning the
infants and toddlers of depressed women is insecure attachment, presumably

due to depressed mothers' insensitivity and negativity. In a later section, the role of attachment as a potential mediator of the effects of parental depression is reviewed. Young children of depressed women displayed higher rates of insecure attachment (e.g., Cohn, Matias, Tronick, Connell, & Lyons-Ruth, 1986; DeMulder & Radke-Yarrow, 1991; Lyons-Ruth, Zoll, Connell, & Grunebaum, 1986; Radke-Yarrow, Cummings, Kuczynski, & Chapman, 1985). Murray (1992) found that postpartum depression was associated with increased rates of insecure attachment 16 months later. In view of the importance of secure attachment as a foundation for the child's self-concept, perceptions of the reliability of others, and for the ability to regulate emotion and explore the world effectively, disturbances of attachment may have profound and enduring consequences. It should be noted, however, the insecure mother–child attachment is by no means a universal outcome with depressed mothers, nor is it specific to maternal depression.

Studies of School-Age Children and Adolescents

Table 1 summarizes the results of a handful of studies that improved on early offspring studies by including direct interview techniques for diagnosing children's disorders. These studies yield three consistent results: children of

Table 1. Diagnostic Outcomes of Children of Clinically Depressed Women

Study	Percent receiving diagnosis by category				
	Any	Major depression	Disruptive behavior	Substance use	Anxiety
Hammen (1991a) (ages 8–16)					
Unipolar	82	45	32	23	27
Bipolar	72	22	22	11	11
Medically ill	43	29	14	7	7
Normal	32	11	8	3	8
Keller et al. (1986); Beardslee et al. (1988) (ages 6–19)					
Unipolar	65	24	30	13	19
Normal	NR[a]	NR	NR	NR	NR
Klein et al. (1988) (ages 14–22)					
Unipolar	51	9	13	11	15
Medically ill	21	0	6	6	3
Normal	24	0	0	8	5
Orvaschel et al. (1988) (ages 6–17)					
Unipolar	41	15	NR	NR	20
Normal	15	4	NR	NR	9
Weissman et al. (1987) (ages 6–23)					
Unipolar	73	38	22	17	37
Normal	65	24	17	7	27

[a]NR, not reported; children may have more than one disorder.

depressed parents have elevated rates of diagnoses compared with normal comparison families; children of depressed parents have higher rates of affective disorders, particularly major depression, than any other disorders; such offspring also have elevated rates of other disorders and commonly experience multiple disorders, including anxiety, substance use, and disruptive behavior disorders. Two of the diagnostic interview studies included additional comparison groups besides nonpsychiatric normal samples. Hammen (1991a) found significantly higher rates of current diagnoses in the 8- to 16-year-old offspring of unipolar women compared to bipolar, medically ill, and normal women. Klein, Clark, Dansky, and Margolis (1988) found higher rates of diagnosis in offspring of unipolar depressed parents compared with medically ill and normal family offspring.

A number of other offspring studies have employed additional indicators of children's functioning besides diagnosis. Lee and Gotlib (1991) compared 7- to 13-year-old children of depressed women with children of women with other nondepressive psychiatric diagnoses, medical illness, and community controls. They found that the offspring of depressed women were more likely than those of control mothers and medically ill mothers to have clinically significant problems on the Child Behavior Checklist and other measures of symptoms. However, they did not differ from the children of psychiatric comparison mothers. Hirsch, Moos, and Reischl (1985) studied adolescent offspring of parents with depression or arthritis, or normal controls; they found that the children of depressed parents were the most impaired on measures of self-esteem, school satisfaction, and symptomatology. However, unlike the results of Lee and Gotlib (1991), the depressed and medical groups did not differ. A large-scale study of 333 mother–child pairs studied child- and mother-reported symptoms as a function of maternal depression diagnosis (Breslau, Davis, & Prabucki, 1988). They found that the 8- to 23-year-old children of depressed women reported higher levels of depressive symptoms than children of nondepressed mothers; mothers not only rated the children as higher on depression symptoms but also on a variety of other domains such as anxiety and conduct problems. Finally, it should be noted that studies of psychosocial functioning of the school-age offspring of depressed women have also reported academic and social problems (e.g., Anderson & Hammen, 1993; Weissman, 1988), intellectual impairment (Kaplan, Beardslee, & Keller, 1987; but see Weissman, 1988, for discrepant results), and negative cognitions about the self (e.g., Jaenicke et al., 1987).

Relatively few studies have followed up children of depressed parents to determine the stability of their diagnoses or dysfunctions over time, but those that have been conducted indicate continuing impairment. For example, Hammen, Burge, Burney, and Adrian (1990) followed 8- to 16-year old children for up to 3 years and found that the children of unipolar women were highly likely (between 63% and 81% over the 3 years) to receive a diagnosis; approximately 60% of the unipolar offspring had disorders characterized as chronic (e.g., dysthymic disorder, overanxious disorder, conduct disorder). The rate of recurrence of major depression was also high; 23% of the children of unipolar women had a recurrent episode at some point during the 3 years (Hammen et al., 1990). The rates of both chronic and recurrent disorders were higher than for bipolar, medically ill, or normal offspring of similar ages. The Weissman offspring study, notable for its large sample size of unipolar parents, examined offspring 2 years after the initial evaluation (when they had been between the ages of 6 and 21). Among children of depressed parents, major depression had a recurrence rate of 16%, and the incidence of new cases of major depression was 8.5% (Warner, Weissman, Fendrich, Wickramaratne, & Moreau, 1992). One follow-up study is of particular interest because it demonstrates that the negative effects of parental depression are not limited to the period of parental depression; Billings and Moos (1985) reported that even though parental depression had remitted, at a 1-year follow-up their children were still functioning more poorly than children of nondepressed parents on measures of psychological symptoms and behavioral problems. The prevalence of disturbance was nearly three times higher (26.5%) among children of remitted depressed parents compared with the children of nondepressed controls (9.5%). Similarly, a 10-month follow-up of the 7- to 13-year-old children of depressed, nondepressed psychiatric, and nondepressed community control women found that despite the remission of the mothers' depressive symptoms, their children continued to display internalizing symptoms, although they improved on externalizing symptoms and other signs of psychosocial adjustment (Lee & Gotlib, 1991).

Conclusions and Implications

Taken together, the studies focusing on children of unipolar depressed women uniformly indicate impairments in the functioning of the children at all ages and across samples of women with depression ranging from mild self-reported symptoms to clinically diagnosed, treatment samples. The problems include both high rates of significant disorders including both depressive and nondepressive diagnoses, as well as academic, cognitive, and social difficulties. The limited longitudinal data suggest that the children's dysfunctions persist even when maternal symptoms have remitted, although little research has specifically examined the influence of depression severity, frequency or chronicity, and timing of maternal symptoms in relation to children's adjustment. It may be hypothesized, however, that even relatively mild but persisting or recurring child symptoms may exert long-lasting effects, since disruptions of children's development of normal skills put the children at a disadvantage in dealing with age-appropriate challenges and may impair the acquisition of subsequent developmental tasks.

The research also suggests that the impact of parental depression is considerable compared to families of nondepressed parents and may exceed the negative effects experienced by children of parents who suffer from other stressful conditions such as medical illness (Hammen et al., 1990; Klein et al., 1988; Lee & Gotlib, 1991; but no differences were found by Hirsch et al., 1985). Less resolved is the question of whether parental depression exerts a more negative influence on children's adjustment compared to other psychiatric groups. However, given the relatively negative consequences of even mild persisting depression—so widespread in the community and especially among young women—the impact of depression is enormous.

Finally, the research on children's outcomes as a function of parental depression is limited by various methodological issues involving measurement and design, but the greatest gap is theoretical: the matter of accounting for the mechanisms by which depression exerts its toll. This is the issue to which we turn next.

CHILDREN OF DEPRESSED PARENTS AND EXPOSURE TO STRESS

There are at least three different components of the stress situation to which children of depressed parents are exposed. These include parental depression itself as the stressor, ongoing stressful conditions to which the child is exposed because of parental depression, and the child's own episodic and chronic stressors. The research on these topics is variable, but in the following sections each is discussed and analyzed, and the particular challenges for the child are explored.

Parental Depression as a Stressor for Children

The constellation of depressive symptoms presents a variety of challenges for a child. In this section, two overlapping aspects of the symptoms are discussed: the potential impact of the symptoms themselves and the impact of depression on the parent's behavior toward the child.

Depressive Symptoms

Consider the symptoms of depression, as shown in Table 2. These experiences indicate a number of potentially difficult situations for a child to face.

Table 2. Features of Depression

Mood symptoms
Sad, down, feels empty, depressed, cries easily
Irritable, short-tempered, oversensitive
Cognitive symptoms
Loss of pleasure and interest in previously pleasurable experiences
Sense of hopelessness, pessimism, futility, bleak future
Feels worthless, self-critical, guilty, inadequate, low self-esteem
Helplessness, easily overwhelmed
Exaggerates misfortunes or construes minor or neutral events negatively
Indecisive
Lack of motivation
Impaired concentration and memory
Thoughts of death or suicide
Somatic symptoms
Change in sleeping, too much sleep or insomnia
Change in appetite, weight gain or loss
Loss of energy
Easily fatigued
Behavioral symptoms
Wants to be left alone, may avoid social interactions
Increased dependency, neediness, reassurance-seeking
Psychomotor change: may move and talk slowly, or may be agitated and restless

The mood symptoms, for example, might be particularly challenging for children, varying by developmental levels. Ample research evidence points to the negative impact that emotional distress in the family has on children, based largely on studies of marital conflict and divorce and spousal and child abuse (Cole & Zahn-Waxler, 1992).

Among the symptoms of depression, sadness, crying, and irritability are likely to be especially stressful, because they raise issues for a child, depending on his or her age, about emotion regulation, disruption of adaptive patterns of interaction, understanding or explaining the "cause" of parental emotions, and trying to restore the parent to a more neutral state. Research on infants of depressed mothers, for example, has shown that face-to-face interactions with a sad or unreactive mother is upsetting to infants, and they respond by becoming wary, upset, and unhappy (Cohn et al., 1986; Field, 1984). Maternal displays of withdrawal or negativity and intrusiveness have been shown to elicit infant responses of anger, withdrawal, and dysphoria (Cohn & Campbell, 1992; Cohn et al., 1986; Field, Healy, Goldstein, & Guthertz, 1990). Thus, very young children may experience distress and problems with their own emotion regulation.

Children might experience parental sadness or crying as signals of something wrong that needs to be explained and dealt with. As with most negative events, one of the initial responses is to ask why this is happening. The causal attributions of young children are not unbiased, and it might be speculated that very young children often blame themselves and feel bad as a result of holding themselves responsible. Children also might hold themselves responsible for the solution to the problem of parental emotional distress. A small amount of research has indeed suggested that some children of depressed mothers are overinvolved and overresponsible in their responses to maternal distress (see Cole & Zahn-Waxler, 1992, for a discussion).

The display of parental irritability is also frightening and upsetting to most children. Both overt hostility and suppressed anger in the form of nonverbal anger are characteristic of some depressed adults. The impact of even nonverbal anger on children appears to be negative, inducing distress and negative responding. As Cummings and Davies (1994) note,

> the ambiguity and chronic tenseness in adults associated with nonverbal anger may act as a stressor for children, increasing their arousal levels, feelings of anger, and uncertainties with regard to how to behave. Because feelings are not clear, out in the open, or resolved when adults express anger nonverbally, these environments may prevent children from safely releasing their own anger and feelings of high arousal and tension, so that children resort to internalizing their feelings. (p. 86)

In our own UCLA study of children of depressed mothers, youngsters were interviewed to determine their awareness of maternal depression and what features they recognized as a sign that she was depressed. Interestingly, irritability was the change in their mothers that the children most associated with her depression; and the more they perceived that she became irritable when depressed, the more they were likely to experience depression themselves. Older children in particular reported that they got angry (Hammen, 1991a).

Probably the other major category of depressive symptoms that might be most problematic for children concerns depressive cognitions: the hopelessness, self-criticism, helplessness, and lack of motivation. As a source of stress, the impact of depressive cognitions might be greatest in its effect on parental interactions with children, based on dysfunctional expectations, attributions, and interpretations of the child's behaviors as discussed below. However, negative cognitions might also have a more direct effect on shaping the way children learn about themselves and their worlds as a result of observing parental cognitive style. Again, the research on the impact of such cognitions has been scarce in comparison to speculation. Most theorists have predicted that depressed parents who display characteristic negative thinking such as self-blame, catastrophizing, and hopeless and helpless cognitions will create depressogenic cognitions in their children through observational learning (e.g., Gelfand & Teti, 1990). Limited data have been gathered on similarity of the depressogenic cognitions of depressed parents and their children (e.g., Seligman et al., 1984, found significant correlations between parent and child attribution style). Whether children pick up their depressed parents' cognitive styles through observational learning is difficult to determine, since such cognitions cannot be measured in isolation from the parent–child interaction style. For instance, in the UCLA Family Study, we found that depressed mothers and their children both made self-critical comments, but the association was probably due to the depressed mothers' critical statements toward the child as well. There were higher correlations between negative self-cognitions in children and maternal criticism directed toward them during interaction tasks than between counts of self-critical cognitions of the mothers and children. That is, the children may have learned to be self-critical because they were criticized and not just in imitation of maternal self-deprecation (e.g., Jaenicke et al., 1987).

All of the other symptoms of the depression syndrome that a depressed parent may display could also represent potentially stressful experiences for children. A parent who does not like to play, go out and do things with the family, who lacks energy to complete tasks, or who has poor memory, all such experiences are potentially distressing. While no study of the impact of specific symptoms on children has been conducted, a survey of adults living with a depressed person is instructive: Coyne and colleagues (1987) found that 40% of the companions and spouses experienced emotional disorders needing treatment as a result of living with a depressed person. They were particularly bothered by the depressed other's lack of interest in social activities, hopelessness, fatigue, and worrying.

Other research on depressed adults has similarly suggested a negative impact of depression on others. A large body of research (too extensive for review here) has clearly indicated that strangers, acquaintances, and roommates find interactions with depressed people to be aversive, often eliciting dysphoria and hostility and rejection from others (e.g., reviewed in Gotlib & Hammen, 1992). Over time, depressed roommates, for example, perceived less social contact with their nondepressed roommates, while the latter were indeed becoming progressively more dysphoric themselves, with less enjoyment and more aggressive reactions toward their depressed roommates (e.g., Hokanson, Hummer, & Butler, 1991; Hokanson, Rubert, Welker, Hollander, & Hedeen, 1989). While research on the negative effects of interactions with depressed adults does not fully clarify the mechanisms by which depression elicits such negative reactions from others, we can speculate that the symptoms themselves are difficult to deal with.

Effects of Ongoing Stressful Conditions to Which Offspring of Depressed Parents Are Exposed

In addition to the effects of exposure to depressive symptoms themselves, there are stressful conditions typically associated with depression that might affect the child. In this section, several are discussed: characteristics of the parent–child relationship, marital conflict and relationship disruption, and other chronic stressors associated with the debility of depression.

Parent–Child Interactions

Perhaps the most obvious stressor for children of depressed parents is the nature and quality of parent–child interactions. A considerable amount of research has documented evidence of dysfunctional interactions and deficient parenting skills (reviewed in Downey & Coyne, 1990; Gelfand & Teti, 1990; Hammen, 1991a; Cummings & Davies, 1994). Early clinical studies indicated that depressed mothers reported increased friction with their families, decreased involvement, lack of affection, and resentment toward children (Weissman, Paykel, & Klerman, 1972). Depressed woman were seen as overwhelmed, anxious, and unresponsive with their infants (e.g., Anthony, 1983; Cohler, Grunebaum, Weiss, Hartmen, & Gallant, 1977; Sameroff, Seifer, & Zax, 1982). These themes of hostility, detachment, and unresponsiveness are the most typical characteristics reported in the large volume of direct observation studies.

Observations of depressed women with their infants and toddlers, for example, have shown that the women display flat affect, provide less touching, contingent responding, and less positive affection compared with nondepressed women interacting with infants (e.g., Field et al., 1990; Fleming, Ruble, Flett, & Shaul, 1988). Maternal depression has also been associated with increased anger and hostility and intrusiveness during mother–infant interactions (e.g., Cohn et al., 1986). Similar problems also characterize depressed mothers with preschool-age children. Compared with nondepressed women, depressed mothers engage in less frequent verbalization, show less responsiveness to children's speech (e.g., Breznitz & Sherman, 1987), display less reciprocity in interactions (Mills, Puckering, Pound, & Cox, 1985), and show more difficulty in asserting control and achieving compromise with their youngsters (Kochanska, Kuczynski, Radke-Yarrow, & Welsh, 1987). In one of the relatively few studies designed to study the specificity of parenting deficits among depressed women, Goodman and Brumley (1990) observed schizophrenic, depressed, and control mothers with their 3-month to 5-year-old children. The depressed mothers were less impaired overall than the schizophrenic mothers, but compared to normal women they displayed significantly less responsiveness, involvement, structure, or discipline.

Studies of older children and adolescents have been somewhat more scarce. In the UCLA Family Study comparing interactions of mothers and 8- to

16-year-old children, groups of unipolar depressed, bipolar, medically ill, and normal families were compared. The unipolar women showed significantly higher rates of criticism and negativity toward their children, less positive comments, and more off-task (uninvolved) comments compared to the other groups (except that they were not less positive than the bipolar women) (Gordon et al., 1989). Hops and colleagues (1987) employed an elaborate and extensive home observation design, specifically assessing verbal interaction sequences. They found evidence of mutually aversive interchanges in which maternal dysphoric affect suppressed family members' aggressive responses, while aggressive affect also suppressed maternal dysphoric affect. The authors interpret the pattern as functional in the short run but overall likely to be maladaptive. Two additional studies of depressed women with school-age children indicated that the mothers made more critical statements directed toward their youngsters than did the nondepressed women (e.g., Webster-Stratton & Hammond, 1988) and displayed more disapproval and aversive interactions (Panaccione & Wahler, 1986). One exception to the general negativity of depressed mothers was reported in the NIMH study of depressed women interacting with their young offspring (preschoolers and their average age 6-year-old siblings), which found that unipolar depressed women were relatively withdrawn and disengaged rather than negative, a difference that might be attributable in part to interactions with younger children (Inoff-Germain, Nottelmann, & Radke-Yarrow, 1992). A later study included many of the same sample when they were preadolescent or adolescents, and did find greater critical and irritable behavior between the depressed mothers and their children, especially when the child also had a psychiatric disorder (Tarullo, DeMulder, Martinez, & Radke-Yarrow, 1994).

Consequences and Mechanisms of Dysfunctional Parent–Child Interactions

In general, the research on direct observation of mother–child dyads reveals that the depressed women are typically unresponsive or negative (or both). What is the effect of these interaction styles on the children? In addition to the problems in general adjustment and the presence of diagnostic conditions reviewed earlier, researchers have noted a variety of impairments specifically associated with or observed during dysfunctional interactions (see reviews in Cummings & Davies, 1994; Gelfand & Teti, 1990). These include disturbances in affect regulation, decreased verbalization, negativity, and off-task behaviors during interactions with their mothers, as well as various indicators of social maladjustment, defiance, conflict, and withdrawal (e.g., Breznitz & Sherman, 1987; Hammen, 1991a; Orvaschel, Weissman, & Kidd, 1980).

Investigators have posited several possible mechanisms by which dysfunctional interaction patterns may have negative consequences for the children. One mechanism is attachment quality (e.g., Cummings & Cicchetti, 1990; Gelfand & Teti, 1990). According to Bowlby's model of mother–infant attachment (Bowlby, 1969, 1980), secure attachment is a consequence of responsive, sensitive, and nurturant reactions of the mother. A woman who is preoccupied, disinterested in, or even hostile toward her baby and fails to respond sensitively and contingently may have a child who grows to conceive of him- or herself as unworthy and the world and other people as untrustworthy, uncaring, or unpredictable. A limited amount of research suggests that depressed women indeed may be at risk for having insecurely attached infants (e.g., Gaensbauer, Harmon, Cytryn, & McKnew, 1984; Lyons-Ruth et al., 1986; Murray, 1992; Radke-Yarrow et al., 1985; reviewed in Cummings & Davies, 1994). Insecure attachment, in turn, may be speculated to interfere with youngsters' development of capacities to regulate affect, behavior, and arousal (Cummings & Davies, 1994). Children exposed to inconsistent and emotionally fluctuating mothers may themselves have difficulty in managing their emotions and acquiring and displaying appropriate behaviors under stressful conditions. Insecurity of attachment has also been linked to a variety of maladaptive social and cognitive characteristics in children and adolescents (e.g., reviewed in Cummings & Davies, 1994).

Another process by which maladaptive parenting associated with depression might have a negative impact on children is through the use of dysfunctional parenting skills (e.g., Cummings & Davies, 1994; Gelfand & Teti, 1990). Parental depression may reduce the parent's attentiveness and energy and increase irritability and hostility that arouse and provoke the child. From a cognitive social learning perspective, a parent who is noncontingent in responding with appropriate rewards for positive behavior, who attends to and rewards aversive behavior, and who is ineffectual in discipline and limit setting is likely to generate and sustain a cycle of child noncompliance and disruptive behaviors (e.g., Patterson, 1982). Depressed parents have indeed been found to be not only more negative and less positive in verbal interactions with their children as noted earlier, but also more inconsistent and ineffectual in child discipline (e.g., Forehand, Lautenschlager, Faust, & Graziano, 1986; Zahn-Waxler, Iannotti, Cummings, & Denham, 1990). They use more forceful control strategies (Fendrich, Warner, & Weissman, 1990) or avoidant, less effortful discipline and conflict resolution strategies (e.g., Kochanska et al., 1987).

Effects of Marital Conflict and Disruption

One of the common interpersonal correlates of depression is difficulty in relationships. High rates of divorce among those with mood disorders have been reported (e.g., Barnett & Gotlib, 1988). Hammen (1991a) found that 75% of the intermittently depressed mothers of her unipolar sample were divorced or separated (compared with 25% of those in the normal comparison group). Some have argued that divorce and marital conflict may account for some of the negative consequences on children of having a depressed parent (e.g., Downey & Coyne, 1990). Several studies have specifically analyzed for the effects of parental divorce on offspring adjustment in high-risk samples. Emery, Weintraub, and Neale (1982) found that parental depression added little to the prediction of child adjustment when marital discord was taken into account. Similarly, children of depressed parents whose parents had severe marital conflict had significantly worse functioning and more diagnoses than offspring not exposed to marital problems (Keller, Beardslee et al., 1986). Billings and Moos (1985) also found that even when parental depression remitted, poor marital and family cohesion continued to predict maladjustment in children 1 year later. The course of major depression in the children of depressed parents may also be affected by marital adjustment; one of the risk factors for protracted depressive episodes in offspring of depressed parents was exposure to parental divorce (Warner et al., 1992).

In view of the large research literature demonstrating child maladjustment as a function of marital discord (e.g., Hetherington, Stanley-Hagen, & Anderson, 1989), the question of depression's role and the mechanisms of effect arises. Downey and Coyne (1990) present five different models of the causal relationships among parental depression, marital conflict, and children's adjustment. For example, one model predicts that marital discord mediates the link between parental depression and child maladjustment; another is that parental depression mediates the link between marital discord and child maladjustment. Research provides some support for each of the models. For instance, some research suggests that marital discord increases the likelihood of ineffective child management practices and that poor skills might be exacerbated by depression (reviewed in Cummings & Davies, 1994). Moreover, children who are repeatedly exposed to parent conflict may become sensitized to conflict and thereby be more likely to experience greater distress, anger, and insecurity (Cummings & Zahn-Waxler, 1992). Children of depressed mothers experiencing marital conflict may also witness poor social problem solving as their parents fail to resolve their difficulties; studies of the problem-solving skills of depressed adults have indicated that they are indeed impaired, at least during depressive periods (e.g., Nezu, 1987). Exposed to depressed maritally conflicted parents, therefore, children's dysfunctional adjustments may reflect a complex combination of poor parental child-rearing skills, sensitization to conflict leading to behavioral and emotional problems, and failure to acquire adaptive social problem-solving skills (or acquisition of maladaptive ones).

Additional Exposure to Chronic and Episodic Stressors in the Family

Many studies of children of depressed parents have focused solely on the parent–child or marital relationship aspects of family life as stressors contributing to negative outcomes. Rarely have studies examined the occurrence of other stressors. One of the realities of chronic or recurrent depression (or other psychopathologies for that matter) is that they commonly occur in the context of ongoing stressful conditions in a variety of domains. As noted earlier, depression is associated with diminished role functioning in social and work life as well. In general, depressed patients have higher levels of both negative events and chronic stressors than do nondepressed individuals (Billings & Moos, 1984). In one of the few studies to examine coexisting stressors in families with a depressed parent, Billings and Moos (1983) found that such families had significantly higher levels of social stressors, as well as less cohesive and more disorganized family environments, than did nondepressed families. The UCLA study of children of unipolar, bipolar, medically ill, and normal women developed an interview measure of maternal chronic strain (ongoing difficulties over at least the last 6 months), covering seven areas (marital/social, occupation, finances, relations with extended family, relations with children, personal health, and health of family members) (Hammen et al., 1987). On every dimension the unipolar women were significantly more stressed than the normal women, and their difficulties were especially pronounced in the realms of social relationships, occupation, finances, and, of course, relations with children. Psychiatric disability and chronic strain go hand in hand, both exerting causal influences on the other. Thus, an important but often-neglected aspect of children's adjustment is their exposure to such conditions.

Not only do individuals with depressive disorders experience various chronic strains, but they also appear to experience an elevated rate of episodic stressors as well (e.g., Billings & Moos, 1984). Although the role of stressors in precipitating depressive episodes has been well documented (e.g., reviewed in Gotlib & Hammen, 1992), the reverse direction of influence is also noteworthy. A study of the occurrence of stressors over a 1-year period in the four groups of women in the UCLA offspring study found that the unipolar women were significantly more likely overall to experience episodic stressors than were the normal women, and of particular note they were significantly more likely than all other groups to experience negative events that were at least partly dependent on their own behaviors or characteristics (Hammen, 1991b). Unipolar depressed women were particularly likely to experience interpersonal conflict events involving not just their children but also other adult relatives, friends, co-workers, and neighbors. It appears that one of the potential vulnerability mechanisms for depression is that depressed people—either by virtue of their depression or of preexisting cognitions and behaviors—actually generate stressful events that in turn may precipitate or exacerbate depression.

If the depressed mothers are experiencing elevated rates of chronic and episodic stressors, their children are likely to suffer the ill effects of exposure to the same stressors. Indeed, Adrian and Hammen (1993) demonstrated that the children of unipolar depressed women were exposed to significantly higher rates of maternal chronic strain. Moreover, chronic strain experienced by the mothers emerged as a more significant and consistent predictor of children's symptoms and psychosocial adjustment that did maternal psychiatric history (Hammen et al., 1987).

In an attempt to explore the mechanism by which chronic strain exerts its deleterious influence on children, Burge and Hammen (1991) hypothesized that it disrupts parent–child communication quality; chronic strain was a significant predictor, beyond the contribution of depressive symptoms, of the relative negativity of interactions with the child during a conflict discussion task. Because it is demoralizing and potentially preoccupying, chronic stress appears to deplete mothers' patience and make them more irritable and less tolerant and supportive of their children. Somewhat similar conclusions were reached in a study of depressed mothers of infants, who reported higher levels of perceived stress as well as more distress associated with their parenting role (Gelfand, Teti, & Fox, 1992). Besides affecting the quality of the parent–child relationship, chronic stressors may also affect the availability of other supportive relationships, such as the other parent or siblings. If also stressed because of chronic family problems, they may be unavailable to help the child cope with the consequences of the stressors. Finally, as we note in a later section, mothers whose chronic stressors create symptoms may be less available to support their children in the face of the children's own stressors and difficulties. Hammen, Burge, and Adrian (1991) showed that when faced with high levels of stressors, only those children who also had a currently symptomatic mother became depressed, a finding that is consistent with the idea of her unavailability to help buffer the ill effects of stress.

Effects of Children's Own Stressors

Even apart from stress associated with parental events and circumstances, the children of depressed parents themselves experience elevated levels of stressors. Comparing adolescent children of depressed, arthritic, and normal parents, Hirsch et al. (1985) found that the offspring of depressed parents reported significantly higher levels of negative events than did the children of normal parents. Moreover, those with the highest stressor levels were more likely to have elevated symptom levels than those with low rates of stress. Using methods of assessing stress based on interviewing both the children and their mothers, a system that yields a very comprehensive picture of the child's environment, the UCLA Family Study found that children of unipolar mothers differed significantly from children of normal mothers on total stress (chronic plus episodic) and episodic stress (Adrian & Hammen, 1993). They also differed significantly on total stress from children of bipolar mothers and of medically ill mothers (Adrian & Hammen, 1993). Thus, children of unipolar depressed women experienced substantial exposure to stress, both their own stressful events and those experienced by their mothers.

Pursuing the particular content areas in which children's stressors occurred provides further clues about the children's risks. Table 3 presents the mean objective stress total scores (based on team ratings of each event by judges who were blind to the child's actual reactions) for several content categories of life events during a 3-year period, adjusted for the covariate of age. Based on results noted earlier concerning the occurrence of stressors in the mothers (Hammen, 1991b), Adrian and Hammen (1993) hypothesized that offspring of unipolar mothers might show similar patterns of "generating" stressors, partic-

Table 3. Children's 3-Year Stress Totals by Content Category[a,b]

	Group			
	Unipolar	Bipolar	Medical	Normal
Loss, bereavement	11.2_a	9.7_{ab}	8.2_{ab}	7.2_b
Family conflict	11.0_a	6.3_b	7.2_{ab}	2.8_c
Peer conflict	4.9_a	3.5_a	1.4_b	1.6_b
Change/move/adjustment	7.6_a	3.6_b	3.7_b	5.5_{ab}
Failures	1.7_a	1.5_a	2.5_a	0.9_a
Other (accidents, health, legal problems)	14.3_a	12.9_a	19.8_a	7.0_b

[a]Adapted from Adrian and Hammen (1993), with permission.
[b]Means are adjusted for the covariate of age. For each content category, means with the same subscripts do not differ significantly from each other based on planned comparisons between the unipolar and each other's group.

ularly conflict events. One analysis not shown in Table 3 compared overall stress totals separately for events that were judged by the rating team to have occurred independent of the child's behavior or characteristics (fateful events, such as illness or things that happened to other people beyond the youngster's control) and for events at least partly due to the child (e.g., had a fight with a friend). In general, the unipolar, bipolar, and medical illness groups did not differ on independent events, although the unipolar offspring had significantly higher levels than the children of normal mothers. Most strikingly, however, the children of unipolar mothers differed significantly from the other groups on stress to which they had contributed (the comparison with bipolar offspring was borderline significant). Furthermore, in terms of the categories presented in Table 3, children of unipolar women had the highest stress levels of all groups in four of the six categories, three of them involving interpersonal relationships. While some of these stressors were beyond the children's control (e.g., loss, bereavement), the high level of peer conflict events suggests that, like their mothers, offspring of unipolar depressed women are contributing to conflictual relationships that in turn might trigger further symptom exacerbations or onsets. The offspring, like their mothers, appear to be generating stressors with which they may be ill-equipped to cope.

Gaps in Research on the Stressful Effects of Maternal Depression

Thus far, we have noted that there are various ways in which children may be exposed to stressors in the context of living with a depressed parent. In this section, additional unresolved issues are raised: heterogeneity of depressive experiences and their impact, and whether depression is associated with unique characteristics that affect children.

The first issue is the relative paucity of research considering the multiple manifestations of depression. Depression may differ somewhat from person to person, as recognized in the prototype features method of the *Diagnostic and Statistical Manual of Mental Disorders* (American Psychiatric Association, 1994). Thus, one person may be tearful, slow, withdrawn, and quiet, while another might be irritable, restless, complaining, and demanding. Thus, youngsters may face highly variable experiences with a depressed parent. Certainly one of the important gaps in the field has been to treat depression as a unitary phenomenon rather than to explore the impact of particular depressive phenomena on children. As Downey and Coyne (1990) and Gelfand and Teti (1990) have pointed out, the differences between a withdrawn and hostile depressed parent are potentially important. Gelfand and Teti (1990) state the issue succinctly: "a depressed mother whose caregiving is manifested by anger, rejection, and harsh, capricious discipline might have a different impact on a child's self-esteem and behavior than one [who] is characteristically apathetic, self-absorbed, tearful, and irresolute as a disciplinarian" (p. 342). A woman with a lack of energy and negativistic beliefs about her abilities may be less persistent and patient and unwilling to persevere or be assertive in conflict resolution. On the other hand, hostility and irritability may reflect not only negative attitudes about herself and her children, but also reflect less tolerance for imperfections or noncompliance in the children. Explorations of the different phenomenol-

ogy of depressive experiences are needed to help characterize the diverse outcomes for children of depressed parents.

A related issue concerns the heterogeneity of the course of depression, and
specifically the effects of severity, chronicity, and timing of depression experiences. The samples of depressed parents studied in offspring research are extremely heterogeneous, some using elevated self-report scores to assess level of
depression and others using clinically diagnosed, treatment-seeking populations. Groups selected in these ways differ on more than just severity, since
even diagnosed women may differ considerably in the extent of impairment
and in the extent of recurrence of their episodes. As noted earlier, even low-
grade symptoms, especially if they are persisting, may be associated with considerable debility and might be even more disruptive than a single episode of
treated depression that remits to a normal mood state with no further symptoms. In view of the heterogeneity of what is meant by a "depressed parent,"
research is clearly needed to determine children's adjustment as a function of
variability in parental depression. Only a few such studies have been reported,
but are generally consistent with the idea that diagnostic status and clinical
history are less critical factors in children's outcomes than current impairment
of functioning (commonly related to chronic symptoms) (e.g., Hammen et al.,
1987; Keller et al., 1986; Richters, 1987; Rutter & Quinton, 1984; Sameroff,
Barocas, & Seifer, 1984).

The matter of timing of parental experiences of depression in relation to
age of the child is also a matter needing further study. Theoretically, maternal
disturbances during the attachment phase of the child's development might be
expected to be particularly disruptive. On the other hand, there may be other
periods of a child's life that represent stressful developmental transitions during which maternal unavailability due to depression might be problematic. In
one of the few studies examining timing of maternal depression, type of child
maladjustment was differentially associated with timing of maternal depressive symptoms. Postpartum-only depression was more associated with anxiety
symptoms, recent depression-only predicted hyperactivity symptoms, and
chronic depression predicted children's aggressiveness (Alpern & Lyons-Ruth,
1993). The sample was drawn from low-income women only, and therefore
needs to be replicated, but the study provides an intriguing example of the
effects of maternal symptoms at specific points in the child's life.

Finally, the issue of the specificity of the effects of maternal depression has
not been fully addressed. There are actually two related questions. One is
whether certain child outcomes are specific to experiences with a depressed
parent, and the other is whether some forms of dysfunctional parenting are
specific to depression. Few studies have addressed the questions with appropriate designs or methods. Studies using various psychopathology or other
high-risk comparison groups such as maternal illness have generally found few
outcomes to be specific to type of parental disorder, and, if anything, children
of depressed parents fare worse on a variety of indicators (e.g., Hammen et al.,
1990). The question of the specificity of parenting experiences associated with
depression has been less often addressed, and indeed is difficult because so
many other conditions to be compared are often accompanied by depressive
symptoms (e.g., child maltreatment, parental alcoholism, divorce). Neverthe-

less, it remains to be seen whether the experiences faced by children of depressed parents represent unique stressors, or more likely, whether they differ mainly in degree and constellation of factors (e.g., Downey & Coyne, 1990).

Conclusions and Implications

Although researchers studying families with depressed parents have identified parental discord as an important psychosocial mediator of the negative outcomes typically shown by children, the neglect of other stressors in the family is striking. As we have argued elsewhere (e.g., Hammen et al., 1987), the diagnosis of a psychiatric disorder is more than a statement of a condition suffered by the individual; it also is a statement that the person's life is disrupted and impaired in various arenas, resulting in the experience of stress and the need to cope with not only the psychological disorder itself but also with its consequences. Moreover, people may contribute to the occurrence of episodic stressors, so that the lives of many diagnosed patients are marked by higher than normal levels of negative events (e.g., Hammen, 1991b). Children of depressed parents show similar patterns; if symptomatic, they typically display deficits in academic and social functioning—not to mention family relationships—and even display higher levels of episodic stressors than children of nondepressed normal parents (e.g., Adrian & Hammen, 1993; Anderson & Hammen, 1993). Future studies not only of offspring of depressed parents but also of children with psychological dysfunctions should expand their scope to include further study of the stressors such youngsters are exposed to and generate, as well as how they cope with them.

CHILDREN'S COPING WITH PARENTAL DEPRESSION

This section explores research on coping behaviors and coping resources in children of depressed parents. Coping is broadly defined as emotional or behavioral responses to stressors that one could infer were intended to deal with the stressor, but at the outset it must be emphasized that there are very few data on the topic of coping among children of depressed parents, and virtually no studies in which offspring have been asked what they did to try to deal with parental disturbance or related stressors. Thus, the section is relatively brief owing to the paucity of research in this area. Most of the relevant research has been conducted by investigators intrigued by the variability of outcomes among offspring of depressed parents, attempting to explore the protective or resilience factors that might help some children to escape relatively unharmed. Two broad areas of focus concern children's characteristics, behaviors, and attributes and family and social support.

Children's Characteristics

Certainly some of the maladaptive behaviors that children of depressed parents display could be construed as dysfunctional efforts to cope with parental disorder. Insecure–avoidant attachment in an infant, for example, has been hypothesized to be an effort to protect the self from insensitive, inconsistent, or rejecting caretaking by withdrawing from or avoiding intimate contact (e.g., Cummings & Davies, 1994). After infancy, young children may resort to non-compliance and disruptive behaviors to cope with frustrations and respond to stress, and as they get older it might be speculated that they increasingly use maladaptive cognitive coping mechanisms, such as self-blaming, depressogenic attribution styles of explaining the causes of negative events, and ruminative self-analysis. Such cognitive patterns have been shown to be associated with, or possibly result in, depression (e.g., Nolen-Hoeksema, 1990). Children of depressed women are indeed more likely to have negative cognitions about themselves (Jaenicke et al., 1987). When such children encounter stressors in their lives, they are more likely to become depressed or to experience other forms of psychopathology than offspring who do not have such negative cognitions (e.g., Hammen, 1991a; Hammen, Adrian, & Hiroto, 1988). Children of unipolar depressed mothers who had more positive levels of self-concept had better current and follow-up diagnostic outcomes than children with lower self-concept (Conrad & Hammen, 1993).

In addition to their potential lack of coping resources in the form of adaptive cognitions about the self or interpretations of causes of negative events, offspring of depressed parents may also be hampered by relatively poor social skills to cope instrumentally with stressors (e.g., Adrian & Hammen, 1993; Anderson & Hammen, 1993), although the precise nature of such deficits has yet to be clarified. Conversely, however, good social competence may be a protective factor in the face of risk due to parental disorder according to research on children of depressed parents (Beardslee, Schultz & Selman, 1987; Conrad & Hammen, 1993; Radke-Yarrow & Sherman, 1990). Other areas of child competence that potentially provide good or dysfunctional coping resources linked with outcomes of children of depressed parents include academic competence (e.g., Conrad & Hammen, 1993) and social problem-solving skills (e.g., Beardslee et al., 1987).

Family and Social Supports

As noted earlier, one of the potential stresses of having a parent with depression is disruption or negative quality of parent–child relationships. Children are thus not only stressed directly by such interactions, but deficient parent–child relationships may also represent the lack of an important emotional and instrumental coping resource. Hammen, Burge, and Adrian (1991) explored depression level in children as a function of the children's own level of stressors and the presence or absence of maternal depression. We found a striking interaction effect such that even under high stress conditions, children did not show depression so long as their mothers were not currently depressed, but were depressed if their mothers were also symptomatic. We interpreted the finding to suggest that maternal availability to help the child buffer the ill effects of stressors is reduced when the mother is depressed, contributing to depressive reactions.

Other studies have similarly suggested that high levels of family cohesion predict better outcomes for children of depressed parents (e.g., Holahan &

Moos, 1987). A good relationship with one or both parents may be a protective factor (Rutter, 1989), although the limited research on children of depressed parents suggests that for some youngsters there is an additional danger of becoming overinvolved or hyperresponsible for the parent's well-being (e.g., Radke-Yarrow, Richters, & Wilson, 1988; Zahn-Waxler et al., 1990). In the UCLA study we found that having a good relationship with a father who lived at home was a resource factor for children of depressed women, but only if he was healthy in the sense of no diagnosable psychological disorder [and unfortunately, such healthy fathers were a minority compared to the typical finding of major psychopathology in the father (Hammen, 1991a)]. Having a good relationship with the mother was also a positive factor related to better outcomes, and we found that depressed mothers tended to interact more positively with their children who were less symptomatic than with youngsters who had diagnosed conditions (Conrad & Hammen, 1989). Indeed, in a small sample of families with siblings who were both included in the study, mothers interacted significantly more positively with those who were nonsymptomatic (Hammen, 1991a). Although the transactional process makes direction of causality difficult to determine, it appears that having a positive relationship with a parent is probably a factor that facilitates coping with the mother's depression.

External supportive relationships may also provide coping resources for offspring of depressed women. Availability of friends, for example, appeared to be associated with better outcomes among children of depressed women in the UCLA study (Conrad & Hammen, 1993). However, as noted earlier, many such children have difficulties in their peer relationships. Also, the families may sometimes be somewhat estranged or isolated from adult relatives who could provide external supports for children (Hammen, 1991a).

A STRESS AND COPING MODEL: IMPLICATIONS FOR INTERVENTION

From a perspective emphasizing the stressors and coping assets of children of depressed parents, the results of this brief review yield a disquieting conclusion. Many of these children are exposed to excessive stress that may overwhelm their coping capacities and available resources; in some children such coping skills and resources may be relatively limited or dysfunctional. The actual stress circumstances are highly problematic: parental symptoms, dysfunctional parent–child relationships, marital discord or disruption, family strain and episodic events, and children's stressors arising in part from their own characteristics, symptoms, and failed coping efforts. The accumulation of such stressful circumstances would be difficult for any child to deal with, but the coping efforts of children or depressed parents may be particularly inadequate to the task because of two additional factors: dysfunctional mastery of developmentally appropriate skills and limited resources for supporting coping activities.

Dysfunctional mastery of developmentally appropriate skills refers to the problems in emotion regulation, attachment security, and behavioral skills that may occur at young ages if exposed to depressed parents during the earliest years. Such deficits may further impair children's acquisition of social and academic skills, creating additional stressors, and may be compounded by exposure to parents who themselves are poor role models for solving problems and coping with stress. Although we have emphasized that there are potentially high levels of objective stress faced by children, it should be noted that youngsters' appraisals of stress and resources, and hence their emotional and behavioral coping responses, may be distorted and negativistic due to the acquisition of cognitive schemas accentuating personal worthlessness and incompetence.

Unfortunately, despite widespread recognition that being a child of a depressed parent is one of the strongest predictors of risk for depression and other disorders, to date few interventions have been developed and extensively tested to deal with these high-risk youngsters. One program, developed by Beardslee et al. (1993), for example, has presented preliminary data based on 20 families of a clinician-based intervention for affectively ill parents and their 8- to 14-year-old children. It shows promise in reducing children's and families' concerns about parental problems, and hopefully such programs will help reduce adjustment problems in the high-risk youngsters. Several programs for the treatment of depressed children and adolescents have been developed and shown to be effective (e.g., Lewinsohn, Clark, Hops, & Andrews, 1990). However, a stress-coping approach to working with high-risk children would seem to require a much greater focus on family relationships and dealing with parental disorders than is typically the case of interventions aimed primarily at cognitive–behavioral skillbuilding. For instance, treatments would need to include components to help the family members accurately understand the features of depression and their influence on parental behavior and to facilitate the parents' effectiveness in child management skills. Such programs would also need to be tailored to appropriate developmental levels of children, since obviously the things that help mother–infant interactions are irrelevant to dealing with a teenager and her mother.

In some ways the greatest challenge to intervention is to identify the appropriate targets. The easiest step would be to develop adjunctive treatments for adults who are already in treatment for depression and who have children. It should now be known by clinicians that if there is a depressed parent, the entire family is feeling the effects, and that children are at high risk especially if the depression is chronic or recurrent. Unfortunately, however, this step is still missing in most clinical care, due in part to the medical model's emphasis on intraindividual disease processes or psychodynamic therapy's emphasis on intrapsychic disorders and the resulting failure to understand the enormous psychosocial correlates and sequelae of depressive disorders. Thus, even the easiest possible intervention target is nonetheless a great challenge.

The limitation in treating children of identified patients is that the vast majority of depressions do not result in treatment seeking, and this may be even more true of the mild, chronic subclinical forms that are nonetheless debilitating. We can only speculate on the negative impact of irritable, demoralized, preoccupied, and lethargic parents on children. Such problems on a large scale and the ideal of bolstering children's stress resistance at early ages seem to call for preventive interventions based on families recruited through schools or pediatric medical services. It is likely that many of the psychological disorders of children—not just depression but also conduct disorder, anxiety disorders, and substance abuse—problems that seemingly have increased enormously in recent years, have been contributed to in part by parental depression. Thus, the toll of parental depression may be enormous. Whether our communities can afford or are willing to face such challenges, however, is a greater issue than the comparatively simpler task of designing preventive interventions.

REFERENCES

Adrian, C., & Hammen, C. (1993). Stress exposure and stress generation in children of depressed mothers. *Journal of Consulting and Clinical Psychology, 61,* 354–359.

Alpern, L., & Lyons-Ruth, K. (1993). Preschool children at social risk: Chronicity and timing of maternal depressive symptoms and child behavior problems at school and at home. *Development and Psychopathology, 5,* 371–387.

American Psychiatric Association. (1994). *Diagnostic and statistical manual of mental disorders* (4th ed.). Washington, DC: Author.

Anderson, C. A., & Hammen, C. L. (1993). Psychosocial outcomes of children of unipolar depressed, bipolar, medically ill, and normal women: A longitudinal study. *Journal of Consulting and Clinical Psychology, 61,* 448–454.

Anthony, E. (1983). An overview of the effects of maternal depression on the infant and child. In H. L. Morrison (Ed.), *Children of depressed parents* (pp. 1–6). New York: Grune & Stratton.

Barnett, P. A., & Gotlib, I. H. (1988). Psychosocial functioning and depression: Distinguishing among antecedents, concomitants, and consequences. *Psychological Bulletin, 104,* 97–126.

Beardslee, W., Keller, M., Lavori, P., Klerman, G., Dorer, D., & Samuelson, H. (1988). Psychiatric disorder in adolescent offspring of parents with affective disorder in a nonreferred sample. *Journal of Affective Disorders, 15,* 313–322.

Beardslee, W., Schultz, L., & Selman, R. (1987). Level of social–cognitive development, adaptive functioning, and DSM-III diagnoses in adolescent offspring of parents with affective disorders: Implications of the development of the capacity for mutuality. *Developmental Psychology, 23,* 807–815.

Beardslee, W., Salt, P., Porterfield, K., Rothberg, P., van de Velde, P., Swatling, S., Hoke, L., Moilanen, D., & Wheelock, I. (1993). Comparison of preventive interventions for families with parental affective disorder. *Journal of the American Academy of Child and Adolescent Psychiatry, 32,* 254–263.

Billings, A., & Moos, R. (1983). Comparisons of children of depressed and nondepressed parents: A social–environmental perspective. *Journal of Abnormal Child Psychology, 11,* 463–485.

Billings, A., & Moos, R. (1984). Coping, stress, and social resources among adults with unipolar depression. *Journal of Personality and Social Psychology, 46,* 877–891.

Billings, A. G., & Moos, R. H. (1985). Children of parents with unipolar depression: A controlled 1-year follow-up. *Journal of Abnormal Child Psychology, 14,* 149–166.

Blazer, D., Kessler, R., McGonagle, K., & Swartz, M. (1994). The prevalence and distribution of major depression in a national community sample: The National Comorbidity Survey. *American Journal of Psychiatry, 151,* 979–986.

Bowlby, J. (1969). *Attachment and loss: Vol. I. Attachment.* New York: Basic Books.

Bowlby, J. (1980). *Loss: Sadness and depression.* New York: Basic Books.

Breslau, N., Davis, G., & Prabucki, K. (1988). Depressed mothers as informants in family history research: Are they accurate? *Psychiatry Research, 24,* 345–359.

Breznitz Z., & Sherman, T. (1987). Speech patterning of natural discourse of well and depressed mothers and their young children. *Child Development, 58,* 395–400.

Broadhead, W., Blazer, D., George, L., & Tse, C. (1990). Depression, disability days, and days lost from work in a prospective epidemiologic survey. *Journal of the American Medical Association, 264,* 2524–2528.

Burge, D., & Hammen, C. (1991). Maternal communication: Predictors of outcome at follow-up in a sample of children at high and low risk for depression. *Journal of Abnormal Psychology, 100,* 174–180.

Cohler, B. J., Grunebaum, H. U., Weiss, J. L., Hartmen, C. R., & Gallant, D. H. (1977). Child care attitudes and adaptation to the maternal role among mentally ill and well mothers. *American Journal of Orthopsychiatry, 46,* 123–133.

Cohn, J., & Campbell, S. (1992). Influence of maternal depression on infant affect regulation. In D. Cicchetti & S. Toth (Eds.), *Rochester Symposium on Developmental Psychopathology. Vol. 4: A developmental approach to affective disorders* pp. 103–130). Rochester, NY: University of Rochester Press.

Cohn, J. F., Matias, R., Tronick, E., Connell, D., & Lyons-Ruth, K. (1986). Face-to-face interactions of depressed mothers and their infants. In E. Tronick & T. Field (Eds.), *Maternal depression and infant disturbance (New Directions for Child Development,* No. 34, pp. 31–46). San Francisco: Jossey-Bass.

Cole, P., & Zahn-Waxler, C. (1992). Emotional dysregulation in disruptive behavior disorders. In D. Cicchetti & S. Toth (Eds.), *Rochester Symposium on Developmental Psychopathology. Vol. 4: Developmental perspectives on depression* (pp. 173–209). Rochester, NY: University of Rochester Press.

Conrad, M., & Hammen, C. (1989). Role of maternal depression in perceptions of child maladjustment. *Journal of Consulting and Clinical Psychology, 57,* 663–667.

Conrad, M., & Hammen, C. (1993). Protective and resource factors in high- and low-risk children: A comparison of children with unipolar, bipolar, medically ill, and normal mothers. *Developmental Psychopathology, 5,* 593–607.

Cox, A., Puckering, C., Pound, A., & Mills, M. (1987). The impact of maternal depression in young children. *Journal of Child Psychology and Psychiatry, 28,* 917–928.

Coyne, J. C., Kessler, R. C., Tal, M., Turnbull, J., Wortman, C. B., & Greden, G. F. (1987). Living with a depressed person. *Journal of Consulting and Clinical Psychology, 55,* 347–352.

Cross-National Collaborative Group. (1992). The changing rate of major depression. Cross-national comparisons. *Journal of the American Medical Association, 268,* 3098–3105.

Cummings, E. M., & Cicchetti, D. (1990). Toward a transactional model of relations between attachment and depression. In M. Greenberg, D. Cicchetti, & E. M. Cummings (Eds.), *Attachment in the preschool years: Theory, research, and intervention* (pp. 339–372). Chicago: University of Chicago Press.

Cummings, E. M., & Davies, P. (1994). Maternal depression and child development. *Journal of Child Psychology and Psychiatry, 35,* 73–112.

Cummings, E., & Zahn-Waxler, C. (1992). Emotions and the socialization of aggression: Adults' angry behavior and children's arousal and aggression. In A. Fraczek & H. Zumkley (Eds.), *Socialization and aggression* (pp. 61–84). New York and Heidelberg: Springer.

DeMulder, E. K., & Radke-Yarrow, M. (1991). Attachment with affectively ill and well mothers: Concurrent behavioral correlates. *Development and Psychopathology, 3,* 227–242.

Depue, T. A., & Monroe, S. M. (1986). Conceptualization and measurement of human disorder and life stress research: The problem of chronic disturbance. *Psychological Bulletin, 99,* 36–51.

Downey, G., & Coyne, J. (1990). Children of depressed parents: An integrative review. *Psychological Bulletin, 108,* 50–76.

Emery, R., Weintraub, S., & Neale, J. (1982). Effects of marital discord on the school behavior of children of schizophrenia, affectively disordered, and normal parents. *Journal of Abnormal Child Psychology, 10,* 215–228.

Fendrich, M., Warner, V., & Weissman, M. M. (1990). Family risk factors, parental depression, and psychopathology in offspring. *Developmental Psychology, 26,* 40–50.

Field, T. (1984). Early interactions between infants and their postpartum depressed mothers. *Infant Behavior and Development, 7,* 517–522.

Field, T., Healy, B., Goldstein, S., & Guthertz, M. (1990). Behavior–state matching and synchrony in mother–infant interactions of nondepressed versus depressed dyads. *Developmental Psychology, 26,* 7–14.

Fleming, A., Ruble, D., Flett, G., & Shaul, D. (1988). Postpartum adjustment in first-time mothers: Relations between mood, maternal attitudes, and mother–infant interactions. *Developmental Psychology, 24,* 71–81.

Forehand, R., Lautenschlager, G. J., Faust, J., & Graziano, W. G. (1986). Parent perceptions and parent–child interactions in clinic-referred children: A preliminary investigation of the effects of maternal depressive moods. *Behaviour Research and Therapy, 24,* 73–75.

Gaensbauer, T. J., Harmon, R. J., Cytryn, L., & McKnew, D. H. (1984). Social and affective development in infants with a manic–depressive parent. *American Journal of Psychiatry, 141,* 223–229.

Gelfand, D. M., & Teti, D. M. (1990). The effects of maternal depression on children. *Clinical Psychology Review, 10,* 320–354.

Gelfand, D., Teti, D., & Fox, C. (1992). Sources of parenting stress for depressed and nondepressed mothers of infants. *Journal of Clinical Child Psychology, 21,* 262–272.

Goodman, S. H., & Brumley, H. E. (1990). Schizophrenic and depressed mothers: Relational deficits in parenting. *Developmental Psychology, 26,* 31–39.

Gordon, D., Burge, D., Hammen, C., Adrian, C., Jaenicke, C., & Hiroto, D. (1989). Observations of interactions of depressed women with their children. *American Journal of Psychiatry, 146,* 50–55.

Gotlib, I. H., & Hammen, C. L. (1992). *Psychological aspects of depression: Toward a cognitive–interpersonal integration.* London: Wiley.

Hammen, C. (1991a). *Depression runs in families: The social context of risk and resilience in children of depressed mothers.* New York: Springer-Verlag.

Hammen, C. (1991b). The generation of stress in the course of unipolar depression. *Journal of Abnormal Psychology, 100,* 555–561.

Hammen, C., Adrian, C., Gordon, D., Burge, D., Jaenicke, C., & Hiroto, D. (1987). Children of depressed mothers: Maternal strain and symptom predictors of dysfunction. *Journal of Abnormal Psychology, 96,* 190–198.

Hammen, C., Adrian, C., & Hiroto, D. (1988). A longitudinal test of the attributional vulnerability model in children at risk for depression. *British Journal of Clinical Psychology, 27,* 37–46.

Hammen, C., Burge, D., & Adrian, C. (1991). Timing of mother and child depression in a longitudinal study of children at risk. *Journal of Consulting and Clinical Psychology, 59,* 341–345.

Hammen, C., Burge, D., Burney, E., & Adrian, C. (1990). Longitudinal study of diagnoses in children of women with unipolar and bipolar affective disorder. *Archives of General Psychiatry, 47,* 1112–1117.

Hetherington, E. M., Stanley-Hagen, M., & Anderson, E. (1989). Marital transitions: A child's perspective. *American Psychologist, 44,* 303–312.

Hirsch, B., Moos, R., & Reischl, T. (1985). Psychosocial adjustment of adolescent children of a depressed, arthritic, or normal parent. *Journal of Abnormal Psychology, 94,* 154–164.

Hokanson, J., Hummer, J., & Butler, A. (1991). Interpersonal perceptions by depressed college students. *Cognitive Therapy and Research, 15,* 443–457.

Hokanson, J., Rupert, M., Welker, R., Hollander, G., & Hedeen, C. (1989). Interpersonal concomitants and antecedents of depression among college students. *Journal of Abnormal Psychology, 98,* 209–217.

Holahan, C., & Moos, R. (1987). Risk, resistance, and psychological distress. A longitudinal analysis with adults and children. *Journal of Abnormal Psychology, 96,* 3–13.

Hops, H., Biglan, A., Sherman, L., Arthur, J., Friedman, L., & Osteen, V. (1987). Home observations of family interactions of depressed women. *Journal of Consulting and Clinical Psychology, 55,* 341–346.

Horwath, E., Johnson, J., Klerman, G., & Weissman, M. (1992). Depressive symptoms as relative and attributable risk factors for first-onset major depression. *Archives of General Psychiatry, 49,* 817–823.

Inoff-Germain, G., Nottelmann, E. D., & Radke-Yarrow, M. (1992). Evaluative communications between affectively ill and well mothers and their children. *Journal of Abnormal Child Psychology, 20,* 189–212.

Jaenicke, C., Hammen, C., Zupan, B., Hiroto, D., Gordon, D., Adrian, C., & Burge, D. (1987). Cognitive vulnerability in children at risk for depression. *Journal of Abnormal Child Psychology, 15,* 559–572.

Johnson, J., Weissman, M., & Klerman, G. (1992). Service utilization and social morbidity associated with depressive symptoms in the community. *Journal of the American Medical Association, 267,* 1478–1483.

Kaplan, B., Beardslee, W., & Keller, M. (1987). Intellectual competence in children of depressed parents. *Journal of Clinical Child Psychology, 16,* 158–163.

Keller, M. (1988). Diagnostic issues and clinical course of unipolar illness. In A. Frances & R. Hales

(Eds.), *American Psychiatric Pulse Review of Psychiatry,* Vol. 7 (pp. 188–212). Washington, D.C.: American Psychiatric Press, Inc.

Keller, M. B., Beardslee, W. R., Dorer, D. J., Lavori, P. W., Samuelson, H., & Klerman, G. R. (1986). Impact of severity and chronicity of parental affective illness on adaptive functioning and psychopathology in children. *Archives of General Psychiatry, 43,* 930–937.

Keller, M. B., Lavori, P. W., Rice, F., Coryell, W., & Hirschfeld, R. M. A. (1986). The persistent risk of chronicity in recurrent episodes of nonbipolar major depressive disorder: A prospective follow-up. *American Journal of Psychiatry, 143,* 24–28.

Kessler, R., McGonagle, K., Zhao, S., Nelson, C., Hughes, M., Eshleman, S., Wittchen, H.-U., & Kendler, K. (1994). Lifetime and 12-month prevalence of DSM-III-R psychiatric disorders in the United States: Results from the National Comorbidity Study. *Archives of General Psychiatry,, 51,* 8–19.

Klein, D., Clark, D., Dansky, L., & Margolis, E. (1988). Dysthymia in offspring of parents with primary unipolar affective disorder. *Journal of Abnormal Psychology, 97,* 265–274.

Klerman, G. L., Lavori, P. W., Rice, J., Reich, T., Endicott, J., Andreason, N. C., Keller, M. C., & Hirschfeld, R. M. A. (1985). Birth-cohort trends in rates of major depressive disorder among relatives of patients with affective disorder. *Archives of General Psychiatry, 42,* 689–695.

Kochanska, G., Kuczynski, L., Radke-Yarrow, M., & Welsh, J. D. (1987). Resolutions of control episodes between well and affectively ill mothers and their young children. *Journal of Abnormal Child Psychology, 15,* 441–456.

Lee, C., & Gotlib, I. (1991). Adjustment of children of depressed mothers: A 10-month follow-up. *Journal of Abnormal Psychology, 100,* 473–477.

Lewinsohn, P., Clark, G., Hops, H., & Andrews, J. (1990). Cognitive-behavioral treatment for depressed adolescents. *Behavior Therapy, 21,* 385–401.

Lewinsohn, P. M., Hoberman, H. M., & Rosenbaum, M. (1988). A prospective study of risk factors for unipolar depression. *Journal of Abnormal Psychology, 97,* 251–264.

Lewinsohn, P. M., Roberts, R. E., Seeley, J. R., Rohde, P., Gotlib, I. H., & Hops, H. (1994). Adolescent psychopathology: II. Psychosocial risk factors for depression. *Journal of Abnormal Psychology, 103,* 302–315.

Lyons-Ruth, K., Zoll, D., Connell, D., & Grunebaum, H. U. (1986). The depressed mother and her one-year-old infant: Environment, interaction, attachment, and infant development. In E. Tronick & T. Field (Eds.), *Maternal depression and infant disturbance* (*New Directions for Child Development, No. 34,* pp. 41–82). San Francisco: Jossey-Bass.

Mills, M., Puckering, C., Pound, A., & Cox, A. (1985). What is it about depressed mothers that influences their children's functioning? In J. E. Stevenson (Ed.), *Recent research in developmental psychopathology* (pp. 11–17). Oxford, England: Pergamon Press.

Murray, L. (1992). The impact of postnatal depression on infant development. *Journal of Child Psychology and Psychiatry, 33,* 543–561.

Nezu, A. (1987). A problem-solving formulation of depression: A literature review and proposal of a pluralistic model. *Clinical Psychology Review, 7,* 121–144.

Nolen-Hoeksema, S. (1990). *Sex differences in depression.* Stanford, CA: Stanford University Press.

Orvaschel, H., Walsh-Allis, G., & Ye, W. (1988). Psychopathology in children of parents with recurrent depression. *Journal of Abnormal Child Psychology, 16,* 17–28.

Orvaschel, H., Weissman, M. M., & Kidd, K. K. (1980). Children and depression: The children of depressed parents; the childhood of depressed patients; depression in children. *Journal of Affective Disorders, 2,* 1–16.

Panaccione, V. F., & Wahler, R. G. (1986). Child behavior, maternal depression, and social coercion as factors in the quality of child care. *Journal of Abnormal Child Psychology, 14,* 263–278.

Patterson, G. R. (1982). *Coercive family process.* Eugene, OR: Castalia Press.

Pound, A., Cox, A., Puckering, C., & Mills, M. (1985). The impact of maternal depression on young children. In J. E. Stevenson (Ed.), *Recent research in developmental psychopathology* (pp. 3–10). Oxford, England: Pergamon Press.

Radke-Yarrow, M., Cummings, E. M., Kuczynski, L., & Chapman, M. (1985). Patterns of attachment in two- and three-year-olds in normal families and families with parental depression. *Child Development, 56,* 884–893.

Radke-Yarrow, M., Richters, J., & Wilson, W. (1988). Child development in the network of relationships. In R. Hinde & J. Stevenson-Hinde (Eds.), *Relationships within families: Mutual influences* (pp. 48–67). Oxford, England: Clarendon Press.

Radke-Yarrow, M., & Sherman, T. (1990). Hard growing: Children who survive. In J. Rolf, A. Masten, D. Cicchetti, K. Nuechterlein, & S. Weintraub (Eds.), *Risk and protective factors in the development of psychopathology* (pp. 97–119). New York: Cambridge University Press.

Richters, J. E. (1987). Chronic versus episodic stress and the adjustment of high-risk offspring. In K. Hahlweg & M. J. Goldstein (Eds.), *Understanding major mental disorder: The contribution of family interaction research* (pp. 74–90). New York: Family Process Press.

Rutter, M. (1989). Intergenerational continuities and discontinuities in serious parenting difficulties. In D. Cicchetti & V. Carlson (Eds.), *Research on the consequences of child maltreatment* (pp. 317–348). New York: Cambridge University Press.

Rutter, M., & Quinton, P. (1984). Parental psychiatric disorder: Effects on children. *Psychological Medicine, 14,* 853–880.

Sameroff, A. J., Barocas, R., & Seifer, R. (1984). The early development of children born to mentally ill women. In N. Watt, E. J. Anthony, L. Wynne, & J. Rolf (Eds.), *Children at risk for schizophrenia* (pp. 482–514). New York: Cambridge University Press.

Sameroff, A. J., Seifer, R., & Zax, M. (1982). Early development of children at risk for emotional disorder. *Monographs of the Society for Research in Child Development, 47,* (7, Serial No. 199).

Seligman, M. E. P., Peterson, C., Kaslow, N. J., Tanenbaum, R. L., Alloy, L. B., & Abramson, L. Y. (1984). Attributional style and depressive symptoms among children. *Journal of Abnormal Psychology, 93,* 235–238.

Tarullo, L. B., DeMulder, E. K., Martinez, P. E., & Radke-Yarrow, M. (1994). Dialogues with preadolescents and adolescents: Mother–child interaction patterns in affectively ill and well dyads. *Journal of Abnormal Child Psychology, 22,* 33–51.

Warner, V., Weissman, M., Fendrich, M., Wickramaratne, P., & Moreau, D. (1992). The course of major depression in the offspring of depressed parents. *Archives of General Psychiatry, 49,* 795–801.

Webster-Stratton, C., & Hammond, M. (1988). Maternal depression and its relationship to life stress, perceptions of child behavior problems, parenting behaviors, and child conduct problems. *Journal of Abnormal Child Psychology, 16,* 299–315.

Weissman, M. (1988). Psychopathology in the children of depressed parents: Direct interview studies. In D. L. Dunner, E. S. Gershon, & J. E. Barrett (Eds.), *Relatives at risk for mental disorders* (pp. 143–159). New York: Raven Press.

Weissman, M., Gammon, G., John K., Merikangas, K., Warner, V., Prusoff, B., & Sholomskas, D. (1987). Children of depressed parents: Increased psychopathology and early onset of major depression. *Archives of General Psychiatry, 44,* 847–853.

Weissman, M. M., Paykel, E. S., & Klerman, G. L. (1972). The depressed woman as a mother. *Social Psychiatry, 7,* 98–108.

Wells, K., Burnam, M. A., Rogers, W., Hays, R., & Camp, P. (1992). The course of depression in adult outpatients: Results from the Medical Outcomes Study. *Archives of General Psychiatry, 49,* 788–794.

Wells, K., Stewart, A., Hays, R., Burnam, M. A., Rogers, W., Daniels, M., Berry, S., Greenfield, S., & Ware, J. (1989). The functioning and well-being of depressed patients: Results from the Medical Outcomes Study. *Journal of the American Medical Association, 262,* 914–919.

Whiffen, V., & Gotlib, I. (1989). Infants of postpartum depressed mothers: Temperament and cognitive status. *Journal of Abnormal Psychology, 98,* 274–279.

Zahn-Waxler, C., Cummings, E. M., Iannotti, R., & Radke-Yarrow, M. (1984). Young offspring of depressed parents: A population at risk for affective problems. *New Directions for Child Development, 26,* 81–105.

Zahn-Waxler, C., Cummings, E. M., McKnew, D., & Radke-Yarrow, M. (1984). Altruism aggression, and social interactions in young children with a manic–depressive parent. *Child Development, 55,* 112–122.

Zahn-Waxler, C., Iannotti, R. J., Cummings, E. M., & Denham, S. (1990). Antecedents of problem behaviors in children of depressed mothers. *Development and Psychopathology, 2,* 271–291.

Zahn-Waxler, C., McKnew, D., Cummings, E. M., Davenport, Y., & Radke-Yarrow, M. (1984). Problem behavior and peer interactions of young children with a manic–depressive parent. *American Journal of Psychiatry, 141,* 236–240.

6

Children's Adaptation to Divorce
From Description to Explanation

JOHN H. GRYCH and FRANK D. FINCHAM

Divorce has become a common experience for children in the United States, where one out of every two is likely to undergo a parental divorce before the age of 18 (see Emery, 1988; Furstenberg, 1990). The high divorce rate has been viewed with alarm by many because there long has been a perception that "broken" homes adversely affect children's adjustment. Early investigations of the effects of divorce on children appeared to support the idea that children from divorced homes were more poorly adjusted than those from intact families, but more recent investigations have gone beyond this simple comparison to investigate processes that lead to better or worse outcomes. In this chapter we examine research on children's adaptation to divorce. To provide a context for our analysis, we begin by summarizing the epidemiology of divorce in the United States and research on the effects of divorce on children. The bulk of the chapter then examines children's adaptation to divorce in relation to four important questions: What increases the stressfulness of divorce for children? What helps children cope more effectively? What interventions exist to facilitate children's adjustment after divorce? What do we still need to learn about children's adaptation after divorce?

WHO GETS DIVORCED?

The divorce rate has shown a steady increase over the course of the twentieth century, with a dip in the 1950s and more rapid increases occurring in the

JOHN H. GRYCH • Department of Psychology, Marquette University, Milwaukee, Wisconsin 53233.   FRANK D. FINCHAM • Department of Psychology, University of Wales, Cardiff CF1 3YG, Great Britain.

Handbook of Children's Coping: Linking Theory and Intervention, edited by Wolchik and Sandler. Plenum Press, New York, 1997.

1960s and 1970s (Cherlin, 1981). Some demographers report that the rate lev-
eled off in the 1980s, but others argue that it has continued to rise (see Castro
Martin & Bumpass, 1989). Estimates of the proportion of current marriages
likely to end in divorce vary from 50 to 66%, a rate considerably higher than
other Western cultures (see Furstenberg, 1990). However, not all couples are
equally likely to divorce. Several factors are associated with an increased probability that a marriage will end in divorce, including race, age at marriage,
whether the couple cohabited prior to marriage, family history of divorce,
education, and the presence and age of children (for a discussion, see Sweet &
Bumpass, 1992). Briefly, divorce rates are almost twice as high for black as for
white families (e.g., Castro Martin & Bumpass, 1989) and for individuals who
marry while in their teens (Norton & Glick, 1979), about 50% higher for couples
who lived together prior to marriage (Sweet & Bumpass, 1992), and about 25%
higher for individuals whose own parents were unmarried at their birth or were
separated prior to age 16. Higher education levels are correlated with lower
divorce rates, which is due in part to the tendency for more highly educated
individuals to marry later and to have been raised in intact families (Sweet &
Bumpass, 1992). Families with one or two children are less likely to divorce
than those without children or those with more than two children (Thornton,
1977). Rates also are lower in families with preschool children compared to
childless families or those with school-aged children (Waite, Haggstrom, &
Kanouse, 1985). Thus, the likelihood of a child experiencing a divorce depends
on a number of social and demographic factors.

Moreover, for many children, divorce marks the beginning of a series of
family transitions. Most adults who divorce later remarry, and thus many children also experience the stressful changes involved in forming a stepfamily.
Since second marriages are more likely to end in divorce than are first marriages (McCarthy, 1978; Castro Martin & Bumpass, 1989), some children will go
through more than one divorce before they reach age 18 (see Furstenberg,
1990). Given the instability of family life in the United States, it is particularly
important to clarify how marital dissolution affects children and to identify the
factors that increase or decrease its stressfulness.

WHAT ARE THE EFFECTS OF DIVORCE ON CHILDREN?

Although much of the research on children's adaptation to divorce has been
criticized on methodological grounds (for a discussion, see Emery, 1988; Kurdek,
1987), it consistently has shown that children from divorced families exhibit
greater maladjustment than children from intact families (for reviews, see Amato
& Keith, 1991; Emery, 1988; Grych & Fincham, 1992a). However, a meta-analysis
of 95 studies comparing children from divorced and intact families showed that
these differences are small, particularly in studies of greater methodological rigor
(Amato & Keith, 1991). The largest difference has been found for externalizing
problems (e.g., aggression, delinquency), with a mean effect size of $-.23$, indicating that the average externalizing score in divorced samples was about one
quarter of a standard deviation higher than in intact samples (Amato & Keith,
1991). Significant but smaller effects also have been found for academic achieve-

ment (mean effect size, −.16), social adjustment (mean effect size, −.12), self-concept (mean effect size, −.09), and internalizing problems such as depression and anxiety (mean effect size, −.08) (Amato & Keith, 1991).

An important question is whether the differences found between children from divorced and intact families are clinically significant. Several studies bear on this issue. For example, in a study of young adolescents who had experienced parental divorce 4 to 6 years earlier, Hetherington and colleagues (1992) found that approximately 20% of boys and 25–30% of girls exceeded the cutoff for clinical levels of behavior problems on the Child Behavior Checklist (Achenbach & Edelbrock, 1981), compared to approximately 10% of children from intact families. Evidence for the clinical significance of adjustment problems in these children is provided by studies showing higher rates of referral for mental health services (e.g., Guidubaldi, Perry, & Cleminshaw, 1984; Kalter & Rembar, 1981). For example, in a large nationally representative sample, 13% of children whose parents had divorced had seen a mental health professional compared to 5.5% of children from intact families. These data suggest that children from divorced families are at increased risk to develop clinical syndromes, but also indicate that the majority of these children do not evidence significant psychopathology.

One of the primary lessons to be learned from the vast body of research on children from divorced families is that there is considerable variation in their functioning and that many (perhaps most) are as well adjusted as their counterparts from intact families (Hetherington, 1988; Hetherington, Stanley-Hagen, & Anderson, 1989). This conclusion opens the door to a new set of questions focused on the processes that account for better or worse outcomes. Mean differences between groups mean very little; to gain a deeper understanding of how divorce affects children, we must go beyond group comparisons to investigate the time course, moderators, and mediators of children's adaptation after divorce. In the remainder of this section, we will review evidence on several factors that may be related to children's adjustment. First, we will examine children's functioning over time and then consider whether gender or age moderates the impact of divorce. Then, we turn our attention toward processes that may account for variability in postdivorce adaptations.

Children's Adaptation over Time

To better understand the impact of divorce on children, it is important to distinguish between short- and long-term effects. Unfortunately, most studies have been cross-sectional and have not specifically examined the length of time that parents have been separated. Other studies note the time elapsed since the final divorce but not the actual separation of the parents. The physical separation of the parents is a more accurate index of the breakup of the family than the legal divorce because of its salience for children. Many children can remember with exquisite detail the events that occurred the day their parents separated but have little or no awareness of when the divorce became final. Considering time since separation is critical to differentiate between children's reaction to the changes that typically occur with divorce (e.g., reduced contact with one parent, moving) from long-lasting effects of marital disruption.

It is common for children to experience sadness, anxiety, anger, sleep disturbances, and other symptoms in the months following a separation (e.g., Hetherington et al., 1989; Kelly, 1988; Wallerstein & Kelly, 1980). Bowlby (1973) used the term "acute distress syndrome" to describe children's reaction to being separated from an attachment figure for a prolonged period of time. He proposed that children first go through a protest phase in which feelings of anger and anxiety predominate, followed by a period of despair in which they exhibit depression, withdrawal, and passivity. Eventually children enter a detachment phase and appear to lose interest in the missing parent. Although Bowlby developed this theory after studying young children housed in residential nurseries in London in the 1940s and 1950s, parallels to children's experience with divorce are clear. An important difference, however, is that most children do not lose contact with the noncustodial parent, at least not right away, and thus many children may not go through a detachment phase. In fact, many children remain intensely connected to the noncustodial parent, to the point of idealizing that parent and fantasizing about living with the parent or the reunification of the whole family. Bowlby's work underscores the normalcy of short-term perturbations in adjustment following parental separation. Most children do not want their parents to divorce, even in highly conflictual families (Kurdek, 1986), and these symptoms are expectable reactions to a stressful event that do not necessarily portend continuing problems in adaptation. How and why some children develop long-term adjustment problems is a critical question for the field, and is best addressed by longitudinal research.

One of the most detailed longitudinal investigations of children's adaptation to divorce was conducted with a sample of preadolescent children by Hetherington and colleagues (Hetherington, 1989; Hetherington et al., 1989; Hetherington, Cox, & Cox, 1982). They found that the first 1 to 2 years after divorce were marked by behavioral and emotional disturbances for both boys and girls. Children who experienced a divorce were more oppositional, did more poorly in school, and had difficulties getting along with peers. After this "crisis" period abated, however, adjustment problems tended to decline, especially for girls. In fact, after 2 years, girls from divorced families were largely indistinguishable from girls living in intact families (Hetherington et al., 1982). Though the group differences were less marked for boys after this 2-year period, those from divorced families continued to exhibit elevated levels of behavior problems. More recent investigations indicate that the differences between children from intact and divorced families are maintained for several years after the divorce (Cherlin et al., 1991; Hetherington et al., 1992; Peterson & Zill, 1986). For example, Hetherington and colleagues (1992) found that young adolescents (average age 11.5 years) whose parents had divorced 4 to 6 years earlier (and separated 6–8 years earlier) showed considerable stability in internalizing and externalizing problems and social and academic competence, with test–retest correlations ranging from .38 to .80 over 2 years. In contrast to their earlier work, both boys and girls showed greater maladjustment than their counterparts from intact families.

Whether the experience of parental divorce continues to affect individuals into adulthood is an interesting but relatively unexplored question. Differences have been found in educational attainment, with children from divorced families doing more poorly than those from intact families, even after controlling for variables such as socioeconomic status and race (Krein & Beller, 1988). The source of this difference is unclear, however (see Furstenberg, 1990). As noted above, individuals whose parents divorce are more likely to get divorced themselves (Sweet & Bumpass, 1992), which may reflect difficulties in developing satisfying interpersonal relationships or simply a greater tendency to see divorce as a viable option when marital difficulties arise. There also is some evidence that girls may exhibit so-called "sleeper effects" in the form of earlier sexual activity or difficulties with romantic relations in adolescence and early adulthood. For example, Wallerstein and Blakesee (1989) reported that young women whose parents had divorced indicated that they had difficulties forming committed emotional relationships. However, the lack of a comparison group in Wallerstein's well-known work makes it difficult to interpret the observations made in this research. Finally, college-aged men and women from divorced families reported more frequent dating, sexual activity, and cohabitation (Booth, Binkerhoff, & White, 1984). Thus, it appears that experiencing divorce in childhood affects later relationships, but the mechanism by which this occurs is not clear. It is possible that divorce shapes children's attitudes, expectations, or "working models" about close relationships, which in turn influence their behavior in these relationships, but this issue has only recently become a focus of study and has not yet generated a systematic body of data (see Hazan & Shaver, 1992).

Gender

More favorable outcomes for girls than boys from divorced families have been reported frequently in research on divorce (see Zaslow, 1988, 1989). However, recent studies have found little evidence of gender differences in children's adjustment after divorce (e.g., Allison & Furstenberg, 1989) and Amato and Keith's (1991) meta-analysis failed to document sex differences on all adjustment problems except social adjustment, where boys evidenced more negative effects than girls. It also has been argued that the type of custody arrangement may be important in determining whether divorce affects boys and girls differently. Specifically, boys show fewer behavior problems than girls when their father has primary custody, which suggests that children adapt better when placed with the same sex parent (e.g., Camara & Resnick, 1988; Peterson & Zill, 1986, Santrock & Warshak, 1979). However, caution should be exercised in generalizing these results to divorced families as a whole because fathers who have primary custody tend to have higher incomes, education levels, and a spouse with psychological difficulties (Emery, 1988).

Although the existence of gender differences in adjustment is questionable, there is evidence that boys and girls interact differently with their parents after divorce. For example, custodial mothers have more conflict with preadolescent boys than girls (Hetherington et al., 1982), whereas custodial fathers are less likely to become involved in coercive exchanges with their sons (Emery, Hetherington, & DiLalla, 1984). Differences in mothers' relationships with their sons and daughters appear to decrease as the children reach adolescence, when the level of mother–daughter conflict increases to match that between mothers and their sons (Hetherington et al., 1992). Whether these differences in parent–child relationships affect children's global adjustment remains an open question.

Age

Children's age at the time of divorce also has been examined as a potential moderator of adjustment. It has been argued that younger children are particularly vulnerable to the effects of divorce due to their stage of personality (e.g., Meissner, 1978) or cognitive (e.g., Wallerstein & Kelly, 1980) development. However, the data on age as a moderating factor have been inconsistent. Some studies have reported more adverse effects on younger children (e.g., Allison & Furstenberg, 1989; Kalter & Rembar, 1981), but others have failed to find age differences in behavioral or emotional problems (Guidubaldi, Perry, & Nastasi, 1987; Stolberg, Camplair, Currier, & Wells, 1987). In their meta-analysis, Amato and Keith (1991) found roughly equal effect sizes in preschool-, elementary-, and high school-aged samples for measures of academic achievement, conduct, and psychological adjustment problems; however, because of a small number of studies involving preschoolers, the effects for this age group were not significant. Elementary school-aged children evidenced the strongest deficits in social adjustment and high school students showed the greatest deficit in self-concept. In general, college students exhibited the best adjustment. In sum, there is no clear evidence that a child's age makes him or her particularly vulnerable to the effects of divorce.

The variability found in children's long-term adjustment raises important questions about the mechanisms by which divorce affects children. This issue is made even more salient by studies that have assessed children prior to the divorce. These studies indicate that children in to-be-divorced families exhibit poorer adjustment than children in families whose parents stay together even years before the separation (Block, Block, & Gjerde, 1986; Cherlin et al., 1991; but see Shaw, Emery, & Tuer, 1993, for contrasting results). For example, using large samples in Great Britain and the United States, Cherlin et al. (1991) found that boys from divorced families exhibited more behavior problems than children from intact families. However, these differences decreased when children's predivorce functioning was controlled, and became nonsignificant when measures of family dysfunction prior to the divorce were taken into account. Results were somewhat different for girls. In the British sample, girls from divorced families also showed more maladjustment than girls from intact families, but these differences did not disappear entirely when predivorce child and family functioning were controlled. In contrast, the adjustment of girls from divorced families in the United States was not significantly different from those in intact families.

The fact that some children show no long-term ill effects of divorce whereas others exhibit adjustment problems before and after the separation underscores the idea that divorce is not a unitary event but rather a multifaceted process that may begin years prior to the physical separation and continue for years after. Divorce has been viewed from a transitional events perspective in which its effects are considered a function of the stressors that occur during the process of marital dissolution and the coping resources available to the child (Felner, Terre, & Rowlison, 1988). Examining which aspects of this process are most closely linked to children's adjustment provides a promising approach to understanding how marital dissolution adversely affects children. In the next section we discuss research on the factors likely to increase the stressfulness of the divorce and then examine factors that promote healthy adaptation.

WHAT IS MOST STRESSFUL ABOUT DIVORCE?

Adopting the perspective that the divorce process begins well before parents separate focuses attention on changes that occur in the family as marital dissatisfaction develops or increases. Separation typically occurs only after months or years of marital discord and does not always serve to end it, and it has been argued that interparental conflict, rather than divorce, best accounts for adjustment difficulties in children (e.g., Emery, 1982). Divorce also sets in motion a series of life changes that can adversely impact both parents and children. Changes in residence, contact with parents, and economic status provide additional stress that may continue to affect children years after the divorce is final.

To assess children's perspective on what is most stressful about divorce, Wolchik, Sandler, Braver, and Fogas (1989) surveyed 11- to 15-year-old children whose parents had divorced within the previous 30 months (mean, 14.6 months) and had them rate the stressfulness of a variety of events that may occur after a divorce. The event rated as most stressful was being blamed by the parents for the divorce. The next two most stressful events had to do with interparental conflict: specifically, parents hitting or hurting each other and parents arguing in front of the child. The next four events all involve children hearing negative things about one or both parents, either from the other parent, relatives, or neighbors. Other highly rated events centered around children's interactions with their parents, such as their mother or father getting mad at them and the noncustodial parent moving out of town, and changes in the child's day-to-day life, including giving up pets or other things they like and making fewer friends. Children's self-report of the most stressful aspects of divorce thus overlaps with the focus of empirical research on interparental conflict, parent–child relationships, and changes in lifestyle. We address each of these in turn.

Interparental Conflict

A large number of studies have indicated that the level of marital conflict present before and after the divorce is a better predictor of children's adjustment than is parents' marital status (e.g., Hetherington et al., 1982; Long, Forehand, Fauber, & Brody, 1987; Shaw et al., 1993). For example, Hetherington et al. (1982) found that decreased conflict after divorce was associated with decreased externalizing behavior in boys; in fact, boys from low-conflict divorced families exhibited lower levels of behavior problems than children in highly conflictual intact families. However, even though an association between marital conflict and child adjustment has been well documented (for reviews, see Cummings & Davies, 1994; Grych & Fincham, 1990), the process by which conflict affects children is not known and a causal relation between the two constructs has not been documented (Fincham, Grych, & Osborne, 1994).

Research in this area has turned from investigating whether marital conflict is related to child adjustment to investigating how it affects children. It has been argued that marital conflict has only indirect effects on children by adversely affecting parenting or parent–child relations (Fauber & Long, 1991). Some studies support this view (e.g., Fauber, Forehand, Thomas, & Wierson, 1990; Johnston, Kline, & Wallerstein, 1989), whereas others indicate that marital conflict also has independent effects (e.g., Jenkins & Smith, 1990; Peterson & Zill, 1986). Marital quality and parenting clearly are interrelated (e.g., Cox, Owen, Lewis, & Henderson, 1989; Easterbrooks & Emde, 1988; Fauber et al., 1990; Hetherington et al., 1992) and examining either factor in isolation necessarily is an oversimplification of a complex system. However, considering the direct or immediate effects of marital conflict on children is useful for illustrating how discord between parents contributes to the stressfulness of divorce for children.

Witnessing conflict between parents (Cummings, Zahn-Waxler, & Radke-Yarrow, 1981) and even between strangers (Cummings, Ballard, El-Sheikh, & Lake, 1991) can cause emotional distress in children from toddlerhood through adolescence (Cummings & Davies, 1994). However, children's response to conflict depends on how it is expressed. Conflict that is aggressive (e.g., Cummings et al., 1989; Grych & Fincham, 1993), child-related (Grych & Fincham, 1993), and poorly resolved (Cummings et al., 1989, 1991) is more upsetting than conflict that is expressed without animosity, concerns a topic unrelated to the child, and is resolved by the parties involved. Interparental conflict is not invariably disturbing for children; its impact appears to depend on whether it is perceived to threaten their sense of well-being (see Davies & Cummings, 1994; Grych & Fincham, 1990). Conflict occurring in the context of divorce is likely to be particularly stressful for children for at least two reasons. First, parents unhappy enough to end their marriage can become embroiled in precisely the kind of conflicts that are most distressing to children: hostile, unresolved, and child-related (e.g., custody). Second, family harmony and stability is integral to a sense of security and well-being for most children, and so conflict associated with divorce should be particularly threatening.

Since marital conflict can be a significant stressor for children, divorce has the potential to improve children's well-being by eliminating this stressor from their lives. Viewed this way, it may be better to break up "for the children's sake" than to stay together for that reason. Unfortunately, divorce does not always bring marital conflict to an end. Parents often continue to fight old battles in new arenas. Postdivorce conflict often revolves around issues such as child support payments, child custody, and visitation arrangements; consequently, continuing hostilities between ex-spouses are particularly likely to be expressed through the link that still unites them, namely, the children. This is especially disconcerting in light of evidence indicating that conflict involving children or parenting issues may be particularly problematic for children. Recent research indicates that children are more likely to blame themselves when the topic of a conflict concerns them (Grych & Fincham, 1993) and that self-blame for parental conflict correlates significantly with child reports of internalizing problems after controlling for the frequency, intensity, and resolution of conflict (Grych, Seid, & Fincham, 1992). Camara (Camara & Resnick, 1989; Hess & Camara, 1979) provides additional support for this idea in showing that children's postdivorce adaptation was predicted by parents' level of agreement about childrearing issues and how they resolved their conflicts but not by the amount of interparental conflict that did not concern the child.

A related way in which continued postdivorce hostilities may adversely affect children is by putting them in a situation where they feel torn between their parents. Children's loyalty and devotion to each parent may be threatened when they are asked to pass on information about one parent to another, hear disparaging remarks about one parent from the other, or receive pressure to side with one parent against the other. Feeling "caught in the middle" between parents has been identified as an important predictor of children's postdivorce adaptation (Buchanan, Maccoby, & Dornbusch, 1991; Johnston, Kline, & Tschann, 1989). Buchanan and colleagues (1991) found that adolescents were more likely to feel caught in the middle when cooperative communication between parents was low and conflict was high. In turn, feeling caught in the middle was associated with greater self-reported depression, anxiety, and deviant behavior. Similarly, in a sample of couples in conflict over custody arrangements, Johnston et al. (1989) found that the effects of interparental aggression on child behavior were mediated by children's experience of being drawn into parental conflicts. Thus, the important factor may not be simply the occurrence of conflict but the extent to which it involves children or creates loyalty conflicts for them. This possibility illustrates the interconnectedness of the marital and parent–child relationships, and we turn next to examine the role of parent–child interaction in divorced families in greater detail.

Parent–Child Relationships

Links between marital discord and parenting have been well documented in intact families (e.g., Cox et al., 1989; Easterbrooks & Emde, 1988; Goldberg & Easterbrooks, 1984; Stoneman, Brody, & Burke, 1989). The strain of tension and conflict in the marriage may reduce parents' capacity to be available and responsive to their children, and differences between parents in childrearing attitudes may be accentuated, resulting in inconsistencies in discipline and increased potential for parent–child conflict. Whether or not difficulties in parent–child relationships exist before the divorce, they are common in the period after separation as both parents and children adapt to changes in the structure of the family. One of the most salient and significant changes is reduced contact with one parent. Although the last decade witnessed increased shared custody, the vast majority of children continue to reside with one parent, usually their mother. Even in states that emphasize shared custody, it is estimated that 80–85% of children reside primarily with one parent (Emery, 1994). The relationship between the custodial parent and child also changes as parental and child roles and responsibilities change. Some of these changes may be positive, whereas others may be a significant source of stress. In the remainder of this section, we first address how separation from the noncustodial parent may affect children and then discuss changes in children's relationship with their custodial parent.

The first question to be addressed concerns fathers' involvement in their children's lives after divorce. Do children really lose a parent when a divorce occurs? Using the National Survey of Children (NSC), Furstenberg and Nord (1985) provide sobering data on this issue by showing that the degree of contact between children and noncustodial fathers drops off dramatically in the years following the separation. For example, they reported that almost half of children in families divorced for less than 2 years saw their fathers at least four times in a typical month compared to 25% of children whose parents divorced 2 to 9 years prior and only 13% whose parents had divorced over 10 years prior. Three quarters of the children in the last group do not see their fathers at all in a typical month (compared to 31% whose parents divorced within 2 years). Noncustodial mothers tend to maintain more frequent contact with their children and, by definition, children in joint physical custody have more contact with both parents, but the percentage of children in these two groups is quite small. Whereas some fathers maintain a vital involvement in their children's lives, the most common experience for children whose parents divorce is gradual loss of contact with their fathers. However, it is notable that half of the children in the NSC still considered their fathers to be members of the family (Furstenberg & Nord, 1985).

The impact of decreased contact with their fathers is difficult to evaluate. A number of studies have failed to find a relationship between frequency of contact with the noncustodial parent and child adjustment (e.g., Furstenberg, Morgan, & Allison, 1987; Kurdek, Blisk, & Siesky, 1981; Luepnitz, 1982), whereas others have shown a positive effect of more frequent visitation on children's functioning, provided that the father is emotionally stable and interparental conflict is not extreme (Hetherington et al., 1982; Wallerstein & Kelly, 1980). Perhaps more important than how often children see their fathers is the nature of their relationship with their father. Surprisingly, however, research examining the association between the quality of children's relationship with the noncustodial parent and their adjustment is rare. Thomas and Forehand (1993) recently reported a significant association between fathers' reports of positive parent–child interactions and teacher reports of lower levels of anxiety/withdrawal and conduct problems in a sample of adolescents whose parents had been divorced an average of 12 months. In contrast, frequency of visitation was not related to child adjustment. Brody and Forehand (1990) also reported positive associations between male adolescents' relationship with their fathers and internalizing (but not externalizing) problems. For both boys and girls the nature of the relationship interacted with degree of interparental conflict: Internalizing problems were highest when conflict was high and relationships with the noncustodial parent were poor, but were reduced by either a positive father–adolescent relationship or lower conflict. Although the quality of the relationship between the noncustodial parent and child appears to be more important for children's adaptation than the quantity of time spent together, quantity is not irrelevant. Maintaining a relationship requires time and consequently frequency of contact may be best understood as necessary but not sufficient for good parent–child relationships after divorce.

Children's relationships with their custodial parent have received much more attention in the literature. This research has suggested that the time following divorce is one of "diminished parenting" in which overburdened, emotionally drained parents can become "temporarily erratic, uncommunicative, nonsupportive, and inconsistently punitive in dealing with their children" (Hetherington et al., 1992). Unfortunately, this is a time when children are in particular need of comfort, consolation, and consistency from their parents, and so the lack of emotional support can exacerbate an already stressful situation. Hetherington and colleagues (1982, 1992) closely examined mother–child relationships in both preadolescent and adolescent samples. Particularly in the first year following divorce, custodial mothers of preadolescents had difficulty controlling and monitoring their children, especially boys, and expressed fewer demands for mature behavior, poorer communication, and less affection. Coercive cycles developed between mothers and sons in which mother's attempts at control or discipline were met by an escalation of noncompliant behavior. Boys received less positive reinforcement than girls and more commands, both positive and negative. The direction of effects is difficult to untangle here, because, as discussed above, girls were better behaved and thus presented less of a challenge to the mother. By 2 years postdivorce, mothers exhibited better communication, consistency, nurturance, and control over their children. Conflict with boys continued to be more frequent than with girls; in fact, divorced mothers and their daughters often formed close relationships.

More recently, the nature of relationships between adolescents and their custodial mothers was investigated (Hetherington et al., 1992), with a somewhat different pattern of results emerging. Compared to nondivorced families, mothers and adolescents engaged in more activities together but also exhibited higher levels of conflict, negativity, and punishment. More difficulties existed with sons than daughters when the children were between 9 and 13 years, but 2 years later few gender differences remained; when they did occur they were in the direction of greater positivity, monitoring, and control with daughters than with sons. Interestingly, compared to those in intact families, adolescents in single-parent homes rated their mothers as warmer and more involved with them but also more negative and coercive. It may be that mothers' relationships with their children become more intense, in positive and negative ways, when they are the sole parent in the household.

Even though existing research underscores the difficulties faced by parents and children after divorce, it should be noted that deterioration in parent–child relationships is not inevitable. Hetherington et al. (1982) found that 25% of fathers and 50% of mothers reported that their relationships with their children improved after the divorce. Clearly, parenting alone during a stressful time is a challenge, and both parents and children experience difficulties as they make the transition to a new living situation. Other factors, such as the amount of change and support families experience may play important moderating roles in this process.

Environmental Changes

Divorce can lead to a number of other changes, large and small, in children's lives. Major changes, such as moving to a new residence, obviously are stressful, but smaller changes in daily routines may also be significant. Experiencing more negative changes tends to be associated with poorer adjustment. For example, Sandler, Wolchik, Braver, and Fogas (1991) found that an increase in negative events was correlated with children's adjustment, but that the continued occurrence of "old" negative events was not. The occurrence of positive stable events seemed to reduce stress and was related to lower levels of maladjustment. Sandler et al. concluded that the combination of experiencing an increased number of negative events and a decreased number of positive events was most highly associated with children's self-reported adjustment problems. This "change for the worse" index did not correlate with parent reports of adjustment, however, suggesting that children's subjective experience of the events may be more important than their occurrence per se. Other studies also have documented a correlation between negative life events and poorer adjustment (Sandler, Wolchik, & Braver, 1988; Stolberg & Anker, 1983; Walsh & Stolberg, 1989). These studies typically examine only the total number of events that occur, and so it is not known if certain changes may be associated with certain problems (e.g., moving with peer difficulties).

The one type of change that occurs to many children that has been studied directly is the loss of income that many custodial mothers experience. Almost half of women have their total family income cut by 50% 1 year after the divorce, and therefore there is considerably less money available for raising the children (Duncan & Hoffman, 1985). Black women and white women whose predivorce income was below the median are hit especially hard: About 40% of the children in these families are living below the poverty line 1 year following the divorce. Compared to married women, single mothers remain economically disadvantaged and their financial situation often improves only with remarriage (Furstenberg, 1990). Although child support and spousal maintenance are intended to redress this imbalance, they often are paid in part or not at all (Weitzman, 1985).

The effects of economic disadvantage on children are broad and will not be reviewed here. Generally, less money is likely to mean poorer housing in a poorer neighborhood, poorer schooling, and poorer quality day care. Moving also may mean losing contact with friends and other individuals who could have provided help and support. The power of economic disadvantage is illustrated by the finding in one study that many of the differences between children from divorced and intact families disappeared when family income level was accounted for (Guidubaldi et al., 1984).

All of these factors—interparental conflict, parent–child difficulties, environmental changes, economic hardship—serve to increase the stress experienced by children whose parents divorce. In a recent review of proposed mediators of postdivorce adjustment, Amato (1993) concluded that interparental conflict has received the strongest empirical support but that no single factor can fully account for the data on child outcomes. In fact, focusing solely on risk factors will provide an incomplete understanding of why some children are more poorly adjusted than others after divorce. It is equally important to examine factors that protect children from the ill effects associated with divorce or enhance their functioning. Although many children from divorced families adapt successfully, research on the processes that lead to good outcomes is relatively sparse. In the next section, we attempt to flesh out the picture of children's adaptation to divorce by examining factors that appear to facilitate good adjustment.

WHAT FACILITATES HEALTHY ADAPTATION?

Work on psychological resiliency in children has identified three classes of variables that appear to protect children in vulnerable or stressful situations (see Garmezy, 1983): personal characteristics (e.g., self-esteem), family support, and supportive social organizations (e.g., schools). Of these factors, the role of support from parents and other family members in promoting children's adaptation to divorce has received the most attention by researchers. Although interventions for children from divorced families often target their cognitions and coping strategies, there is little basic research documenting how these individual factors relate to postdivorce adjustment, and even less on schools or other social organizations.

Social Support

By its very nature, divorce threatens children's relationships with important people in their lives. Separation may sharply reduce their contact with one parent, and, as noted above, marital discord can lead to negative changes in parents' interactions with their children. It seems logical that the presence of supportive individuals would be particularly important for children going through a divorce. Parents may be the most important source for such support, but children also may find attention, caring, and comfort from others, including relatives, nonfamilial adults (e.g., neighbors, teachers), siblings, and peers. Few studies, however, have examined the influence of supportive others on children's postdivorce adaptation. Most have focused on parents as sources of support, and consequently less is known about how other adults and children may help children cope with divorce. We review what is known about the effects of social support by considering the different sources of support that have been investigated: parents, siblings, other relatives, adults outside of the family, and peers.

Before turning to this research, it is helpful to consider how support from others might relate to children's functioning during and after divorce. Theory and research on coping suggests two ways that social support may facilitate coping with the stress of divorce. The first proposes that involvement with supportive others will have a general, positive "main effect" on children's adjustment. That is, receiving support from others improves children's adaptation regardless of the level of stress that they are experiencing. The alternative model posits that support will have a positive effect when children are experiencing a high level of stress but will not be related to adjustment when stress is low (Cohen & Wills, 1985). This buffering hypothesis thus predicts a moderating role or interaction effect for social support.

A second issue to consider in examining social support is the function(s) it serves. What do other people do that is helpful during a time of stress? In developing a measure to assess children's level of social support, Wolchik and colleagues (1989) described five functions that support can fulfill: recreation, advice, provision of goods/services, emotional support, and positive feedback. Depending on their age and relationship to the child, different individuals will be more or less likely to provide each function, and this scheme presents a useful framework for understanding how the groups reviewed below can be a help to children whose parents divorce.

Parents

As discussed above, children's relationships with parents have been shown to play an important role in mediating their adaptation to divorce. Given that the divorce threatens a child's bond with an attachment figure, there is likely to be no adequate substitute for consistent support from parents. Indeed, warm, supportive relationships with parents are consistently associated with better postdivorce adjustment (Camara & Resnick, 1988; Hess & Camara, 1979; Hetherington et al., 1982; Peterson & Zill, 1986). Maintaining good relationships with both parents clearly is associated with better outcomes, but whether a supportive relationship with only one parent is sufficient to reduce the stressful effects of divorce is less certain.

Research on this issue has produced inconsistent findings. For example, Hetherington and colleagues (1982) found a positive effect of one good parent–child relationship only if it was with the custodial parent and only if it was rated as very good rather than moderately good. In contrast, Camara and Resnick (1987) reported that a warm, affectionate, and close relationship with the noncustodial parent attenuated most of the effects of having a negative relationship with the custodial parent. Finally, Hess and Camara (1979) found that a positive affective relationship with either parent was related to better social interaction with peers and academic performance and lower stress and aggression than poor relationships with both parents.

One possible explanation for these discrepant results involves the amount of time children spent with their noncustodial parent. In Hetherington's sample, some of the children had little or no contact with their fathers, whereas children in Hess and Camara's research had more frequent contact. Children who do not see their fathers very often are unlikely to profit much from having good relationships with them. Since noncustodial mothers tend to stay in closer contact with their children, it may be expected that support from noncustodial mothers is more highly related to child adjustment than is father support. However, when noncustodial parents are involved, they may well play an important role in mediating children's adaptation.

These studies describe "main effects" of positive parent–child relationships on child adjustment. Supportive interactions with parents appear to have a direct effect on children's well-being after divorce, though the possibility that these relationships take on added importance when stress is high cannot be ruled out. Parents can provide each of the support functions listed earlier, and thus are particularly important in helping their children adjust to the changes associated with divorce. However, parents typically are under enormous strain themselves and may not be as available (emotionally or physically) as their children would like. Further, children who are angry at one or both parents for causing the divorce may be less likely to turn to the parent for support and guidance.

Other Adults

Adults other than children's parents also may be important sources of support after divorce. Grandparents, aunts and uncles, neighbors, and teachers who are involved with the child can help children in a number of direct ways (Wolchik, Ruehlman, Braver, & Sandler, 1989). They may reduce the fears often experienced by younger children that their basic needs will not be met or that they will be abandoned. They also may take over some of the recreational or educational activities usually assumed by parents. Finally, they may help children to understand the divorce and correct misconceptions about why their parents have less time for them (Wolchik et al., 1989). As discussed in more detail below, children may blame themselves for the divorce and other adults can provide an important corrective to such beliefs (see Grych & Fincham, 1992b). Nonparental adults also can provide indirect help for children by supporting their parents (e.g., by helping with household or child care tasks or providing emotional support), thereby making it easier for parents to be available to their children.

The little research that exists in this area indicates that support from nonparental adults can help attenuate the stress of divorce for children. Wolchik and colleagues (1989) reported that children with higher overall levels of adult support reported lower levels of adjustment problems. Interestingly, neither maternal or paternal support had direct or indirect effects on children's adjustment; only support from extended family predicted better adaptation. The type of effect differed depending on who rated children's adjustment. When parent reports were used, nonparental adult support was related directly to child adjustment. In contrast, child reports of adjustment showed indirect or stress-buffering effects of support. When children had experienced a larger number of "changes for the worse" (increased undesirable events plus decreased desirable events), support from nonparental adults led to decreased reports of anxiety, depression, and aggressiveness. When they reported little change for the worse, support from nonfamily adults was associated with poorer adjustment. This counterintuitive finding may reflect the possibility that children functioning more poorly after divorce may receive additional attention (wanted or unwanted) from adults. For example, parents may seek out more help when their children are more difficult to handle.

The supportive role of other adults, particularly grandparents, also has been investigated, but with mixed results. Guidubaldi and Cleminshaw (1983) found that more contact with the custodial parent's parents was associated with better academic performance, whereas Hetherington (1989) reported that grandparents did not appear to play a significant role unless the children lived in the home with them. She did find, however, that contact with the noncustodial parents' relatives was related to better social and academic adjustment.

Siblings

Siblings are in a unique position to provide support to each other because they share similar experiences going through a divorce. Depending on their ages and the age difference between them, they can provide several types of support to each other, including shared recreational activities, emotional support, and advice. However, a number of factors may mitigate against siblings being a source of support for each other. First, younger children may not have attained the level of empathy needed to recognize that their sibling is in distress nor the resources to provide the kind of help needed, particularly when they need support themselves. Second, children may compete for the decreased amount of parental attention available or be pulled in different directions by loyalties to their parents. Thus, even though siblings are a potential source of support, they also are potential rivals (see Gano-Phillips & Fincham, 1995).

Although there has been little empirical research on siblings as providers of support, there are some data to suggest that sibling relations may be more a source of stress than support. Hetherington and colleagues (1992) provided the most detailed data on this issue in their study of early adolescents from divorced, remarried, and intact families. Overall, siblings from divorced families tended to be more negative toward each other than those in intact families, though not as negative as siblings in remarried families. This finding applied more to boys than to girls, however. Girls from divorced families were much like children in intact families in that they showed greater empathy, support, and involvement than boys. These findings were consistent over the 2-year course of the study, suggesting that going through a marital transition does not necessarily draw children together; in fact, it appeared that children in early adolescence began distancing or disengaging from siblings earlier than those from intact families. Similar results were found with preadolescent children (Hetherington, 1988): Siblings in divorced and remarried families had more problematic relationships than those in intact families, with boys generally demonstrating higher levels of aggressive, coercive behavior than girls in these families. Sibling interactions among these younger children did improve over time in the remarried families, though they never attained the level of siblings in intact, never-divorced families. Moreover, the quality of sibling relationships was linked to parent–child interaction in all types of families. When parents were punitive, unaffectionate, or demonstrated preferential treatment toward one sibling over another, sibling relationships suffered (Hetherington, 1988). In contrast, siblings in divorced families where both parents were involved and consistent often exhibited considerable warmth and loyalty toward one another.

The next question to be addressed is whether the quality of sibling relationships is related to children's adjustment. Hetherington et al. (1992) found with their adolescent sample that the level of negative interaction between siblings was associated with greater externalizing behavior and lower social competence and that positive interactions were correlated in the opposite direction. However, it did not appear that the quality of sibling relationships directly affected later adjustment (although it did in remarried families). Similarly, Kempton, Armistead, Wierson, and Forehand (1991) found that children without siblings exhibited more externalizing problems than those with siblings, but suggested that the quality of the sibling relationship determines whether it is beneficial. Consistent with the developmental hypothesis above, Hetherington (1989) indicates that positive sibling relationships exerted more of a buffering role for older than younger children in a preadolescent sample. She also reports that sibling support played a larger role in later rather than earlier stages of marital transitions, perhaps reflecting the stabilization that tends to occur a couple of years after the divorce. It may be only then, when their own level of distress has decreased and some consistency has returned to their lives, that siblings can turn to each other for support.

Peers

Children's friends also represent a possible source of support. Peers are likely to be particularly appropriate for sharing fun activities, but as children get older their friends can become an important source of advice and emotional support as well. The small amount of research in this area has failed to show much effect of peer support on children's adaptation to divorce (e.g., Wolchik et al., 1989). Lustig, Wolchik, and Braver (1992) did find a significant interaction between age and support from "chums" (same sex, roughly same-age peers) in predicting adjustment: Older children (average age 13.7 years) with high support reported fewer adjustment problems than those with low support. There was no association between support and adjustment for younger children (average age 9.3 years), and no significant results were found when parent reports of adjustment were used. Although Lustig et al. had hypothesized a buffering effect for peer support, no stress by support interaction was found. The age differences they reported may be due to developmental differences in the nature of friendship relations. Intimate disclosure becomes more important in close friendships as children age, and so the older children in the sample may have benefited from receiving emotional support as well as sharing play activities (Lustig et al., 1992).

An important issue to consider when examining the role of social support is whether children can mobilize and make use of potentially supportive others. As described earlier, many children exhibit disruptive behavior problems that could push away others who might otherwise be helpful to them. Boys in particular may end up isolating themselves because of aggressive or obnoxious behavior (Emery, 1988). In addition to the presence of behavior problems, a child's ability to engage others is likely to be important. This type of social skill may be an important predictor of children's level of support from others as well as their overall functioning. Those who have difficulty enlisting others to help them may be particularly likely to develop longer-term adjustment problems. Older children are likely to be better at requesting and utilizing support than are young children, which may account for the age differences found in the Lustig et al. (1992) study described above.

Individual Differences

Individual characteristics such as personality traits and self-esteem have been identified as important factors in understanding why some individuals appear more resilient in the face of stress than others (e.g., Garmezy, 1983). Such factors have received little attention in divorce research, which has tended to focus more on circumstances and events external to the child. However, a growing body of work on children's coping strategies and cognitions suggests that children's perceptions and responses to divorce-related circumstances are important for understanding variability in postdivorce adaptation. Finally, although it has rarely been examined empirically, child temperament has been proposed to be a moderator of their adjustment. We examine each of these factors in turn.

Given that divorce presents children with a variety of stressful experiences that challenge their everyday functioning, investigating their efforts to cope with these stressors provides a promising approach for understanding their adaptation. Several studies have examined relations between coping strategies and postdivorce adjustment (Armistead et al., 1990; Kliewer & Sandler, 1993; Krantz, Clark, Pruyn, & Usher, 1985; Kurdek & Sinclair, 1988; Sandler, Tein, & West, in press). The most conceptually and methodologically sophisticated of these used a factor analytically derived scheme for classifying children's coping efforts and a longitudinal design to test both cross-sectional and predictive associations between the coping strategies, negative life events, and psychological symptoms (Sandler et al., 1994). Sandler and colleagues found considerable stability in both the level of stress experienced and the types of coping strategies reported by 8- to 12-year-olds over a 5½-month period. They reported that active coping, defined as use of positive cognitive or behavioral strategies to understand and solve a problem, had stress-buffering effects on concurrent child conduct problems and predicted lower levels of depression 5½ months later. Similarly, the use of distraction (avoiding thinking about the problem by engaging in another activity) predicted lower levels of depression and anxiety. In contrast, avoidance (trying not to think about the problem, wishful thinking) and seeking support from others was related to greater adjustment problems. Other studies similarly have linked active coping with social competence and adjustment (Kliewer & Sandler, 1993; Krantz et al., 1985) and avoidance with psychological maladjustment (Armistead et al., 1990; Kliewer & Sandler, 1993), though differences in defining and measuring coping strategies make comparisons across studies difficult.

Finding that support seeking correlated with poorer adjustment is surprising considering the emphasis given to social support in other research. However, the quality of the support received is an important factor in determining the efficacy of support seeking as a coping strategy, and Sandler et al. (1994) did not assess children's perception of the adequacy of the help they received. Thus, it is possible that the results reflect a need for support that is not adequately met by the individuals from whom they sought help (Sandler et al., 1994). As noted above, children who turn to overwhelmed parents may not find the support they need, whereas seeking help from different individuals may have more positive results. This point underscores the importance of the match between the type of coping strategy used and the child's specific environmental circumstances. Which coping strategies are most adaptive may depend on the type of problem children are facing, the resources available to them, and the point in the divorce process that the stressor occurs. For example, distraction may be more effective than active problem solving for situations in which the child has little control or where children's efforts lead to parental resentment.

Work on coping indicates that children's cognitions may be quite important for understanding the impact of divorce. Parental separation often is very confusing for children, and their ability to understand what has transpired and why is thought to be important for healthy adjustment (Grych & Fincham, 1992b; Wallerstein, 1983). Cognitive processes in children's adaptation to divorce have been examined in a variety of ways. First, several studies have investigated children's thoughts about the divorce and its consequences. For example, Kurdek and Berg (1983) found that certain attitudes about the divorce (e.g., blame, hope of reunification, fear of abandonment) were associated with parent and teacher ratings of adjustment. However, they later failed to find a relation between "problematic beliefs" about divorce and teacher ratings of behavior problems, although these beliefs were correlated with child self-reports of adjustment (Kurdek & Berg, 1987). One of the problematic beliefs examined by Kurdek and his colleagues—self-blame for the divorce—has been emphasized in clinical writings as a mediator of children's adjustment to divorce, but the empirical data on this question are sketchy (see Grych & Fincham, 1992b). Thus, at present it is not clear whether children's attributions for divorce serve as either risk or protective factors.

Other studies have examined whether characteristic ways of thinking affect children's adjustment to divorce. Mazur, Wolchik, and Sandler (1992) assessed "cognitive errors" (catastrophizing, overgeneralizing, and personalizing) and "positive illusions" (high self-regard, illusion of personal control, and optimism for the future) for negative divorce-related events in a sample of children whose parents had divorced within the previous 2 years. They found that cognitive errors correlated positively with self-reported anxiety and self-esteem and maternal reports of behavior problems, and that positive illusions were related to lower levels of self-reported aggression. Moreover, they showed that these appraisals accounted for variance in children's adjustment beyond that attributable to the occurrence of negative events. The role of locus of control has been emphasized in other studies. Because children going through a divorce often experience negative changes, many of them beyond their control, it has been proposed that their belief in their ability to exert control over their lives may decrease, which may adversely impact their adjustment. Fogas, Wolchik, Braver, Freedom, and Bay (1992) found support for such a mediational model in a sample of children between the ages of 8 and 15. That is, negative events led to decreased internal locus of control, which in turn correlated with poorer adjustment. Thus, having a sense of personal control over events may serve as a protective factor for children undergoing divorce. Kurdek et al. (1981) also found that locus of control, along with level of interpersonal reasoning, significantly correlated with adolescents' report of their feelings about the divorce and parental report of overall adjustment.

A final individual characteristic proposed to influence children's adaptation to divorce is temperament (Hetherington, 1989; Kurdek, 1987). In one of the only empirical reports on the role of temperament, Hetherington (1989) found that children's temperament had an indirect, moderating effect on their adjustment. Specifically, it did not appear to be related to adjustment when the level of stress in children's lives was low and social support was high. However, when social support was less available, temperamentally easy children were better adjusted than were temperamentally difficult children. Difficult temperament thus may serve as a vulnerability factor that comes into play only if the level of stress children experience reaches a certain threshold.

Societal Support

The role of social organizations in facilitating children's adaptation to divorce also has received very little attention. Organizations and institutions such as schools, day care centers, and athletic or social groups potentially afford children a source of stability and access to concerned, caring individuals. Involvement in such groups also may provide a sense of connection for children experiencing a disruption in their families and of consistency amid change. In one of the few examinations of social organizations, Guidubaldi and colleagues (1984, 1987) have reported that stable and supportive school environments are related to better adaptation. The potential benefit of this kind of support requires further elaboration and is an important area of future study.

In sum, several factors that facilitate healthy adjustment after divorce have been identified. Supportive relationships with other adults—especially parents—appear to have direct positive effects on children's adaptation, but siblings and peers do not appear to play a similar role, at least until adolescence. Much more work is needed to describe how and when other adults such as relatives, teachers, and neighbors can become significant sources of support for children going through a divorce. In addition, examining children's ability to seek out and utilize support will be critical for understanding the linkage between support and adjustment. Individual characteristics, particularly children's coping strategies and cognitions, also appear to be important for explaining why some children adapt to divorce better than others. Continued investigation of the cognitions that are most pertinent for mediating adjustment and which coping strategies are likely to be most adaptive for different kinds of events will further elaborate the role of intrapersonal factors.

Studies on potential protective factors have important implications for intervention efforts because they identify resources and strengths that can be enhanced through appropriate treatment or prevention programs. In the next section, we examine interventions developed for children from divorced families.

WHAT INTERVENTIONS ARE AVAILABLE FOR CHILDREN FROM DIVORCED FAMILIES?

The potential adverse effects of divorce on children have led to the development of a number of interventions designed to meet the needs of these children. These interventions attempt to enhance children's functioning either by reducing factors associated with adverse outcomes or by increasing factors associated with positive outcomes, or both. Many children experiencing divorce also are treated in individual or family therapy (see Hodges, 1991), but our focus will be on programs developed specifically for addressing the problems faced by children from divorced families. The most common intervention approach discussed in the literature is a child-focused, time-limited education/therapy group that focuses on helping children better understand and cope with the divorce. Groups for parents also have been developed that may have an indirect effect on children by facilitating the parents' postdivorce adaptation. The emphasis on involving children directly may be somewhat surprising in light of the paucity of data on child characteristics associated with better adjustment, but it reflects the individual-centered approach of traditional clinical psychology (for a community-oriented approach to divorce intervention, see Humphreys, Fernandes, Gano-Phillips, Bhana, & Fincham, 1993). At the same time, the success reported by some of these groups suggests that basic research may profit by concentrating more effort on understanding individual variables in children's adaptation to divorce. In this section, we describe and evaluate the efficacy of child- and parent-focused groups.

Child-Focused Interventions

The intervention programs for children from divorced families that have been evaluated in the past decade share a common core of features. These programs use a structured group format that typically lasts 8–14 sessions. The group format is preferred over individually oriented treatment because it normalizes the experience of divorce and provides a supportive network of peers who are undergoing similar stress. Although groups have been run in mental health centers, conducting them in community settings like schools and religious facilities allows children to remain in familiar surroundings and rely on or build an already existing support system. A final advantage of using a group format is that more children can be served, more economically, than individually oriented treatment approaches. Groups for children from divorced families also tend to share similar goals. First, they attempt to help clarify children's perceptions and interpretations of divorce-related events so that they can better understand why the divorce happened and make sense of their role in it. Second, they help children to learn new coping strategies for dealing with upsetting feelings, parent–child conflict, visitation problems, and other stressors. Finally, they attempt to increase children's level of social support.

Several intervention groups have been designed, but few have been systematically evaluated. The program that has been studied most extensively is the Children of Divorce Intervention Project (CODIP) (Alpert-Gillis, Pedro-Carroll, & Cowen, 1989; Pedro-Carroll, Alpert-Gillis, & Cowen, 1992; Pedro-Carroll & Cowen, 1985; Pedro-Carroll, Cowen, Hightower, & Guare, 1986). In addition to its focus on understanding the divorce and improving children's coping strategies, this program strives to enhance children's regard for themselves and their families. The program has documented positive effects on children's adaptation. For example, a sample of white, middle-class, fourth through sixth grade children whose parents had divorced an average of 2 years earlier were compared to demographically matched children in a delayed-treatment group (Pedro-Carroll & Cowen, 1985). Two weeks after the group ended participants rated themselves as less anxious but did not evidence changes in attitudes about the divorce or self-perceived competence. Notably, teachers rated group participants as demonstrating less shyness/anxiety, increased frustration tolerance, and greater "adaptive assertiveness," and parent ratings similarly showed greater increases in overall adjustment following the group.

The CODIP group also has been adapted for a racially mixed urban population (Alpert-Gillis et al., 1989; Pedro-Carroll et al., 1992) and for younger children (Alpert-Gillis et al., 1989). Modifications for the urban group included a greater emphasis on the extended family and on the acceptability of diverse types of families. Similar positive results have been documented for these groups: Compared to children from divorced families not participating in the program and children from intact families, group participants reported feeling more positive about themselves and their parents and greater confidence in their coping abilities; parents viewed the children as exhibiting better overall adjustment; and teachers rated the children as higher in assertiveness, task orientation, and frustration tolerance. However, teacher reports did not reveal changes in externalizing, internalizing, or learning problems (Alpert-Gillis et al., 1989).

Research on other intervention programs is less thorough and the results are more mixed. Some programs report positive effects on certain outcome variables, but they have not documented consistent, general effects on the adjustment of children who participated (Bornstein, Bornstein, & Walters, 1988; Kalter, Pickar, & Lesowitz, 1984; Kalter, Schaefer, Lesowitz, Alpern, & Pickar, 1988; Roseby & Deutsch, 1985). Several of these studies are marked by serious methodological flaws, such as the absence of a comparison group, use of measures of unknown reliability and validity, and nonrandom assignment to groups. Even when groups have demonstrated positive outcomes, the proposed mediators of change rarely have been evaluated, and consequently the process by which change occurs is not known. Further, most evaluation studies have assessed children shortly after the end of the groups but have not conducted longer term follow-ups to test whether positive effects are maintained.

Parent-Focused Interventions

Based on theory and research documenting that many of the stressors associated with divorce are under the parents' rather than the child's control, a group specifically for custodial parents was developed and evaluated by Wolchik et al. (1993). The intervention targeted several of the factors proposed to mediate children's adaptation to divorce: mother–child relationships, discipline, negative divorce events (including interparental conflict), contact with fathers, and support from nonparental adults. The intervention program consisted of ten group sessions and two individual sessions for custodial mothers and emphasized skill acquisition or enhancement. Participants included 70 mothers, separated an average of 23 months, who had a child between the ages of 8 and 15. Children's adjustment and change in the proposed mediators were assessed 10–12 weeks after the end of the group and process measures were obtained during the group to evaluate the integrity of the intervention. The group was designed as a preventive intervention, and thus families in which either the mother or the child reported clinical levels of depression were excluded and referred for clinical treatment.

The intervention led to improvements in some of the proposed mediators targeted. The most consistent effects involved positive changes in the quality of mother–child relationships for the program group. Negative life events, discipline, and contact with fathers did not show consistent changes across mother and child reports, and, contrary to prediction, program children reported less support from nonparental adults than children in the control condition. This last finding may be due to program mothers and children spending more time together, leaving less time (and perhaps less need) for support from other adults. Results pertaining to the benefits of the group for children's adjustment were mixed. Children of group mothers reported lower levels of aggression but did not differ from waiting list controls on self-reported anxiety, conduct disorder, or depression. Maternal reports of child adjustment indicated that program children who had higher initial scores showed greater improvement than those in the waiting list group that had high scores, whereas program and waiting list children who exhibited better adjustment at pretest did not differ in outcome. Moreover, Wolchik and her colleagues found that changes in mother–child relationships partially mediated the impact of the group on child adjustment.

The effectiveness of the intervention in enhancing the mother–child relationship relative to the other targeted mediators may reflect the fact that much more group time was devoted to this factor than any other and/or that it is the mediator over which mothers have the most direct control. Significant changes in father–child relations, interparental conflict, and support from nonparental adults may require the participation of fathers and other adults in the intervention. This evaluation thus indicates that targeting parents is an effective way to ameliorate some of the adverse effects of divorce on children because it directly addresses factors found to be related to postdivorce adaptation.

Interventions Including Parents and Children

Stolberg's (Stolberg & Cullen, 1983; Stolberg & Garrison, 1985) Divorce Adjustment Project adopts a systemic approach to intervention by including both children and their custodial parents in intervention groups. The group for parents includes a focus on learning more effective parenting methods and on the parent's own adjustment to the divorce. It teaches child management techniques as well as communication strategies for reducing conflict both with children and former spouses. In addition, it addresses children's and adults' typical responses to divorce to help parents better understand what their children are going through. Evaluation of the efficacy of the 12-week group presented a mixed picture. Stolberg and Garrison (1985) studied 82 7- to 13-year-old children and their mothers, who had been divorced between 9 and 33 months. Participants were divided into four groups: child-only participation, parent-only participation, child and mother participation, and a no-treatment control group. In addition to measuring adjustment at the end of the group and 5 months later, proposed mediators of the change in adjustment (e.g., parental support, discipline) were assessed.

The results were somewhat counterintuitive. Children in the child-only group showed greater improvement in self-esteem (at end of group) and adaptive social skills (at 5 months posttest) than those in the combined or no treatment condition. Mothers in the mother-only group also showed greater gains in adjustment than did those in the combined condition. However, mothers in the intervention groups did not show greater gains in parenting skills than the mothers who were not in a group, and the children in the mother-only group did not show any benefits from having their mothers in a group. The failure of the combined intervention for mothers and children to prove superior to either group alone may be due to preexisting differences between the participants in different conditions. Participants were not randomly assigned to groups, and children in the combined condition were better adjusted at the outset and therefore would not be expected to show as much positive change. Mothers in the mother-only group and combined groups also differed in the length of time they had been separated and in their occupation.

Stolberg and Mahler (1994) recently reported a follow-up study that manipulated the components of the children's group. Children from 8 to 12 years of age whose parents had been separated an average of 3 years took part in a group that provided either social support, support plus skill building (primarily understanding and labeling feelings, self-control strategies), or support, skill building, and limited parental involvement designed to enhance the transfer of skills from group to home. Changes in these children's adjustment were compared to groups of children from divorced and intact families who did not receive the intervention. Compared to the divorced controls, children in the support plus skills group showed significant improvement in parent ratings of internalizing and externalizing problems and children in the support, skills, and transfer group reported decreased trait anxiety at the end of group. In a 1-year follow-up, both of these intervention groups showed improvement on parent ratings of behavior problems but were not significantly different from each other or the support only group. Teacher reports of academic and behavioral functioning and children's perceptions of competence did not show similar gains.

Interventions for children and parents from divorced families thus present promising, if limited, evidence of their efficacy. The programs differ on several dimensions that may be important for understanding their effectiveness, particularly the degree to which the interventions are based on empirical findings from basic research on divorce and the clarity with which they identify and assess the targets of change. The majority of intervention programs appear to draw little on generative research in determining their goals and methods of change and fail to assess the mediators targeted by the intervention. Consequently, they reveal only whether the program helped children, not how it helped them. Clearly, there is value in learning whether a program "works," but to advance understanding about how divorce affects children and how best to facilitate their adjustment, we need to know why they work. Only by evaluating whether change in the proposed mediators is linked to changes in child adjustment can valid claims be made regarding the process of change. Moreover, such evidence in turn enriches basic research by providing quasi-experimental or, if random assignment is used, experimental tests of proposed mediators (see section below on using intervention research to test theory). The mediators targeted by various programs differ with, for example, the CODIP program focusing on individual child characteristics and Wolchik and colleagues' group focusing on parent–child relationships. The fact that both groups provide some evidence of effectiveness increases confidence that individual and family factors are important for shaping children's adaptation to divorce.

FUTURE DIRECTIONS

The last two decades have provided a wealth of information about the adjustment of children whose parents divorce. Research in this area began by studying whether children from divorced families differed from those in intact families and now has turned to investigate why some children exhibit continued problems after divorce while others appear to adapt successfully. A complex picture is emerging that highlights the contribution of interparental conflict, parent–child relationships, environmental changes, coping efforts, and social support in shaping children's adjustment to divorce, but much is yet to be learned about the factors that influence the stress children experience and their ability to cope with divorce. In this final section we briefly discuss issues that we believe are most important to address as we continue to investigate how marital dissolution affects children.

Tracking Adaptation over Time

Studies that assess children at one point in time are useful for exploring group differences but shed little light on the process of adapting to divorce. Research that examines child and family functioning prior to divorce and follows children for years after the divorce has the most potential for illuminating the developmental trajectory of children's adaptation. Hetherington and colleagues' detailed longitudinal studies have provided the richest data on children's adjustment after divorce, but they were conducted with samples limited in terms of race and socioeconomic status. Even though they are very labor-intensive and expensive to conduct, in-depth prospective studies with multiple waves of assessment are invaluable for disentangling the various factors that lead to child maladjustment (parent–child relationships, sibling relationships, interparental conflict). The measurement and analysis of change is a complex endeavor, however, and existing research has not yet exploited the potential of sophisticated analytic techniques for examining changes in children's functioning over time.

Understanding Resiliency

Much more attention has been paid to the stressful aspects of divorce than to the factors that help children adapt successfully. A shift in emphasis from pathology to resiliency would pave the way for new research into intrapsychic, interpersonal, and societal influences on healthy adaptation. Of the three classes of resiliency factors identified by Garmezy (1983), only family relationships have been studied extensively, and that research is limited by its emphasis on custodial parents. Sources of strength and support in family relationships have been studied less than discipline practices or the amount of time parents spend with children, but ultimately they may be more important in understanding what helps children through the stress of divorce. The second class of resiliency factors—individual child characteristics—has been emphasized in interventions developed for children from divorced families but has received less attention by basic researchers. How children interpret and understand the divorce, their ability to enlist others for support, and the extent and facility of their coping repertoire all may be important factors mediating their adjustment. Similarly, support provided by nonfamily members, such as grandparents and neighbors, and by institutions, such as schools and day care, has been studied little. Drawing on the resiliency literature may provide other possibilities for application to divorce.

Developing Theory

Much of the research on children's adaptation to divorce has been descriptive in nature. Although important for establishing the existence and parameters of a phenomenon, it does not explain the phenomenon. Most theoretically based studies adopt a stress and coping perspective, which has been useful for conceptualizing how certain events and interactions may serve as either risk or protective factors in children's adaptation. This perspective also has been useful for incorporating multiple levels of analysis (individual, familial, societal) into a coherent model of adaptation over time. However, more complete understanding of how divorce affects children will be facilitated by broadening the theoretical orientations used to study it. For example, as divorce typically involves the disruption of parent–child relationships, attachment theory may be particularly pertinent for understanding children's adaptation.

There are at least three ways in which attachment theory could inform the study of divorce. First, assessing attachment security provides an index of children's adjustment that has been linked to later social and personal functioning. This approach would be especially useful for assessing the adaptation of toddler and preschool-aged children, for whom the establishment of secure attachment represents a critical developmental task. Second, children's attachment history may be an important moderator of their adjustment to divorce. It might be predicted, for instance, that insecurely attached children would be particularly disturbed by changes in their relationships with their parents and evidence greater anxiety than securely attached children. Third, exploring how divorce may affect children's working models of relationships may enhance understanding of longer-term outcomes such as the higher divorce rate for children from divorced families. Attachment theory could easily be integrated with the stress and coping perspective to investigate issues such as whether children with different attachment histories have different perceptions of divorce-related events or use different types of strategies to cope with them (e.g., active coping vs. avoidance).

Cognitive developmental theory also is pertinent for understanding how children of different ages may perceive and respond to divorce. Although the likely existence of developmental differences in children's beliefs and interpretations of divorce has been noted, there has been little empirical work beyond Wallerstein and Kelly's (1980) description of age changes in children's perceptions and emotional responses to divorce. Like attachment theory, work on cognitive development could add to a stress and coping approach by detailing how children of different ages interpret and respond to changes in the family. Such a perspective would be particularly important for tailoring interventions to children of different ages as children's perceptions of the most salient aspects of divorce and their ability to cope with them will depend on their level of cognitive development.

Examining Relations among Proposed Mediators

Several factors now have been consistently supported as mediators of children's postdivorce adjustment, but rarely have more than one of these factors been examined in the same study. Consequently, little is known about the relations among variables such as interparental conflict, parent–child relationships, and nonpayment of child support and their relative ability to predict child outcomes. The handful of studies that have examined multiple mediators indicate that prediction of child adjustment is improved by the inclusion of more than one risk factor and that the interrelations among mediators are likely to be complex (e.g., Pillow et al., 1991; Simons, Whitbeck, Beaman, & Conger, 1994; Stolberg & Bush, 1985). For example, in their longitudinal study of adolescents, Simons and colleagues (1994) found that both maternal and paternal parenting, and to a lesser extent interparental conflict, accounted for unique variance in child adjustment, though associations among the variables were not consistent across reporters. Their findings also underscore the importance of controlling for associations among mediators in showing that family income and child support did not have a significant effect on child adjustment once parenting practices and parental conflict were taken into account. Stolberg and Bush (1985) similarly found support for the importance of interparental conflict and parenting. They reported that interparental hostility and parenting skills correlated with internalizing problems, whereas externalizing problems were predicted by interparental hostility and number of life changes, and social competence was associated with all three mediators. Finally, Braver and colleagues (1993) found that visitation by the noncustodial parent and child support compliance were predicted by a third variable: fathers' perceptions of control in their children's lives. Fathers who felt integral to their children's lives visited more frequently and paid child support more reliably than fathers who felt disenfranchised from family life, who appeared to withdraw from the obligations of parenthood. By examining multiple mediators, these studies go beyond simply identifying variables related to child adaptation to exploring the processes by which events and circumstances unfold over time and mutually influence each other and child adjustment.

Viewing Children as "Independent Variables"

Research on divorce tends to view child adjustment as an outcome measure and to ignore the role that children play in shaping events. Children are active participants in their environment and can have positive or negative effects on others. For example, children's behavior may serve to increase parental stress and contribute to family problems in a number of ways: Aggressive,

defiant children are more difficult to parent and can undermine parental attempts at discipline, and many children respond to being triangulated between
parents by playing the parents off each other, which may exacerbate interparental conflict. A recent longitudinal study of adolescents provides some evidence
for the role of "child effects" in family functioning after divorce (Simons et al.,
1994). Simons and colleagues found that elevated levels of externalizing problems predicted poorer quality parenting 1 year later for mothers and fathers of
boys. Internalizing problems did not affect later parenting, and the effects for
externalizing problems held only for the first 2–3 years after separation; follow-
up 1 year later failed to show a significant effect. Children also are instrumental
in determining the level of support they receive. Some children are skilled at
engaging others and mobilizing support networks, while others may fail to
attract help from others or actually repel potential support givers. At the intraindividual level, children's own coping resources and strategies are likely to
play an important role in their adjustment to divorce. Investigating questions of
causality requires longitudinal designs, preferably including at least three time
points, that can track the timing of changes in child and parental functioning.

Using Intervention Research to Test Theory

Unfortunately, basic research on divorce and evaluation studies of interventions have had little influence on each other (see Grych & Fincham, 1992a).
Findings from basic research on the role of family interactions have not been
well-integrated into most child-focused interventions and most evaluation
studies do not appear to have been informed by basic research. The potential
for productive cross-fertilization between these two approaches is substantial,
however. Most outcome studies have focused on documenting changes in children's adjustment following participation in the program, which is necessary
for assessing the efficacy of the intervention but only scratches the surface of
what evaluation research can investigate. Such studies also can provide valuable information about the mediators of divorce adjustment. The goals of intervention programs presumably reflect hypotheses about the factors that promote
healthy adaptation to divorce. For example, interventions that target children's
understanding of the divorce are hypothesizing that such cognitions are important for shaping their functioning. This hypothesis can be tested by measuring
the variables of interest (here cognitions) and testing whether (1) the program
changes them and (2) change is related to child functioning (see Wolchik et al.,
1993, for an example). Thus, investigating the therapeutic process and outcome
also can test theory about adaptation to divorce. Of course, factors that improve
children's adjustment after divorce are not necessarily those responsible for the
onset or even maintenance of adjustment problems, but positive relations between changes in these factors and adaptation provides evidence for what can
mediate improvement after divorce.

Clarifying What Works for Whom

Echoing a goal of research on psychotherapy with adults, evaluations of
divorce interventions may profit from detailed analysis of the components of

the intervention as well as who the intervention helps most. Understanding which elements of the interventions are most closely related to outcome will help interventionists better focus their programs on what works. For example, presently it is not known how many sessions are needed to produce positive changes or which activities facilitate attainment of the program goals. Addressing such issues comprises a more advanced stage of evaluation research that is contingent on demonstrating that the intervention does actually help. Similarly, assessing whether groups of children (e.g., those whose parents divorced within a year prior vs. more than 2 years) vary in the benefits they gain may help tailor interventions for particular groups.

Another approach to matching interventions with participants' needs involves use of a screening procedure to select participants (see Pillow et al., 1991, Wolchik et al., 1993). For example, Wolchik and colleagues used an empirically derived questionnaire battery to identify families for their custodial parent group. They obtained scores on measures of the mediators targeted in the intervention program and selected those families whose scores indicated difficulties in these areas. This approach maximizes the effectiveness (both cost and therapeutic) of interventions by selecting those who need it the most and excluding those who appear to be functioning well in the areas addressed by the intervention.

CONCLUSION

In this chapter we have tried to answer a number of important questions about the impact of divorce on children. Not surprisingly, the answers are complex and reflect the interplay of many different factors in a child's life. In brief, experiencing parental separation and divorce often, but not invariably, leads to an array of behavioral and emotional disturbances in children. For many children this reaction is temporary, lasting perhaps 1 to 2 years, and is followed by a return to healthy functioning. However, for some children marital dissolution sets in motion a variety of stressors that are ongoing. Children whose parents continue to fight, whose relationships with their parents are conflictual or distant, who experience a number of negative life changes, and who suffer from economic hardships are more likely to evidence continued signs of maladjustment. On the other hand, children's adaptation to divorce is facilitated when parents cooperate with each other over childrearing issues, resolve conflicts that arise between them, and maintain close relationships with the children; when children use active coping strategies; and when children's lives remain relatively stable. Thus, children's adaptation is shaped by both adverse events and circumstances and the positive resources and support available to them.

Interventions have been developed for children who experience problems adjusting to divorce, and there are promising reports of the effectiveness of programs designed for both children and their parents. However, more research is needed to determine what kinds of interventions work and especially how they work. Unfortunately, there has been a gap between basic research on the consequences of divorce for children and the intervention programs designed to help them. Narrowing this gap by integrating basic research into the design of interventions and using evaluation research to provide evidence about mediators of children's adaptation will be mutually beneficial for these two lines of inquiry and ultimately for the children they serve.

REFERENCES

Achenbach, T. M., & Edelbrock, C. (1983). *Manual for the Child Behavior Checklist and Revised Child Behavior Profile*. Burlington, VT: University Associates in Psychiatry.

Allison, P. D., & Furstenberg, F. F. (1989). How marital dissolution affects children: Variations by age and sex. *Developmental Psychology, 25*, 540–549.

Alpert-Gillis, L. J., Pedro-Carroll, J. L., & Cowen, E. L. (1989). The children of divorce intervention program: Development, implementation, and evaluation of a program for young urban children. *Journal of Consulting and Clinical Psychology, 57*, 583–589.

Amato, P. R. (1993). Children's adjustment to divorce: Theories, hypotheses, and empirical support. *Journal of Marriage and the Family, 55*, 23–38.

Amato, P. R., & Keith, B. (1991). Consequences of parental divorce for the well-being of children: A meta-analysis. *Psychological Bulletin, 110*, 26–46.

Armistead, L., McCombs, A., Forehand, R., Wierson, M., Long, N., & Fauber, R. (1990). Coping with divorce: A study of young adolescents. *Journal of Clinical Child Psychology, 19*, 79–84.

Block, J. H., Block, J., & Gjerde, P. F. (1986). The personality of children prior to divorce: A prospective study. *Child Development, 57*, 827–840.

Booth, A., Binkerhoff, D. B., & White, L. K. (1984). The impact of divorce on courtship. *Journal of Marriage and Family, 46*, 85–94.

Bornstein, M. T., Bornstein, P. H., & Walters, H. A. (1988). Children of divorce: Empirical evaluation of a group-treatment program. *Journal of Clinical Child Psychology, 17*, 248–254.

Bowlby, J. (1973). *Attachment and loss. Vol. 2: Separation*. New York: Basic Books.

Braver, S. L., Wolchik, S. A., Sandler, I. N., Sheets, V. L., Fogas, B., & Bay, C. (1993). A longitudinal study of noncustodial parents: Parents without children. *Journal of Family Psychology, 7*, 9–23.

Brody, G. H., & Forehand, R. (1990). Interparental conflict, relationship with the noncustodial father, and adolescent post-divorce adjustment. *Journal of Applied Developmental Psychology, 11*, 139–147.

Buchanan, C. M., Maccoby, E. E., & Dornbusch, S. M. (1991). Caught between parents: Adolescents' experience in divorced homes. *Child Development, 62*, 1008–1029.

Camara, K. A., & Resnick, G. (1987). Marital and parental subsystems in mother-custody, father-custody, and two-parent households: Effects on children's social development. In J. P. Vincent (Ed.), *Advances in family intervention, assessment, and theory* (Vol. 4, pp. 165–196). Greenwich, CT: JAI.

Camara, K. A., & Resnick, G. (1988). Interpersonal conflict and cooperation: Factors moderating children's post-divorce adjustment. In E. M. Hetherington & J. Aratesh (Eds.), *Impact of divorce, singleparenting, and stepparenting on children* (pp. 169–195). Hillsdale, NY: Erlbaum.

Camara, K. A., & Resnick, G. (1989). Styles of conflict, resolution and cooperation between divorced parents: Effects on child behavior and adjustment. *American Journal of Orthopsychiatry, 59*, 560–575.

Castro Martin, T., & Bumpass, L. L. (1989). Recent trends and differentials in marital disruption. *Demography, 26*, 37–51.

Cherlin, A. J. (1981). *Marriage, divorce, remarriage: Changing patterns in the postwar United States*. Cambridge, MA: Harvard University Press.

Cherlin, A. J., Furstenberg, F. F., Chase-Lansdale, P. L., Kiernan, K. E., Robins, P. K., Morrison, D. R., & Teitler, J. O. (1991). Longitudinal studies of the effects of divorce on children on Great Britain and the United States. *Science, 252*, 1386–1389.

Cohen, S., & Wills, T. A. (1985). Stress, social support, and the buffering hypothesis. *Psychological Bulletin, 98*, 310–317.

Cox, M. J., Owen, M. T., Lewis, J. M., & Henderson, V. K. (1989). Marriage, adult adjustment, and early parenting. *Child Development, 60,* 1015–1024.

Cummings, E. M., Ballard, M., El-Sheikh, M., & Lake, M. (1991). Resolution and children's responses to interadult anger. *Developmental Psychology, 27,* 462–470.

Cummings, E. M., & Davies, P. (1994). *Children and marital conflict.* New York: Guilford.

Cummings, E. M., Vogel, D., Cummings, J. S., & El-Sheikh, M. (1989). Children's responses to different forms of expression of anger between adults. *Child Development, 60,* 1392–1404.

Cummings, E. M., Zahn-Waxler, C., & Radke-Yarrow, M. (1981). Young children's responses to expressions of anger and affection by others in the family. *Child Development, 52,* 1274–1282.

Davies, P. T., & Cummings, E. M. (1994). Marital conflict and child adjustment: An emotional security hypothesis. *Psychological Bulletin, 116,* 387–411.

Duncan, G. J., & Hoffman, S. D. (1985). Economic consequences of marital instability. In M. David & T. Smeeding (Eds.), *Horizontal equity, uncertainty, and economic well-being* (pp. 112–131). Chicago: University of Chicago Press.

Easterbrooks, M. A., & Emde, R. N. (1988). Marital and parent–child relationships: The role of affect in the family system. In R. A. Hinde & J. Stevenson-Hinde (Eds.), *Relationships within families: Mutual influences* (pp. 83–103). Oxford, England: Oxford University Press.

Emery, R. E. (1982). Interpersonal conflict and the children of discord and divorce. *Psychological Bulletin, 92,* 310–330.

Emery, R. E. (1988). *Marriage, divorce, and children's adjustment.* Newbury Park, CA: Sage.

Emery, R. E. (1994). *Renegotiating family relationships.* New York: Guilford.

Emery, R. E., Hetherington, E. M. & DiLalla, L. F. (1984). Divorce, children and social policy. In H. W. Stevenson & A. E. Siegel (Eds.), *Child development research and social policy* (pp. 189–266). Chicago: University of Chicago Press.

Fauber, R., & Long, N. (1991). Children in context: The role of the family in child psychotherapy. *Journal of Consulting and Clinical Psychology, 59,* 813–820.

Fauber, R., Forehand, R., Thomas, A. M., & Wierson, M. (1990). A mediational model of the impact of marital conflict on adolescent adjustment in intact and divorced families: The role of disrupted parenting. *Child Development, 61,* 1112–1123.

Felner, R. D., Terre, L., & Rowlison, R. T. (1988). A life transition framework for understanding marital dissolution and family reorganization. In S. A. Wolchik & P. Karoly (Eds.), *Children of divorce: Empirical perspectives on adjustment* (pp. 35–66). New York: Gardner.

Fincham, F. D., Grych, J. H., & Osborne, L. (1994). Does marital conflict cause child maladjustment? Directions and challenges for longitudinal research. *Journal of Family Psychology, 8,* 128–141.

Fogas, S., Wolchik, S. A., Braver, S. L., Freedom, D. S., & Bay, R. C. (1992). Locus of control as a mediator of negative divorce-related events and adjustment problems in children. *American Journal of Orthopsychiatry, 62,* 589–598.

Furstenberg, F. F. (1990). Divorce and the American family. *Annual Review of Sociology, 16,* 379–403.

Furstenberg, F. F., Morgan, S. P., & Allison, P. D. (1987, April). Parental participation and children's well-being after marital disruption. Paper presented at the annual meeting of the Population Association of America, Chicago.

Furstenberg, F. F., & Nord, C. W. (1985). Parenting apart: Patterns of childrearing after marital disruption. *Journal of Marriage and the Family, 47,* 893–904.

Gano-Phillips, S., & Fincham, F. D. (1995). Family conflict, divorce, and children's adjustment. In M. Fitzpatrick & A. Vangelisti (Eds.), *Perspectives on family communication* (pp. 206–231). Newbury Park, CA: Sage.

Garmezy, N. (1983). Stressors of childhood. In N. Garmezy & M. Rutter (Eds.), *Stress, coping and development in children* (pp. 43–84). New York: McGraw-Hill.

Goldberg, W. A., & Easterbrooks, M. A. (1984). Role of marital quality in toddler development. *Developmental Psychology, 20,* 504–514.

Grych, J. H., & Fincham, F. D. (1990). Marital conflict and children's adjustment: A cognitive–contextual framework. *Psychological Bulletin, 108,* 267–290.

Grych, J. H., & Fincham, F. D. (1992a). Interventions for children of divorce: Toward greater integration of research and action. *Psychological Bulletin, 110,* 434–454.

Grych, J. H., & Fincham, F. D. (1992b). Marital dissolution and family adjustment: An attributional analysis. In T. Orbuch (Ed.), *Close relationship loss: Theoretical perspectives* (pp. 157–173). New York: Springer-Verlag.

Grych, J. H., & Fincham, F. D. (1993). Children's appraisals of marital conflict: Initial investigations of the cognitive–contextual framework. *Child Development, 64,* 215–230.

Grych, J. H., Seid, M., & Fincham, F. D. (1992). Assessing marital conflict from the child's perspective: The Children's Perception of Interparental Conflict Scale. *Child Development, 63,* 558–572.

Guidubaldi, J., & Cleminshaw, H. (1983, August). Impact of family support system on children's academic and social functioning after divorce. Paper presented at the annual meeting of the American Psychological Association, Anaheim, CA.

Guidubaldi, J., Perry, J. D., & Cleminshaw, H. K. (1984). The legacy of parental divorce. In B. B. Lahey & A. E. Kazdin (Eds.), *Advances in clinical child psychology* (Vol. 7, pp. 109–151). New York: Plenum Press.

Guidubaldi, J., Perry, J. D., & Nastasi, B. K. (1987). Assessment and intervention for children of divorce: Implications of the NASP-KSU nationwide survey. In J. Vincent (Ed.), *Advances in family intervention, assessment, and theory* (Vol. 4, pp. 33–69). Greenwich, CT: JAI Press.

Hazan, C., & Shaver, P. R. (1992). Broken attachments: Relationship loss from the perspective of attachment theory. In T. Orbuch (Eds.), *Close relationship loss: Theoretical perspectives* (pp. 174–192). New York: Springer-Verlag.

Hess, R. D., & Camara, K. A. (1979). Post-divorce relationships as mediating factors in the consequences of divorce for children. *Journal of Social Issues, 35,* 79–96.

Hetherington, E. M. (1988). Parents, children, and siblings: Six years after divorce. In R. Hinde & J. Stevenson-Hinde (Eds.), *Relationships within families* (pp. 311–331). Oxford, England: Clarendon Press.

Hetherington, E. M. (1989). Coping with family transitions: Winners, losers, and survivors. *Child Development, 60,* 1–14.

Hetherington, E. M., Clingempeel, W. G., Anderson, E. R., Deal, J. E., Hagen, M. S., Hollier, E. A. & Linder, M. S. (1992). Coping with marital transitions: A family system perspective. With commentary by Eleanor E. Maccoby. *Monographs of the Society for Research in Child Development, 57,* 1–206.

Hetherington, E. M., Cox, M., & Cox, R. (1982). Effects of divorce on parents and children. In M. Lamb (Ed.), *Nontraditional families* (pp. 233–288). Hillsdale, NJ: Erlbaum.

Hetherington, E. M., Stanley-Hagen, M., & Anderson, E. R. (1989). Marital transitions: A child's perspective. *American Psychologist, 44,* 303–312.

Hodges, W. F. (1991). *Interventions for children of divorce.* New York: Wiley.

Hoyt, L. A., Cowen, E. L., Pedro-Carroll, J. L., & Alpert-Gillis, L. J. (1990). Anxiety and depression in youth children of divorce. *Journal of Clinical Child Psychology, 19,* 26–32.

Humphreys, K., Fernandes, L. O., Gano-Phillips, S., Bhana, A. E., & Fincham, F. D. (1993). A community oriented approach to divorce intervention. *Family Journal, 1,* 4–12.

Jenkins, J. M., & Smith, M. A. (1990). Factors protecting children living in disharmonious homes: Maternal reports. *Journal of the American Academy of Child and Adolescent Psychiatry, 29,* 60–69.

Johnston, J. R., Kline, M., & Tschann, J. M. (1989). Ongoing post-divorce conflict in families contesting custody: Effects on children of joint custody and frequent access. *American Journal of Orthopsychiatry, 59,* 576–592.

Kalter, N., Pickar, J., & Lesowitz, M. (1984). School-based developmental facilitation groups for children of divorce: A preventive intervention. *American Journal of Orthopsychiatry, 54,* 613–623.

Kalter, N., & Rembar, J. (1981). The significance of a child's age at the time of parental divorce. *American Journal of Orthopsychiatry, 51,* 85–100.

Kalter, N., Schaefer, M., Lesowitz, M., Alpern, D., & Pickar, J. (1988). School-based support groups for children of divorce. In B. H. Gottlieb (Ed.), *Martialing social support: Formats, processes and effects* (pp. 165–185). Newbury Park, CA: Sage.

Kelly, J. B. (1988). Longer-term adjustment in children of divorce: Converging findings and implications for practice. *Journal of Family Psychology, 2,* 119–140.

Kempton, T., Armistead, L., Wierson, M., & Forehand, R. (1991). Presence of a sibling as a potential buffer following parental divorce: An examination of young adolescents. *Journal of Clinical Child Psychology, 20,* 434–438.

Kliewer, W., & Sandler, I. N. (1993). Social competence and coping among children of divorce. *American Journal of Orthopsychiatry, 63,* 432–440.

Krantz, S. E., Clark, J., Pruyn, J. P., & Usher, M. (1985). Cognition and adjustment among children of separated or divorced parents. *Cognitive Therapy and Research, 9,* 61–77.

Krein, S. F., & Beller, A. H. (1988). Educational attainment of children from single-parent families: Differences by exposure, gender, and race. *Demography, 25,* 221–234.

Kurdek, L. A. (1986). Children's reasoning about parental divorce. In R. D. Ashmore & D. M. Brodzinsky (Eds.), *Thinking about the family: Views of parents and children* (pp. 233–276). Hillsdale, NJ: Erlbaum.

Kurdek, L. A. (1987). Children's adjustment to parental divorce: An ecological perspective. In J. P. Vincent (Ed.), *Advances in family intervention, assessment and theory* (Vol. 4, pp. 1–31). Greenwich, CT: JAI Press.

Kurdek, L. A., & Berg, B. (1983). Correlates of children's adjustment to their parent's divorces. In L. A. Kurdek (Ed.), *New directions in child development. Vol. 19: Children and divorce* (pp. 47–60). San Francisco: Jossey-Bass.

Kurdek, L. A., & Berg, B. (1987). Children's beliefs about parental divorce scale: Psychometric characteristics and concurrent validity. *Journal of Consulting and Clinical Psychology, 55,* 712–718.

Kurdek, L. A., & Sinclair, R. J. (1988). Adjustment of young adolescents in two-parent nuclear, stepfather, and mother-custody families. *Journal of Consulting and Clinical Psychology, 56,* 91–96.

Kurdek, L. A., Blisk, D., & Siesky, A. E. (1981). Correlates of children's long-term adjustment to their parent's divorce. *Developmental Psychology, 17,* 565–579.

Long, N., Forehand, R., Fauber, R., & Brody, G. (1987). Self-perceived and independently observed competence of young adolescents as a function of parental marital conflict and recent divorce. *Journal of Abnormal Child Psychology 15,* 15–27.

Luepnitz, D. A. (1982). *Child custody: A study of families after divorce.* Lexington, MA: Lexington Books.

Lustig, J. L., Wolchik, S. A., & Braver, S. L. (1992). Social support in chumships and adjustment in children of divorce. *American Journal of Community Psychology, 20,* 393–399.

Mazur, E., Wolchik, S. A., & Sandler, I. N. (1992). Negative cognitive errors and positive illusions for negative divorce events: Predictors of children's psychological adjustment. *Journal of Abnormal Child Psychology, 20,* 523–542.

McCarthy, J. (1978). A comparison of the probability of the dissolution of first and second marriages. *Demography, 15,* 345–359.

Meissner, W. W. (1978). Conceptualization of marriage and family dynamics from a psychoanalytic perspective. In T. J. Paolino & B. S. McCrady (Eds.), *Marriage and marital therapy* (pp. 25–88). New York: Brunner/Mazel.

Norton, A. J., & Glick, P. C. (1979). Marital instability in America. Past, present and future. In G. Levinger & O. C. Moles (Eds.), *Divorce and separation* (pp. 6–19). New York: Basic Books.

Pedro-Carroll, J. L., Alpert-Gillis, L. J., & Cowen, E. L. (1992). An evaluation of the efficacy of a preventive intervention for 4th–6th grade urban children of divorce. *Journal of Primary Prevention, 13,* 115–130.

Pedro-Carroll, J. L., Cowen, E. L., Hightower, A. D., & Guare, J. C. (1986). Preventive intervention with latency-aged children of divorce: A replication study. *American Journal of Community Psychology, 14,* 277–289.

Pedro-Carroll, J. L., & Cowen, E. L. (1985). The children of divorce intervention program: An investigation of the efficacy of a school-based prevention program. *Journal of Consulting and Clinical Psychology, 53,* 603–611.

Peterson, J. L., & Zill, N. (1986). Marital disruption, parent–child relationships, and behavior problems in children. *Journal of Marriage and the Family, 48,* 295–307.

Pillow, D. R., Sandler, I. N., Braver, S. L., Wolchik, S. A., & Gersten, J. C. (1991). Theory-based screening for prevention: Focusing on mediating processes in children of divorce. *American Journal of Community Psychology, 19,* 809–836.

Roseby, V., & Deutsch, R. (1985). Children of separation and divorce: Effects of a social-role taking group intervention on fourth and fifth graders. *Journal of Clinical Child Psychology, 14,* 55–60.

Sandler, I. N., Tein, J., & West, S. G. (1994). Coping, stress and the psychological symptoms of children of divorce: A cross-sectional and longitudinal study. *Child Development, 65,* 1744–1763.

Sandler, I. N., Wolchik, S. A., Braver, S. L., & Fogas, B. (1991). Stability and quality of life events and psychological symptomatology in children of divorce. *American Journal of Community Psychology, 19,* 501–520.

Sandler, I. N., Wolchik, S. A., & Braver, S. L. (1988). The stressors of children's postdivorce environments. In S. A. Wolchik & P. Karoly (Eds.), *Children of divorce: Empirical perspectives on adjustment* (pp. 185–232). New York: Gardner.

Santrock, J. W., & Warshak, R. A. (1979). Father custody and social development in boys and girls. *Journal of Social Issues, 35,* 112–135.

Shaw, D. S., Emery, R. E., & Tuer, M. D. (1993). Parental functioning and children's adjustment in families of divorce: A prospective study. *Journal of Abnormal Child Psychology, 21,* 119–134.

Simons, R. L., Whitbeck, L. B., Beaman, J., & Conger, R. D. (1994). The impact of mothers' parenting, involvement by nonresidential fathers, and parental conflict on the adjustment of adolescent children. *Journal of Marriage and the Family, 56,* 356–374.

Stolberg, A. L., & Bush, J. P. (1985). A path analysis of factors predicting children's divorce adjustment. *Journal of Clinical Child Psychology, 14,* 49–54.

Stolberg, A. L., Camplair, C., Currier, K., & Wells, M. J. (1987). Individual familial and environmental predictors of children's post-divorce adjustment and maladjustment. *Journal of Divorce, 11,* 51–70.

Stolberg, A. L., & Anker, J. M. (1983). Cognitive and behavioral changes in children resulting from parental divorce and consequent environmental changes. *Journal of Divorce, 7,* 23–41.

Stolberg, A. L., & Cullen, P. M. (1983). Preventive interventions for families of divorce: The divorce adjustment project. In L. A. Kurdek (Ed.), *New directions in child development. Vol. 19: Children and divorce* (pp. 71–81). San Francisco: Jossey-Bass.

Stolberg, A. L., & Garrison, K. M. (1985). Evaluating a primary prevention program for children of divorce: The divorce adjustment project. *American Journal of Community Psychology, 13,* 111–124.

Stolberg, A. L., & Mahler, J. (1994). Enhancing treatment gains in a school-based intervention for children of divorce through skill training, parental involvement, and transfer procedures. *Journal of Consulting and Clinical Psychology, 62,* 147–156.

Stoneman, Z., Brody, G. H., & Burke, M. (1989). Marital quality, depression, and inconsistent parenting: Relationship with observed mother–child conflict. *American Journal of Orthopsychiatry, 59,* 105–117.

Sweet, J. A., & Bumpass, L. L. (1992). Disruption of marital and cohabitation relationships: A social demographic perspective. In T. Orbuch (Ed.), *Close relationship loss: Theoretical perspectives* (pp. 67–89). New York: Springer-Verlag.

Thomas, A. M., & Forehand, R. (1993). The role of parental variables in divorced and married families: Predictability of adolescent adjustment. *American Journal of Orthopsychiatry, 63,* 126–135.

Thorton, A. (1977). Children and marital stability. *Journal of Marriage and Family, 39,* 531–540.

Tschann, J. M., Johnston, J. R., Kline, M., & Wallerstein, J. S. (1989). Family process and children's functioning during divorce. *Journal of Marriage and the Family, 51,* 431–444.

Waite, L. J., Haggstrom, G. W., & Kanouse, D. E. (1985). The consequences of parenthood for the marital stability of young adults. *American Sociological Review, 50,* 850–857.

Wallerstein, J. S. (1983). Children of divorce: Stress and developmental tasks. In N. Garmezy & M. Rutter (Eds.), *Stress, coping, and development in children* (pp. 265–302). New York: McGraw-Hill.

Wallerstein, J. S., & Blakeslee, S. (1989). *Second chances: Men, women, and child a decade after divorce.* New York: Ticknor & Fields.

Wallerstein, J. S., & Kelly, J. B. (1980). *Surviving the breakup: How children actually cope with divorce.* New York: Basic.

Walsh, P. E., & Stolberg, A. L. (1989). Parental and environmental determinants of children's behavioral, affective, and cognitive adjustment to divorce. *Journal of Divorce, 12,* 265–282.

Weitzman, L. J. (1985). *The divorce revolution.* New York: Free Press.

Wolchik, S. A., Ruehlman, L. S., Braver, S. L., & Sandler, I. N. (1989). Social support of children of divorce: Direct and stress buffering effects. *American Journal of Community Psychology, 17,* 485–501.

Wolchik, S. A., Sandler, I. N., Braver, S. L,. & Fogas, B. (1989). Events of parental divorce: Stressfulness ratings by children, parents, and clinicians. *American Journal of Community Psychology, 14,* 59–74.

Wolchik, S. A., West, S. G., Westover, S., Sandler, I. N., Martin, A., Lustig, J., Tein, J., & Fisher, J. (1993). The children of divorce parenting intervention: Outcome evaluation of an empirically based program. *American Journal of Community Psychology, 21,* 293–331.

Zaslow, M. J. (1988). Sex differences in children's response to parental divorce: 1. Research methodology and postdivorce family form. *American Journal of Orthopsychiatry, 58,* 355–378.

Zaslow, M. J. (1989). Sex differences in children's response to parental divorce: 2. Samples, variables, ages, and sources. *American Journal of Orthopsychiatry, 59,* 118–141.

7

Children's Coping with Parental Illness

NANCY L. WORSHAM, BRUCE E. COMPAS, and SYDNEY EY

What happens to children when their mother or father is seriously ill? What is the impact of parental illness on their psychological and behavioral adjustment? Are children faced with certain types of stressors as a result of specific parental illnesses such as diabetes, arthritis, heart disease, or cancer? And how do children cope with the stress of having an ill parent? Are some coping responses associated with better psychological adjustment and others related to poorer adaptation? These questions form the basis for a growing interest in the consequences of parental physical illness for the psychological well-being of children (e.g., Compas et al., 1994; Lewis, Hammond, & Woods, 1993).

Interest in the impact of parental medical illness on children's psychological adjustment and coping behavior is not new. For example, Rutter's (1966) original research on this topic suggested that children were at risk for psychological maladjustment when faced with a chronic or recurrent (as opposed to acute) medical illness in a parent. Concern about the psychological well-being of children of ill parents has continued, both among professionals and laypersons (e.g., Leventhal, Leventhal, & Nguyen, 1985; Turk & Kerns, 1985). It is a widely held impression that children with a medically ill parent are under significant stress and that they may lack the necessary resources to cope effectively with this stress. Therefore, these children are seen as at risk for psychological maladjustment. Many of the assumptions that are held about children of ill parents are tenuous, however, as they are based on clinical case observations and may not be supported by empirical research.

NANCY L. WORSHAM • Department of Psychology, Gonzaga University, Spokane, Washington 99258.   BRUCE E. COMPAS • Department of Psychology, University of Vermont, Burlington, Vermont 05405.   SYDNEY EY • Department of Psychology, University of Memphis, Memphis, Tennessee 38152.

Handbook of Children's Coping: Linking Theory and Intervention, edited by Wolchik and Sandler. Plenum Press, New York, 1997.

Our purpose is to review the literature investigating the impact of parental medical illness on children, communicate current knowledge regarding children's coping with this stressful experience, and review existing interventions targeting children's adaptation to parental medical illness. We first present an overview of medical illness among young and middle-aged adults of parenting age. Second, we review the literature targeting the children's psychological adjustment to parental medical illness, including consideration of methodological problems in this area. Third, we review the research that has examined children's coping and social support in response to parental medical illness. Fourth, we provide an overview of the few existing interventions targeting children's adjustment to parental medical illness. Finally, directions for future research are suggested.

PREVALENCE OF PARENTAL MEDICAL ILLNESS

Definitive figures of the number of children exposed to serious physical illness in a parent are difficult to obtain. Incidence and prevalence data for most diseases are based on age and other sociodemographic characteristics that do not include status as a.parent. However, it is clear that a number of acute and chronic diseases are quite prevalent among young and middle-aged adults (ages 18–50) who are likely to have children living in the home.

Prevalence rates for a variety of different forms of cancer indicate that many children may be faced with a parent who is diagnosed with a malignancy. For example, roughly one third of cancer patients are 55 years or younger, indicating that hundreds of thousands of adults of parenting age are diagnosed with cancer each year (Biegel, Sales, & Schulz, 1991). With regard to other medical conditions, the US National Center for Health Statistics provides information regarding rates of conditions for different age ranges and for both genders. For example, arthritis affects 25.8 per 1000 males and 35.8 per 1000 females under the age of 45 years. Furthermore, 27.3 per 1000 males and 34.2 per 1000 females are affected by heart conditions. Rates regarding the prevalence of diabetes among 17- to 44-year old young adults and adults are 7.7 per 1000 males and 10.4 per 1000 females (National Center for Health Statistics, 1993). Extrapolating from these data, it can be estimated that as many as 5–15% of children and adolescents may have parents who suffer from a significant medical condition. These figures in combination with data on other acute and chronic illnesses among adults suggest that millions of adults who are of child-rearing age suffer from a significant disease. Therefore, we can project that millions of children each year are exposed to the stress associated with a serious parental illness.

IMPACT OF PARENTAL MEDICAL ILLNESS ON CHILDREN'S PSYCHOLOGICAL ADJUSTMENT

In spite of the pervasiveness of acute and chronic illness among adults of parenting age and the general concern expressed for children who are exposed to the stress of parental illness, surprisingly little empirical research has directly assessed the short- and long-term effects of this stressor. We were able to identify only seven empirical studies that examined the relationship between parental medical illness and child and adolescent psychological adjustment, and four additional studies that examined adjustment to parental medical illness by way of comparison to parental psychopathology. The following criteria were used in selecting relevant studies for this review: (1) documentation of an acute or chronic parental medical illness, (2) inclusion of standardized measures of children's psychological adjustment (e.g., self-report, parental report), and (3) children of the medically ill parents ranging in age from 0 to 18 years at the time of parents' illness. Publications were excluded that relied solely on case studies (e.g., Grandstaff, 1976), empirical studies that included adult children only or did not differentiate between majority-aged and minority-aged children (e.g., Wellisch, Gritz, Schain, Wang, & Siau, 1991), empirical studies addressing family issues that did not include children (e.g., Cassileth et al., 1984), studies focused on bereavement following a parent's death (e.g., Berman, Cragg, & Kuenzig, 1988), or publications that were solely theoretical in nature (e.g., Lewandowski, 1992). We will draw extensively on our own longitudinal investigation of the psychological adjustment of cancer patients, their spouses, and their children (e.g., Compas et al., 1994; Welch, Wadsworth, & Compas, 1996; Compas, Worsham, Ey, & Howell, 1996; Epping-Jordan, Compas, & Howell, 1994; Ey, Compas, Epping-Jordan, & Worsham, 1996; Grant & Compas, 1995; Malcarne, Compas, Epping-Jordan, & Howell, 1995).

Children's adjustment to parental illness may vary as a function of a number of parameters and potential moderating factors, and these factors are important to consider in reviewing the existing research. These include (1) the type and severity of the parent's disease, (2) whether the disease is acute or chronic in nature, (3) gender of the ill parent and child, (4) age of the child, (5) time of the onset of the parent's illness (prior to child's birth, during childhood, during adolescence), (6) degree of physical impairment in the patient, (7) whether the illness is heritable versus nonheritable, (8) degree of the patient's cognitive impairment and emotional distress related to the illness, and (9) characteristics of treatment (e.g., lengthy hospitalizations, presence of severe side effects).

Parental Medical Illness

Seven studies have directly investigated the impact of parental medical illness on children's and adolescents' psychological adjustment (Compas et al., 1994; Dura & Beck, 1988; Lewis, Woods, Hough, & Bensley, 1989; Moguilner, Bauman, & De-Nour, 1988; Rickard, 1988; Siegel et al., 1992; Wellisch, Gritz, Schain, Wang, & Siau, 1992). Parental cancer was the focus in four of these studies (Compas et al., 1994; Lewis et al., 1989; Siegel et al., 1992; Wellisch et al., 1992), with the remaining studies examining a heterogeneous set of diseases and conditions.

Several studies have examined the psychological adjustment of children whose parents suffer from chronic diseases. Dura and Beck (1988) compared self-report measures of depression and anxiety and parental reports of children's psychological adjustment among three groups of children (age range, 7–13 years; mean = 9.7 years): children of mothers experiencing chronic pain (n = 7), children of mothers diagnosed with diabetes (n = 7), and children of mothers experiencing no medical illness ($n = 7$). The authors reported significant differences between the three groups on self-reports of depression; children of parents with chronic pain had significantly greater self-reported symptoms of depression than control children. Self-reported symptoms of depression for children of diabetic parents fell between the other two groups and were not significantly different from either. Although there were significant differences between groups, none of the mean group scores were clinically elevated; the authors did not report the proportion of children who scored above a clinical cutoff on the depressive symptoms measure. There were no significant differences between groups on children's self-reported anxiety. In addition, there were no significant differences between groups on parents' report of their children's emotional–behavioral problems.

Moguilner et al. (1988) studied 25 children from 11 families in which one parent was undergoing chronic hemodialysis. The children were distinguished with regard to age, with 13 children between the ages of 8 and 12 years (mean = 9.7) and 12 adolescents between the age of 13 and 17 years (mean = 15.2). The authors formed three groups of "well-adjusted" families ($n = 3$ with 5 children), "moderately adjusted" families ($n = 4$ with 10 children), and "maladjusted" families ($n = 4$ with 10 children). Comparisons of these three groups indicated that children from maladjusted families had significantly poorer self-concepts than children from well-adjusted families. The authors concluded that children's and adolescents' adjustment was quite varied, but they did not cite the numbers of children who fell into a clinical range. In addition, the authors speculated that the two age groups of children did not differ in overall adjustment, but that the younger group of children showed a consistent relationship between their adjustment and their parents' emotional adjustment, while this pattern was not true of the adolescents.

Rickard (1988) studied the occurrence of maladaptive health-related behaviors and teacher-rated conduct problems between three groups of children (age range 8–12 years; mean = 9.6 years): children of fathers with chronic low back pain ($n = 21$), children of parents with diabetes ($n = 21$), and control children ($n = 21$). Results indicated that children of fathers with chronic pain had significantly more conduct problems according to teacher reports. Additional measures indicated significant differences between children of fathers with chronic pain and both children of diabetic fathers and control children, with children of fathers with chronic pain reporting significantly more pain-related behaviors themselves in response to the scenarios and greater external locus of control. It is noteworthy that children of diabetic fathers did not differ significantly from control children.

The most extensive data are available on children whose parents have been diagnosed with cancer (Northouse, 1995). Lewis and colleagues have reported on the process of children's adjustment to maternal breast cancer in a series of papers (e.g., Issel, Ersek, & Lewis, 1990; Lewis, 1990; Lewis, Ellison, & Woods, 1985; Lewis et al., 1989, 1993; Stetz, Lewis, Primomo, 1986). Lewis et al. (1989) presented data on the adjustment of 48 children ranging in age from 6 to 12 years whose mothers had been diagnosed with breast cancer, diabetes, or fibrocystic breast disease (control group). None of the mothers were currently undergoing treatment and the mean duration since diagnosis was 3 years. Fathers completed standardized measures of their relationship with their children and their children's psychosocial functioning in terms of peer relations. Results indicated that frequent father–child interactions coupled with higher marital adjustment were associated with more positive child psychosocial functioning. Unfortunately, specific data were not provided regarding numbers of children functioning within a clinical range nor describing direct comparisons of the three groups of children. Lewis et al. (1985) reported on the adjustment of children of mothers with nonmetastatic breast cancer. They found that mothers' ratings of children's behavioral–emotional problems did not differ from a normative sample. Similarly, interviewers' ratings of children's adaptive functioning were also within the normal range. Children's self-reports, however, reflected lower levels of self-esteem in comparison with normative data. Follow-up with this sample after the death of a parent provided some unexpected findings, as children who lost a parent due to cancer did not differ from controls in self-reports of symptoms of depression and anxiety (Siegel, Karus, & Raveis, 1996).

The psychological adjustment of children faced with a terminal diagnosis (expected survival time of approximately 4 to 6 months) in a parent was examined by Siegel et al. (1992). Parent and child self-report measures of adjustment were obtained for 62 children aged 7 to 16 years (mean = 11.1) and compared with data from a large community sample of children whose parents were not terminally ill. Children whose parents were dying of cancer reported more symptoms of depression and anxiety and lower self-esteem than did children in the comparison sample. Furthermore, children of terminally ill parents were rated by their parents as higher in both internalizing and externalizing behavior problems than were children in the comparison sample. Analyses of child gender or age or whether the mother or father was ill were not reported.

Wellisch and colleagues (1992) reported on a retrospective investigation of the psychological functioning of daughters of breast cancer patients with a consideration for the age of the child at the time of maternal diagnoses and illness. Participants were 60 adult daughters ranging in age from 22 to 63 years (mean = 42.4 yr) of women who had experienced breast cancer. With regard to age at the time of maternal illness, 9 of the 60 were children (age 0–10 years) at the time of diagnosis and 15 were adolescents (age 11–20 years). The authors targeted the relationship between daughters' age at time of maternal diagnosis and five life experience variables (long-range life plans, daily activity, role change with mother, feelings about degree of involvement with mother's illness, and daughter's perception of mother's reaction to mastectomy). The authors identified statistically significant differences for two of the variables: children's and adolescents' long-range life plans were more likely to have been changed and adolescents were more likely to feel discomfort regarding their involvement with the mother's illness. The authors conclude that "those who were children (at the time of diagnosis) had moderate adjustment problems, and those who were adolescents had the greatest adjustment problems" (p. 177).

In our own research we have examined the impact of parental cancer in a study of 26 children, 50 adolescents, and 34 young adults (total $N = 110$) whose mother (72%) or father (28%) had been recently diagnosed (mean of 4 months postdiagnosis) with cancer (Compas et al., 1994). Parents varied in the type and severity of their cancer, with the most frequent diagnoses being breast cancer, gynecologic cancer, brain tumors, and hematologic malignancies. They also differed in the severity of their disease, as 33% had stage I cancer, 28% stage II, 22% stage III, and 17% stage IV cancer. This study offered the opportunity to examine the effects of maternal versus paternal cancer, age of the child, and gender of the child on children's psychological adjustment. Children's adjustment was measured by their self-reports of symptoms of anxiety and depression and stress response syndrome symptoms (intrusive thoughts and avoidance), and subsequent analyses have examined parental reports of the adjustment of these children (Welch et al., 1996). Standardized measures of children's emotional and behavioral problems were used for comparison to representative norms.

For all age groups, children's adjustment was unrelated to the type or severity of their parents' cancer, but poorer adjustment was associated with children's perceptions of the seriousness of their parents' illness. Furthermore, self-reported symptoms of anxiety/depression and stress response syndrome symptoms varied as a function of the child's age, gender, and whether the mother or father had cancer (Compas et al., 1994). Adolescents reported more anxiety/depression symptoms than children or young adults, with adolescent girls reporting the highest levels of distress. Adolescent girls whose mothers had cancer reported significantly more symptoms of anxiety and depression than girls whose fathers had cancer or boys with ill mothers or fathers. Stress response symptoms displayed a somewhat different pattern, as children reported higher levels of intrusive thoughts about their parent's cancer than did adolescents or young adults. Stress response symptoms differed among adolescents, however, in a pattern similar to that found for symptoms of anxiety/depression; that is, adolescent girls whose mothers had cancer reported more intrusive thoughts than girls whose fathers were ill or boys whose mothers or fathers had cancer.

The clinical significance of these findings was further considered by examining the proportion of children who exceeded clinical cutoffs on the measures of anxiety/depression symptoms. Using a criterion of a T score of 63 (corresponding to the 90th percentile), significantly more adolescent girls of mothers with cancer (25%) were in the clinical range than would be expected from the normative data on this scale. The percentage of children in the clinical range did not differ from expected rates for preadolescent children.

Subsequent analyses with this sample have examined the processes that may contribute to the relatively high levels of distress experienced by the adolescent daughters of women with cancer (Grant & Compas, 1995). It is noteworthy that children's and adolescents' self-reports of anxiety/depression symptoms were not related to their parents' reports of emotional distress (Compas et al., 1994). That is, emotional distress of children in these families was not the consequence of parents' emotional distress over their illness. Grant and Compas (1995) examined two other processes that may specifically account for the heightened distress of adolescent girls whose mothers were ill: increased levels of family stress (cf. Compas & Wagner, 1991) and girls' use of ruminative as compared with distraction coping (cf. Nolen-Hoeksema, 1990). Adolescent girls reported significantly more family responsibility stress (e.g., taking care of younger siblings, increased responsibilities at home) than girls whose fathers were ill and than boys whose parents had cancer. Results of multiple regression analyses showed that levels of family responsibility stress fully accounted for the interaction of gender of the child and gender of the parent with cancer in predicting symptoms of anxiety/depression in these girls. Although girls used more ruminative coping than boys, their use of rumination did not account for their increased distress. Thus, disruptions in family roles when a mother had cancer and the chronic strains generated by these changes led to adverse effects on adolescent daughters.

Finally, parents' reports of their children's psychological adjustment were examined in this sample (Welch et al., 1996). Mean scores for parents' reports of their children's symptoms of anxiety/depression were all within the normal range. With regard to preadolescent children, parent and child reports did not differ, since both reports indicated relatively low levels of anxiety/depression symptoms. Adolescents' self-reports of anxiety/depression symptoms were significantly higher than parents' ratings of these symptoms for their adolescents. Thus, the strikingly high levels of distress reported by adolescent girls were either not observed or not reported by their parents.

Parental Medical Illness versus Parental Psychopathology

Four groups of researchers have incorporated parental medical illness as a comparison group in their research targeting the impact of parental psychopathology on children and adolescents. Two groups of researchers identified an adverse and/or mixed effect (Adrian & Hammen, 1993; Hammen, Adrian, Gordon, Burge, Jaenicke, & Hiroto, 1987; Hammen, Burge, & Adrian, 1991; Hammen, Burge, Burney, & Adrian, 1990; Hammen, Gordon, Burge, Adrian, Jaenicke, & Hiroto, 1987, Hirsch, Moos, & Reischl, 1985); two did not identify an adverse effect (Klein, Clark, Dansky, & Margolis, 1988; Lee & Gotlib, 1989a, 1989b, 1991).

Hammen and colleagues have investigated maternal affective disorders, medical illness, and stress as risk factors for child and adolescent psychopathology in a variety of ways (Adrian & Hammen, 1993; Anderson & Hammen, 1993; Hammen, Adrian, et al., 1987; Hammen et al., 1990, 1991). Although typically not comparing the differences between medical controls and normal controls, Hammen and colleagues' overall results suggest that a parent's medical illness increases children's (age range, 8 to 16 years) risk of psychological maladjustment in comparison to normal controls on some measures of child functioning. Nevertheless, children of medically ill parents tend to fare better than children of parents with psychopathology.

Hirsch et al. (1985) compared three groups of adolescents ranging in age from 12 to 18 years (mean = 14.8): Children of depressed parents ($n = 16$), children of a parent with rheumatoid arthritis ($n = 16$), and children of parents free from psychological or physical disability ($n = 16$). The depressed but not the arthritic group reported significantly more symptoms than the comparison group. Both the depressed and arthritic group reported significantly poorer self-esteem. The only significant difference on school adjustment between groups indicated that control group children engaged in significantly more school activities than children of depressed and arthritic parents. No significant differences on reports of family environment were found.

Klein et al. (1988) compared three groups of children ranging in age from 14 to 22 years, 47 children of unipolar depressed parents (mean = 18.3 years), 33 children of parents hospitalized for chronic orthopedic or rheumatological conditions (mean = 17.7 years), and 38 control group children from 18 families (mean = 17.4 years). Results indicated that the children of medically ill parents did not differ significantly from controls in lifetime rates of affective disorders or in terms of social impairment. The children of unipolar depressed parents differed significantly from both the medical and control groups in terms of lifetime rates of disorder and social impairment.

Lee and Gotlib (1989a) reported the results of a cross-sectional comparison of children of unipolar depressed mothers ($n = 20$), children of nondepressed psychiatric patients ($n = 13$), children of nondepressed arthritis patients ($n = 8$), and control children ($n = 30$) (age range, 7 to 13 years). Children of mothers with arthritis did not differ significantly from control children on clinician ratings or on maternal reports of emotional–behavioral problems. None of the children of medically ill mothers were rated as functioning in the clinical range on maternal reports. Longitudinal follow-up analyses of 61 of these mother–child dyads were reported by Lee and Gotlib (1989b). No significant differences were found between the children of medically ill mothers and the control children on either the interview or the maternal reports of problems. Overall, the "medically ill" group did not display clinical elevations of emotional and behavioral problems. In addition, the medically ill and control mothers did not differ significantly in terms of self-reported and clinician-rated depression. Both groups were within the "normal" range on these measures. Due to attrition rates, Lee and Gotlib (1991) in their 10-month follow-up study did not include nondepressed medical controls.

Summary

Although research on children's adjustment to parental medical illness is still in its early stages, two general impressions can be drawn at this point. First, parental illness is associated with moderate levels of psychological distress and maladjustment in children. The majority of studies have found that there is at least some indication that parental medical illness has an adverse impact on children's adjustment, most often in the form of internalizing problems or negative affect (Compas et al., 1994; Dura & Beck, 1988; Hammen et al., 1991; Lewis et al., 1989; Moguilner et al., 1988; Rickard, 1988; Siegel et al., 1996; Wellisch et al., 1992). Evidence of distress in these children is much more consistent from children's self-reports than from parental reports of their children's adjustment. Levels of distress in these children appear to be greater than in community control samples or normative base rates but less than the levels of distress and maladjustment found in children of parents with an identified form of psychopathology. The clinical significance of these symptom levels is more difficult to evaluate, since proportions of children exceeding clinical criteria are often not reported. Those instances in which such criteria have been employed suggest that levels of distress in these children should not be trivialized as "subclinical" (Compas et al., 1994).

The second impression that can be formed from this research is that there is considerable variation in the adjustment of children whose parents are ill. Age or developmental level appears to be an important moderating factor, with adolescents reporting higher level of maladjustment than younger children. Lewandowski (1992) has suggested that the impact of a parent's illness on children should be understood within a developmental context. For example, adolescents may be more cognitively aware of risks associated with their parent's illness and also may be called upon to fulfill tasks associated with the ill parent's role. In addition, as suggested by Carter and McGoldrick (1988), families may cope differently at different stages in their development (e.g., new parents as compared to parents of adolescents). Findings reported by Grant and Compas (1995) suggest that stressful processes within families may differ for adolescents as compared with children and for girls versus boys. That is, parental cancer contributed to more ongoing stress in the form of family responsibilities for adolescent girls. Furthermore, maternal versus paternal illness may have a different effect on the adjustment of sons and daughters in these families; girls of ill mothers may be an especially vulnerable group. Aggregate or group-level analyses may disguise such individual differences in children's adjustment, highlighting the need to develop and test a priori hypotheses about factors that moderate levels of distress.

Methodological Issues

Considering that research in this area is in its early stages, it is not surprising that studies have suffered from a variety of methodological problems (Biegel et al., 1991). First, the sample sizes in most studies have been quite small, with total samples ranging from 21 (Dura & Beck, 1988) to 110 (Compas et al., 1994). Analyses of subgroups have involved even smaller samples, e.g., seven children per group in the study by Dura and Beck (1988). We acknowledge the challenges that are involved in obtaining samples of children whose parents are ill, especially when trying to contact families near the time of the parent's diagnosis and to obtain a sample that is homogeneous with regard to type of disease. Nonetheless, the effect of small samples has been to limit statistical power and to raise questions about the representativeness of the samples in this research. The lack of adequate statistical power has limited the ability to detect effects that are small or moderate in magnitude. This is particularly problematic with regard to analyses of moderator variables such as age, gender, and paternal versus maternal illness. There may be differences in children's adjustment as a function of these variables that have gone undetected.

Second, studies have used cross-sectional rather than longitudinal designs, with only one study offering initial analysis from longitudinal data (Welch et al., 1996). Reliance on cross-sectional designs is a reasonable first step for research in this area. Prospective designs are needed, however, to determine how children's adjustment may change over the course of their parents' illness. Data reported by Welch et al. (1996) indicate that levels of children's emotional distress decline in the months following their parent's cancer diagnosis. A related problem involves the use of retrospective reports from parents or children on their adjustment at a prior point in time (e.g., Wellisch et al., 1992). Retrospective reports are subject to a variety of sources of error and need to be corroborated by further research in which children's adjustment is assessed at the time of their parent's illness.

Third, interpretation of these findings is limited by concerns about the measurement of children's adjustment, both in terms of the aspects of children's functioning that have been assessed and the informants who have provided the data. Most studies have assessed child and adolescent internalizing problems (e.g., symptoms of depression, anxiety, low self-esteem), while some have also included measures of externalizing problems (e.g., symptoms of aggression or conduct problems). Evaluation of the clinical significance of these symptoms has not been consistent across studies, yet this represents an important step in interpreting the meaning of these symptoms. Furthermore, problems in adaptive functioning in peer relationships, school performance, and developmentally appropriate activities should be measured, since these areas could also be affected by parental illness as a result of disruptions in family roles and relationships. The need to include multiple perspectives on children's adjustment is also evident, as different informants are likely to offer quite different perspectives on children's functioning and well-being (e.g., Welch et al., 1996).

Finally, greater attention to potential moderators and mediators of the impact of parental illness on child adjustment is needed. Analyses of moderator variables will involve further consideration of those factors that account for individual differences in children's responses to parental illness. Mediator variables are those that account for the processes through which parental illness affects children's adjustment. We will now turn our attention to coping processes as one of the primary factors that may account for children's adjustment to parental illness.

CHILDREN'S COPING WITH PARENTAL MEDICAL ILLNESS

Children's coping responses are assumed to play a central role in their emotional adjustment to a wide range of stressful experiences, including the stress of parental illness. Some types of coping responses may be effective in helping children change some aspect of the stress of their parent's illness or to manage or palliate their emotional distress, whereas other forms of coping may unintentionally increase children's emotional distress.

Research on children's coping with parental illness needs to be grounded in a sound conceptual model of the coping process. It is important to recognize that coping refers to only a subset of responses to stress; specifically, coping includes effortful or volitional responses and does not include involuntary reactions to stress (Compas, Connor, Osowiecki, & Welch, in press; Lazarus & Folkman, 1984). Coping efforts are most often distinguished on the basis of the function or goal that they serve for the individual. The broadest functional distinction of coping strategies has been made between problem-focused coping (efforts to change or solve some aspect of the stressor) and emotion-focused coping (efforts to manage or palliate negative emotions that arise from the stressor). The relative efficacy of problem- and emotion-focused coping is dependent on the actual or perceived controllability of the stressor: problem-focused coping has been shown to be more efficacious in controllable situations and emotion-focused coping better matched with uncontrollable situations (e.g., Compas, Malcarne, & Fondacaro, 1988; Forsythe & Compas, 1987). Psychological distress is lower when control appraisals and coping efforts are matched and higher when there is a mismatch between these two factors.

When considering coping efforts of children, it is further important to account for developmental differences in coping efforts. Findings from studies of children's coping with a wide range of stressors indicate that the use of problem-focused coping is relatively stable with age, whereas use of emotion-focused coping increases during childhood and adolescence (for reviews, see Compas, Malcarne, & Banez, 1992; Compas, Worsham, & Ey, 1992). Children's competency in employing these different types of coping may also change developmentally, although little attention has been given to this issue in prior research.

The empirical literature addressing children's coping with parental medical illness is limited to investigations of children who are coping with parental cancer by Lewis and colleagues and Compas and associates. Issel et al. (1990) investigated how 81 children (ranging in age from 6 to 20 years) coped with their mother's breast cancer. Children completed semistructured interviews targeting their individual- and family-based coping efforts. Responses were content analyzed and classified into four broad domains: being "in her shoes" (e.g., help around the house), carrying on "business as usual" (e.g., acting normal), tapping into "group energy" (e.g., spending time together), and putting the cancer "on the table" (e.g., talking about it). Children also reported the individuals on whom they relied for social support (parents, other family members, friends, other adults). Although no statistical analyses were reported, the authors did compare the percentages of 6- to 12-year-old children and 13- to 20-year-old adolescents who reported these various coping strategies. For example, more younger children than adolescents turned to their fathers for support (46% vs. 17%); more adolescents than children received support from friends (57% vs. 23%). However, the selection of categories was not empirically based, nor was it drawn directly from a review of prior conceptualizations of coping strategies. Furthermore, the relationship between coping and psychological adjustment was not addressed.

Lewis et al. (1993) reported on coping at the level of family processes in a sample of 40 women with breast cancer and their spouses. Children's psychosocial functioning (as reflected in a measure of peer relationships) was related to more frequent interactions with the nonill parent and to the family's use of introspective coping responses. The measure of introspective family coping reflected the degree to which the family worked together to try to generate solutions to problems and family members provided feedback to one another about their coping. Effective family coping was disrupted, however, by the presence of marital distress and depressive symptoms in the nonill parent.

In our own research we have examined perceptions of control, coping responses, and social support in children, adolescents, and young adults whose parents have cancer (Bolton, 1995; Compas et al., 1996). Data were obtained near the time of the parents' cancer diagnosis in individual structured interviews. In response to a semistructured interview, participants described their use of problem-focused coping efforts, emotion-focused coping, coping intended to serve both problem- and emotion-focused goals (dual-focused coping), and the provision and receipt of social support. After generating a list of the ways that they had coped with their parent's cancer, children rated each of their responses as dealing with their emotions (emotion-focused coping), dealing with the problem or situation (problem-focused coping), or both (dual-focused coping). Examples of emotion-focused coping generated by these children included "watching television to get my mind off of it," "spending time with my friends to forget about it," and "spending time in my room to think about my feelings." Problem-focused responses included "helping out with chores around the house" and "trying to be good so he doesn't have to get upset and feel worse." Reports of symptoms of anxiety/depression were obtained using age-appropriate measures and stress response syndrome symptoms (intrusive thoughts and avoidance) were obtained on a modified version of the Impact of Event Scale (Horowitz, Wilner, & Alvarez, 1979) at the time of the interviews.

Children generally considered their parents' illness as beyond their personal control, with a mean rating of 1.8 on a scale of 1 (no control) to 5 (high control). In contrast, ratings of control of powerful others (e.g., medical professionals) were significantly higher (mean = 2.8). Perceptions of personal or external control did not vary with age (Compas et al., 1996). Thus, children's coping with parental cancer is an example of coping under conditions of relatively low personal control.

Age differences were found in the use of emotion-focused and dual-focused coping, whereas the use of problem-focused coping was not related to age. Specifically, adolescents reported using more emotion-focused and dual-focused coping than did younger children; adolescents and young adults did not differ in their reports of coping (Compas et al., 1996). Intrusive thoughts about parents' cancer were inversely related to age: preadolescent children reported higher levels of intrusive thoughts than adolescent or young adults, and adolescents reported more intrusion than young adults. In contrast, avoidance increased with age, as adolescents and young adults reported more avoidance of thoughts about their parents' cancer than did young children.

Correlational analyses were conducted to examine the associations of coping with perceptions of control and with stress response symptoms and symptoms of anxiety/depression (Compas et al., 1996). The three types of coping were unrelated to perceptions of personal or external control. Emotion-focused coping was related to more avoidance ($r = .29$, $p < .001$) and to higher levels of anxiety/depression symptoms ($r = .32$, $p < .001$). Dual-focused coping was related to greater avoidance ($r = .25$, $p = .002$) but lower levels of intrusive thoughts ($r = -.23$, $p = .006$). Problem-focused coping was not related to any of the measures of symptoms of distress. Furthermore, there were no interactions between perceptions of control and coping in predicting the stress response or anxiety/depression symptoms in multiple regression analyses. That is, the match between control beliefs and coping was not found in predicting distress.

Bolton (1995) examined the provision and receipt of social support by children within these families. Children, adolescents, and young adults responded to questions in a structured interview asking about the ways in which they had helped others in their family to cope with their parent's cancer (provision of support) and the ways that others had helped them to cope (receipt of support). Responses were then coded by external raters into four categories of support based on the framework of Cohen and Wills (1985): esteem support, instrumental support, informational support, and social companionship. Both adolescents and children reported that they provided significantly more instrumental support than they received, and they received more informational support than they provided. The reports of esteem support and social companionship reflected a balance between provision and receipt of these categories of support.

Based on previous analyses that showed that adolescent girls were the most distressed subgroup of children in these families (Compas et al., 1994), additional analyses examined the association of adolescents' reports of symptoms of anxiety/depression and their reports of providing and receiving support. For both adolescent boys and girls, providing informational support was correlated with higher distress ($r = .31$, $p = .026$) and receiving informational support was correlated with lower distress ($r = -.38$, $p = .036$). For adolescent girls, the correlation of symptoms of anxiety/depression and the receipt of social companionship support approached significance ($r = .32$, $p = .077$). That is, there was a trend for girls who received social companionship from others in their family to be more distressed.

These two studies represent the initial steps in research on the ways that children cope with parental illness, and interpretations of these early findings must be made cautiously. The results suggest three patterns that are worthy of continued investigation. First, emotion-focused coping was related to more emotional distress and more avoidance of thoughts about their parents' cancer in these children (Compas et al., 1996). This is consistent with findings from the larger literature on coping in which coping efforts that focus on one's emotional state are typically associated with greater distress. Second, parental cancer appears to offer children very little opportunity to experience a sense of personal control. Consistent with the absence of personal control, there was no evidence that matching the use of problem-focused coping to appraisals of control was beneficial for these children. As in other studies, no interaction of perceived control and the use of emotion-focused coping was found. This is particularly noteworthy in light of separate analyses of their parents' coping that found that high perceived control and the use of problem-focused coping was associated with lower emotional distress for their parents who had cancer (Osowiecki & Compas, 1996). Third, processes of family coping and social support offer both resources for coping and sources of increased distress. Adolescents who are called on to provide informational support about their parents' cancer to other family members experience more distress, perhaps because this is a task that exceeds their personal resources. Furthermore, adolescent girls may receive certain types of companionship from others in the family that actually serves to increase their distress. One possibility is that adolescent girls may spend time with their mothers discussing their mothers' illness and unintentionally increasing their own concerns and distress.

Rather than providing definitive findings, these studies are better considered in terms of their contributions to the methodology in this new area of research. First, it is noteworthy that both studies used semistructured interviews to obtain children's reports of coping, rather using questionnaires as is most common in research on adults' coping. Interviews were required because there are no self-report questionnaires available that assess coping across a wide age range of children, adolescents, and young adults. Semistructured interviews have a number of strengths in this context, including their sensitivity to individual differences in the experience of children coping with parental illness. Standardized questionnaires may be somewhat insensitive to the unique demands placed on children by this experience. On the other hand, interviews have several limitations as well. Most importantly, interviews appear to undersample the coping efforts that are used by children in response to parental illness. In our own research, children and adolescents generated an average of only two to three coping responses. If they had been provided with an inventory of several dozen coping items, it is likely that they would have reported more strategies for coping with their parents' cancer. A second methodological concern is reflected in the use of cross-sectional designs in these studies. Cross-sectional analyses present problems in interpreting the association between coping and distress. Specifically, the finding that emotion-focused coping was related to more emotional distress may indicate that children used certain types of coping that actually increased their negative affect (Compas et al., 1996). It is equally plausible, however, that this correlation indicates that those children who were more distressed responded with greater efforts to manage and palliate their negative emotions. Only prospective analyses will help to disentangle these relationships.

INTERVENTIONS TO FACILITATE CHILDREN'S ADJUSTMENT TO PARENTAL ILLNESS

As recognition of the psychological impact of illness has increased, provision of psychosocial support to adult patients and their families has become a component of services in many comprehensive health organizations. Unfortunately, no controlled evaluations of psychosocial interventions for children of parents with serious illness have been reported in the literature. The few studies that have appeared are primarily qualitative in nature. We will briefly describe these reports and evaluate them in light of the studies of the impact of parental illness on children's adjustment that were reported above.

Greening (1992) described the "Bear Essentials" program, which targeted 4- to 8-year-old children of parents with cancer. The program involved a group treatment for children and parents (seen in separate groups) addressing their adjustment to and coping with parental cancer. Group sessions targeted a variety of issues (e.g., visiting the hospital, affective responses) and were conducted weekly for 90 minutes. Although no standardized assessment of psychological adjustment or coping behaviors was conducted, Greening (1992) concludes that "the data did demonstrate that we were proceeding in the right direction" (p. 55). The basis of this determination was not specified. Greening identifies this lack of standardized assessment as a limitation of the study and states that an outcome-based evaluation instrument is being developed for future use.

Walsh-Burke (1992) describes the impact of the "We Can Weekend" treatment program with 14 cancer patients and their families. The program was designed to promote communication among cancer patients and their families. The children ranged in age from childhood to adulthood (no details with regard to age or other demographic characteristics of the sample were provided). Assessment instruments were developed for use in the study and included a problem checklist, a coping strategies checklist, a cancer information inventory, open-ended questions, and self-ratings of the respondent's communication and coping. Unfortunately, a description of the intervention was not provided. Furthermore, only half ($n = 7$) of the families completed all assessment instruments. According to the author, results suggested that family communication strategies and use of coping strategies were higher following treatment; however, specific details describing these results were not provided.

Nicholson et al. (1993) examined the impact of children's visitation to adult critical care units on 20 children's (age range, 5–17 years; mean = 10.3) emotional and behavioral responses. The authors employed a quasi-experimental design in the comparison of children who participated in a visit to their parent's ($n = 4$) or grandparent's ($n = 6$) critical care unit and children who were not given the opportunity to visit their parent ($n = 2$) or grandparent ($n = 8$). Behavioral and emotional responses of children were assessed with both parent and child reports on the Perceived Change Scale (Craft, 1986) and child reports on the Revised Children's Manifest Anxiety Scale (R-CMAS) (Reynolds & Richmond, 1978). Results suggested that there were no significant differences between the groups on the R-CMAS and parent reports on the Perceived Change Scale. Significant differences were found on the child report of the Perceived Change Scale, suggesting that children who participated in facilitated visitation reported significantly less change in behavioral and emotional responses associated with the stressor or hospitalization. The authors conclude that facilitated visitation was beneficial, resulting in fewer perceived behavioral and emotional changes for children of hospitalized parents or grandparents.

This brief summary of research on interventions to enhance children's coping illustrates the very preliminary status of this work. Interventions have been developed based primarily on clinical observations and experience and are not necessarily consistent with empirical research on children's adjustment to parental illness. For example, Greenberg (1992) described a program to facilitate the adjustment of young children whose parents have cancer. Findings from several recent studies suggest that young children are not adversely affected by parental cancer, as they may not be cognitively aware of the seriousness or the implications of their parents' illness (e.g., Compas et al., 1994). In contrast, adolescents appear to be a much more vulnerable group, and no interventions have been described that focus on their unique needs when faced with an ill parent. Therefore, the highest priority is for the development of interventions that are informed by the small but growing literature on children's adjustment to and coping with parental illness.

Future interventions can build on previous research in several ways. First, interventions can be used to assist families in managing family responsibilities and the redistribution of roles. Particular attention needs to be given to protecting adolescent girls from the burdens of increased caretaking and other responsibilities, especially when their mothers are ill. Second, processes of the provision and receipt of social support within families are also a target for interventions. Adolescents appear to be poorly equipped to provide informational support to others within the family, while they appear to benefit, as reflected in lower levels of psychological distress, from receiving informational support. Third, it appears that adolescents can benefit from interventions that facilitate the development of more effective methods of managing their emotional distress. Current data indicate that adolescents may rely on avoidant methods of coping that are ineffective in managing their distress. Facilitating more effective individual coping may be accomplished either in family, group, or individual interventions.

FUTURE DIRECTIONS

When an area of research is at such an early stage in development, the directions for future research are many. Four broad steps are of highest priority. First, there is a clear need for more longitudinal data on the psychological adjustment of children whose parents are suffering from a serious illness. The relative absence of longitudinal data on children's adjustment makes it difficult to consider the course and process of adaptation to parental illness.

Second, researchers need to attend to individual differences in the adjustment of children to the stress of parental illness. Group-level analyses are likely to indicate that children experience moderate levels of emotional distress and maladjustment associated with parental illness. Group-level analyses, however, may well disguise significant variations among children in their adaptation. The use of standardized measures that can be used to identify those children with clinically significant levels of maladjustment will be important. Current research suggests that adolescents may be particularly vulnerable to the stress of parental illness, and these initial findings warrant further examination.

Third, the processes through which parental illness exerts an impact on children's adjustment warrants further research. Children's coping efforts may both facilitate their adjustment to parental illness in some instances and actually contribute to poorer adjustment in others. Furthermore, ongoing processes of stress within families in the weeks and months following a parent's diagnosis appear to be important.

Finally, interventions need to be developed that reflect the findings from descriptive studies of emotional distress and coping in children whose parents are ill. It appears that interventions will need to target high-risk groups of children rather than being delivered to all children whose parents are seriously ill. Moreover, these interventions can draw on the larger literature on enhancing children's skills in coping with stress.

REFERENCES

Adrian, C., & Hammen, C. (1993). Stress exposure and stress generation in children of depressed mothers. *Journal of Consulting and Clinical Psychology, 61,* 354–359.

Anderson, C. A., & Hammen, C. L. (1993). Psychosocial outcomes of children of unipolar depressed, bipolar, medically ill, and normal women: A longitudinal study. *Journal of Consulting and Clinical Psychology, 61,* 448–454.

Berman, H., Cragg, C. E., & Kuenzig, L. (1988). Having a parent die of cancer: Adolescents' reactions. *Oncology Nursing Forum, 15,* 159–163.

Biegel, D. E., Sales, E., & Schulz, R. (1991). *Family caregiving in chronic illness.* Newbury Park, CA: Sage.

Bolton, D. A. (1995). *Social support in families: Examining the provision and receipt of social support in families when a parent has cancer.* Unpublished doctoral dissertation, University of Vermont.

Carter, B., & McGoldrick, M. (1988). *The changing family life-cycle: A framework for family therapy.* Needham Heights, MA: Allyn & Bacon.

Cassileth, B. R., Lusk, E. J., Strouse, T. B., Miller, D. S., Brown, L. L., & Cross, P. A. (1984). A psychological analysis of cancer patients and their next-of-kin. *Cancer, 55,* 72–76.

Cohen, S., & Wills, T. A. (1985). Stress, social support, and the buffering hypothesis. *Psychological Bulletin, 98,* 310–357.

Compas, B. E., Connor, J., Osowiecki, D., & Welch, A. (in press). Effortful and involuntary responses to stress: Implications for coping with chronic stress. In B. H. Gottlieb (Ed.), *Coping with chronic stress.* New York: Plenum Press.

Compas, B. E., Malcarne, V. L., & Banez, G. A. (1992). Coping with psychosocial stress: A developmental perspective. In B. Carpenter (Ed.), *Personal coping: Theory, research, and application* (pp. 47–64). New York: Praeger.

Compas, B. E., Malcarne, V., & Fondacaro, K. (1988). Coping with stress in older children and young adolescents. *Journal of Consulting and Clinical Psychology, 56,* 405–411.

Compas, B. E., & Wagner, B. M. (1991). Psychosocial stress during adolescence: Intrapersonal and interpersonal processes. In S. Gore & M. Colton (Eds.), *Adolescence, stress, and coping* (pp. 67–85). New York: Aldine de Gruyter.

Compas, B. E., Worsham, N., Epping-Jordan, J. E., Howell, D. C., Grant, K. E., Mireault, G., & Malcarne, V. (1994). When mom or dad has cancer: Markers of psychological distress in cancer patients, spouses, and children. *Health Psychology, 13,* 507–515.

Compas, B. E., Worsham, N. L., & Ey, S. (1992). Conceptual and developmental issues in children's coping with stress. In A. LaGreca, L. Siegel, J. Wallander, & C. E. Walker (Eds.), *Advances in pediatric psychology: Stress and coping with pediatric conditions* (pp. 7–24). New York: Guilford Press.

Compas, B. E., Worsham, N., Ey, S., & Howell, D. C. (1996). When mom or dad has cancer: II. Coping, cognitive appraisals, and psychological distress in children of cancer patients. *Health Psychology, 15,* 167–175.

Craft, M. J. (1986). Validation of responses reported by school-aged siblings of hospitalized children. *Children's Health Care, 15,* 6–13.

Epping-Jordan, J. E., Compas, B. E., & Howell, D. C. (1994). Predictors of cancer progression in young adult men and women: Avoidance, intrusive thoughts, and psychological symptoms. *Health Psychology, 13,* 539–547.

Ey, S., Compas, B. E., Epping-Jordan, J. E., & Worsham, N. (1997). *Stress responses and psychological adjustment in cancer patients and their spouses.* Manuscript submitted for publication.

Forsythe, C. J., & Compas, B. E. (1987). Interaction of cognitive appraisals of stressful events and coping: Testing the goodness of fit hypothesis. *Cognitive Therapy and Research, 11,* 473–485.

Grandstaff, N. W. (1976). The impact of breast cancer on the family. In J. M. Vaeth (Ed.), *Frontiers of radiation therapy and oncology* (Vol. 11, pp. 146–156). Basel, Switzerland: Karger.

Grant, K. E., & Compas, B. E. (1995). Stress and anxious–depressed symptoms of anxiety/depression among adolescents: Searching for mechanisms of risk. *Journal of Consulting and Clinical Psychology, 63*, 1015–1021.

Greening, K. (1992). The "Bear Essentials" program: Helping young children and their families cope when a parent has cancer. *Journal of Psychosocial Oncology, 10*, 47–61.

Hammen, C., Adrian, C., Gordon, D., Burge, D., Jaenicke, C., & Hiroto, D. (1987). Children of depressed mothers: Maternal strain and symptom predictors of dysfunction. *Journal of Abnormal Psychology, 96*, 190–198.

Hammen, C., Burge, D., & Adrian, C. (1991). Timing of mother and child depression in a longitudinal study of children at risk. *Journal of Consulting and Clinical Psychology, 59*, 341–345.

Hammen, C., Burge, D., Burney, E., & Adrian, C. (1990). Longitudinal study of diagnoses in children of women with unipolar and bipolar affective disorder. Archives of General Psychiatry, 47, 1112–1117.

Hammen, C., Gordon, D., Burge, D., Adrian, C., Jaenicke, C., & Hiroto, D. (1987). Maternal affective disorders, illness, and stress: Risk for children's psychopathology. *American Journal of Psychiatry, 144*, 736–741.

Hirsch, B. J., Moos, R. H., & Reischl, T. M. (1985). Psychosocial adjustment of adolescent children of a depressed, arthritic, or normal parent. *Journal of Abnormal Psychology, 94*, 154–164.

Horowitz, M. J., Wilner, N., & Alvarez, W. (1979). Impact of Event Scale: A measure of subjective stress. *Journal of Consulting and Clinical Psychology, 41*, 209–218.

Issel, L. M., Ersek, M., & Lewis, F. M. (1990). How children cope with mother's breast cancer. *Oncology Nursing Forum, 17*, 5–12.

Klein, D. N., Clark, D. C., Dansky, L., & Margolis, E. T. (1988). Dysthymia in the offspring of parents with primary unipolar affective disorder. *Journal of Abnormal Psychology, 97*, 265–274.

Lazarus, R. S., & Folkman, S. (1984). *Stress, appraisal, and coping.* New York: Springer.

Lee, C. M., & Gotlib, I. H. (1989a). Clinical status and emotional adjustment of children of depressed mothers. *American Journal of Psychiatry, 146*, 478–483.

Lee, C. M., & Gotlib, I. H. (1989b). Maternal depression and child adjustment: A longitudinal analysis. *Journal of Abnormal Psychology, 98*, 78–85.

Lee, C. M., & Gotlib, I. H. (1991). Adjustment of children of depressed mothers: A 10-month follow-up. *Journal of Abnormal Psychology, 100*, 473–477.

Levanthal, H., Levanthal, E. A., & Nguyen, T. V. (1985). Reactions of families to illness: Theoretical models and perspectives. In D. C. Turk & R. D. Kerns (Eds.), *Health, illness, and families: A lifespan perspective* (pp. 108–145). New York: Wiley.

Lewandowski, L. A. (1992). Needs of children during the critical illness of a parent or sibling. *Critical Care Nursing Clinics of North America, 4*, 573–585.

Lewis, F. M. (1990). Strengthening family supports. *Cancer, 65*, 752–759.

Lewis, F. M., Ellison, E. S., & Woods, N. F. (1985). The impact of breast cancer on the family. *Seminars in Oncology Nursing, 1*, 206–213.

Lewis, F. M., Hammond, M. A., & Woods, N. F. (1993). The family's functioning with newly diagnosed breast cancer in the mother: The development of an explanatory model. *Journal of Behavioral Medicine, 16*, 351–370.

Lewis, F. M., Woods, N. G., Hough, E. E., & Bensley, L. S. (1989). The family's functioning with chronic illness in the mother: The spouse's perspective. *Social Science and Medicine, 29*, 1261–1269.

Malcarne, V. L., Compas, B. E., Epping-Jordan, J. E., & Howell, D. C. (1995). Cognitive factors in adjustment to cancer: Attributions of self-blame and perceptions of control. *Journal of Behavioral Medicine, 18*, 401–417.

Moguilner, M. E., Bauman, A., & De-Nour, A. K. (1988). The adjustment of children and parents to chronic hemodialysis. *Psychosomatics, 29*, 289–294.

National Center for Health Statistics. (1993). *Advance data from vital and health statistics: Numbers 111–120.* (National Center for Health Statistics Vital Health Stat 16(12)). Washington, DC: US Government Printing Office.

Nicholson, A. C., Titler, M., Montgomery, L. A., Kleiber, C., Craft, M. J., Halm, M., Buckwalter, K., &

Johnson, S. (1993). Effects of child visitation in adult critical care units: A pilot study. *Heart and Lung, 22*, 36–45.

Nolen-Hoeksema, S. (1990). *Sex differences in depression.* Stanford, CA: Stanford University Press.

Northouse, L. L. (1995). The impact of cancer in women on the family. *Cancer Practice, 3*, 134–142.

Osowiecki, D., & Compas, B. E. (1997). *Coping and control beliefs in adjustment to cancer.* Manuscript submitted for publication.

Reynolds, C. R., & Richmond, B. (1978). What I Think and Feel: A revised measure of children's manifest anxiety. *Journal of Abnormal Child Psychology, 6*, 271–280.

Rickard, K. (1988). The occurrence of maladaptive health-related behaviors and teacher-rated conduct problems in children of chronic low back pain patients. *Journal of Behavioral Medicine, 11*, 107–116.

Rutter, M. (1966). *Children of sick parents: An environmental and psychiatric study.* London: Oxford University Press.

Siegel, K., Karus, D., & Raveis, V. H. (1996). Adjustment of children facing the death of a parent due to cancer. *Journal of the American Academy of Child and Adolescent Psychiatry, 35*, 442–450.

Siegel, K., Mesagno, F. P., Karus, D., Christ, G., Banks, K., & Moynihan, R. (1992). Psychosocial adjustment of children with a terminally ill parent. *Journal of the American Academy of Child and Adolescent Psychiatry, 31*, 327–333.

Stetz, K., Lewis, F. M., & Primomo, J. (1986). Family coping strategies and chronic illness in the mother. *Family Relations, 35*, 515–522.

Turk, D. C., & Kerns, R. D. (1985). The family in health and illness. In D. C. Turk & R. D. Kerns (Eds.), *Health, illness, and families: A life-span perspective* (pp. 1–22). New York: Wiley.

US Bureau of the Census. (1993). *Statistical abstract of the United States: 1993* (113th ed.). Washington, DC: US Government Printing Office.

Walsh-Burke, K. (1992). Family communication and coping with cancer: Impact of the We Can Weekend. *Journal of Psychosocial Oncology, 10*, 63–81.

Welch, A. S., Wadsworth, M. E., & Compas, B. E. (1996). Adjustment of children and adolescents to parental cancer. *Cancer, 77*, 1409–1418.

Wellisch, D. K., Gritz, E. R., Schain, W., Wang, H.-J., & Siau, J. (1991). Psychological functioning of daughters of breast cancer patients. Part I: Daughters and comparison subjects. *Psychosomatics, 32*, 324–336.

Wellisch, D. K., Gritz, E. R., Schain, W., Wang, H.-J., & Siau, J. (1992). Psychological functioning of daughters of breast cancer patients. Part II: Characterizing the distressed daughter of the breast cancer patient. *Psychosomatics, 33*, 171–179.

8

Risks and Interventions for the Parentally Bereaved Child

JANELLE R. LUTZKE, TIM S. AYERS,
IRWIN N. SANDLER, and ALICIA BARR

There are few other stressful events that occur in a child's or adolescent's life that have as potentially profound and lasting impact as the death of a parent. Yet, what evidence is there to support this statement? What, if any, kinds of mental health or adjustment problems might these children experience? And if the death of a parent does indeed put children or adolescents at risk, what are the important risk and protective factors that mediate or moderate the relationship between parental death and children's adjustment? Finally, what kinds of preventive interventions have been or need to be developed for the parentally bereaved child? Some initial answers to these questions are provided in this chapter. We begin by discussing the epidemiology of parental death in children and adolescents. Next, we review the research literatures examining the risks of adjustment problems and other developmental outcomes in children and the mental health outcomes in adulthood. As part of these reviews, we use meta-analytic methods to begin to explore the strength of the findings across studies and at the same time offer critiques and point to some of the methodological limitations of these studies. We then turn to a review the literatures that have examined some of the factors associated with the effects of parental bereavement. We discuss the interventions that have been developed and experimentally evaluated for these children, and finally we conclude the chapter with some recommendations for further research in this area.

JANELLE R. LUTZKE and ALICIA BARR • Department of Psychology, Arizona State University, Tempe, Arizona 85287-1104.   TIM S. AYERS and IRWIN N. SANDLER • Department of Psychology and Program for Prevention Research, Arizona State University, Tempe, Arizona 85287-1108.

Handbook of Children's Coping: Linking Theory and Intervention, edited by Wolchik and Sandler. Plenum Press, New York, 1997.

EPIDEMIOLOGY

To understand the potential implications of parental bereavement for the mental health problems of children it is useful to take an epidemiological perspective. According to the 1990 US Census, 2,2132,000 (3.4%) of children under the age of 18 had experienced the death of a parent (73% death of a father, 25% death of a mother, 1.2% death of both parents) (US Bureau of the Census, 1990). Unfortunately, census data are not available on the entire population to describe the occurrence of parental death across demographic categories such as age of child, gender, or ethnicity. However, the occurrence of parental death across children who differ on these demographic characteristics can be obtained for a subgroup of bereaved children: children who live in a single-parent household with a widowed parent. Of the 809,000 bereaved children who live in a single-parent household, 85.5% live with their mothers and 14.5% live with their fathers; 56% are male; 12.2% are under age 6, 32% are 6 to 12 years of age, and 55% are between 12 and 18 years of age; and 56.7% are white non-Hispanic, 21.3% are Hispanic, and 21.9% are African American (US Bureau of the Census, 1994). It is interesting to note, however, that since only 809,000 of the 2,213,200 bereaved children in 1994 were living with a single parent, many bereaved children are living in blended families or are in the care of people other than their surviving parents.

RELATIONS OF PARENTAL DEATH TO MENTAL HEALTH PROBLEMS AND OTHER DEVELOPMENTAL OUTCOMES

While parental death is clearly a traumatic and painful experience for children, there have been relatively few methodologically sound studies investigating the relations of this event to the development of mental health problems or other negative developmental outcomes. This section will review studies to address the following three questions: What is the relation between parental death and children's mental health problems and other developmental outcomes? How do the mental health or other problems of bereaved children change over time? What is the relation between parental death that occurs in childhood and mental health problems in adulthood?

All of the studies reviewed in this section met two minimal methodological criteria. First, the studies compared a bereaved sample with a comparable nonbereaved sample of children or adolescents. Studies that simply describe problems or reactions in community or clinic-based samples of bereaved children were omitted. Second, all studies utilized measures with acceptable psychometric properties. The studies differed, however, in other methodological features, including methods of sampling the bereaved and comparison children, sample size, and time since parental death. The potential effects of these methodological issues on the inferences that can be drawn concerning the effects of parental death will be discussed following the review of the findings. Table 1 describes the sample characteristics, design, outcomes assessed, and major findings that were observed. The review is organized to summarize ef-

Table 1. Studies Examining the Relations between Parental Death and Child and Adolescent Mental Health Problems

Author	Sample and study characteristics[a]	Outcomes assessed and findings
Ambert & Saucier (1984)	Age = 12–19 N(b) = 312 N(c) = 4227 School survey sample Time since death: not stated Cross-sectional	Adolescent report: bereaved adolescents rated themselves as having significantly poorer academic performance and lower educational aspirations There were no significant differences on ratings of liking in school

Felner et al. (1975)	Age = 5–10
	Study 1:
	    N(b) = 32
	    N(c) = 30
	Study 2:
	    N(b) = 38
	    N(c) = 38
	Bereaved and comparison children were drawn from a pool of children identified by teachers as having significant early school adjustment problems
	Time since death: not stated
	Cross-sectional
		Teacher report: bereaved children significantly higher overall maladjustment and moodiness/withdrawal; no significant differences for acting out or learning problems

Gregory (1965)	Age = 9th grade[b] N(b) = 800 N(c) = 9617 Statewide sample of Minnesota school children Time since death: not stated	Police and court files: bereaved children who had a father die had significantly higher levels of delinquency
Gersten et al. (1991)	Age = 8–15 N(b) = 92 N(c) = 20 Bereaved children from community sample; matched control group of children who had not experienced major stressor Time since death: 3–30 months Cross-sectional	Child report: bereaved children had significantly higher levels of depression; conduct disorder, n.s. Parent report: depression, n.s., conduct disorder, n.s.
Hainline & Feig (1978)	Age = 17–23 N(b) = 12 N(c) = 24 Bereaved subjects were volunteers from the community; two comparison groups: (1) divorce, (2) intact Time since death: not stated Cross-sectional	Self-report: self-esteem, n.s.; anxiety, n.s. Observational measures: behavior toward males, n.s.

(continued)

Table 1. *(Continued)*

Author	Sample and study characteristics[a]	Outcomes assessed and findings
Hetherington (1972)	Age = 13–17 N(b) = 24 N(dv) = 24 N(c) = 24 Bereaved adolescents from a community recreation center with matched comparison groups: (1) divorce (dv), (2) intact (in) Time since death: not stated Cross-sectional	Interview with adolescent: bereaved adolescents had significantly lower self-esteem and higher anxiety Observational measures: bereaved girls were more anxious around males
Kranzler et al. (1990)	Age = 3–6 N(b) = 26 N(c) = 40 Bereaved children referred for study by school and health professionals; comparison group drawn from preschool programs from intact families Time since death: 1–6 months Cross-sectional	Parent report: bereaved children were significantly higher on measures of depression, anxiety, and conduct disorder Teacher report: bereaved children were significantly higher on measures of depression, anxiety, and conduct disorder
Partridge & Kotler (1987)	Age = 15–17 N(b) = 18 N(dv) = 18 N(in) = 18 Community sample of bereaved; two comparison groups: (1) divorce (dv), (2) intact (in) Time since death: not stated Cross-sectional	Adolescent report: self-esteem, n.s. Parent report: overall adjustment, n.s.
Sandler et al. (1996)	Age = 8–15 N(b) = 92 N(c) = 20 Bereaved children from community sample; matched control group of children who had not experienced major stressor Time since death: 3–30 months Cross-sectional	Child report: bereaved children rated themselves significantly lower on academic success than controls; self-esteem n.s.; locus of control n.s. Parent report: bereaved children were rated significantly lower on academic success than controls
Saucier & Ambert (1982)	Age = 12–19 N(b) = 312 N(c) = 4227 School survey sample Time since death: not stated Cross-sectional	Adolescent report: bereaved adolescents rated themselves as being significantly less optimistic about their future and chance of being successful
Silverman & Worden (1993)	Age = 6–17 N(b) = 120 N(c) = 73 Bereaved and comparison children from a community sample[c] time since death: assessments at 4 months and 1 year reported; longitudinal	Child report: bereaved children has significantly more somatic complaints

Table 1. *(Continued)*

Author	Sample and study characteristics[a]	Outcomes assessed and findings
Sood et al. (1992)	Age = 5–12 N(b) = 38 N(dp) = 38 N(c) = 19 Bereaved children from community sample; two comparison groups: (1) depressed inpatient (dp), (2) nonclinic (nc) Time since death: 3–12 weeks Cross-sectional	Child report: overall somatic complaints, n.s.; headaches and gastrointestinal tract disturbances most commonly endorsed
Van Erdewegh et al. (1982)	Age = 2–17 N(b) = 105 N(c) = 80 Bereaved children from community sample with matched control Time since death: assessments were conducted at 1 month and 13 months since death Longitudinal	Child report: bereaved children had significantly higher levels of depressive mood symptoms, withdrawn behavior, and significantly poorer school performance
Worden & Silverman (1996)	Age = school-aged (6–17)[d] N(b) = 70 N(c) = 70 Matched by age, gender, school grade, and socioeconomic background; bereaved children from community sample Time since death: bereaved children were assessed at three points; 4 months, 1 year, and 2 years after death of parent Control children assessed at the 1st and 2nd anniversary of bereaved child's loss Longitudinal	Child report: at 1 year, bereaved children viewed themselves as less well-behaved and having poorer scholastic abilities than their matched controls; at 2 years, bereaved children viewed themselves as less well-behaved, poorer social abilities, and lower overall self-worth; at 1- and 2-year assessments, bereaved children had significantly higher external locus of control Parent report: at 2-year assessment, bereaved children had significantly higher social withdrawal, anxiety/depression; n.s. differences on somatic complaints, delinquent, aggressive, or attention-seeking behaviors at 1- or 2-year assessments; at 2-year assessment, significantly more of the bereaved children (21%) were at subclinical levels on the CBCL than control children (3%)

[a] N(b) = number of subjects in the bereaved group, N(c) = number of subjects in the control group.
[b] Gregory conducted an anterospective study of a statewide sample of Minnesota ninth-grade children (n = 11,329). The number of subjects in the bereaved and control groups presented here reflect the total number of subjects (collapsed over sex) that could be included in the calculation of the ES (i.e., n = 10,417).
[c] See Worden and Silverman (1996) for another description of this study.
[d] Ages of the children were not reported in this article; however, Silverman and Worden (1993), which is also based on this sample, provide this information.

fects of parental death on internalizing and externalizing problems, beliefs, and academic success.

To help summarize the findings, effect sizes (ESs: specifically Cohen's *d*) were calculated for each dependent variable measured when sufficient information was available. When more than one dependent variable for a particular study measured overlapping constructs (i.e., moody, crying, sad), a mean ES was calculated for these measures. In calculating the ES, the bereaved and control group means were coded such that a positive Cohen's *d* indicated that the bereaved subjects experienced more of the measured construct.*

Internalizing Problems

Depression

The most consistent finding in the literature is the association between parental bereavement and depression in childhood. Four well-designed studies found that parental bereavement is related to depressive symptoms in children, including clinical levels of depressive disorder. Gersten, Beals, and Kallgren (1991) studied a community-based sample of 92 bereaved children, ages 8 through 15, recruited from health department records of deaths that occurred in the past 2 years. The comparison sample was a demographically matched control group selected from the same neighborhood, who had not experienced parental death, parental divorce, or parental alcoholism. They found that bereaved children had higher levels of depressive symptoms than the comparison group as assessed by a structured diagnostic interview. Using *Diagnostic and Statistical Manual of Mental Disorders,* 3rd edition (DSM-III) (American Psychiatric Association, 1980) diagnostic criteria to assess major depression from the structured diagnostic interview, Gersten et al. (1991) found a 9.8% preva-

---

*All ES measures and homogeneity tests were calculated via DSTAT, version 1.11, software for the meta-analytic review of research literatures (Johnson, 1993). Typically, each study reported bereaved versus control comparisons on several dependent variables. Cohen's *d* was calculated for each dependent variable within each study. Cohen's *d* represents the difference between means divided by a standard deviation. Bereaved and control group means were coded such that a positive *d* indicated that bereaved subjects experienced more of the measured construct (somatic symptoms, depressive mood, etc.) than control subjects.

If two or more dependent variables for a particular study measured overlapping constructs (i.e., disinterest in school, learning problems, school dropout), a mean ES was calculated for those measures and then categorized within the overall construct (i.e., school problems). To be consistent with this strategy of producing one ES per construct within each study, in the longitudinal investigations the ESs were averaged across the two assessments. This admittedly masks potential effects that emerge over time, but these findings are noted elsewhere in the text. If a dependent variable for a particular study did not measure a construct that overlapped with other measures within that study, the single Cohen's *d* was used in subsequent analyses.

Once all ESs for each study were organized into distinct construct categories, a weighted mean ES for the construct was calculated to represent the average bereaved/control difference. Effect sizes for each study were weighted by the sample size for the study. Additionally, homogeneity tests were conducted on the ESs within each construct. When homogeneity tests indicated that the ES for a particular study differed greater than chance from the other effect sizes, a weighted mean ES was recalculated for the construct, excluding the case that was heterogeneous. These cases are reported in the main body of the text. Complete details about the procedures used and the ESs that were calculated for each study can be obtained from the authors.

lence of major depression among the bereaved children compared to a 1.3% prevalence among the control children. Based on this, they calculated the risk ratio of parental death for major depression to be 7.5.

Kranzler, Shaffer, Wasserman, and Davies (1990) studied bereaved pre-school-aged children 1 to 3 months following parental death. They found that both parents and teachers rated the bereaved children as having significantly higher levels of depression on a subscale that reflected the DSM-III-R criteria when compared to controls. Bereaved children themselves also reported significantly more fear and less happiness than control children.

Van Eerdewegh, Bieri, Parrilla, and Clayton (1982) conducted a longitudinal study with a community sample of children aged 2 to 17 in which children's mental health problems were assessed 1 month and 13 months after the parent's death using a structured interview with the surviving parent. They found that at both assessments bereaved children displayed significantly more depressive mood symptoms including sadness, crying, and irritability compared to controls. When a depressive syndrome was defined as three or more symptoms from the depression checklist, the group of bereaved children had a significantly higher rate of depression (14%) than controls (4%).

Bereaved and nonbereaved children in the Harvard Child Bereavement Study were assessed 1 and 2 years after the death of their parent. Bereaved children scored significantly higher on the anxiety/depression scale of the Achenbach Child Behavior Checklist (CBCL) than nonbereaved children at the 2-year follow-up assessment, although there were no differences between the groups at the 1-year assessment (Worden & Silverman, 1996).

In terms of depressive mood and symptoms, the studies reviewed yielded a wide range of effect sizes from 1.23 observed in the Kranzler et al. (1990) study to .25 in Van Eerdewegh et al. (1982) study. The weighted mean ES (weighted by the sample size) for all studies investigating depressive symptoms (Gersten et al., 1991; Kranzler et al., 1990; Van Eerdewegh et al., 1982; Worden & Silverman, 1996) was .48. After removing the one study that yielded an ES that was not homogeneous with the others (i.e., Kranzler et al., 1990), the weighted mean ES for depressive mood was .37. An ES represents the difference in means between two groups divided by the pooled standard deviation; thus, an ES of .37 suggests that on the average the mean of the bereaved group on measures of depressive mood is more than a third of a standard deviation higher than the mean of the comparison group.*

A much larger mean weighted ES was found (ES = .79) when combining the studies (i.e., Felner, Stolberg, & Cowen, 1975, Study 1 and 2; Van Eerdewegh et al., 1982) that examined variables measuring overall negative affect (e.g., moody, irritable, crying, sad). In summary, the evidence from these stud-

---

*It is important to note that the practice by some investigators of not reporting the results of statistical tests (i.e., *F, t,* etc.) when findings are not significant in their studies thereby does not allow the ESs to be calculated for these findings. These lack of findings, and probable small and potential ESs that are of an opposite sign, then are not included in the mean weighted ES that is calculated for that construct. The degree to which the studies reviewed do not provide information on nonsignificant findings could result in some inflation of the calculated ES, relative to the population of studies. Circumstances where these practices might influence the calculation of the weighted mean ESs are indicated in the text.

ies indicates that relatively large differences between bereaved and non-bereaved children are generally observed when investigating overall negative affect (e.g., sad, crying, irritable, and/or moody symptoms), while those studies that have investigated the types of depressive symptoms that are typically more indicative of clinical depression yield a moderate effect size of .37.

Anxiety and Withdrawal

Five studies provide evidence that bereaved children are more anxious and withdrawn than controls. Kranzler et al. (1990) found that bereaved children aged 3 to 6 were rated by their teachers and parents as displaying significantly more anxiety than control children 1 to 6 months following the death. Saucier and Ambert (1986) found that bereaved adolescents aged 12 to 15 rated themselves as being nervous significantly more often than nonbereaved adolescents. Using observational measures, Hetherington (1972) reported that bereaved adolescent girls became significantly more withdrawn in the presence of males than nonbereaved adolescents. Felner et al. (1975) found that teachers rated bereaved students as being more moody and withdrawn than nonbereaved students. Bereaved children in the Harvard Child Bereavement Study also scored significantly higher on the withdrawn scale of the CBCL than nonbereaved children 2 years following the death (Worden & Silverman, 1996).

There were only two studies in which an effect size could be calculated for anxiety (Kranzler et al., 1990; Partridge & Kotler, 1987). The weighted mean ES was .70. However, as a summary statement, this weighted mean ES should be taken very cautiously, since the ESs for these two studies differed so greatly (ES 1.08 and .03). The mean weighted ES for withdrawal behaviors was .35 (based on Silverman & Worden, 1993; Van Eerdewegh et al., 1982; Worden & Silverman, 1996), but increases to .44, after removing the one study that yielded an ES not homogeneous with the others (i.e., Silverman & Worden, 1993). It is interesting to observe that the ES for withdrawal behaviors was very comparable to the mean weighted ES obtained for depressive mood. These behaviors are often associated features of depressive symptomatology.

Somatic Symptoms

There is inconsistent evidence from four studies on the relationship between parental death and children's somatic complaints. Sood, Weller, Weller, Fristad, and Bowes (1992) found no significant differences in self-reported somatic complaints between bereaved children aged 5 to 12 and a nonbereaved comparison group. Van Eerdewegh et al. (1982) found very few differences between parental report of bereaved children's somatic problems as compared to nonbereaved controls. Of the nine somatic symptoms they assessed, the only significant difference found was that bereaved children had a higher incidence of bed-wetting. Silverman and Worden (1992) reported that bereaved children had significantly more somatic symptoms than nonbereaved children, and that approximately 10% of their sample had suffered from a serious illness within a year after the parent's death. However, in a later report utilizing other data from this same sample, Worden and Silverman (1996) found no differences between the bereaved and nonbereaved children on the somatic subscale of the CBCL at either the 1- or 2-year follow-up assessments. In those studies that provided data to allow calculation of an ES (Silverman & Worden 1993; Sood et al., 1992; Van Eerdewegh et al., 1982), the weighted mean ES for somatic symptoms was .19, suggesting small differences between the bereaved and comparison children.

Externalizing Symptomatology

There is inconsistent evidence for the association between parental death and increased externalizing problems for bereaved children or adolescents. Gersten et al. (1991) found that bereaved children were not significantly different from controls on conduct problems on parental or self-ratings or a structured psychiatric diagnostic interview. However, there was a nonsignificant trend for bereaved children to have more conduct problems on the psychiatric diagnostic interview.

Van Eerdewegh et al. (1982) found no differences between parental reports of externalizing behavior problems between bereaved children and controls either immediately following the death or 1 year after the death. In a preschool-aged sample, teachers and parents rated bereaved children as displaying significantly higher conduct problems than controls; however, this finding held only for boys (Kranzler et al., 1990). In the Harvard Child Bereavement Study there were no significant differences for bereaved and nonbereaved children on parental report on either the aggressive or delinquent scales of the CBCL (Worden & Silverman, 1996). Interestingly, bereaved children's self-report on Harter's behavioral conduct subscale (Harter, 1979) indicated that they are less well behaved than their nonbereaved matched controls 1 and 2 years after the death of their parent. Additional evidence for the relationship of bereavement and conduct problems is reported by Gregory (1965), who examined police and court files and found that children who had experienced the death of a father had significantly higher rates of delinquency.

Weighted mean ESs were calculated for studies that investigated externalizing symptomatology in two different but related areas: acting out–disruptive behaviors and delinquent behaviors. In addition, a mean ES for all studies exploring externalizing behavior problems was calculated. In terms of acting out–disruptive behaviors, a moderate ES of .29 was obtained. Excluding one study that had a mean ES that was not homogeneous with the others (Felner et al., 1975, Study 2), the mean weighted ES for the remaining studies was .33. A small mean weighed ES of .10 was obtained for the two studies that examined delinquent behavior (Gregory, 1965; Silverman & Worden, 1993). Finally, a mean weighted ES of .11 was obtained for all studies that examined externalizing behaviors (based on Felner et al., 1975, Study 1 and 2; Gersten et al., 1991; Gregory, 1965; Kranzler et al., 1990; Partridge & Kotler, 1987; Silverman & Worden, 1993; Van Eerdewegh et al., 1982). One cautionary statement should be made about this summary ES. After removing the study by Gregory (1965) that had an extremely large sample and a small ES (.10) and which investigated more severe signs of delinquency (i.e., police records), the ES increases to .23. Thus, the evidence appears to be small to moderately strong for differences between bereaved and nonbereaved children in acting out and disruptive behaviors but much weaker when more extreme delinquent behaviors are assessed.

Developmental Outcomes: Attitudes, Beliefs, and Success in Developmental Tasks

Several theoretical models propose that the experience of major stressors such as bereavement affects a wide range of beliefs about the self and the world and success on developmental tasks (Janoff-Bulman, 1985; Brown & Harris, 1978; Brown, Harris, & Bifulco, 1986). This section will review those studies that examine locus of control beliefs, self-esteem, and academic success. In examining the effects of bereavement on children's locus of control, Worden and Silverman (1996) found that children who had experienced the death of a parent have significantly more external locus of control at 1 and 2 years following the death than nonbereaved children. Two studies have found no significant differences between bereaved and nonbereaved children on self-report measures of self-esteem (Hainline & Feig, 1978; Partridge & Kotler, 1987). However, 2 years following the death of a parent, bereaved children in the Harvard Child Bereavement Study had significantly lower levels of self-esteem than nonbereaved children (Worden & Silverman, 1996). Saucier and Ambert (1982) also found that bereaved adolescents reported having significantly less optimism for success in later life than nonbereaved adolescents.

Felner et al. (1975) and Felner, Ginter, Boike, and Cowen (1981) found no significant differences in level of teacher-reported learning problems between bereaved and nonbereaved children. However, Van Eerdewegh et al. (1982) found that bereaved children had significantly poorer school performance based on academic records. In another study, bereaved adolescents rated themselves as having significantly poorer academic performance and lower educational aspirations than their nonbereaved peers (Ambert & Saucier, 1984). Worden and Silverman (1996) reported that 1 year after the death, bereaved children had significantly lower scores on their perceived scholastic abilities, but these differences were not significant at the 2-year follow-up.

Recently, we compared the locus of control, self-esteem, and academic success of a sample of 92 bereaved children and a matched sample of 20 nonbereaved controls (Sandler, Barr, Ayers, & Lutzke, 1996). Bereaved children had significantly lower academic success as rated on parent and self-report measures, but they were not significantly different from controls on locus of control beliefs or self-esteem.

In the two studies that investigated locus of control and where there was sufficient information to calculate ES, the mean weighted ES was −.28 (Sandler et al., 1996; Worden & Silverman, 1996). A mean weighted ES of −.36 was obtained for studies on self-esteem (Partridge & Kotler, 1987; Hetherington, 1972; Sandler et al., 1996; Worden & Silverman, 1996). However, removing the one study with an ES that was not homogeneous (i.e., Worden & Silverman, 1996) results in a mean ES of −.18, suggesting more modest differences in self-esteem between bereaved and nonbereaved children. The ESs for school problems varies as a function of the type of problem assessed. As an example, the two studies that investigated high school dropout rate, as a measure of school problems (e.g., Gregory, 1965; Van Eerdewegh et al., 1982), yielded a mean ES of .26, which is of moderate size. In contrast, the study by Sandler et al. (1996) investigating parent and children's report of academic success yielded large ESs of .73 and .60, respectively. These differences aside, the overall mean weighted ES for school problems was a moderate .27 (based on Felner et al., 1975, Study 1 and 2; Gregory, 1965; Partridge & Kotler, 1987; Sandler et al., 1996; Van Eerdewegh et al., 1982). In summary, although not all studies have resulted in significant findings, there appears to be small to moderate differences between bereaved and nonbereaved children on their self-esteem, locus of control beliefs, and academic success.

Limitations of Current Research

Several significant methodological problems limit the interpretation or generalizability of the findings of these studies: potential sampling bias, small sample size, and reliance on only parent and/or teacher reports of child outcomes (cf. Cook, 1990; Worden & Silverman, 1996). One common problem is the use of nonrepresentative samples of bereaved children. Several studies rely exclusively on samples of children referred for psychological services (e.g., Kranzler et al., 1990; Felner et al., 1981) who may have a higher rate of symptomatology than bereaved children from community samples. While other studies (e.g., Gersten et al., 1991; Worden & Silverman, 1996) utilized community samples (either school or community based), very few reported on representativeness of their samples as compared to the population of bereaved children. Using death certificates of adults likely to be survived by a child aged 8 through 15, Gersten et al. (1991) were able to contact an estimated 73% of potentially eligible families; of those who were contacted, 53.8% agreed to be interviewed. Those who were interviewed did not differ from refusers on ethnicity, neighborhood social class, or cause of death. However, more surviving mothers than fathers agreed to be interviewed. Because gender of surviving parent did not relate to outcome measures, it is not likely that this variable affected their results. However, even this study, which carefully assessed representativeness of the bereaved population, did not obtain data from a large and significant subgroup of bereaved families: those who moved or could not be located.

An additional problem is that many studies have used very small sample sizes, with most including fewer than 50 subjects (Kranzler et al., 1990; Sood et al., 1992; Weller, Weller, Fristad, & Bowes, 1990). Such small samples reduce the statistical power to detect differences between groups.

Use of a limited number of methods of data collection is another common problem. Many studies only obtained parent and teacher reports of children's outcomes (i.e., Felner et al., 1981; Van Eerdewegh et al., 1982; Kranzler et al., 1990) and failed to obtain child self-report, behavioral observations, or structured diagnostic interviews. Parents, teachers, and children differ significantly in how they rate children's symptomatology, with their ratings being based on observation of child behavior in different settings and being affected by different systematic biases (Achenbach, McConaughy, & Howell, 1987). Because parent ratings are affected by level of psychological distress (Breslau, Davis, & Prabucki, 1988), bereaved parents are more likely to view their children as being more symptomatic than nonbereaved parents.

Because of reporter biases, studies that rely exclusively on a single reporter are somewhat limited. It is interesting to note that Weller et al. (1990) used a physiological measure, the dexamethasone suppression test (DST), and two paper-and-pencil measures to assess depression with a sample of bereaved children aged 7 to 18 years, 4 weeks following parental death. The DST involves assessing level of cortisol secretion. Nonsuppression on the DST has been associated with depression in the general literature, and the bereaved group had a significantly higher number of nonsuppressors on the DST than did the control group. Nonsuppression on the DST was also associated with higher self-report of depressive symptoms.

CHANGES IN CHILDREN'S MENTAL HEALTH PROBLEMS OVER TIME FOLLOWING PARENTAL DEATH

One critical issue is understanding how the effects of parental death on children change over time. Parental death is clearly a traumatic event for children, so that early emotional distress, somatic problems, cognitive disturbances, and problems in school might be expected as manifestations of a normal grief response (Silverman & Worden, 1992). However, two contrasting models can be postulated for how the effects of parental death change over time. A stress dissipation model would predict that the effects of stress lessen over time. According to this model, parental death is a trauma that brings an immediate grief response, the effects of which become less intense as the child is temporally removed from the event. An exacerbation model would predict that the effects grow stronger and perhaps more pervasive over time. According to this model, the death has reverberating effects that bring about other stressors in the child's environment, such as increased demoralization in the surviving parent, economic problems for the family, loss of ties with other family members, and so on, and that the negative effects grow as these new stressors accumulate.

Five longitudinal studies have examined changes in the effects of parental death over time. Using a sample of 105 bereaved children aged 2 to 17, Van Eerdewegh et al. (1982) conducted assessments 1 month and 13 months after parental death. At the 13-month assessment they found a significant increase in abdominal pain and fights with siblings and a decreased interest in school. However, they also found a significant decrease in dysphoric mood and an increased interest in nonacademic activities over time.

Elizur and Kaffman (1983) conducted assessments 6, 18, and 42 months following parental death in a sample of 25 Israeli children aged 2 to 10. Their outcome variable was pathological bereavement, which included symptoms of overdependent behavior, sleep disorders, learning difficulties, anxiety, and conduct disorder. They found that 45% of the children displayed pathological bereavement 6 months after the death, 48% at 18 months, and 39% at 42 months following the death. They also found that affective grief reactions were most frequent at the 6-month assessment and steadily declined over the subsequent assessments. In contrast, behavior problems were most frequent at the 18-month assessment and subsided 42 months postloss.

A study of 11 adolescents was conducted to describe bereavement reactions 6 weeks, 7 months, and 13 months following the death of a parent (Harris, 1991). At the initial assessment all adolescents reported crying and feeling sad. Ruminations about the death, sleep disturbances, and impaired school performance were also common. The onset of depression, alcohol abuse, and delinquency occurred after 7 months in 64% of the sample. After 13 months, the intrusive ruminations had decreased and most adolescents reported lower levels of distress. However, the generalizability of these findings is questionable because of the small sample size and lack of quantitative analysis.

Silverman and Worden (1992) assessed typical reactions and experiences of children immediately following the death of their parent and changes from 4 months to 1 year following the death. They reported that on the day children found out about the death, 91% cried; however, 4 months after the death only 33% reported frequent crying and after 1 year only 13% cried regularly. Twenty percent of children reported having trouble concentrating in school 4 months after the death, and 16% still had trouble concentrating in school 1 year following the death. In general, they found that crying, problems sleeping, and difficulty concentrating in school significantly decreased over time, but accidents and health problems significantly increased. No significant differences were found for frequency of headaches across time.

Weller and colleagues (cited in Clark, Pynoos, & Goebel, 1994) studied a sample of bereaved children and depressed and normal controls from 1 month until 13 months after the death. They reported that bereaved children had significantly more depressed symptoms than controls at 1 month but not at the follow-ups. However, bereaved children had less interest in school and more conduct problems than controls for up to 1 year following the death.

In summary, the evidence from these five studies provided mixed evidence for the changes in psychological symptoms of bereaved children over time. There is evidence that measures of distress decrease over time, consistent with a stress dissipation model. However, other problems such as acting-out behavior, accidents, and lack of interest in school may follow a more complicated trajectory and may increase over time. There is, however, a paucity of evidence to allow a clear understanding of changes in psychological problems over time in bereaved children.

MENTAL HEALTH OUTCOMES IN ADULTHOOD

The six studies that have examined the relation between parental death during childhood and adult psychopathology have yielded mixed results. Characteristics of these studies are presented in Table 2.

Barnes and Prosen (1985) asked 1250 adults to fill out a questionnaire during a visit to their general practitioners' offices. Participants completed a depression scale and reported whether they had experienced the death of a parent during childhood and if so, their age when the death occurred. They

Table 2. Retrospective Studies Examining the Relations between Parental Death during Childhood and Adult Psychopathology

Author	Sample and study characteristics	Outcomes assessed and findings
Adam et al. (1982)	Age = adults N = 98 N(c) = 102 Subjects were 98 adults admitted to the emergency room after attempting suicide and 102 matched controls	Self-report: participants who had attempted suicide had a significantly higher incidence of bereavement during childhood than in the comparison group
Barnes & Prosen (1985)	Age = adults N = 1250 Subjects were adults who visited their general practitioners' offices and filled out a questionnaire	Self-report: patients who had experienced the death of a parent during childhood had a significantly higher level of depression in adulthood
Hallstrom (1987)	Age = 38–54 N = 60 N(c) = 400 Subjects were 60 women who had been diagnosed with major depression compared to 400 nondepressed women	Self-report: there were no significant differences in rate of childhood bereavement between the depressed and comparison group
Kendler et al. (1992)	Age = 17–55 N = 1018 twin pairs N(b) = 62 N(s) = 123 Subjects were female twins who had either experienced the death of a parent or separation from a parent during childhood; community-based sample	Subject report: parental death was not related to an increased risk for major depression or generalized anxiety disorder; parental death was related to increased risk for panic disorder and phobias
Thyer et al. (1989)	Age = adults N = 43 N(c) = 39 Subjects were 43 adults who had been diagnosed with panic disorder or agoraphobia, compared to 39 adults without panic disorder or agoraphobia	Self-report: there was no significant difference in the rate of childhood bereavement between panic disorder/agoraphobic group and comparison group
Zall (1994)	Age = adults N(b) = 28 N(c) = 23 Subjects were women who had experienced the death of a parent before the age of 13 and who currently had at least one child under the age of 10; 23 women who had not lost a parent were used for comparison	Self-report: bereaved women had significantly higher levels of depression and suicidality, were significantly more worried about their own death, were more overprotective with their children, and pushed harder to be perfect than nonbereaved women; no significant differences were found on measures of parental functioning

found that patients who had experienced the death of a parent during childhood had a significantly higher level of depression in adulthood (ES = .07) than patients who had not lost a parent.

In a study of 51 women, Zall (1994) also found that women who had experienced the death of a parent before the age of 13 had significantly higher levels of depression and suicidality and were significantly more worried about their own death than women who had not lost a parent in childhood. Adam, Bouckoms, and Streiner (1982) assessed rates of childhood bereavement in 98 adults who were admitted to the emergency room following suicide attempts and compared them to rates of childhood bereavement in 102 adults from a general practice who were matched on age and gender. They found a significantly higher rate of childhood bereavement among the suicide attempters, which yielded an ES of .19.

In contrast, several other studies failed to find a relation between childhood bereavement and adult depression. For example, Hallstrom (1987) compared the incidence of childhood bereavement in 60 depressed and 400 nondepressed women and found no differences. In a study of 1018 female twin pairs, of which 62 twin pairs experienced the death of a parent before the age of 17, Kendler, Neale, Kessler, Heath, and Eaves (1992) found that death of a parent in childhood did not put women at risk for developing major depression in adulthood.

Childhood bereavement has also been examined as a risk factor for adulthood anxiety and panic disorder. Zall (1994) found that women who had a parent die before the age of 13 worried more about their own children, were more overprotective, and felt more pressure to be perfect than women who did not have a parent die in childhood. In their sample of twin pairs, Kendler et al. (1992) found that although childhood bereavement was not a risk factor for generalized anxiety disorder in adulthood, it was significantly related to an increased risk for panic disorder and phobias. Finally, Thyer, Himle, and Miller-Gogoleski (1989) studied 43 adults who had been diagnosed with panic disorder and 39 adults who did not evidence panic disorder and found no significant group differences in the rate of childhood bereavement.

Limitations of the Studies

The primary limitation of these studies is that they all used a retrospective design in which the bereaved group was compared to a control. A prospective longitudinal design involving several assessments before and after the death of the parent would provide a more precise estimate of the long-term effects of bereavement on adult adjustment. Another limitation is that some of these studies used clinical samples where patients had been diagnosed with severe psychological disorders (Adam et al., 1982: suicide attempters; Hallstrom, 1987: major depression; Thyer et al., 1989: panic disorder or agoraphobia). Community samples such as those used by Barnes and Prosen (1985), Kendler et al. (1992), and Zall (1994) provide a clearer, more representative picture of the long-term effects of bereavement in childhood.

PREDICTORS OF THE EFFECTS OF PARENTAL BEREAVEMENT

Major life stressors like bereavement can be conceptualized as processes that are precipitated by a major change but which involve multiple smaller changes that continue over time (Felner, Terre, & Rowlinson, 1988; Sandler, Wolchik, & Braver, 1988). Felner and colleagues (1988) have proposed a transitional events model in which the major event (i.e., bereavement) results in multiple changes in the child's environment, each of which present adaptive coping tasks. Children's adjustment to the stressor depends on several factors, including the number and severity of stressful changes, their interpersonal resources, such as relationships with other family members, and their intrapersonal resources, such as their social and cognitive abilities. Differences in these factors across children account for the variability in the effects of major life stressors on children's psychological symptomatology.

Primary research tasks are to identify the bereavement-related life changes that children experience and study their relations with children's adjustment. Gersten and colleagues developed the Parental Death Events List (PDEL), a measure of the life change events that occur to bereaved children (Program for Prevention Research, 1987). Professionals who worked with bereaved families and people who had experienced the death of a parent generated events that might have an impact on children following the death of a parent. Events were defined as "objectively verifiable occurrences in an individual's environment of which the individual is aware and which have a significant impact on the individual." Thoughts and feelings were not included.

In addition, Sandler, Ramirez, and Reynolds (1986) developed the General Life Events Scale for Children (GLESC), a more general life events inventory that assesses a variety of negative life events that occur in the lives of children. Children's self-reports of negative events utilizing both the GLESC and PDEL were assessed in two separate samples (West, Sandler, Pillow, Baca, & Gersten, 1991; Sandler et al., 1992). In each sample, bereaved children were asked if each event had occurred during the past 3 months. For each of the events endorsed, children also rated how upsetting the event had been when it occurred. The frequency of negative events endorsed and children's ratings of how upsetting the events were are presented in Table 3 for the combined samples. The events are rank-ordered in terms of the percentage of children who reported their occurrence. As can be seen, the most frequent events were: parent worried about brother or sister; sibling very angry or upset; and parent acted very worried, upset, or sad. As shown in the last column, the most upsetting events were: relatives saying bad things about the deceased, neighbors saying bad things about the parent, and moving to a different house than your parent.

As part of a content analysis, Li, Lutzke, Sandler, and Ayers (1995) derived categories that classified some of these events into four distinct categories: changes in child's environment (e.g., people you do not know very well came to visit, a new adult started taking care of you on a regular basis), expectations for the child's behavior following the death (e.g., your relative said you should act differently than you did before your parent died, you are told to be the man/woman of the house), parental distress (e.g., your parent acted worried,

Table 3. Occurrence and Distress Scores for Negative and Ambiguous Events Reported by Bereaved Children and Adolescents[a]

	Occurrence (%)	Distress (mean)
Parental Death Event List (PDEL): Selected negative events[b]		
Parent worried about brother or sister	61.0	4.01
Relatives sad/upset	44.6	3.38
Relatives told you to be more responsible	40.6	3.59
Heard parent arguing with others	25.9	4.16
Pet died or ran away	22.6	5.17
Relatives disagreed about what you should do	21.0	3.83
School peers uneasy since death	20.6	4.35
Relatives told you to act differently than before death	17.5	4.49
Sibling moved to a different house than you	15.4	4.49
Someone told parent to get a new spouse	13.9	4.36
Relatives said bad things about the deceased	6.8	6.14
You moved to a different house than parent	2.5	5.72
General Life Event Scale (GLESC): Selected negative events[c]		
Sibling very angry, upset	51.6	3.44
Parent acted worried, upset, sad	49.7	3.92
Close friend in serious trouble	33.5	3.29
Parent talks about money problems	32.9	4.22
Close friend moved	22.7	4.69
Parent forgot to do promised things	22.7	4.25
Close family member died	18.4	5.21
Sibling in serious trouble	16.8	3.92
Family members hit each other	16.0	5.00
Child ill	15.9	3.85
Parent ill	14.0	5.22
Sibling ill	13.8	3.80
Parent fought or argued with family	13.4	2.92
Relatives say bad things about parent	11.7	4.58
Neighbors say bad things about parent	11.1	6.00
Parent drunk	9.1	3.00
Parent acted badly in front of friends	8.0	4.83
Parent lost job	3.1	3.00
Parent arrested or jailed	0.6	—
GLESC and *PDEL*: Ambiguous items[d]		
Relatives listened to child's ideas	76.5	3.42
Parent answered child's questions about deceased	70.4	3.60
Parent answered child's questions about parents death	66.5	3.71
Adult home when child back from school	59.6	3.58
Child made friends with adult	55.9	3.58
Relatives bought child things	55.6	3.58
Relatives gave family money	12.8	4.21

[a]Frequencies of occurrence for the negative and ambiguous events reflect the compilation of both the Community Survey (Program for Prevention Research, 1987; $n = 92$) and Family Bereavement Program (Sandler et al., 1992; $n = 72$) subjects. The sample numbers for specific items ranged from 143 to 164, due to missing data (e.g., children with no siblings would not respond to certain items). The distress ratings were obtained for the *GLESC* items in only the Family Bereavement Program study. Ratings of distress was measured using a Likert scale. Children or adolescents were asked to rate the event in terms of how upsetting the event was for them on a scale from 1 (a little upsetting), 4 (pretty upsetting), to 7 (very upsetting).
[b]*Parental Death Event List* (Program for Prevention Research., 1987).
[c]*General Life Event Scale* (Sandler et al., 1986).
[d]Events were also rated by an independent panel of ten experts in terms of how stressful (1–7) they would be for an "average" child. Events with a mean rating greater than five were defined as negative events, and events with a mean rating of 3–5 were defined as ambiguous events.

upset, or sad; your mom/dad was concerned or worried about your brothers and/or sisters), and death reminders [e.g., your mom/dad talked about your dad/mom (deceased parent), all of your relatives said your mom/dad (deceased parent) is watching you]. Events were reliably coded by category and event scores in each category were summed to yield measures of these four types of events. Four simultaneous multiple regression analyses were conducted in which measures of symptomatology (depression, anxiety, conduct disorder, and total symptoms) were regressed on the event scores to assess the unique contribution of each event type. For total symptoms and anxiety scores, only parental distress contributed unique variance. Parental distress had a significant relation to higher conduct problems, while death reminders had a significant negative relation with conduct problems. The finding for death reminders is consistent with the theory that talking about the deceased parent with the surviving parent should relate to lower acting out problems.

Child and Environmental Predictors of Adaptive Outcomes in Bereaved Children

Children's adaptation to stressful changes that follow the death of a parent involve complex intrapersonal and environmental processes. Children respond to changes with affective arousal, interpret these events, and attempt to cope with them. While these cognitive, affective, and behavioral responses are rarely studied directly, researchers have begun to investigate individual (e.g., self-esteem) and environmental (e.g., parental warmth) resources that affect the adaptation processes. We review those studies that investigated the relationship between individual and environmental variables and children's adjustment. These studies have generally tested simple models of the direct relationship between personal and environmental resources and adjustment following parental death. Only rarely have more complex models of mediation or moderation been investigated, and these models have only been examined in cross-sectional models (Wheaton, 1985; James & Brett, 1984). After this review, we propose alternative models of the effects of personal and environmental variables on children's adjustment.

Child Characteristics

Many authors have underscored the importance of individual child characteristics in determining children's response to stressors (Felner et al., 1988; Grych & Fincham, 1990; Kurdek, 1988). Children's perceptions of themselves and of the world may lead to significant variability in the types and amount of symptomatology they experience following the death of a parent. The major child characteristics that have been studied in bereaved children are locus of control beliefs and self-esteem.

Two studies have examined the effects of locus of control and self-esteem. Silverman and Worden (1992) looked at the direct correlation of locus of control, as measured on the Nowicki–Strickland scale, and parents' ratings of children's symptomatology on the CBCL in a sample of children aged 6 to 17 years old 4 months after the death. They found that bereaved children with an external locus of control had significantly higher symptomatology than children with an internal locus of control.

Lutzke, Li, Ayers, and Sandler (1995) examined locus of control and self-esteem as mediators of the relation between negative life events and symptomatology in a sample of 92 recently bereaved children. Children's reports of all variables were used. It was found that locus of control significantly mediated the relation between negative life events and depression, anxiety, and conduct disorder. Conceptually, the mediational model is consistent with the idea that children develop a more external locus of control as a function of experiencing multiple stressful events that are beyond their control, such as depression in the surviving parent, family economic problems, and parental remarriage. The external locus of control in turn leads to increased psychological symptomatology.

Lutzke et al. (1995) also found that self-esteem significantly mediated the relation between negative life events and symptomatology for the three types of symptomatology assessed (i.e., depression, anxiety, and conduct disorder). Children's self-esteem might suffer following the death of a parent because the surviving parent may feel too overwhelmed or depressed to reinforce the child for positive things they do, thus leading to feelings of rejection and lower self-worth.

It is interesting to note that while the evidence is mixed as to whether bereaved children have a more external locus of control or lower self-esteem than controls, control beliefs and self-esteem mediate the effects of the smaller postdeath stressful events on mental health problems. It may be that it is the cascade of negative events that sometimes follow parental death rather than the death per se that affects children's beliefs and consequently increases their symptoms.

Another variable that may affect bereaved children's adjustment is their religious beliefs. Religious beliefs may provide a cognitive framework for understanding the death and/or may reflect children's integration in a religious community where they can talk about the death of their parent. As an example, in the adult literature, regular participation in religious ceremonies and rating religion as important have been shown to positively relate to increased perceptions of social support and greater meaning found in the loss of a child. These variables in turn were related to greater well-being and less distress (McIntosh, Cohen, Silver, & Wortman, 1993).

One study has examined the effects of religious beliefs on children's adjustment following the death of a parent (Gray, 1987). Adolescents were asked if they had any beliefs that were religious or spiritual in nature. Adolescents who reported religious or spiritual beliefs had significantly lower depression scores and significantly lower frequency of major depression than adolescents who had no religious beliefs. Although it is difficult to draw conclusions based on one study, this finding suggests that aiding children in finding meaning or conceptualizing the death in an understandable way may reduce some of the negative impact of the death.

It should be noted that these studies investigated the relations between children's general beliefs about themselves or their world and do not directly assess what children report doing to cope with the stressors they experience following the death of their parent. Only one study has assessed the relations between bereaved children's symptoms and their coping. Lawrence (1995) assessed the relations between child and adolescent reports of four dimensions of coping (active, distraction, avoidance, and support), perceived coping efficacy, and self-reported depression and parent-reported conduct problems in a sample of 66 bereaved children and adolescents aged 7 through 14. They found that support coping was significantly related to lower parent-reported conduct problems and perceived efficacy of coping was related to lower self-reported depression. They also found that support coping and active coping were related to higher perceived efficacy of coping.

Social Environmental Resources

The child's social environment may have a significant influence on adjustment following parental death. Theoretically, social environmental influences may directly affect child mental health problems. For example, these influences may present as additional stressors for the child and may overlap with our previously described measure of bereavement-related stressful events. On the other hand, social environmental factors may function as protective resources that counteract the effects of the negative events or moderate (dampen) their negative effects. Four aspects of bereaved children's social environments have been studied: parental depression, parent–child relationships, family environment, and socioeconomic status.

There is good reason to believe that parents' grief and depression following the death of a spouse could lead to increased problems for their children. Five studies have assessed parental demoralization or depression and all of them have found that it is significantly related to increased symptomatology in children following the death of a parent (Kranzler et al., 1990; Sandler et al., 1992; Sood et al., 1992; Van Eerdewegh, Clayton, & Van Eerdewegh, 1985; West et al., 1991).

While the grief is not identical with clinical depression, many of the affective and behavioral symptoms overlap. Thus, the mechanisms by which grief affects child mental health problems may be similar to those reported for depressed parents. Several studies have reported a significant positive relation between parental depression and children's psychological symptomatology in the general literature (e.g., Coopersmith, 1967; Hetherington, Cox, & Cox, 1982; Mash & Johnson, 1983; Shaw & Emery, 1988; Weissman, Leckman, Merikangas, Gammon & Prusoff, 1984). Researchers in this area have proposed several mechanisms by which living with a depressed parent may affect children's mental health: (1) exposure to a distressed parent may directly elicit child negative affect; (2) parental depression might lead parents to communicate more negative, hopeless interpretations of events to their children; and (3) parental depression may affect the parent–child relationships, leading to more irritable interactions and poorer quality parenting (see Chapter 5, this volume).

One of the consequences of parental death may be to negatively impact the relationship between the surviving parent and the child. Parents might be so depressed or absorbed in their own grief that they stop spending positive time with their children and may be less effective in their use of discipline strategies. Such changes in parenting may lead to increased conduct problems and depression (Patterson, 1982; Chapter 5, this volume).

Two aspects of the parent–child relationship—parental warmth and parental support—were measured by Sandler, Gersten et al. (1988). They found that nonbereaved families had a marginally higher level of parental warmth but no group difference on parental support. These researchers reported that parental warmth was significantly negatively related to conduct disorder and marginally negatively related to depression in the bereaved sample. Parental support and children's symptomatology were not significantly related. It has also been found that parental warmth partially mediates the effects of parental death on children's adjustment (West et al., 1991). This provides evidence that one mechanism by which parental death affects children's adjustment involves deterioration in the quality of the parent–child relationship, which in turn leads to increased symptomatology.

Saler and Skolnick (1992) found further evidence for the effects of parent–child relationships on adjustment. In their study of adults who had lost a parent during childhood, participants who reported having a positive relationship with their surviving parents (open communication, high levels of warmth, and quality time together) had lower levels of depression in adulthood than participants who reported negative relationships with their surviving parents.

Three studies have examined the effects of the relationship with a parental replacement figure on adult psychopathology (Bifulco, Brown, & Harris, 1987; Birtchnell, 1980; Parker & Manicavasagar, 1986). Birtchnell (1980) found that the incidence of psychiatric illness was significantly higher among bereaved women who reported having bad relationships with their mother replacements during childhood than among women who had good relationships with their mother replacements. Bifulco et al. (1987) studied the rate of depression in women who had experienced the death of a parent during childhood. They found that lack of adequate care from the surviving parent or the parental substitute served as a vulnerability factor that increased the rate of depression in adulthood. Parker and Manicavasagar (1986) studied women whose mothers died during childhood and whose fathers had remarried. Women who rated their stepmothers and maternal replacement figures as inadequate had a significantly higher rate of depression in adulthood.

The effects of family environment on the mental health of bereaved children has also been studied. Using a community sample, Sandler (1988) compared the family environments of bereaved children and nonbereaved children on the following variables: family cohesiveness, conflict, expression, organization, control, total family environment, and stable positive family events. They found that the two groups differed significantly only on measures of family cohesiveness and stable positive family events, with the nonbereaved group scoring more positively on both measures. Sandler et al. found that the rate of stable positive family events was significantly, negatively related to both depression and conduct disorder in the bereaved group.

Parker and Manicavasagar (1986) used retrospective reports from women who had experienced the death of their mothers during childhood. They found

that women who reported that their remaining family members offered sufficient support over the few months following the death had significantly lower
levels of depression than women who reported insufficient family support.

Several studies have investigated the joint effects of multiple social environmental variables. Using the same sample of children as Sandler et al. (1988),
West et al. (1991) used structural equation-modeling techniques to test a theoretical model of the variables that lead to symptomatology in bereaved children. In their model, parental death leads to changes in family mediators,
which in turn lead to adjustment problems. Using parents' reports of children's
symptomatology and four social environment variables (parental depression,
positive stable events, negative events, and family cohesion), they examined
the standardized path coefficients to determine significant relations. A significant relation was found between parental death and a decrease in family cohesion and an increase in parental distress. Family cohesion, parental distress,
and negative events were significantly related to children's symptomatology. A
similar model was tested using children's reports of their own symptomatology, positive stable events, and negative events. There was a significant relation
between parental death and a decrease in positive stable events, and both
positive stable events and parental warmth were significantly related to lower
symptomatology, while negative events related to higher symptoms.

Partridge and Kotler (1987) created a composite score of the following
family environment variables: family cohesion, support from surviving parent,
coercive discipline, adolescent autonomy in decision making, level of family
stress, parent–adolescent closeness, parental demoralization, and parental encouragement of adolescent autonomy. This composite variable was significantly related to adjustment problems in bereaved adolescents. Family environment accounted for a significant amount of variance in adolescents'
adjustment after family type (bereaved vs. intact) was controlled for; however,
family type was not a significant predictor of adjustment after family environment was controlled for. The results of this study, along with those of other
studies, suggest that parental death leads to changes in the family environment,
which put children at risk for developing symptomatology.

Four studies have examined how the socioeconomic status of the family
following the death of a parent affected the mental health of bereaved children
in adulthood. Three studies reported that lower social class of bereaved families was a significant predictor of adult mental health problems (Birtchnell &
Kennard, 1981; Harris, Brown, & Bifulco, 1987; Parker & Manicavasagar, 1986),
while one study did not find a significant relation between socioeconomic
status of bereaved families and adult mental health problems (McLeod, 1991).
Illustratively, Harris et al. (1987) found that both the social class of the family
following the death of the parent and current social class were related to depression in women who had lost a mother during childhood. They propose that
low social class of the bereaved family sets in motion a series of events that
ultimately lead to depression. Harris et al. found significant associations between low social class and lack of adequate care of the children. Lack of adequate care was significantly related to premarital pregnancy, which related to
lower current social class and selection of a nonsupportive mate, which in turn
led to women's increased vulnerability to depression.

PREVENTIVE INTERVENTION PROGRAMS

The majority of bereavement interventions that have been developed have been designed for adults (Osterweis, Solomon, & Green, 1984), and most of the interventions that have targeted children have not been empirically evaluated (Christ, Siegel, Mesagno, & Langosch, 1991; Lohnes & Kalter, 1994; Zambelli & DeRosa, 1992). Black and Urbanowicz (1985) did collect limited follow-up data on an intervention for bereaved children. Their intervention consisted of six family counseling sessions within 5 months following the death. At the 1-year follow-up assessment, children in the intervention group had significantly fewer behavior problems and sleep disturbances than children in the control group, although significant methodological problems make interpretation of their results difficult. Only posttreatment assessments were conducted and only half of the families in the intervention condition agreed to the 1-year follow-up interview.

Recently, prevention researchers have underscored the importance of developing theory-based preventive interventions (Coie et al., 1993; Gersten et al., 1991; Sandler et al., 1992). Consistent with the model of theory-based interventions, the Family Bereavement Program (FBP) was designed to modify variables identified as mediators of the relationship between parental death and children's symptomatology (West et al., 1991). The mediators targeted were parental demoralization, parental warmth, stable positive events, and negative events (for more details, see Sandler et al., 1992). The FBP was divided into two phases: the Family Grief Workshop and the Family Advisor Program. The Family Grief Workshop was a structured three-session workshop that provided an opportunity for bereaved families to meet other families who had similar experiences and to improve the warmth of the parent–child relationship. The Family Advisor Program involved 12 sessions in which a family advisor met with families to help decrease parental demoralization and negative events and increase the occurrence of positive events in the home and the warmth of the parent–child relationship (Sandler et al., 1992). The family advisor met with the family in their home once a week to teach them the skills necessary to modify the mediators.

Evaluation of a randomized experimental trial found that the program led to parental ratings of increased warmth in the parent–child relationships, increased satisfaction with their social support, and the maintenance of family discussion of grief-related issues. The program also led to parent ratings of decreased conduct disorder, depression, and overall problems in older but not younger children. The program did not significantly change children's reports of the family environment or adjustment problems.

The results from this first experimental trial are seen as encouraging, but two modifications were seen as needed to strengthen program effects. First, the intervention program was changed to a group format to provide group support, increase the fidelity of the implementation of the intervention, and make dissemination more efficient. Separate groups were developed for children and parents to have them learn and apply complementary skills to improve family functioning and child coping with bereavement-related stressors. Second, the interventions was designed to target two additional putative mediators: children coping with bereavement-related stressors and parent's use of consistent discipline. Our analyses showed that both locus of control and self-esteem mediated the effects of bereavement-related stress on children's adjustment (Lutzke et al., 1995). Coping skills were taught so that children could learn how to deal with negative life events while maintaining a positive self-esteem and a sense of control and efficacy in dealing with life stress. Discipline was added as a mediator, because the use of consistent discipline has been found to be an important predictor of children's adjustment in general samples (Gardner, 1989; Lempers, Clark-Lempers, & Simons, 1989; Vicary & Lerner, 1986; Vuchinich, Bank, & Patterson, 1992; Wentzel, Feldman, & Weinberger, 1991) and bereaved samples (Strength, 1991; Worden, 1994). The program is now being subject to a randomized experimental evaluation that involves extensive evaluation of the effects of the program on coping, family functioning, and children's psychological problems.

DIRECTIONS FOR FUTURE RESEARCH

Through our review of the literature, we believe, as has been suggested by others (Clark et al., 1994), that regional and national epidemiological studies of parental bereavement would help describe the demography and psychosocial settings of these children. The significant methodological problems in studies investigating the risk status of parentally bereaved children still limits the generalizability of some findings. Further longitudinal investigations are needed with large, representative samples and appropriate comparison groups and that focus on the immediate and longer-term effects of parental bereavement. An alternative research design that might be useful in this context is one that compares bereaved children with children who have experienced a parental divorce and who have lost all contact with the noncustodial parent. Such a design would allow the investigator to identify experiences and risks that are unique for the parentally bereaved child. This discussion highlights what is one of the most difficult aspects of the design of studies in bereavement-related research; that is, the selection of appropriate comparison groups.

Another significant problem in the study of bereaved children is the common lack of pretest data in bereavement research. This limits the conclusions as to how the status of the children or family, prior to the death, may affect the grief process or mental health outcomes of the children or family. Recent advances in research design could help address some of the limitations of existing bereavement research. To address some of these issues in their work on pregnancy loss, Toedter, Lasker, and Campbell (1990) have offered a new research design they label as the "retrospective pretest design with a surrogate comparison group." In this design, they select a group that has not experienced the traumatic event but is as similar as possible to what the experimental group was prior to the event. This group is the "surrogate" for the pretest and serves as a check for the accuracy of retrospective data. Both groups are followed longitudinally and are assessed at multiple points, with the surrogate and experimental group providing current and retrospective reports at various assessments. Such a design can address some of the threats to validity that other studies utilizing retrospective reports might confront. In order to circumvent some of the difficult methodological problems in this area, researchers will have to continue to be innovative in their design of future studies.

Changes in bereaved children and adolescents over time need more research attention. Descriptive information is needed on how affective, cognitive, and behavioral responses to parental death change over time. Such research would address significant questions concerning the normative and pathological courses of grief. To accomplish this, more work needs to be done in developing reliable and valid measures that assess various aspects of the grief process (cf. Clark et al., 1994, for a description of work assessing the phenomenology of adolescent bereavement). Such instruments can also be used to explore relations between the grief process and more distal mental health outcomes.

While a greater number of studies have examined the direct relations between child, family, or social environment characteristics and mental health problems of bereaved children, very few studies have systematically tested alternative prospective models of how these variables interrelate. How do effective parenting, coping, and social support interact to predict mental problems of bereaved children and adolescents? What aspects of the family environment make a difference in the developmental pathways of bereaved children? Does talking about grief and/or expression of affect in the early months following the death have prognostic significance for mental health problems later in childhood, adolescence, or adulthood?

Methodologically sound, theoretically based preventive intervention trials of bereavement programs are needed (Coie et al., 1993; Lipsey, 1992; Sandler et al., 1992; Schneiderman, Winders, Tallett, & Feldman, 1994). The evaluation of these interventions needs to use psychometrically sound measures of adjustment and measures that assess the putative program mediators. If the interventions are successful in targeting and changing the putative program mediators, one also needs to establish that these changes lead to better adjustment in the children who have received the intervention (cf. Sandler et al., 1992). In bereavement research, a theory-based approach to a preventive intervention trial not only provides for a test of the efficacy of the preventive intervention, but also can further our understanding of the processes and mechanisms by which the death of a parent affects the developmental outcomes for bereaved children and adolescents.

ACKNOWLEDGMENTS

Support for this chapter was provided by NIMH Grant #P50-MH39246 to support the Preventive Intervention Research Center and NIMH Grant #P50-MH49155 to support the Family Bereavement Program at Arizona State University, which is gratefully acknowledged. The authors also wish to gratefully acknowledge the helpful comments for and review of this chapter by Sharlene Wolchik and Sarah Jones.

REFERENCES

Achenbach, T., McConaughy, S., & Howell, C. (1987). Child/adolescent behavioral and emotional problems: Implications of cross-informant correlations for situational specificity. *Psychological Bulletin, 101,* 213–232.

Adam, K., Bouckoms, A., & Streiner, D. (1982). Parental loss and family stability in attempted suicide. *Archives of General Psychiatry, 39,* 1081–1085.

Ambert, A., & Saucier, J. (1984). Adolescents' academic success and aspirations by parental marital status. *Canadian Review of Sociology and Anthropology, 21,* 62–74.

American Psychiatric Association. (1980). *Diagnostic and statistical manual of mental disorders* (3rd ed.). Washington, DC: Author.

Barnes, G., & Prosen, H. (1985). Parental death and depression. *Journal of Abnormal Psychology, 94,* 64–69.

Bifulco, A., Brown, G., & Harris, T. (1987). Childhood loss of parent, lack of adequate parental care and adult depression: A replication. *Journal of Affective Disorders, 12,* 115–128.

Birtchnell, J. (1980). Women whose mothers died in childhood: An outcome study. *Psychological Medicine, 10,* 699–713.

Birtchnell, J., & Kennard, J. (1981). Early mother-bereaved women who have and have not been psychiatric patients. *Social Psychology, 16,* 187–197.

Black, D., & Urbanowicz, M. A. (1985). Bereaved children family intervention. In J. E. Stevenson (Ed), *Recent research in developmental psychopathology* (pp. 179–187). Oxford, England: Pergamon.

Breslau, N., Davis, G., & Prabucki, K. (1988). Depressed mothers as informants in family history research—Are they accurate? *Psychiatry Research, 24,* 345–359.

Brown, G. W., & Harris, T. (1978). *Social origins of depression.* New York: Free Press.

Brown, G. W., Harris, T. O., & Bifulco, A. (1986). Long-term effects of early loss of parent. In M. Rutter, C. E. Izard, & P. B. Reid (Eds.), *Depression in young people: Developmental and clinical perspectives* (pp. 251–297). New York: Guilford Press.

Christ, G., Siegel, K., Mesagno, F., & Langosch, D. (1991). A preventive intervention program for bereaved children. *American Journal of Orthopsychiatry, 61,* 168–178.

Clark, D. C., Pynoos, R. S., & Goebel, A. E. (1994). Mechanisms and processes of adolescent bereavement. In R. J. Haggerty, L. R. Sherrod, N. Garmezy, & M. Rutter (Eds.), *Stress, risk, and resilience in children and adolescents: Processes, mechanisms, and interventions* (pp. 100–146). New York: Cambridge University Press.

Coie, J. D., Watt, N. F., West, S. G., Hawkins, J. D., Asarnow, J. R., Markman, H. J., Ramey, S. L., Shure, M. B., & Long, B. (1993). The science of prevention: A conceptual framework and some directions for a national research program. *American Psychologist, 48,* 1013–1022.

Cook, T. D. (1990). The generalization of causal connections: Multiple theories in search of clear practice. In L. Sechrest, E. Perrin, & J. Bunker (Eds.), *Research methodology: Strengthening causal interpretations of non-experimental data, AHCPR Conference Proceedings* (pp. 9–31). US Department of Health and Human Services, Agency for Health Care Policy and Research.

Coopersmith, S. (1967). *The antecedents of self-esteem.* San Francisco: W. H. Freeman.

Elizur, E., & Kaffman, M. (1983). Factors influencing the severity of childhood bereavement reactions. *American Journal of Orthopsychiatry, 53,* 668–676.

Felner, R., Ginter, M., Boike, M., & Cowen, E. (1981). Parental death or divorce and the school adjustment of young children. *American Journal of Community Psychology, 9,* 181–191.

Felner, R., Stolberg, A., & Cowen, E. (1975). Crisis events and school mental health referral patterns of young children. *Journal of Consulting and Clinical Psychology, 43,* 305–310.

Felner, R., Terre, L., & Rowlinson, R. (1988). A life transition framework for understanding marital dissolution and family reorganization. In S. A. Wolchik & P. Karoly (Eds.), *Children of divorce: Empirical perspectives on adjustment* (pp. 35–65). New York: Gardner Press.

Gardner, F. (1989). Inconsistent parenting: Is there evidence for a link with children's conduct problems? *Journal of Abnormal Child Psychology, 17,* 223–233.

Gersten, J., Beals, J., & Kallgren, C. (1991). Epidemiology and preventive interventions: Parental death in childhood as a case example. *American Journal of Community Psychology, 19,* 481–499.

Gray, R. (1987). Adolescent response to the death of a parent. *Journal of Youth and Adolescence, 16,* 511–525.

Gregory, I. (1965). Anterospective data following childhood loss of a parent. *Archives of General Psychiatry, 13,* 99–109.

Grych, J., & Fincham, F. (1990). Marital conflict and children's adjustment: A cognitive contextual framework. *Psychological Bulletin, 108,* 267–290.

Hainline, L., & Feig, E. (1978). The correlates of childhood father absence in college-aged women. *Child Development, 49*, 37–42.

Hallstrom, T. (1987). The relationships of childhood socio-demographic factors and early parental loss to major depression in adult life. *Acta Psychiatrica Scandinavica 75*, 212–216.

Harris, E. (1991). Adolescent bereavement following the death of a parent: An exploratory study. *Child Psychiatry and Human Development, 21*, 267–281.

Harris, T., Brown, G., & Bifulco, A. (1987). Loss of parent in childhood and adult psychiatric disorder: The role of social class position and premarital pregnancy. *Psychological Medicine, 17*, 163–183.

Harter, S. (1979). *Manual: Perceived Competence Scale for Children*. Denver, CO: University of Denver.

Hetherington, E. (1972). Effects of father absence on personality development in adolescent daughters. *Developmental Psychology, 7*, 313–326.

Hetherington, E., Cox, M., & Cox, R. (1982). Effects of divorce on parents and children. In M. Lamb (Ed.), *Nontraditional families: Parenting and child development*. Hillsdale, NJ: Erlbaum.

James, L. R., & Brett, J. M. (1984). Mediators, moderators and tests for mediation. *Journal of Applied Psychology, 69*, 307–321.

Janoff-Bulman, R. (1985). The aftermath of victimization: Rebuilding shattered assumptions. In C. Figley (Ed.), *Trauma and it's wake: The study and treatment of posttraumatic stress disorder* (pp. 15–35). New York: Brunner/Mazel.

Johnson, B. T. (1993). DSTAT software for the meta-analytical review of research literatures (version 1.11) [Computer software]. Hillsdale, NJ: Erlbaum.

Kendler, K., Neale, M., Kessler, R., Heath, A., & Eaves, L. (1992). Childhood parental loss and adult psychopathology in women. *Archives of General Psychiatry, 49*, 109–116.

Kranzler, E., Shaffer, D., Wasserman, G., & Davies, M. (1990). Early childhood bereavement. *Journal of the American Academy of Child and Adolescent Psychiatry, 29*, 513–520.

Kurdek, L. A. (1988). Cognitive mediators of children's adjustment to divorce. In S. A. Wolchik & P. Karoly (Eds.), *Children of divorce: Empirical perspectives on adjustment* (pp. 233–267). New York: Gardner.

Lawerence, G. B. (1995). *The impact of coping and perceived control on adjustment in children who have lost a parent*. Unpublished doctoral dissertation, Columbia University, New York.

Lempers, J., Clark-Lempers, D., & Simons, R. (1989). Economic hardship, parenting, and distress in adolescence. *Child Development, 60*, 25–39.

Li, S., Lutzke, J., Sandler, I., & Ayers, T. S. (1995, June). Structure and specificity of negative life event categories for bereaved children. Poster presented at the Biennial Conference of the Society for Community Research and Action, Chicago, IL.

Lipsey, M. W. (1992). Theory as method: Small theories of treatments. In L. B. Sechrest & A. G. Scott (Eds.), *New directions for program evaluation* (No. 57, pp. 5–38). San Francisco: Jossey-Bass.

Lohnes, K., & Kalter, N. (1994). Preventive intervention groups for parentally bereaved children. *American Journal of Orthopsychiatry, 64*, 594–603.

Lutzke, J., Li, S., Ayers, T., & Sandler, I. (1995, June). Self-esteem and locus of control as mediators of the effects of bereavement stress on children's adjustment. Poster presented at the Biennial Conference of the Society for Community Research and Action, Chicago, IL.

Mash, E., & Johnson, C. (1983). Parental perceptions of child behavior problems, parenting self-esteem, and mother's reported stress in younger and older hyperactive and normal children. *Journal of Consulting and Clinical Psychology, 51*, 86–99.

McIntosh, D., Cohen Silver, R., & Wortman, C. (1993). Religion's role in adjustment to a negative life event: Coping with the loss of a child. *Journal of Personality and Social Psychology, 65*, 812–821.

McLeod, J. (1991). Childhood parental loss and adult depression. *Journal of Health and Social Behavior, 32*, 205–220.

Osterweis, M., Solomon, F., & Green, M. (1984). *Bereavement reactions, consequences and care*. New York: Raven Press.

Parker, G., & Manicavasagar, V. (1986). Childhood bereavement circumstances associated with adult depression. *British Journal of Medical Psychology, 59*, 387–391.

Partridge, S., & Kotler, T. (1987). Self-esteem and adjustment in adolescents from bereaved, divorced, and intact families: Family type versus family environment. *Australian Journal of Psychology, 39*, 223–234.

Patterson, G. (1982). *Coercive family process*. Eugene, OR: Castalia.

Program for Prevention Research. (1987). *Documentation of scales: PIRC community survey*. Tempe: Arizona State University.

Saler, L., & Skolnick, N. (1992). Childhood parental death and depression in adulthood: Roles of surviving parent and family environment. *American Journal of Orthopsychiatry, 62*, 504–516.

Sandler, I. N., Barr, A., Ayers, T. S., & Lutzke, J. R. (1996). Unpublished data analysis. Program for Prevention Research, Arizona State University, Tempe, AZ.

Sandler, I., Gersten, J., Reynolds, K., Kallgren, C., & Ramirez, R. (1988). Using theory and data to plan support interventions: Design of a program for bereaved children. In B. H. Gottlieb (Ed.), *Marshaling social support: Formats, processes, and effects* (pp. 53–83). Newbury Park, CA: Sage.

Sandler, I. N., Rameriz, R., & Reynolds, K. D. (1986, August). Life stress for children of divorce, bereaved and asthmatic children. Poster presented at the American Psychological Association Convention, Washington, DC.

Sandler, I., West, S., Baca, L., Pillow, D., Gersten, J., Rogosch, F., Virdin, L., Beals, J., Reynolds, K., Kallgren, C., Tien, J., Kriege, G., Cole, E., & Ramirez, R. (1992). Linking empirically based theory and evaluation: The Family Bereavement Program. *American Journal of Community Psychology, 20*, 491–521.

Sandler, I., Wolchik, S., & Braver, S. (1988). The stressors of children's postdivorce environments. In S. A. Wolchik & P. Karoly (Eds.), *Children of divorce: Empirical perspectives on adjustment* (pp. 111–144). New York: Gardner Press.

Saucier, J., & Ambert, A. (1982). Parental marital status and adolescents' optimism about their future. *Journal of Youth and Adolescence, 11*, 345–354.

Saucier, J., & Ambert, A. (1986). Adolescents' perception of self and of immediate environment by parental marital status: A controlled study. *Canadian Journal of Psychiatry, 31*, 505–512.

Schneiderman, G., Winders, P., Tallett, S., & Feldman, W. (1994). Do child and/or parent bereavement programs work? *Canadian Journal of Psychiatry, 39*, 215–218.

Shaw, D., & Emery, R. (1988). Chronic family adversity and school-aged children's adjustment. *Journal of American Academy of Child and Adolescent Psychiatry, 27*, 200–206.

Silverman, P., & Worden, W. (1992). Children's reactions in the early months after the death of a parent. *American Journal of Orthopsychiatry, 62*, 93–104.

Silverman, P., & Worden, W. (1993). Children's reactions to the death of a parent. In M. Stroebe, W. Stroebe, & R. Hansson (Eds.), *Handbook of bereavement: Theory, research and intervention* (pp. 300–316). New York: Cambridge University Press.

Sood, B., Weller, E., Weller, R., Fristad, M., & Bowes, J. (1992). Somatic complaints in grieving children. *Comprehensive Mental Health Care, 2*, 17–25.

Strength, J. M. (1991). *Factors influencing the mother–child relationship following the death of the father and how that relationship affects the child's functioning*. Unpublished doctoral dissertation, Rosemead School of Psychology, La Mirada, CA.

Thyer, B., Himle, J., & Miller-Gogoleski, M. A. (1989). The relationship of parental death to panic disorder: A community-based replication. *Phobia Practice and Research Journal, 2*, 29–36.

Toedter, L. J., Lasker, J. N., & Campbell, D. T. (1990). The comparison group problem in bereavement studies and the retrospective pretest. *Evaluation Review, 14*, 75–90.

US Bureau of the Census. (1990). *Statistical abstracts of the US, 1990* (110th ed.). Washington, DC: US Government Printing Office.

US Bureau of the Census, Current Population Reports. (1994). *Marital status and living arrangements: March, 1994* Washington, DC: US Government Printing Office.

Van Eerdewegh, M., Bieri, M., Parrilla, R., & Clayton, P. (1982). The bereaved child. *British Journal of Psychiatry, 140*, 23–29.

Van Eerdewegh, M., Clayton, P., & Van Eerdewegh, P. (1985). The bereaved child: Variables influencing early psychopathology. *British Journal of Psychiatry, 147*, 188–194.

Vicary, J., & Lerner, J. (1986). Parental attributes and adolescent drug use. *Journal of Adolescence, 9*, 115–122.

Vuchinich, S., Bank, L., & Patterson, G. (1992). Parenting, peers, and the stability of antisocial behavior in preadolescent boys. *Developmental Psychology, 28,* 510–521.

Weissman, M., Leckman, J., Merikangas, K., Gammon, G., & Prusoff, B. (1984). Depression and anxiety disorders in parents and children. *Archives of General Psychiatry, 41,* 845–852.

Weller, E., Weller, R., Fristad, M., & Bowes, J. (1990). Dexamethasone suppression test and depressive symptoms in bereaved children: A preliminary report. *The Journal of Neuropsychiatry and Clinical Neurosciences, 2,* 418–421.

Wentzel, K., Feldman, S., & Weinberger, D. (1991). Parental child rearing and academic achievement in boys: The mediational role of social–emotional adjustment. *Journal of Early Adolescence, 11,* 321–339.

West, S., Sandler, I., Pillow, D., Baca, L., & Gersten, J. (1991). The use of structural equation modeling in generative research: Toward the design of a preventive intervention for bereaved children. *American Journal of Community Psychology, 19,* 459–489.

Wheaton, B. (1985). Models for the stress-buffering functions of coping resources. *Journal of Health and Social Behavior, 26,* 352–354.

Worden, J. W. (1994, November). What really helps in the long run? New findings of a longitudinal study of school-aged children who lose a parent to death. Paper presented at the National Conference on Loss and Transition/West, Scottsdale, AZ.

Worden, J. W., & Silverman, P. R. (1996). Parental death and the adjustment of school-age children. *Omega Journal of Death and Dying, 33,* 91–102.

Zall, D. (1994). The long-term effects of childhood bereavement: Impact on roles as mothers. *Omega Journal of Death and Dying, 29,* 219–230.

Zambelli, G., & DeRosa, A. (1992). Bereavement support groups for school-age children: Theory, intervention, and case example. *American Journal of Orthopsychiatry, 62,* 484–493.

9

Understanding Stress Associated with Adolescent Pregnancy and Early Childbearing

PAUL A. LANGFIELD and KAY PASLEY

In addition to the typical demands placed on today's adolescents, young women who find themselves pregnant at this stage of life encounter a barrage of additional challenges. The stress of pregnancy is heaped upon an existing transitional period wrought with its own developmental stressors. The combination of pregnancy and adolescence creates stress that is greater than the sum of either pregnancy or adolescence alone, which can result in damaging consequences for the teen mother, her children, and society in general. Researchers have focused significant attention on the stress and adaptation of pregnant adolescents to the multiple demands inherent in this situation. In this chapter, we examine the extant literature on stress among pregnant and parenting adolescents, emphasizing the complexity of these phenomena and assessing the effectiveness of current interventions.

ADOLESCENT STRESS

The storm-and-stress conceptualization of adolescence has been widely debated since its introduction in 1904 by G. Stanley Hall. However, most schol-

PAUL A. LANGFIELD • Rocky Mountain Neuropsychological Sciences, P.C., Ft. Collins, Colorado 80524.   KAY PASLEY • Human Development and Family Studies, University of North Carolina, Greensboro, Greensboro, North Carolina 27412.
Handbook of Children's Coping: Linking Theory and Intervention, edited by Wolchik and Sandler. Plenum Press, New York, 1997.

ars concur that adolescence is accompanied by stress comparable to that experienced at other points of developmental transition (for reviews, see Compas, 1987; Johnson, 1986). From an adaptation perspective (McCubbin & Patterson, 1981), stress results from an imbalance between an actual or perceived demand and an individual's actual or perceived capability to meet that demand. Thus, stress emerges in adolescence from demands that are inherent in the typical adolescent transition and are considered normative. For example, potential stress results from the normal demands from the academic, psychosocial, physical, and developmental arenas at this time. Many adolescents also must cope with less normative demands related to poverty, disability, minority status, and other specialized life circumstances. Early pregnancy and childbearing are nonnormative life circumstances that present challenges for which most adolescents are not prepared.

The literature suggests that while most adolescents engage in sexual activity before they graduate high school (Moore, Snyder, & Daly, 1992), the majority also report that pregnancy is an unintended outcome of this activity (Moore, 1992). The trend toward a higher incidence of adolescent childbearing, especially out-of-wedlock childbearing, is complicated by a concomitant increase in women who elect to parent their offspring. In past decades, 90% of single mothers placed their children for adoption. Now, less than 4% of unintended live births to adolescents are legally released for adoption (Bachrach, London, & Stolley, 1992).

Parenthood is inherently stressful at any age. Sources of stress unique to first parenthood include the pregnancy and birth experiences, problems associated with redefining adult roles to incorporate that of parent, and financial strain (Olson et al., 1983). These stresses are further complicated by changes in one's self-definition and in relationships with significant others and social institutions (Cowan & Hetherington, 1991). When the transition to parenthood is coupled with the stress of the adolescent transition, cumulative stress is greater (Langfield, 1992). The combination of changes results in an exponential increase in stress from role ambiguity (Boss, 1977), competing developmental tasks (Codega, 1988; Cowan & Hetherington, 1991), and negotiating multiple transitions simultaneously (Pasley, Langfield, & Kreutzer, 1993).

INCIDENCE OF ADOLESCENT PREGNANCY AND PREGNANCY OUTCOMES

The rates of adolescent pregnancy in the United States are higher and have increased more rapidly than in any other industrialized nation. Estimates indicate that the percent of females 15–19 who ever had sexual intercourse rose from 28.6% in 1970 to 51.5% in 1988 (Centers for Disease Control, 1992). More recent evidence suggests that by 19 years of age, at least 80% report having experienced intercourse (Moore et al., 1992). Further, each year more than one million adolescents in the United States become pregnant, and half of the pregnancies result in live births (Furstenberg, Brooks-Gunn, & Chase-Landsdale, 1989; Testa, 1992). As of 1992, nearly one of every three births in the United States was to a single woman (Bumpass & Raley, 1995), and one of ten was to an adolescent (National Center for Health Statistics, 1993).

The 1970s saw a decrease in births to adolescent mothers, and this trend continued through 1986. A resurgent increase in adolescent births occurred through 1990 when 533,000 live births to females under 20 were reported, up from 472,000 in 1986. Figures currently available show a slight decrease in 1991 (US Bureau of the Census, 1993). Important concomitant changes have occurred with the trend in high adolescent pregnancy rates. These include higher rates of out-of-wedlock pregnancy (US Bureau of the Census, 1993) and more frequent decisions on the part of adolescent mothers to raise their children rather than give them up for adoption (Bachrach et al., 1992; Roosa, Fitzgerald, & Carson, 1982). For example, since 1970, there has been a steady increase in the rate of births to unmarried women 15 to 19 years of age per 1000 unmarried women 15 to 44 years of age from 22.4 in 1970 to 44.8 in 1991 (US Bureau of the Census, 1993).

Part of the concern stems from the increase in the rate of pregnancy and resulting births to adolescents 15 years of age and younger. While many fewer young adolescents give birth to a child, more pregnancies are occurring among this younger age group (Freeman & Rickles, 1993). Figures show that in 1980, the rate per 1000 women 15 to 44 years old was 1.1 for those younger than 15 and 53.0 for women 15 to 19 years of age. These numbers had increased to 1.4 and 62.1 by 1991. A steady annual increase in pregnancies to younger adolescents began in 1984 and continued to climb, as with older adolescents. Interestingly, figures show a gradual increase in the rate of births to younger adolescents since 1970, but a decrease in the rate for older adolescents. In 1970, the rate per 1000 was 1.2 for adolescents under 15 years of age and 68.3 for 15- to 19-year-olds (US Bureau of the Census, 1993).

The United States Compared to Other Countries

Adolescent pregnancy continues to affect the United States to a greater degree than any other industrialized nation in the world (Senderowitz & Paxman, 1985). Even with similar rates of adolescent intercourse, England, France, and Canada have less than half the incidence of adolescent pregnancy found in America. The state with the lowest rates of teenage pregnancy in the United States is North Dakota (US Bureau of the Census, 1993). Yet, this rate is equivalent to the highest provincial rate in Canada (Henshaw, 1993). The rate of adolescent pregnancy in the United States is three times higher than that noted for Sweden and nine times higher than that noted for the Netherlands (Allan Guttmacher Institute, 1994). Despite the similarity of these countries' economic and cultural norms, the United States continues to experience more teenage pregnancy. What we know is that teens in these countries report about the same level of sexual intercourse. However, US teens are less effective in preventing pregnancy (e.g., poorer use of contraception and less sex education) and have less access to abortion (Henshaw, 1993).

Racial Variations

Much of the concern over adolescent pregnancy in the United States arises from the marked differences among racial groups in both its occurrence and consequences. Consider first that the increase in births to unmarried women is especially pronounced for white females. Data show that in 1970 there were 26.4 births to unmarried women for every 1000 unmarried female aged 15 to 44 years. In 1991, this figure had increased to 45.2 births. For white women, the rate per 1000 went from 13.9 in 1970 to 34.6 in 1991 (120% increase). For African-American women the rate went from 95.5 to 189.5 over the same time, representing a 50% increase (US Bureau of the Census, 1993).

When we look at the figures for unmarried births to adolescent women, especially those 15 to 19 years old, African-American teens are more than twice as likely to become adolescent mothers than are white teens (42% vs. 19%, respectively). This difference is especially pronounced under the age of 15, when a birth is six times more likely in African Americans than in whites (Kahan & Anderson, 1992).

The highest birthrate to adolescents is among Americans of Hispanic origin, with Mexican Americans being the dominant group (National Center for Health Statistics, 1991, 1993). Estimates show that 9% of adolescent births nationally are to Mexican Americans, even though they represent just 6% of the total female population (Warrick, Christianson, Walruff, & Cook, 1993).

CONSEQUENCES OF TEEN PREGNANCY AND PREMATURE CHILDBEARING

Having a child as an adolescent can have negative implications for all aspects of the young mother's life, including financial, social, educational, physical, occupational, psychological, and developmental well-being. These effects also can extend to the child, the young father, and society in general. We focus here on those consequences that (1) are consistently found across studies and (2) that have the highest social impact. Certainly, neither the outcomes discussed here include all possible outcomes nor are the citations exhaustive, but are used as examples of the literature.

In general, teenage pregnancy has a number of potentially negative consequences for both the teen mother and her child (Furstenberg, 1991; Hayes, 1987; Hollander, 1995). The adolescent runs the risk of health complications during pregnancy and birth, school dropout, persistent poverty, marital difficulties, and single parenthood (Adams, Adams-Taylor, & Pittman, 1989; Furstenberg, 1991; Miller & Moore, 1990). Her child may suffer poor cognitive development, and social–behavioral adjustment problems are noted (Furstenberg et al., 1989; Halsey, Collins, & Anderson, 1993; Hayes, 1987; Spencer, 1985). Society also feels the burden of adolescent pregnancy. Burt (1986) estimated that adolescent pregnancy cost society $5.16 billion through food stamps and Aid to Families with Dependent Children (AFDC) over a 20-year period. Recent figures suggest that meeting the needs of pregnant and parenting adolescents costs the nation between 7 and 8.9 billion dollars annually (Holmes, 1996; Passell, 1996). Further, Bane and Elwood (1986) noted that adolescent mothers spend more time on welfare than any other group. Harris (1991) demonstrated that the histories of 288 teen mothers some 17 years later showed a dependence on welfare, although most were employed continuously and became self-supporting. Such realities have fueled public concern of the costs of early childbearing in human and financial terms (ABC/Washington Post, 1982; CBS News, 1994; Coombs-Orme, 1993).

We concur with Miller (1992) that the stress of adolescent pregnancy can have devastating consequences for the teen parent, her child, and society at least in the short run. For many, negative consequences are not short-lived. As such, research directed at understanding and enhancing the coping skills and resiliency of this population continues to be of paramount importance to reducing the consequences.

Consequences to Teenage Mothers

Of the many negative consequences of teen pregnancy and premature childbearing for the mother, decreased educational attainment, lower employment opportunities, and poverty are the most persistent. Other consequences include poorer parenting (see, for example, Passino et al., 1993; Vukelich & Kliman, 1985), increased likelihood of divorce (Pasley, 1995), and increased vulnerability to health problems (Auvenshine & Enriquez, 1985; Geronimus, 1991). Few studies have examined the psychological risks of teen pregnancy and parenting to the adolescent. Findings from an early study (Barth, Schinke, & Maxwell, 1983) compared 62 teen mothers, 63 pregnant teens, and 60 non-pregnant, nonparenting teens and found no differences in reported levels of anxiety or depression. Data from 2152 female adolescents receiving services from seven health clinics throughout the nation compared responses from sexually inactive, never-pregnant, pregnant, and child-rearing adolescents (Stiffman, Powell, Earls, & Robins, 1990). These researchers found that adolescent parents and sexually inactive adolescents had the lowest number of mental health problems (they did not differ from each other), while the never-pregnant and pregnant had similarly the highest numbers of problems.

Outcomes are affected by other factors as well (e.g., race), and they also affect other outcomes (e.g., repeat pregnancy). Regarding race, differences exist in the consequences of adolescent pregnancy. African Americans are more likely than either whites or Hispanics to complete schooling after giving birth. On the other hand, Hispanic adolescents are most likely to parent and marry simultaneously, resulting in the highest dropout rate of all racial groups (Pasley, 1995). Furthermore, the stressful circumstances surrounding adolescent childbearing are often exacerbated by another birth, since over half of adolescent mothers have a second child within 2 years. Estimates suggest that 31% of teenagers who gave birth prior to age 17 and 24% of those who gave birth at age 18 or 19 had a second child within 2 years (Allan Guttmacher Institute, 1994).

That each of these outcomes is frequently associated with teen pregnancy and premature childbearing is indisputable. However, it is difficult to determine how many of these consequences are actually due to the mother's age or due to other factors. From a macrosociological perspective, a multitude of factors contribute to one's adjustment to a disruptive life event such as teen pregnancy. For example, the relationship between adolescent pregnancy, early marriage, and subsequent divorce is entangled because for some groups early pregnancy is highly correlated with early marriage, and both early marriage and pregnancy are associated with marital difficulties. While an additive model seems to be logical and one that is commonly advanced, Teti and Lamb (1989) argued that the presence of children in an adolescent marriage acts to stabilize the marriage. We believe that linear hypothesizing does little to further our understanding of the complex and varied trajectories that result in undesirable consequences of adolescent pregnancy. For example, when decreased education, financial instability, and impoverished backgrounds are considered (factors associated with early marriage) (Trend & Harlan, 1990), the extent of financial hardship (both past and current) may be a prime contributor to eventual divorce among adolescent marriages, rather than either early marriage or early childbearing per se. However, the focus of much of the outcome research has compared adolescent marriages (those contracted before 20 years of age) with adult marriages (those contracted after 19 years of age) to identify the factors that contribute to marital instability and the pathways to divorce. In many ways, these typical comparisons are like examining apples and oranges. What is lacking from this literature are comparisons of teen marriages that remain intact with those that terminate. Studies incorporating within-group comparisons would do much to further our understanding of the qualities of early marriages that make them resilient to the multiple stresses inherent in premature childbearing and the resulting life course.

A simplistic view of the causes and consequences of teen pregnancy assumes that the life trajectories of teen mothers are similar. Recent research suggests that many of the consequences typically linked to teen parenting are not characteristics of this population over time (Furstenberg, Brooks-Gunn, & Morgan, 1987). Furthermore, the diversity of the life course of teen mothers suggests that for many the pattern is not linear. In other words, not all teen mothers have lives of poverty and have children who follow their path. Consistent with other social science research, well-designed, longitudinal research on the consequences of adolescent pregnancy is the exception rather than the rule. In place of such studies, researchers have been hasty to generalize short-term outcomes and extend a vision of doom for the futures of adolescent parents. One exception has been the study of African-American teen mothers from Baltimore followed over 20 years. The findings from this work (Furstenberg et al., 1987) paint a less negative picture of adolescent mothers. These authors note that the majority of former adolescent mothers (70.5%) ultimately completed high school and were employed (67.8%).

Other scholars (Horowitz, Klerman, Kuo, & Jekel, 1991) emphasize that certain intervention strategies and a supportive environment can improve the long-term success of these women. Studies show that when pregnant teens receive prenatal, obstetric, and social services (Lawrence & Merritt, 1983; McAnarney & Hendee, 1989; Polit, 1989) and attend special school programs for pregnant and parenting adolescents (Furstenberg et al., 1987), they are more likely to have better outcomes. Thus, the research studies emphasizing short-term effects are important in their own right; however, they are somewhat misleading and do not provide a complete picture of the future life chances of adolescent mothers (Furstenberg, 1991).

The Link between Poverty and Adolescent Pregnancy

Adolescent pregnancy and premature childbearing, lowered educational and occupational attainment, and poverty are intimately tied and represent one pathway to intergenerational poverty in America. Because adolescent child-bearing is more common among those who have the fewest social and econom-ic opportunities (e.g., racial minorities, inner-city dwellers, and isolated rural communities) (Hayes, 1987; National Center for Health Statistics, 1991), ado-lescent pregnancy is central to the intergenerational transmission of poverty. As Moore and associates (1993) intimate, teen parenthood is likely one link in the chain of economic devastation passed from generation to generation, but teen pregnancy and parenting per se do not cause poverty (Males, 1993).

The link between poverty and adolescent pregnancy is neither linear nor simple. While we know that adolescent mothers are likely to come from impov-erished backgrounds (Allan Guttmacher Institute, 1994; Abrahamse, Morrison, & Waite, 1988), to be poor themselves (Caldas, 1993; Trent & Harlan, 1990), and to require public assistance (Bane & Elwood, 1986; Committee on Ways and Means, 1989; Duncan & Hoffman, 1990; Harris, 1991), the path to their own poverty status is not a direct one. Other characteristics associated with teen pregnancy and parenting contribute to the continuation of poverty. For exam-ple, early childbearing is associated with early marriage (Teti & Lamb, 1989), the production of larger families (Hofferth, 1987), and unstable marriages and divorce (Furstenberg et al., 1987; Thornton, & Rogers, 1987). Marrying at a young age is associated with both increased family size (Hofferth, 1987) and lower educational attainment (Kerkhoff & Parrow, 1979; Lowe & Witt, 1984). Large family size contributes to underemployment and the resulting poverty. Similarly, adolescent marriages that end often leave the teen mother as the head of a single-parent family (Garfinkel & McLanahan, 1986); single parenting predicts lower educational attainment and employment (Krein & Beller, 1988), and is associated with the likelihood of living in poverty. Finally, growing up in a single-parent family, especially one that is disadvantaged by underemploy-ment or unemployment, puts the next generation of adolescents at risk for premarital pregnancy (Aquilino, 1996; Astone, 1993; Bumpass & Raley, 1995; Furstenberg et al., 1987). Thus, the cycle of poverty and teen pregnancy contin-ues. Because members of minority groups are most likely to have the fewest social and economic opportunities, they have a much higher risk of remaining in this cycle. The complexity of factors affecting the cycle also means that intervention attempts must address broader contextual issues that promote the intergenerational transmission of poverty.

Effects of Early Childbearing on the Children

Conceptualizing a reciprocal relationship between poverty and early child-bearing has implications for the children of teen parents. For example, children born to adolescent mothers are more likely to be low-birth-weight babies, to experience persistent infections, to die from sudden infant death syndrome, and to be victims of abuse and neglect (Allan Guttmacher Institute, 1994; Bol-ton, 1980; Boyer & Fine, 1992; Field, 1980); some of these outcomes are espe-cially pronounced for children born to teens 10 to 14 years of age (Leland, Petersen, Braddock, & Alexander, 1995). Additional research shows that the children of adolescent mothers are more aggressive, less self-controlled, and perform more poorly on indicators of academic achievement than their peers born to older mothers (Furstenberg & Chase-Landsdale, 1989). However, once again, because the effects seem to be influenced by added stressful conditions, such as poverty, it is difficult to determine the extent to which these negative outcomes are directly attributable to the age of the mother at the time of birth.

Certainly early physical difficulties are related to the less comprehensive prenatal care typical of adolescent mothers (Allan Guttmacher Institute, 1994). Some behavioral outcomes likely stem from poor prenatal care, poor parenting skills, and a number of other environmental conditions such as persistent poverty, living in poor/violent neighborhoods, and being medically/educationally underserviced. Theoretically, outcomes would be less negative under more positive contextual influences. We believe that more studies are needed that address broader contextual influences to further our understanding of the causal factors affecting child outcomes given the current debate among scholars regarding causes (see, for example, Bachrach & Carver, 1992; Furstenberg, 1992; Geronimus, 1991).

Effects of Teenage Parenting on Young Men

Not all teen pregnancies are fathered by teenage boys. In fact, about 74% of teenage pregnancies are fathered by men older than 18 (Allan Guttmacher Institute, 1994). Males (1993) found that the younger the mother, the greater the partner age gap. Using data from California, he reported that among mothers 11 to 12 years of age, the fathers of their children were on average 9.8 years older; among mothers 13 to 14 years of age, the fathers averaged 4.6 years older; and among those mothers 15 to 19 years, the fathers averaged 3.7 years older. However, statements from health agencies continue to portray teenage pregnancy as resulting from intercourse between adolescent partners (Roper, 1993). The reality that most babies born to adolescent mothers are fathered by older men has particular relevance for prevention and intervention that must do more to target the behavior of older men, if decreases in teenage pregnancy are to be realized.

Since many of the fathers of children born to teen mothers are older, by virtue of their increased maturity they should be more able to meet their economic responsibilities than would younger fathers. The association between poverty and early childbearing, however, may mean that many of these older fathers are either underemployed or unemployed, and this limits their ability to provide adequately for their children. Some also may be unwilling to accept financial responsibility for their children (Marsiglio, 1991).

Important to our discussion here is the fact that adolescent fathers have been the focus of limited research, and this has resulted in few definitive statements about the effects of their parenting status on them. We do know that some effects of early childbearing on young men are similar to those reported for teen mothers. For example, they are more likely than their older peers or their same-age, nonfather peers to experience academic difficulties and truncated education and employment instability (Dearden, Hale, & Alvarez, 1992; Hendricks, 1988; Marsiglio, 1995). Also, adolescent fathers demonstrate less competent parenting behaviors (Ketterlinus, Lamb, & Nitz, 1991).

Research also indicates that adolescent fatherhood is associated with vocational instability, health problems, and difficulty establishing and maintaining interpersonal relationships (Ketterlinus et al., 1991). The father's relationship with the teen mother also is characterized by instability and is often a source of stress rather than support to both (Elster, 1991). Teen fathers often disengage from their children over time (Furstenberg & Harris, 1993; Neville & Parke, 1991). Most young, unmarried fathers are highly motivated to be involved in the parenting experience early on. Their disengagement is tied to an inability to provide financially for the child, relationship problems with the mother and/or her family, and societal barriers (e.g., funding guidelines for receiving AFDC and Medicare) (Furstenberg et al., 1987). Disengagement is especially common among young fathers in highly disadvantaged populations (Danziger & Radin, 1990; Marsiglio, 1989).

Clearly, young fathers are less able to economically "do for" their children and maintain the type of commitment men see as part of being a good father (Furstenberg, 1994). Some suggest that the teen father can function as an effective source of support for the teen mother, if he is allowed to do so and receives encouragement by the mother, both families, peers, and social service providers. Thus, the context in which the young father is located must be adequately supportive of his desire for involvement, if involvement is to be realized. In addition, others argue that the definition of good fathering must be broadened to include variations and must recognize and value a wider range of acceptable involvement patterns (Pasley & Minton, 1997).

What is evident here is the need for more research to better understand the process of disengagement of younger (teenage) fathers. We also suggest that failure to examine both adolescent fathers and their older peers who are even more responsible for pregnancies to teenage women results in limited understanding of the contexts that contribute to stress for teenage mothers and their children.

A CLOSER LOOK AT STRESS IN PREGNANT AND PARENTING ADOLESCENTS

We implied earlier that the gestalt of stress related to teen pregnancy and early childbearing stems from the fact that unlike a typical adolescent, the pregnant or parenting adolescent finds herself in more than one life stage (adolescence and young adulthood) and in two family stages (families with adolescents and first parenthood) simultaneously. We argue here that the competing developmental tasks of these life stages are stress inducing for the pregnant and parenting adolescent. Integrating ideas from several theories seems to provide the best explanation of the nature of the stress confronting these adolescents. Theoretically, stress arises from changes in the status quo (Boss, 1988). As a result, one is most vulnerable to stress at points of family transitions (e.g., marriage, birth) and individual transitions (e.g., adolescence). Clearly, the transition to parenthood is stressful in its own right. Researchers (Cowan & Hetherington, 1991; Olson et al., 1983) have highlighted areas of potential stress for first-time parents, including relationships with the self, partners, children, and nonfamily institutions, as well as intergenerational relationships within the family and financial strain. At the same time, a pregnant adolescent may be facing the challenge of balancing her needs for autonomy from and connection to her family. Olson and associates (1983) concluded that "no phase of the family life cycle seems to be more stressful than the adolescent years" (p. 219), a time when 50% of teenagers in their study of 1000 families saw interacting with their family of origin as their biggest stressor and daily hassles involving their parents topped their lists of stressors.

Taking on the role of parent can draw the adolescent back into her family of origin for much needed emotional, financial, and other types of support. Relying on her family for these supports can put her at odds with the normative developmental tasks of gaining autonomy in adolescence. Pile up results because of the demands created by each of these stressful transitions separately. However, separately these transitions do not fully illustrate the gestalt of stress that the multiple transitions create. Teenage pregnancy means that the adolescent must cope with gaining the expected autonomy, while securing the necessary support to care for herself and for her child. Yet, more dependence on her family may be needed, which impedes her autonomy. For the family, teenage pregnancy forces the adolescent simultaneously to straddle multiple developmental transitions and social roles—roles that are sometimes at odds with one another. The adolescent mother is responsible for (1) the care and nurturance of her child (parent role), (2) the economic support of her child (worker role), and (3) her own development as an adolescent (self role). Financially providing for her child means she has less time and energy to devote to the care and nurturance of the child and for fulfilling her educational obligations that have long-term implications for her well-being and that of her child. The adolescent's need to expand her peer network, choose a career, and deal with physical maturation may compete with the need to provide for her newborn. If the teen chooses to get married, the couple faces the challenge of moving forward to an advanced family life stage without adequate time to establish themselves as a dyad prior to the arrival of the baby.

Given the nature and origins of the stress related to adolescent pregnancy, adaptation centers around effectively juggling the demands of various developmental tasks inherent in these family-related and individually based transitions. Thus, stress emerges from role confusion, role strain, and role ambiguity in the simultaneous negotiation of multiple stages. Just as there is wide diversity in outcomes of adolescent pregnancy and parenting, however, the nature of the stress to pregnant teens also varies by other factors as well. Race and pregnancy status are two factors addressed in the literature.

Variations by Race

Evidence suggests that the experience of the pregnant and parenting African-American teen is different from that of a Hispanic or white teen. In fact, some scholars argue that adolescent childbearing may be adaptive and developmentally appropriate (Gabriel & McAnarney, 1983; Sandven & Resnick, 1990), especially for African Americans. From a developmental perspective, the results of a study of sisters showed that African-American mothers in their 20s were more likely than teen mothers to bear low-birth-weight babies and drink and smoke during pregnancy, and less likely to breast-feed or have used the services of well-baby clinics (Geronimus & Korenman, 1991). The reverse pattern applies to whites. Moreover, the long-standing practice of informal adoption (e.g., grandmothers accepting much of the burden of child rearing) within the African-American family means there is less stigma attached to adolescent childbearing (Stack, 1974; Wolf, 1983). Historically, African-American families have been more accommodating to early childbearing because the kin network typically rallies to provide social support (McAdoo, 1988). Some evidence supports McAdoo's observation and finds that teen pregnancy is more acceptable within an extended family where demands of parenting are shared (Swenson, Erickson, Ehlinger, Carlson, & Swaney, 1989; Ladner, 1987). The adaptive pattern of caring for children within an extended kin network provides much needed support for the adolescent who is coping with the multiple transitions discussed earlier.

Since African-American teens are half as likely to get married when pregnant than whites (Kahan & Anderson, 1992), they are more likely to live in an extended family household (Hofferth, 1984; Sweet & Bumpass, 1987). It may be that the value of reciprocal obligations common in African-American families (McAdoo, 1988) prompts them to personally sacrifice on behalf of the welfare of the family (e.g., a grandmother caring for her grandchild). Members of the extended family may be more willing to provide assistance and resources to teen mothers in need. It seems logical that aside from other contextual realities, the African-American adolescent who lives in a supportive kin-focused family system would experience less stress than another teen in a different cultural and familial context, at least in the short run.

Overinvolvement of family members is seen by some scholars (e.g., Watson & Protinsky, 1991) as a contextually adaptive response and one that is positively associated with the development of healthy identity in adolescents. Further, finding from a study of the children of single-parent mothers, using detailed life history data on childhood living arrangements from the National Survey of Families and Households, showed that when grandparents and relatives acted as supplemental rather than substitute parents, children of single-parent mothers had higher educational attainment and slower movement into adult roles (Aquilino, 1996). Thus, it is both the involvement and the nature of that involvement that may make a difference in the lives of young mothers and their offspring.

We cannot ignore, however, the broader context in which many African Americans and other people of color reside. It is this broader context where realities such as poverty lessen the potential positive effects of support provided by kin networks. Still, we believe that overall social support plays a vital role in reducing the potential negative outcomes of stress associated with adolescent pregnancy and early childrearing.

Some evidence shows that regardless of race only a small proportion of teen mothers live with their families after an initial period (Eggebeen, Crockett, & Hawkins, 1990; Hill, 1990). As such, adolescent mothers and their children may experience more instability in their family context than originally believed (Furstenberg, 1991). Also, being young and African American in America places one at risk for poverty, which places one at risk for negative outcomes.

Some research on the outcomes of teen pregnancy for African Americans suggests that they may experience less stress or cope more effectively with the stress than other racial groups. African Americans who parent as teenagers are more likely to finish high school than are either white or Hispanic adolescent parents (Upchurch & McCarthy, 1990). Thus, African-American teen mothers are more often able to accomplish one of the central individual developmental tasks of adolescence. Other evidence suggests that adolescent childbearing has less effect on the overall earnings of African Americans than whites. The income difference between an African American who had a child as a teenager and one who delayed child rearing is less than the difference between whites in these two groups (Moore et al., 1993). Economic advantage is associated with delaying motherhood until age 25 or later among whites but not among African Americans (Astone, 1993). This means that adolescent parenthood is less disruptive to the economic status of African Americans than to whites, primarily because of the differential income advantage linked to minority status.

Whereas the kinship patterns and their implicit values evident in African-American families may alleviate some of the stress experienced by teen mothers, the values inherent in the Hispanic culture may make early parenthood more challenging for the Hispanic teen. As previously mentioned, Hispanics are the most likely of all racial groups to drop out of school in general, and lower education is associated with later negative economic consequences (Mott & Marsiglio, 1985; Upchurch & McCarthy, 1990). The high dropout rate among Hispanic teens may reflect the importance placed on marriage, especially when pregnancy occurs. Recall that Hispanics are more likely than other racial groups to both marry and parent simultaneously (Forste & Tienda, 1992). Choosing to raise the baby and to marry are noted risk factors in the dropout literature independent of one another; together, they seem to have an additive effect and further the risk of truncating one's education. In addition, the religious values emphasizing marriage and traditional gender roles also may prompt young Hispanic fathers to drop out of school and get jobs to support their new family. On the other hand, like African Americans, Hispanic teen mothers are more likely to live in an extended family network during and after pregnancy than are whites, and this source of support may reduce stress. Important within-group differences are noted: Mexican Americans were twice as likely and Puerto Ricans were less likely to live in extended families than were whites (Trent & Harlan, 1994).

We believe that the emergence of cultural differences such as the ones discussed here must serve as ever-present reminders that the experiences of pregnancy and parenting for teenagers are varied and more complicated than much of the literature typically recognizes. These young women are not a homogeneous group (Freeman & Rickles, 1993; Hamburg & Dixon, 1992). Clearly, the complexity of life experience for pregnant and parenting adolescents also is apparent within a specific racial or ethnic group and as a function of the broader context (e.g., socioeconomic factors). However, few studies have focused on teasing out the diversity of experiences.

Variations by Parenting Status

We have argued (Pasley et al., 1993) that the nature of stress for adolescents varies by pregnancy status also, although limited research has examined status. A young woman who is pregnant will experience different emotions and stressors than will a young women who is caring for a 2-week-old child. Similarly, the emotions and stressors for an adolescent mother with an infant will be different from one caring for a 2-year-old child. Because adolescent pregnancy does not always result in birth, and childbirth does not always result in parenthood, a teenager who has just determined that she is pregnant may experience stress around how and when to tell her parent(s). The adolescent who has decided to have an abortion may experience stress related to grieving the loss of the fetus, whereas the adolescent who decides to carry to term may experience stress around adoption decisions. These decisions differ from the adolescent mother who must find reliable child care so she can attend school or secure employment.

Most of the literature has not examined such within-group variations. Instead, scholars commonly treat pregnant and parenting adolescents as if they are a homogeneous group. We believe that these failures reduce the accuracy of research hypotheses and conclusions and may impede the effectiveness of interventions planned with a "typical" adolescent in mind. Thus, there are benefits to viewing the nature of stress for each of the groups separately. Our own evaluation of 15 teen parent programs in Colorado (Pasley & Kreutzer, 1989) showed that the content/curriculum was directed toward students who intend to parent their child. No formal attention was given to examining other options, so these programs implicitly support the single choice of parenthood.

We could find little research that addressed parenting status. One study examined pregnancy resolution by comparing women who relinquish their children for adoption with those who elect to parent their children (Bachrach et al., 1992). Other research more germane here, albeit limited, has addressed differential sources of stress in pregnant and parenting adolescents. Barth and Schinke (1983) found that pregnant adolescents reported more situations as stressful than did parenting adolescents, and they felt less able to cope with their circumstances. Stern and Alvarez (1992) reported that neither pregnant nor parenting adolescents saw school as stressful, whereas nonpregnant adolescents did. Their findings showed differences between pregnant and parenting teens: 75% of pregnant teens reported personal or internal stresses most difficult (e.g., family problems), and 71% of parenting adolescents reported external stresses most difficult (e.g., living conditions, child care). Still other research (Pasley et al., 1993) examined both differences in pregnant and parenting adolescents in terms of the sources of stress and other factors associated with stress (e.g., social support, coping strategies). No differences were found between groups in overall stress. For pregnant adolescents ($n = 60$), good feelings about self were associated with lower levels of overall stress and experiencing less stress from engaging in deviant behaviors (e.g., stealing) and other sources of distress (e.g., getting pimples, running away). More frequent use of coping strategies and being older were predictive of more stress from autonomy (e.g., new friends, deciding about college). For parenting adolescents ($n = 92$), satisfaction with social support was predictive of less overall stress and less stress stemming from issues of autonomy. The authors concluded that the correlates were more predictive of stress for pregnant adolescents and that some differences between the groups were evident. If these results reflect the experiences of other pregnant and parenting adolescents, then intervention programs would need to address the unique issues faced by these groups. For example, self-esteem and self-worth issues could be emphasized for pregnant adolescents, whereas ways of finding satisfaction in one's support network could be emphasized with parenting adolescents.

We believe that continued examination of between-group differences, whether the comparisons are by racial groups or pregnancy status, will not provide the depth of information necessary to further our understanding of the etiology of this social phenomenon or determine effective interventions. Nor will such information enable us to adequately explain variations in adaption. Only by emphasizing within-group (e.g., between pregnant and parenting teens) rather than between-group (e.g., teen mothers and adult mothers) variations will our understanding of the issues faced by pregnant and parenting adolescents grow. Such research will permit us to design and implement more effective interventions that address the existing diversity of the population served.

SOCIAL SUPPORT AS A KEY TO ADAPTATION

The literature on family stress suggests that "resources" help to ameliorate stress. In fact, the use of existing resources and the acquisition and use of new resources are believed to assist one in coping successfully with stress (McCubbin & Patterson, 1981). One such resource can be social support or one's access to resources from one's social network, including material and emotional resources. Unfortunately, in the empirical literature social support tends to be viewed broadly and is often operationalized in ways that disregard its multidimensional nature. Recent research has defined social support in increasingly precise ways that allow comparisons across studies and offer more useful findings.

Social support is one of the most commonly investigated resources in studies of pregnant and parenting adolescents. In the case of teen pregnancy, scholars believe that the acquisition of social support is important to dealing effectively with pregnancy and/or parenting (deAnda et al., 1992; Wasserman, Brunelli, & Rauh, 1990), emphasizing its stress-buffering role. Commonly defined as the frequency of use of certain sources or having access to an increased number of supports, social support has been shown to foster coping and adaptation for adolescent mothers and their children (Barth & Schinke, 1983). Studies show that social support defined in these ways positively affects parenting both directly and indirectly (Boukydis, 1987; Crnic, Greenberg, Ragozin, Robinson, & Basham, 1983; Crockenberg, 1988), increases feelings of love toward the child (Crockenberg, 1987), alleviates stress (McLanahan, 1983), and promotes physical and psychological health of the mother (Whitman, Borkowski, Schellenbach, & Nath, 1987).

Social support also can reflect more than the number of persons in one's support network (size) and includes the sources of support (e.g., family, friends, professionals), the types of support given (e.g., tangible), and the amount of support received. The assumption underlying these objective measures is that larger numbers of support providers and amounts given means better support is provided and more positive outcomes should result. However, Nath, Borkowski, Whitman, and Schellenbach (1991) argued that amount of support is not always directly associated with feeling supported. Where adolescent mothers are concerned, several refinements to the conceptualization of social support have occurred. For example, Barrera (1981) differentiated between desired and actual support, and Pasley et al. (1993) differentiated between support perceived as helpful or unhelpful. Importantly, the amount of support needed or considered acceptable may vary by the context or the characteristics of the adolescent. A teen in need of financial support can go to his or her parent and borrow the needed sum. Here, the parent is the object of support and provides the desired level of support. However, the parent may punish her psychologically afterward by implicitly questioning her financial maturity and personal autonomy. In this case, the desired level of support is provided, but the outcome of gaining this support does not foster coping and, in fact, may make it more difficult for the teen in the long run. Some research supports this scenario (Stockdale, Crase, & Petersen, 1990).

We suggest that continued examination of the multidimensional nature of social support is an important target for future research. Such attention can result in findings that are more meaningful to intervention attempts. What we may find is that certain support is more or less helpful to different parenting statuses and to women who differ by race, age, and socioeconomic status.

Source, Size, Type, and Amount of Support

In the case of adult mothers, spouses are the most important source of support (Belsky, 1984; Crnic et al., 1983). However, the situation is different for adolescent mothers. Since their relationship with the child's father often is unstable, especially over time, family, school personnel, community resources, and friends tend to be more influential sources of support (Colletta, 1981; Whitman et al., 1987), although early on the child's father may play a key role in providing support (Stockdale et al., 1990). Research shows that families are rated by Hispanic and African-Americans teen mothers as their main source of support (Colletta & Lee, 1983; Feiring, Fox, Jaskir, & Lewis, 1987).

Regarding size of social support network, only one study was found. Stockdale and associates (1990) examined data from 77 nonpregnant/nonparenting adolescents and 77 pregnant/parenting adolescents, following the latter group over a 6-month period. They found that for both groups initially the size of the support network included six persons. When negative interaction with their network was controlled, this was reduced to three people who provided positive social support, and this network size was maintained 6 months later.

In addition to source and size, type of support is an important consideration. Just as various woodworking tools are designed for specific purposes and for use under unique circumstances, various types of support may work to greater or lesser degrees for specific stressors. For an adolescent mother who lacks money for food, it is logical that economic support may be most helpful. Economic support, however, may be less relevant for an adolescent whose primary stress stems from underlying emotional issues. Some research supports this hypothesis. Stockdale and associates (1990) found a decrease in overall support, financial support from fathers, advice given by grandparents, and social participation with one's sister when pregnant teens became parents. Interestingly, the mothers and boyfriends of the adolescents were seen as providing as much unconflicted support (positive support) as conflicted support (negative support) during the pregnancy and afterward.

Taken together, the results of these studies suggest that adopting a stressor-specific view of support (Cohen & McKay, 1884; Gottlieb, 1978) may facilitate understanding the complex nature of stress and coping in pregnant and parenting adolescents. Applying this approach to research increases the likelihood that the services provided to these young women, their children, and their families are more relevant. However, we could find no study that did this, and we believe such research is needed.

Still other scholars (Belsky, 1984; Granger, 1983; Sarason & Sarason, 1984) concur with Nath and associates (1991) about possible discrepancies between the objective (amount) and subjective meaning (e.g., satisfaction) and outcomes of social support. Although not using pregnant and parenting adolescents in their studies, some research finds that increased support leads to no change in stress or even increases stress or other negative outcomes due to the adolescent's locus of control (Sandler & Lakey, 1982), level of abstract thought (Granger, 1983), or feelings of conflict with sources of support (Crawford, 1984). Pasley and associates (1993) reported that neither objective nor subjective indicators of social support predicted stress in pregnant adolescents. However, the frequency with which parenting adolescents obtained support (the measure of objective support) was the sole predictor of overall stress and stress associated with gaining autonomy, explaining about 5–6% of the variance. Depending on the nature of other contextual and/or personal variables, higher amounts of support may result in more negative, more positive, or no changes in outcomes.

Further Refinements of Social Support as a Construct

Other refinements of the construct of social support have increased its usefulness in studies of adolescent mothers. Barrera (1981) suggested that adolescents' perceptions about support have a greater effect on their reactions to a stressor than does the actual amount of support received. Barrera (1981) found that satisfaction with the support received was inversely correlated with anxiety, depression, and somatization and not correlated with objective support. Others (Heller, Swindle, & Dusenburg, 1986) concur with this position, although we were unable to confirm these finding in our own work (Pasley et al., 1993), where stress was the outcome measure. However, we believe it would be premature to give up this line of research and assume that one's satisfaction with the support received does not affect outcomes for pregnant and parenting adolescents. As a result, more studies must query pregnant and parenting adolescents about what is and is not helpful to them in addition to gathering information about the type, sources, and amount of support received. Then determining the additional factors that influence the outcomes (e.g., coping strategies) would promote the development of explanatory models that suggest greater specificity, while attending to important within-group variations.

Finally, a developmental assessment of social support is needed. Recall that in the case of adolescent mothers, these teens are attempting to parent their children while achieving autonomy from one's family of origin. Because development is an ongoing process, it makes sense that support would need to change over time. Unger (1985) suggested that gradually reducing the amount of support to the adolescent would be developmentally appropriate, since it would encourage her to assume greater responsibility for the care of her child. Given that research has established the beneficial nature of social support and that more support may not be desirable, Unger's position is unique. Clearly the gradual reduction of support is a simple solution and may be inappropriate to the range of adolescent parents. We believe that far too little is now known about the (1) nature of social support, (2) the way social support needs change over the life course, and (3) the conditions under which needs for social support change for pregnant and parenting teens. Further investigation is warranted in this area to fully understand the role of social support in the adjustment of these adolescents. The key is in answering questions about the nature of social support that is and is not helpful to particular groups of adolescents.

REDUCING ADOLESCENT PREGNANCY AND THE RESULTING COMPLICATION: WHAT INTERVENTION STUDIES TELL US

In 1981, public concern and debate regarding adolescent sexuality resulted in mandating government intervention (Public Health Service Act Amendments of 1981). Thus, the Adolescent Family Life Act (AFLA) came into being in 1988 and is currently the only federal program devoted exclusively to adolescent sexuality and pregnancy (Department of health and Human Services, 1988). The major goal of this act is to prevent or postpone adolescent sexual activity so that adolescent pregnancy and parenthood are reduced. To achieve this goal, interventions that focus on abstinence from sexual activity among adolescents and/or general sex education have been supported. These programs are called primary prevention programs (Miller et al., 1993). Besides promoting abstinence, another key element of these primary prevention programs is family involvement, so many interventions also focus on enhancing parent–adolescent communication around sexuality (White & White, 1991). Meanwhile, secondary prevention programs aim to avoid birth and parenthood, mitigate their negative consequences, and prevent repeat pregnancies (Jorgensen, Potts, & Camp, 1993). Many programs combine both primary and secondary preventions.

In a recent review of some 24 AFLA programs, White and White (1991) discussed the diversity across such programs. Some programs are school based, whereas others are operated by community and/or state agencies. Still others link schools with agencies in the community. The target ages range from kindergartners through high school seniors, and about half of the programs are designed for preadolescents. Populations targeted for services also vary from individual adolescents or parents to entire families and from adolescents who are not yet sexually active to those that are expecting or currently parenting.

Programs directed specifically at pregnant and parenting adolescents vary widely. Our own examination of 15 of the 18 programs operating in Colorado in 1988 is an example of this variation. Programs differed by duration of service (1 month postpartum to high school graduation), location of service (integrated within the regular school program or located off-site in an alternative location), and nature of the services (e.g., personal counseling, child care, transportation). The content (e.g., academic content only vs. academic content plus parenting content, vocational training) and delivery strategies of the programs also varied greatly. Some programs used individualized lessons, whereas others kept the student in her regular classroom/school activities, as if her life would remain unchanged. Some provided many support services (e.g., links with other community agencies/services, personal and job counseling, daycare), whereas others provided nothing beyond that which any ordinary student received.

How Successful Are Our Interventions?

Overall, White and White (1991) concluded that the effectiveness of primary prevention programs has yet to be established convincingly. Others suggest that too few studies have been done that promote understanding of why some program models appear to succeed and others do not (Warrick et al., 1993; Stahler & DuCette, 1991). We know far more about programs that intervene on behalf of already-pregnant and parenting adolescents than we know about programs to prevent the pregnancy, and results from studies of secondary prevention programs are more consistent. Although programs vary by the population served, the nature and duration of the services provided and the content and focus of the program (e.g., vocational training, parenting education) studies show that they make a difference. The findings from several longitudinal studies emphasize the importance of participation in such specialized programs (Furstenberg et al., 1987; Horowitz et al., 1991; Seitz & Apfel, 1993). For example, Seitz and Apfel (1993) found that repeat pregnancy was delayed over the next 5 years when postpartum intervention lasted at least 7 weeks. These authors suggest that the special nature of the program (e.g., small classes, nurturance, personalized guidance, and mentoring) all contributed to the delayed pregnancy, high completion rates for high school, and employment status. A number of studies that focus on facilitating the transition to parenthood for at-risk groups of mothers (e.g., those who are economically disadvantaged, single parents), including adolescent mothers, consistently found that mentoring was a key to positive outcomes for both the mother and her children (Olds, Henderson, Chamberlain, & Tatelbaum, 1986; Olds, Henderson, Kitzman, & Cole, 1995). Another study (Ruch-Ross, Jones, & Musick, 1992) included over 1000 program participants and compared them with a matched sample from a nationally representative study (National Longitudinal Survey of Youth). They found that while the programs in which participants were enrolled varied greatly, two services made a difference: home visiting and parenting groups. Overall, students enrolled in special programs were more likely to remain in school, become employed, and avoid subsequent pregnancy 12 months post-baseline. Other studies show that "mainstreaming" pregnant students so that they have access to all academic courses and are able to remain in the program for an extended period of time, requiring their participation in a parenting class, providing them with extensive outreach efforts, and having strong case management for the provision of services were all associated with positive outcomes for pregnant and parenting students (Horowitz et al., 1991; Polit, 1989; Seitz & Apfel, 1993; Warrick et al., 1993).

Problems with Program Evaluation

The literature is replete with criticisms of existing attempts at program evaluation. Early on there was less public concern for the demonstrated effectiveness of interventions; it sufficed that interventions were available. In a context where resources are restricted, funding organizations are increasingly interested in knowing whether their investment pays off. Thus, the field of program evaluation has grown and standards for evaluations have risen (Peterson, Card, Eisen, & Sherman-Williams, 1994). Scholars (White & White, 1991) noted that evaluation must determine the enduring changes in behavior (e.g., sexual activity, repeat pregnancy) that result from program participation, and that studies with longitudinal designs are needed. Others argue that many evaluations have design flaws and are limited by sample self-selection, the lack of longitudinal follow-up, and absent or inadequate comparison groups (Ruch-Ross et al., 1992).

As a result, Peterson and associates (1994) offered guidelines for program evaluation specific to the assessment of teenage pregnancy prevention/intervention programs. Others have encouraged the use of national data sets as comparison groups when programs are unable to collect data simultaneously from a group of nonparticipants (Ruch-Ross et al., 1992). Still others suggest that outcome measures must include changes in behavior rather than simply assessing changes in attitude or participant satisfaction (Roosa & Christopher, 1990).

How Can We Prevent the Negative Effects of Teenage Pregnancy?

White and White (1991) argued that the field of study lacks adequate knowledge about the factors that contribute to early sexual activity. The literature is replete with correlational studies and those using univariate analyses that fail to address the complex nature of the etiology of adolescent sexual behavior. Few studies have included multiple factors or the examination of how such factors affect outcomes over time. This means that large data sources are necessary for future studies, and studies must include a longitudinal focus. Moreover, when programs are designed, what is known from the empirical literature is often ignored. For example, Roosa and Christopher (1990) criticized short-term prevention programs whose goal it is to enhance self-esteem, because research shows that the relationship between sexual behavior and self-esteem is a complex one. They also showed that many such programs dedicate little time to discussing self-esteem. Under these conditions, assessing changes in self-esteem is inappropriate.

Some scholars have begun to look more closely at some of these issues. Investigators show that the causes of teenage pregnancy are more complex than we acknowledged—a complexity that is further ignored by most of our interventions. For example, research examining the backgrounds of 500 teen mothers indicated that two thirds of them had histories of sexual and physical abuse primarily by adult men about 27 years of age (Boyer & Fine, 1992). Applying these findings to program design suggests that programs may fail because they are not prepared to address such traumatic personal histories. Whereas many intervention programs provide crisis counseling, most programs fail to include longer-term personal and/or family therapy (Warrick et al., 1993). As a result, desired outcomes of program participation may be limited because the programs do not address the traumatic pasts of the participants.

Another interesting finding focuses on the relationship between teen pregnancy and poverty. Using lagged correlations, Males (1993) found that teen parenting did not cause poverty, but poverty seemed to precede high rates of teen childbearing. In fact, "Since 1980, as youth poverty rose and prevention efforts proliferated, birth rates have risen" (Males, 1993, p. 431). This suggests that interventions that ignore broader contextual issues around poverty are less likely to be effective in the long run. Recent policy recommendation to cut AFDC benefits to single mothers (many of whom are teenage parents) will "only increase the deprivation of millions of children and parents and further erode the central income-support function" of such programs (Plotnick, 1993, p. 327).

Other scholars have offered suggestions for improving the quality of our knowledge in this area. For example, some have advocated for a life-course perspective in addressing issues related to adolescent pregnancy and parenthood (Chase-Landsdale, Brooks-Gunn, & Paikoff, 1991). As such, evaluations must include ongoing data collection over the course of a teen parent's life, if we are to understand and address long-term outcomes. Only a few studies have done so (see, for example, Furstenberg et al., 1987). Another recommendation that we advocated earlier is to carefully examine within-group variations. Because researchers often treat all program participants as if they were a homogeneous group, studies have not examined whether certain interventions are more effective with certain groups. (The work of Warrick and associates is a notable exception.)

CONCLUSIONS

Over time we have accumulated a good deal of useful information on adolescent pregnancy and its consequences. The source for much of this information has been data from large, nationally representative samples. However, the knowledge stemming from these studies is primarily descriptive in nature and based on correlational analyses that provide causal hints but not definitive proof. Many of these studies stem from a problem-oriented paradigm where singular cause–effect models prevail. The typical problem-oriented focus uses between-group comparisons that assume homogeneity within groups (i.e., all pregnant teens have the same experiences). From this paradigm, differences are due to some pathology or deficiency in the nonnormative group such as those who bear children prematurely. Thus, the problem-oriented paradigm means that differences would be interpreted as maladaptive.

More recent studies reflect a normative–adaptive paradigm. From this perspective, researchers attempt to describe and understand the processes and mechanisms that place children at risk for problem behaviors (e.g., becoming adolescent parents) without a priori assumptions that these processes and mechanisms are maladaptive or problematic. The normative–adaptive paradigm emphasizes the mechanisms that predispose children both to vulnerability and resilience (Rutter, 1990) and assumes that these mechanisms involve more complex relationships than singular cause–effect models. This newer paradigm considers the broader context in which problem behaviors occur. Here, no assumption is made that the context itself is problematic or pathological. Instead, in this approach, heterogeneity is assumed, transactional models are included that test the reciprocal nature of relationships between variables, and within-group comparisons become a primary analytic strategy.

In this review, more recent studies reflect the normative–adaptive paradigm. The study by Males (1993) is one example where the reciprocal influence of poverty on adolescent parenthood was noted. Other studies have focused on describing and gaining insight into other key areas (e.g., differential stress in pregnant and parenting adolescents). As such, these studies and others met some of the assumptions forwarded by this paradigm. For example, studies have attempted to understand individual variations in response to different degrees of risk by gaining accurate knowledge of risk mechanisms, not just risk indicators. Also, the results of the few longitudinal studies noted here explored the dynamic nature of risk factors (e.g., as circumstances change, the risk alters and the outcomes may differ) and mechanisms that buffer or protect the adolescent from certain negative outcomes. Consider the research on social support that suggests that what is supportive at one period may not be supportive later. Clearly, this paradigm assumes variation by individual, situation, and contextual factors. Future research that continues to tease out these variations is essential, if interventions are to effectively meet the needs of the population of pregnant and parenting adolescents.

Jorgensen (1991) summarized the state of research in this area when he noted that "the solution to the adolescent pregnancy 'puzzle' is far more complex than it once was thought to be, as many formidable barriers continue to inhibit our ability to identify effective pregnancy-prevention interventions" (p. 374). Increased sensitivity to larger contextual issues that affect stress associated with adolescent pregnancy and its consequences is apparent in the literature. Given the diversity of the circumstances of teenage mothers, the key of future research efforts is to determine what conditions increase a particular teen's vulnerability to stress and to design programs based on the empirical findings.

REFERENCES

ABC/Washington Post. (1982). *Roper Center Poll.* Storrs, CT: University of Connecticut.

Allen Guttmacher Institute. (1994). *Facts in brief: Teenage reproductive health in the United States.* New York: Author.

Abrahamse, A. F., Morrison, P. A., & Waite, L. J. (1988). Teenagers willing to consider single-parenthood: Who is at greater risk. *Family Planning Perspectives, 20,* 13–18.

Adams, G., Adams-Taylor, S., & Pittman, K. (1989). Adolescent pregnancy and parenthood: A review of the problems, solutions, and resources. *Family Relations, 38,* 228–229.

Aquilino, W. S. (1996). The lifecourse of children born to unmarried mothers: Childhood living arrangements and young adult outcomes. *Journal of Marriage and the Family, 58,* 293–310.

Astone, N. M. (1993). Are adolescent mother just single mothers? *Journal of Adolescent Research, 3,* 353–371.

Auvenshine, M. A., & Enriquez, M. G. (1985). *Maternity nursing.* Belmont, CA: Wadsworth.

Bachrach, C. A., & Carver, K. (1992). *Outcomes of early childbearing: An appraisal of recent evidence.* Summary of a conference convened by NICHD, May 18–19, 1992, Bethesda, MD.

Bachrach, C. A., London, K. A., & Stolley, K. S. (1992). Relinquishment of premarital births: Evidence from national survey data. *Family Planning Perspectives, 24,* 27–32.

Bane, M. J., & Elwood, D. T. (1986). Slipping into and out of poverty: The dynamics of spells. *Journal of Human Resources, 21,* 1–23.

Barrera, M. J. (1981). Social support in the adjustment of pregnant adolescents: Assessment issues. In B. H. Gottlieb (Ed.), *Social networks and social support* (pp. 69–96). Beverly Hills, CA: Sage.

Barth, R. R., & Schinke, S. P. (1983). Coping with daily strain among pregnant and parent adolescents. *Journal of Social Service Research, 7,* 51–63.

Barth, R. R., Schinke, S. P., & Maxwell, J. S. (1983). Coping strategies of counselors and school age mothers. *Journal of Counseling Psychology, 30,* 346–354.

Belsky, J. (1984). The determinants of parenting: A process model. *Child Development, 55,* 83–96.

Bolton, F. G., Jr. (1980). *The pregnant adolescent: Problems of premature parenthood.* Beverly Hills, CA: Sage.

Boss, P. (1977). A clarification of the concept of psychological father presence in families experiencing ambiguity of boundary. *Journal of Marriage and the Family, 39,* 141–151.

Boss, P. (1988). *Family stress management.* Newbury Park, CA: Sage.

Boukydis, C. F. (1987). *Research on support for parents and infants in the postnatal period.* Norwood, NJ: Ablex.

Boyer, D., & Fine, D. (1992). Sexual abuse as a factor in adolescent pregnancy and child maltreatment. *Family Planning Perspectives, 24,* 4–11, 19.

Bumpass, L. L., & Raley, R. K. (1995). Redefining single-parent families: Cohabitation and changing family reality. *Demography, 32,* 97–109.

Burt, M. R. (1986). Estimating the public cost of teenage childbearing. *Family Planning Perspectives, 18,* 211–226.

CBS News (1994, February 7–11). *Eye on America.*

Caldas, S. J. (1993). Current theoretical perspectives on adolescent pregnancy and childbearing in the United States. *Journal of Adolescent Research, 8,* 4–20.

Centers for Disease Control. (1992). Sexual behavior among high school students. *Morbidity and Mortality Weekly Report, 40,* 885–888.

Chase-Landsdale, P. L., Brooks-Gunn, J., & Paikoff, R. L. (1991). Research and programs for adolescent mothers: Missing links and future promises. *Family Relations, 40,* 396–403.

Colega, S. A. (1988). *Coping behavior of teen mothers: An exploratory study and comparison of Mexican Americans and Anglos.* Unpublished master's thesis, Colorado State University, Ft. Collins.

Cohen, S., & McKay, G. (1984). Social support, stress, and the buffering hypothesis: A theoretical analysis. In A. Baum, S. E. Taylor, & J. E. Singer (Eds.), *Handbook of psychology and health* (Vol. 4, pp. 253–267). Hillsdale, NJ: Erlbaum.

Colletta, N. D. (1981). Social support and the risk of maternal rejection by adolescent mothers. *Journal of Psychology, 109,* 191–197.

Colletta, N. D., & Lee, D. (1983). The impact of support for black adolescent mothers. *Journal of Family Issues, 4,* 127–143.

Committee on Ways and Means. (1989). US House of Representatives. *Background material and data on programs within the jurisdiction of the Committee on Ways and Means.* Washington, DC: Government Printing Office.

Compas, B. E. (1987). Stress and life events during childhood and adolescence. *Clinical Psychology Review, 7,* 275–302.

Coombs-Orme, T. (1993). Health effects of adolescent pregnancy: Implications for social workers. *Families and Society, 74,* 344–354.

Cowan, P. A., & Hetherington, E. M. (Eds.). (1991). *Family transitions*. Hillsdale, NJ: Erlbaum.

Crawford, G. (1984). Critique of social support of teenage mothers. In K. Bernard, P. Brandt, B. Raff, & P. Carroll (Eds.), *Social support and families of vulnerable infants* (pp. 272–279). White Plains, NY: March of Dimes Birth Defect Foundation.

Crnic, K. A., Greenberg, M. T., Ragozin, A. S., Robinson, N. M., & Basham, R. B. (1983). Effects of stress and social support on mothers and premature and full-term infants. *Child Development, 54*, 209–217.

Crockenberg, S. B. (1987). Predictors and correlates of anger toward and punitive control of toddlers by adolescent mothers. *Child Development, 58*, 964–975.

Crockenberg, S. (1988). Social support and parenting. In H. E. Fitzgerald, B. M. Lefter, & M. D. Yogman (Eds.), *Theory and research in behavioral pediatrics* (Vol. 4, pp. 141–174). New York: Plenum Press.

Danziger, S. K., & Radin, N. (1990). Absent does not equal uninvolved: Predictors of fathering in teen mother families. *Journal of Marriage and the Family, 52*, 636–642.

deAnda, D., Darroch, P., Davidson, M., Gilly, J., Javidi, M., Jefford, S., Komorowski, R., & Morejon-Schrobsdorf, M. (1992). Stress and coping among pregnant adolescents. *Journal of Adolescent Research, 7*, 94–109.

Dearden, K., Hale, C., & Alvarez, J. (1992). The educational antecedents of teen fatherhood. *British Journal of Educational Psychology, 62*, 139–147.

Department of Health and Human Services. (1988). *Adolescent family life demonstration projects*. Washington, DC: US Public Health Service.

Duncan, G., & Hoffman, S. (1990). Teenage welfare receipt and subsequent dependence among black adolescent mothers. *Family Planning Perspectives, 22*, 16–20.

Eggebeen, D. J., Crockett, L. J., & Hawkins, A. J. (1990). Patterns of adult male coresidence among young children of adolescent mothers. *Family Planning Perspectives, 22*, 219–223.

Elster, A. R. (1991). Fathers, teenage. In R. M. Learner, A. C. Petersen, & J. Brooks-Gunn (Eds.), *Encyclopedia of adolescence* (pp. 360–364). New York: Garland.

Feiring, C., Fox, N. A., Jaskir, J., & Lewis, M. (1987). The relation between social support, infant risk status, and mother–infant interaction. *Developmental Psychology, 23*, 400–405.

Field, T. M. (1980). Interactions of preterm and term infants with their lower- and middle-class teenage and adult mothers. In T. Field, S. Goldberg, D. Stern, & A. Sostek (Eds.), *High-risk infants and children* (pp. 113–132). New York: Academic.

Forste, R., & Tienda, M. (1992). Race and ethnic variation in the schooling consequences of female adolescent sexual activity. *Social Science Quarterly, 73*, 12–30.

Freeman, E. W., & Rickles, K. (1993). *Early childbearing: Perspectives on pregnancy, abortion, and contraception*. Newbury Park, CA: Sage.

Furstenberg, F. F., Jr. (1991). As the pendulum swings: Teenage childbearing and social concern. *Family Relations, 40*, 127–138.

Furstenberg, F. F., Jr. (1992). Teenage childbearing and cultural rationality: A thesis is search of evidence. *Family Relations, 41*, 239–243.

Furstenberg, F. F., Jr. (1994, August). *Fathering in the inner city: Parental participation and public policy*. Unpublished manuscript.

Furstenberg, F. F., Jr., Brooks-Gunn, J., & Chase-Landsdale, L. (1989). Teenaged pregnancy and childbearing. *American Psychologist, 44*, 452–469.

Furstenberg, F. F., Jr., Brooks-Gunn, J., & Morgan, S. P. (1987). Adolescent mothers and their children in later life. *Family Planning Perspectives, 19*, 142–151.

Furstenberg, F. F., Jr., & Chase-Landsdale, P. L. (1989). Teenage pregnancy and childbearing. *American Psychologist, 44*, 313–320.

Furstenberg, F. F., Jr., & Harris, K. M. (1993). When and why fathers matter: Impacts of father involvement on the children of adolescent mothers. In R. I. Lerman & T. J. Ooms (Eds.), *Young unwed fathers: Changing roles and emerging policies* (pp. 117–138). Philadelphia, PA: Temple University Press.

Gabriel, A., & McAnarney, E. R. (1983). Parenthood in two subcultures. *Adolescence, 18*, 579–966.

Garfinkel, I., & McLanahan, S. S. (1986). *Single mothers and their children: A new American dilemma*. Washington, DC: Urban Institute Press.

Geronimus, A. T. (1991). Teenage childbearing and social reproductive disadvantage: The evolution of complex questions and the demise of simple answers. *Family Relations, 40*, 463–471.

Geronimus, A. T., & Korenman, S. (1991, November). *Maternal youth or poverty? Health disadvantage of infants with teenage mothers.* Paper presented at the annual meeting of the American Public Health Association, Atlanta, GA.

Gottlieb, B. H. (1978). The development and application of a classification scheme of informal helping behaviors. *Canadian Journal of Behavioral Science, 10,* 105–115.

Granger, R. D. (1983). *Effects of early intervention, social supports, and concepts of development on stress experienced by mothers of handicapped children.* Unpublished master's thesis, Graduate College of the University of Illinois at Chicago Circle.

Hall, G. S. (1904). *Adolescence* (Vol. 2). Englewood Cliffs, NJ: Prentice-Hall.

Halsey, C. L., Collins, M. F., & Anderson, C. L. (1993). Extremely low birth weight children and their peers: A comparison of preschool performance. *Pediatrics, 91,* 807–811.

Hamburg, B. A., & Dixon, S. L. (1992). Adolescent pregnancy and parenthood. In M. K. Rosenheim & M. F. Testa (Eds.), *Early parenthood and coming of age in the 1990s* (pp. 17–32). New Jersey: Rutgers University Press.

Harris, K. M. (1991). Teenage mothers and welfare dependency: Working off welfare. *Journal of Family Issues, 12,* 492–518.

Hayes, C. (Ed.). (1987). *Risking the future: Adolescent sexuality, pregnancy and childbearing* (Vol. 1). Washington, DC: National Academy Press.

Heller, K., Swindle, R. W., & Dusenburg, L. (1986). Components of social support processes. *Journal of Consulting and Clinical Psychology, 54,* 466–470.

Hendricks, L. E. (1988). Outreach with teenage fathers: A preliminary report on three ethnic groups. *Adolescence, 23,* 711–720.

Henshaw, S. K. (1993). Teenage abortion, birth and pregnancy statistics by state, 1988. *Family Planning Perspectives, 25,* 122–126.

Hill, M. (1990, May). *Shared housing as a form of economic support for young unmarried mothers.* Paper presented at the annual Population Association of American Meetings, Toronto, Canada.

Hofferth, S. (1984). Kin networks, race, and family structure. *Journal of Marriage and the Family, 46,* 791–806.

Hofferth, S. (1987). Social and economic consequences of teenage childbearing. In S. L. Hofferth & C. D. Hayes (Eds.) *Risking the future* (Vol. 2, pp. 123–144). Washington, DC: National Academy Press.

Hollander, D. (1995). Studies suggest inherent risk of poor pregnancy outcomes for teenagers. *Family Planning Perspectives, 27*(6), 262–268.

Holmes, S. A. (1996, June 13). '96 cost of teen pregnancy is put at $7 billion. *The New York Times,* pp. A11, A19.

Horowitz, S. M., Klerman, L. V., Kuo, H. S., & Jekel, J. F. (1991). School-age mothers: Predictors of long term educational and economic outcomes. *Pediatrics, 87,* 862–868.

Johnson, J. H. (1986). *Life events as stressors in childhood and adolescence.* Beverly Hills, CA: Sage.

Jorgensen, S. R. (1991). Project Taking Charge: An evaluation of an adolescent pregnancy prevention program. *Family Relations, 40,* 373–380.

Jorgensen, S. R., Potts, V., & Camp, B. (1993). Project Taking Charge: Six-month follow-up of a pregnancy prevention program for early adolescents. *Family Relations, 42,* 401–406.

Kahan, J. R., & Anderson, K. E. (1992). Intergenerational patterns of teen fertility. *Demography, 29,* 39.

Kerkhoff, A. C., & Parrow, A. A. (1979). The effect of early marriage on the educational attainment of young men. *Journal of Marriage and Family Therapy, 41,* 97–107.

Ketterlinus, R. D., Lamb, M. E., & Nitz, K. (1991). Developmental and ecological sources of stress among adolescent parents. *Family Relations, 40,* 435–441.

Krein, S., & Beller, A. (1988). Educational attainment of children from single-parent families: Differences by exposure, gender, and race. *Demography, 25,* 221–234.

Ladner, J. (1987). Black teenage pregnancy: A challenge for educators. *Journal of Negro Education, 56,* 53–63.

Langfield, P. A. (1992). *Predictors of pregnant and parenting adolescent educational attainment: A test of the Double ABCX Model.* Unpublished master's thesis, Colorado State University.

Lawrence, R. A., & Merritt, T. A. (1983). Infants of adolescent mothers: Perinatal, neonatal, and infancy outcomes. In E. R. Anarney (Ed.), *Premature adolescent pregnancy and parenthood* (pp. 149–168). New York: Grune and Stratton.

Leland, N. L., Petersen, D. J., Braddock, M., & Alexander, G. R. (1995). Variations in pregnancy outcomes by race among 10–14-year-old mothers in the United States. *Public Health Reports, 110*(1), 53–59.

Lowe, G. D., & Witt, D. D. (1984). Early marriage as a career contingency: The prediction of educational attainment. *Journal of Marriage and Family Therapy, 46*, 689–698.

Males, M. (1993). School-age pregnancy: Why hasn't prevention worked? *Journal of School Health, 63*, 429–432.

Marsiglio, W. S. (1989). Adolescent males' pregnancy resolution preferences and family formation intentions: Does family background make a difference for blacks and whites? *Journal of Adolescent Research, 4*, 214–237.

Marsiglio, W. S. (1991). Men's procreative consciousness and responsibility: A conceptual analysis and research agenda. *Journal of Family Issues, 12*, 323–342.

Marsiglio, W. S. (1995). Young nonresident biological fathers. *Marriage and Family Review, 20*, 325–348.

McAdoo, H. P. (1988). *Black families* (2nd ed.). Newbury Park, CA: Sage.

McAnarney, E. R., & Hendee, W. R. (1989). Adolescent pregnancy and its consequences. *Journal of the American Medical Association, 262*, 74–77.

McCubbin, H. I., & Patterson, J. M. (1981, October). *Family stress and adaptation to crisis: A double ABCX model of family behavior.* Paper presented at the annual meeting of the National Council on Family Relations, Milwaukee, WI.

McLanahan, S. S. (1983). Family structure and stress: A longitudinal comparison of two-parent and female-headed families. *Journal of Marriage and the Family, 45*, 347–357.

Miller, B. C. (1992). Adolescent parenthood, economic issues, and social policies. *Journal of Family and Economic Issues, 13*, 467–475.

Miller, B. C., & Moore, K. A. (1990). Adolescent sexual behavior, pregnancy, and parenting: Research through the 1980s. *Journal of Marriage and the Family, 52*, 1025–1044.

Miller, B. C., Norton, M. C., Jenson, G. O., Lee, T. R., Christopherson, G., & Kling, P. K. (1993). Impact of facts & feelings: A home-based video sex education curriculum. *Family Relations, 42*, 392–400.

Moore, K. A. (1992). *Facts at a glance.* Washington, DC: Child Trends.

Moore, K. A., Myers, D. E., Morrison, D. R., Nord, C. W., Brown, B., & Edmonston, B. (1993). Age at first childbirth and later poverty. *Journal of Adolescent Research, 3*, 393–422.

Moore, K. A., Snyder, N. A., & Daly, M. (1992). *Facts at a glance.* Washington, DC: Child Trends.

Mott, F. L., & Marsiglio, W. (1985). Early childbearing and completion of high school. *Family Planning Perspectives, 17*, 234–237.

Nath, P. S., Borkowski, J. G., Whitman, T. L., & Schellenbach, C. J. (1991). Understanding adolescent parenting: The dimensions and functions of social support. *Family Relations, 40*, 411–420.

National Center for Health Statistics. (1991). Advance report of final natality statistics, 1989. *Monthly Vital Statistics Report, 40*(8), Supplement.

National Center for Health Statistics. (1993). Advance report of final natality statistics, 1991. *Monthly Vital Statistics Report, 42*(3), Supplement.

Neville, B., & Parke, R. D. (1991). Fathers, adolescents. In R. M. Lerner, A. C. Petersen, & J. Brooks-Gunn (Eds.), *Encyclopedia of adolescence* (pp. 354–359). New York: Garland.

Olds, D., Henderson, C. R., Chamberlain, R., & Tatelbaum, R. (1986). Preventing child abuse and neglect: A randomized trial of nurse home visitation. *Pediatrics, 78*, 65–78.

Olds, D., Henderson, C. R., Kitzman, H., & Cole, R. (1995). Effects of prenatal and infancy nurse home visitation on surveillance of child maltreatment. *Pediatrics, 95*, 365–372.

Olson, D. H., McCubbin, H. I., Barnes, H., Larson, A., Muxen, M., & Wilson, M. (1983). *Families: What makes them work?* Beverly Hills, CA: Sage.

Pasley, K. (1995). Teenage parenting. In D. Levinson (Ed.), *Encyclopedia of sociology* (pp. 721–723). New York: Plenum Press.

Pasley, K., & Kreutzer, J. (1989). *Assessing the impact of child care centers on reducing the dropout rate of teen parents enrolled in Colorado's vocational education programs: Final report.* Colorado Community College and Occupational Education System, State Department of Education.

Pasley, K., Langfield, P. A., & Kreutzer, J. A. (1993). Predictors of stress in adolescents: An exploratory study of pregnant and parenting females. *Journal of Adolescent Research, 8*, 326–347.

Pasley, K., & Minton, C. (1997). Generative fathering after divorce and remarriage: Beyond the disappearing dad. In A. J. Hawkins & D. C. Dollahite (Eds.), *Generative fathering: Beyond deficit perspectives* (pp. 118–133). Newbury Park, CA: Sage.

Passell, P. (1996, June 20). Teen-age childbearing: The cost is put at $8.9 billion a year. *The New York Times*, pp. C2, D2.

Passino, A. W., Whitman, T. L., Borkowski, J. G., Schellenback, C. J., Maxwell, S. E., Keogh, D., & Rellinger, E. (1993). Personal adjustment during pregnancy and adolescent parenting. *Adolescence, 28*, 97–122.

Peterson, J. L., Card, J. J., Eisen, M. B., & Sherman-Williams, B. (1994). Evaluating teenage pregnancy prevention and other social programs: Ten stages of program assessment. *Family Planning Perspectives, 26*, 116–121.

Plotnick, R. D. (1993). The effect of social policies on teenage pregnancy and childbearing. *Families in Society, 74*, 324–328.

Polit, D. F. (1989). Effects of a comprehensive program for teenage parents: Five years after Project Redirection. *Family Planning Perspectives, 21*, 164–187.

Roper, W. L. (1993). Kids, health, and the media: What can public health offer? *Journal of School Health, 63*, 273–275.

Roosa, M. W., & Christopher, F. S. (1990). Evaluation of an abstinence-only adolescent pregnancy prevention program: A replication. *Family Relations, 39*, 363–367.

Roosa, M. W., Fitzgerald, H. E., & Carson, N. A. (1982). Teenage parenting and child development: A literature review. *Infant Mental Health Journal, 3*, 4–18.

Ruch-Ross, H. S., Jones, E. D., & Musick, J. S. (1992). Comparing outcomes in a statewide program for adolescent mothers with outcome since a national sample. *Family Planning Perspectives, 24*, 66–71, 96.

Rutter, M. (1990). Psychosocial resilience and protective mechanisms. In J. Rolf, A. S. Masten, D. Cicchetti, K. H. Nuechterlein, & S. Weintraub (Eds.), *Risk and protective factors in the development of psychopathology* (pp. 181–214). Cambridge, MA: Cambridge University Press.

Sandler, I. N., & Lakey, B. (1982). Locus of control as a stress moderator. The role of control perceptions and social support. *American Journal of Community Psychology, 10*, 65–80.

Sandven, K., & Resnick, M. D. (1990). Informal adoption among black adolescent mothers. *American Journal of Orthopsychiatry, 60*, 210–224.

Sarason, I. G., & Sarason, B. R. (1984). Life changes, moderators of stress, and health. In A. Baum, S. E. Taylor, & J. E. Singer (Eds.), *Handbook of psychology and health* (Vol. 4, pp. 279–299). Hillsdale, NJ: Erlbaum.

Seitz, V., & Apfel, N. H. (1993). Adolescent mothers and repeated childbearing. Effects of a school-based intervention program. *American Journal of Orthopsychiatry, 63*, 572–581.

Senderowitz, J., & Paxman, J. (1985). Adolescent fertility: Worldwide concerns. *Population Bulletin, 40*(2), (Population Reference Bureau).

Spencer, C. M. (1985). *Children of teenage parents: A review of the literature*. (Report No. PSO 15300). Springfield, IL: State Board of education, Dept. of Planning, Research, and Evaluation. (ERIC Document reproduction service No. ED 260 830).

Stack, C. B. (1974). *All our kin, strategies for survival in a black community*. New York: Harper & Row.

Stahler, G. J., & DuCette, J. P. (1991). Evaluating adolescent pregnancy programs: Rethinking our priorities. *Family Planning Perspectives, 23*, 129–133.

Stern, M., & Alvarez, A. (1992). Pregnant and parenting adolescents: A comparative analysis of coping response and psychological adjustment. *Journal of Adolescent Research, 5*, 54–66.

Stiffman, A. R., Powell, J., Earls, F., & Robins, L. N. (1990). Pregnancies, childrearing, and mental health problems in adolescents. *Youth and Society, 21*, 483–495.

Stockdale, D. F., Crase, S. J., & Petersen, K. R. (1990, November). *Social support for pregnant or parenting and nonpregnant and nonparenting adolescents*. Paper presented at the annual meeting of the National Council on Family Relations, Seattle, WA.

Sweet, J. A., & Bumpass, L. L. (1987). *American families and households*. New York: Russell Sage.

Swenson, I., Erickson, E., Ehlinger, E., Carlson, G., & Swaney, S. (1989). Fertility, menstrual characteristics, and contraceptive practices among white, black and SE Asian refugee adolescents. *Adolescence, 24*, 647–654.

Testa, M. F. (1992). Racial and ethnic variation in the early life course of adolescent welfare mothers. In M. K. Rosenhiem & M. F. Testa (Eds.), *Early parenthood and coming of age in the 1990s* (pp. 89–112). New Brunswick, NJ: Rutgers University Press.

Teti, D. M., & Lamb, M. E. (1989). Socioeconomic and marital outcomes of adolescent marriage, adolescent childbirth and their co-occurrence. *Journal of Marriage and the Family, 51,* 203–212.

Thornton, A., & Rogers, W. (1987). The influence of individual and historical time on marital dissolution. *Demography, 24,* 1–22.

Trent, K., & Harlan, S. L. (1990). Household structure among teenage mothers in the United States. *Social Science Quarterly, 71,* 439–457.

Trent, K., & Harlan, S. L. (1994). Teenage mothers in nuclear and extended households: Differences by marital status and race/ethnicity. *Journal of Family Issues, 15,* 309–337.

Unger, D. G. (1985). *The relationship of specific social and psychological coping resources with the adjustment of adolescent primiparas.* Unpublished doctoral dissertation, University of South Carolina, Columbia.

Upchurch, D. M., & McCarthy, J. (1990). The timing of first birth and high school completion. *American Sociological Review, 49,* 491–493.

US Bureau of the Census. (1993). *Statistical abstract of the United States* (113th Ed.). Washington DC: US Government Printing Office.

Vukelich, C., & Kliman, D. S. (1985). Mature and teenage mothers' infant growth expectations and use of child development information sources. *Family Relations, 34,* 189–196.

Warrick, L., Christianson, M. B., Walruff, J., & Cook, P. C. (1993). Educational outcomes in teenage pregnancy and parenting programs; Results from a demonstration. *Family Planning Perspectives, 25,* 148–155.

Wasserman, G., Brunelli, S., & Rauh, V. (1990). Social support and living arrangements of adolescent and adult mothers. *Journal of Adolescent Research, 5,* 54–65.

Watson, M. F., & Protinsky, H. (1991). Identity stability of black adolescents. *Adolescence, 26,* 963–966.

Whitman, T. L., Borkowski, J. G., Schellenbach, C. J., & Nath, P. S. (1987). Predicting and understanding developmental delay of children of adolescent mothers: A multi-dimensional approach. *American Journal of Mental Deficiency, 92,* 40–56.

White, C. P., & White, M. B. (1991). The Adolescent Family Life Act: Content, findings, and policy recommendations for pregnancy prevention programs. *Journal of Clinical Child Psychology, 20,* 58–70.

Wolf, A. M. (1983). A personal view of black inner-city foster families. *American Journal of Orthopsychiatry, 53,* 144–151.

III

Physical and Environmental Stressors

10

Children's Coping with Chronic Illness

WENDY KLIEWER

This chapter considers the impacts of chronic physical illness on children and adolescents. As with many of the stressors discussed in this volume, chronic illness is heterogeneous in nature. Chronic illnesses vary in their age of onset, age at diagnosis, the functional impairment involved, prognosis of the disease, treatment demands and regimen, visibility, amount of pain involved, cyclic or constant nature of the symptoms, and predictability and pain of symptoms. This chapter focuses on the most prevalent chronic diseases experienced by children and adolescents, as well as diseases that are less common but present significant coping challenges. Physical disabilities are excluded.

This chapter begins by describing the extent of chronic illness in children and adolescents, then discusses the psychological impact of having a chronic condition. Models of children's adaptation to chronic illness are reviewed next, followed by a discussion of adaptive tasks and developmental issues faced by children with chronic physical conditions. A summary of interventions to facilitate adjustment and suggestions for future directions close out the chapter.

SCOPE OF THE PROBLEM

Chronic illnesses and conditions (including physical disabilities) affect approximately 19% of children less than 18 years of age, or 12 million children nationwide, according to the most recent epidemiological estimates (Newacheck & Stoddard, 1994; Newacheck & Taylor, 1992). Approximately one fourth of all affected children have multiple chronic conditions. Among all

WENDY KLIEWER • Department of Psychology, Virginia Commonwealth University, Richmond, Virginia 23284.
Handbook of Children's Coping: Linking Theory and Intervention, edited by Wolchik and Sandler. Plenum Press, New York, 1997.

Table 1. Estimated Prevalence of Chronic Diseases and
Conditions in Children, Ages 0–20, in the United States

Disorder	Prevalence estimates per 1000
Arthritis	2.20
Asthma	38.00
Moderate to severe	10.00
Chronic renal failure	0.08
Terminal	0.01
Nonterminal	0.07
Cystic fibrosis	0.20
Diabetes mellitus	1.80
Hemophilia	0.15
Acute lymphocytic leukemia	0.11
Phenylketonuria	0.10
Sickle-cell disease	0.46
Sickle-cell anemia	0.28
Spina bifida	0.40

children with chronic conditions, approximately three fourths are mildly to moderately affected. That is, most children report being bothered "not at all," "very little," or "some" by their conditions and have minimal limitations to their usual activities (Newacheck & Taylor, 1992).

Table 1 presents the most common chronic illnesses and their prevalence estimates. Asthma is by far the most common chronic illness, and chronic renal failure the most rare. With regard to demographic differences in prevalence rates, juvenile rheumatoid arthritis is about twice as common in females relative to males, while asthma and leukemia are more common in males. Of course, hemophilia affects males exclusively. Cystic fibrosis, diabetes mellitus, and leukemia are more common among Caucasians relative to other ethnic groups, while sickle cell disease primarily afflicts African Americans, and pediatric acquired immunodeficiency syndrome (AIDS) is more common among minority children (Garrison & McQuiston, 1989).

In addition to variation in their prevalence, chronic illnesses differ in their prognosis. Estimated proportions of children surviving to age 20 range from 25% for children with chronic renal failure to 98% for children with moderate to severe asthma (Gortmaker & Sappenfield, 1984). Spina bifida and acute lymphocytic leukemia have survival rates in the 40–50% range. Recent medical advances have greatly improved the prognoses for children with cancer and cystic fibrosis in particular (American Cancer Society, 1995). Because children with chronic illnesses are surviving longer than in the past, health professionals have shifted their attention away from a singular focus on mortality to consider the range of psychosocial effects of chronic illnesses (Eiser, 1994).

PSYCHOSOCIAL IMPACT OF CHRONIC ILLNESS

Historically, it was commonly believed that most children with chronic illnesses developed some form of psychological disorder. Much of the early work in this area was flawed methodologically, however, suffering from poor instrumentation, definitional inconsistency, and inappropriate (or no) control groups. Recent research has challenged the assumption that the majority of chronically ill children also suffer psychosocial deficits (Eiser, 1990; Garrison & McQuiston, 1989). In general, health professionals and behavioral scientists recognize the vast individual differences that exist in response to chronic illness. Some children with chronic illnesses are well-liked by their peers, excel in school, and appear free from anxiety and depression. Other children are immature for their age, socially awkward, and anxious or depressed. Despite individual variation, however, children with a chronic illness, relative to healthy controls, are about two to four times as likely to have a psychiatric diagnosis some time during their childhood or adolescence (Drotar & Bush, 1985; Eiser, 1990; Garrison & McQuiston, 1989; Lavigne & Faier-Routman, 1992).

Both population-based studies and studies of specific disease groups have addressed the psychosocial costs of chronic illness during childhood. In general, the findings from studies of specific disease groups have been equivocal. Studies comparing children with asthma to controls have reported greater depression in young (3–6 years old) asthmatics (Mrazek, Anderson, & Strunk, 1985) relative to controls, but no differences in self-concept or psychiatric diagnosis in older (7–12 years old) children with asthma (Kashani, Koenig, Shepperd, Wilfley, & Morris, 1988). Parents of children with asthma were more likely to report psychiatric symptoms in their children, relative to control parents (Kashani et al., 1988). A review of the school performance of children with asthma (Celano & Geller, 1993) indicates that children with severe asthma do not differ significantly in their school performance from children without asthma, despite their greater absenteeism. When performance deficits do occur, they may be due to iatrogenic effects of corticosteroid treatment.

Methodologically sound studies of children with cystic fibrosis (Breslau, 1985; Thompson, Hodges, & Hamlett, 1990) have found that children with cystic fibrosis do not demonstrate more adjustment problems overall than non-referred control children, though some differences exist on specific indices of adjustment. Breslau compared children with cystic fibrosis, cerebral palsy, myelodysplasia, multiple physical handicaps, and controls on mother-rated symptoms, and Thompson et al. compared children with cystic fibrosis to psychiatrically referred and nonreferred children on mother-rated symptoms. Of the 18 adjustment indices assessed in the Thompson et al. study, children with cystic fibrosis scored higher than nonreferred controls on four measures: worries, self-image, separation anxiety, and overanxious disorder.

Research with children who have sickle-cell disease has similarly found few differences between these children and appropriate control groups on measures of psychological adjustment (Lemanek, Moore, Gresham, Williamson, & Kelley, 1986) or peer relations (Noll, Ris, Davies, Bukowski, & Koontz, 1992). Lemanek et al. compared 30 children ages 6–16 with sickle-cell disease to 30 healthy controls who attended a family medical clinic for routine care and to established norms. Data were collected from children, parents, and physicians. Lemanek et al. found no significant differences between the two groups of children on self-concept; depression; home, school, or peer adjustment; or on a measure of parental discipline methods. However, when compared to a normative sample with a higher-socioeconomic level, children with sickle-cell disease demonstrated more behavior problems. One area where children with sickle-cell disease do appear to be at risk is learning problems, due to both cerebral vascular accidents and iatrogenic effects of treatments typically prescribed for children with sickle-cell disease (Brown, Armstrong, & Eckman, 1993).

Social isolation and psychological problems appear to characterize some children with juvenile rheumatoid arthritis, particularly adolescents and those with severe forms of the disease (Billings, Moos, Miller, & Gotlieb, 1987; Daltroy et al., 1992; Ungerer, Horgan, Chaitow, & Champion, 1988). Billings and colleagues compared 42 children with severe rheumatic disease to 52 children with a milder or inactive form of rheumatic disease and to 93 healthy, demographically matched controls. Children were compared on physical, psychological, and behavioral adjustment and on the number of school days missed. Children with severe rheumatic disease had more psychological problems, particularly feelings of anxiety and sadness, than either of the other two groups of children. Children with rheumatic disease, regardless of severity, reported fewer activities with friends relative to controls. Daltroy et al. compared the adjustment scores of 102 4- to 16-year-olds with juvenile arthritis to age and sex norms. After adjusting for the effects of disease-related questions, 15% of the children with arthritis had clinical levels of behavior problems, with the highest percentage among male adolescents. Similarly, 19% of the children were in the clinical range on the social competence subscale, with adolescent males demonstrating the lowest levels of competence.

Extensive research has been conducted on children with diabetes mellitus (Delamater, 1992; Hanson, 1992; Hauser et al., 1986; Johnson, 1988), and a number of studies show adjustment problems in youngsters with this disease, particularly adolescents. Hauser et al. (1979) compared the ego development and self-esteem of 163 11- to 19-year-old diabetics to 53 nondiabetics ages 13–14 and to two other samples who had been tested on ego development. Hauser et al. (1979) found that ego development was lower among the diabetics relative to the other groups, and this was not a function of the duration of the illness. Boys were assessed as having lower levels of ego development relative to girls. Self-esteem was not associated with illness per se, but was lower for adolescents whose diabetes was of longer duration and reported lower ego development. Sullivan (1978) also compared diabetics with nondiabetics on self-esteem and self-reported depression. In her sample of girls, there were no differences on self-esteem, and only physiological symptoms of depression were reported more frequently among diabetics versus nondiabetics. In a review of the psychological characteristics of children with diabetes, Rovet, Ehrlich, Czuchta, and Akler (1993) found that children who develop diabetes before age 5, who have severe hypo- and hyperglycemia, or who have frequent hypoglycemic episodes are at increased risk for neurocognitive deficits.

Children's adjustment to cancer has also received considerable attention. Kaplan, Busner, Weinhold, and Lenon (1987) compared the depressive symptomatology of children and adolescents with cancer (leukemia and nonleukemia) to published norms and found that children with cancer did not show higher levels of depressive symptomatology. In fact, younger children had lower levels of depressive symptoms relative to published norms. Worshel et al. (1988) compared children with cancer to psychiatrically referred children and healthy controls. Children with cancer had lower self-reported depression than both control groups. However, comparisons with parents' and nurses' ratings of children's depression suggest that the children with cancer may have been denying their feelings. The psychological adjustment of 81 children with brain tumors was compared to 31 children with malignancies not involving the central nervous system (Mulhern, Carpentieri, Shema, Stone, & Fairclough, 1993). Although these two groups did not differ on parent-rated behavior problems, both groups scored higher on one or more indices of adjustment problems relative to norms.

Several longitudinal studies have also been conducted with children who have cancer. In a longitudinal follow-up of 117 individuals who had survived childhood cancer, Koocher and O'Malley (1981) found that 47% of the survivors showed evidence of psychological maladjustment. When compared to a small group of individuals who had been successfully treated for other chronic illnesses in childhood, the cancer survivors showed higher levels of maladjustment and lower life satisfaction. When compared with general population norms, however, the cancer survivors were not more depressed. In a 2-year study of the peer adjustment of adolescents with cancer, Noll, Bukowski, Davies, Koontz, and Kulkarni (1993) found that these adolescents were perceived as more socially isolated, relative to matched classroom controls, but did not differ on multiple indicators of social acceptance or on self-reported affect.

Concern about potential cognitive deficits associated with cancer treatments (particularly irradiation) has spawned a number of research studies. Cousens, Waters, Said, and Stevens (1988) completed a meta-analysis of 31 studies focused on the effects of irradiation on children with acute lymphoblastic leukemia. Brown and Madan-Swain (1993) critically reviewed irradiation- and chemotherapy-related neurocognitive effects on children with leukemia. Both reviews note that a number of studies have documented a high incidence of neurocognitive deficits associated with radiation therapy. These deficits appear on tasks associated with functioning in the frontal lobe and right hemisphere, and are more deleterious in younger children. Because of the iatrogennic effects associated with irradiation, chemotherapies without radiation are currently used with children who have favorable prognoses. The data on the effects of chemotherapies are sparse and equivocal. As Brown and Madan-Swain (1993) note, the few studies in this area focus on short-term effects and are plagued by methodological problems, thereby preventing definitive conclusions. Butler and Copeland (1993) make several recommendations for improving research in this area, including use of randomized, prospective designs when possible; controls for sociodemographic variables and other potential confounds; use of comparison groups without reported insults to the central nervous system; collection of data from independent measures of brain functioning; evaluation of functions beyond intelligence and academic achievement; and adequate description of administration and scoring techniques.

Although end-stage renal disease is quite rare, it presents enormous coping challenges, given the physical deformities and high rate of mortality associated with this disease (Korsch & Fine, 1985). Garralda, Jameson, Reynolds, and Postlethwaite (1988) compared 22 children with chronic renal failure who were not on dialysis with a matched control group of 22 children on dialysis and 31 healthy controls. Composite psychiatric ratings were based on data from parent and teacher interviews and child self-report. Definite psychiatric disturbance was most common in the dialysis group, while mild psychiatric problems were most common in the nondialysis group. Both groups of renal patients had higher rates of disturbance compared with healthy controls.

In addition to the above chronic illnesses, the literature suggests that children and adolescents with spina bifida (Tew & Laurence, 1985) and isolated growth hormone deficiency (Allen, Warzak, Greger, Bernotas & Huseman, 1993) experience more adjustment problems than healthy controls. Tew and Laurence (1985) compared 44 10-year-olds with spina bifida to 53 nondisabled children who were matched on sex, birth order, and socioeconomic status (SES). Children with spina bifida reported more feelings of personal inferiority, heightened social maladjustment with peers, and greater levels of family maladjustment relative to controls, even when the severity of the handicap was controlled. The fact that the children with spina bifida had significantly lower IQs than the control children may partially explain these findings.

Allen et al. (1993) studied 56 3- to 16-year-olds with isolated growth hormone deficiency, and compared their sample to established norms for psychological adjustment. Severity of the stature problem was strongly associated with social skill impairment. Preadolescents had more parent-rated behavior problems than either clinical or nonclinical norms. Boys ages 12–16 had more behavior problems and lower social competence scores than nonclinical norms, and both boys and girls ages 6–11 had lower social competence scores relative to clinic norms. However, on all other measures, children with isolated growth hormone deficiency were not different from norms. Allen et al. argue that the disease-specific features of isolated growth hormone deficiency are what underlie the psychosocial difficulties children experience.

As the above review indicates, studies that focus on children with specific diseases have yielded equivocal findings. Many studies do find differences between children with chronic illnesses and either appropriate controls or published norms. Differences in depression, anxiety, and other psychiatric symptoms and ego development are a few areas in which chronically ill children, as a group, fare worse than healthy controls. However, a significant number of studies report no significant differences between chronically ill youth and controls on many of these same variables, and there is less evidence for group differences on measures of self-concept, self-esteem, and peer relationships.

In a meta-analytic review of 87 studies that focused on psychological adjustment to pediatric physical disorders, Lavigne and Faier-Routman (1992) evaluated the effects of chronic illness on overall adjustment problems, internalizing and externalizing disorders, and self-concept. They also compared studies by the type of control procedures used (comparison with normative data vs. with study-recruited controls) and across raters and disease group. Lavigne and Faier-Routman concluded that children with physical disorders did show increased risk for overall adjustment problems and internalizing and externalizing symptoms; however, their conclusions are qualified. Effect sizes were smaller when comparisons were made to study-recruited controls versus normative data. In the case of self-concept, when careful matching procedures were used, chronically ill children did not differ from controls. Teachers were more likely to report differences on internalizing symptoms, while parents were more likely to report differences on externalizing symptoms. Although the small number of studies of some diseases made cross-disease comparisons difficult, the authors found greater psychosocial impairment in diseases characterized by neurological and sensory impairments than diseases without these features.

One of the few population-based studies of psychosocial risk supports the conclusions of Lavigne and Faier-Routman. Cadman, Boyle, Szatmari, and Offord (1987) surveyed nearly 1900 families in Ontario, Canada, including almost 3300 4- to 16-year-old children. Their study compared children with chronic diseases and physical disabilities, chronic diseases only, and healthy controls. Types of psychological dysfunction assessed included neurosis, conduct disorder, attention deficit disorder and hyperactivity, and other psychiatric disorders such as anxiety disorders. Relative to healthy controls, children with chronic illnesses (without physical disabilities) were twice as likely to have a psychological diagnosis, but were not more likely to show social impairments such as being isolated, getting along with peers, having low levels of competence, or having academic difficulties.

The lack of consistency between some of the disease-specific studies and meta-analytic studies or the Cadman et al. (1987) study may be partially due to sample size. Chronically ill children and their families are difficult to recruit; therefore, sample sizes are often small. In some disease–specific studies the samples may be too small to show higher rates of psychiatric disorder in chronically ill children than in comparison children. Further, the outcome measures used in studies may not be sensitive enough to detect differences in the behavior or functioning of chronically ill children relative to controls.

In a recent issue of the *Journal of Pediatric Psychology,* leading pediatric researchers were invited to comment on the state of the research in the areas of pediatric chronic disease and how research can be advanced. Glasgow and Anderson (1995), writing about diabetes, make a number of points that apply to many of the disease-specific studies reviewed above. First, they suggest that much of the research on pediatric chronic conditions to date is either atheoretical or does not integrate research findings with the literature. Although this has begun to change during the past 5 years, more innovative conceptual models and variables are needed. Second, most studies ignore the social contexts in which adjustment is occurring. There are family, neighborhood, and broader cultural influences that may affect psychosocial adjustment to chronic conditions. Recently, developmental psychologists have renewed their attention to contextual influences on development and are designing some innovative approaches to assess these influences. Pediatric psychologists may benefit from some of these approaches. A third shortcoming is that most studies do not have representative samples. Obtaining pediatric samples is difficult, and it may not be possible to collect information from representative groups. If that is the case, then these limitations should be noted. Glasgow and Anderson (1995) argue that population-based samples are needed to advance the field. It may be the case that convenience samples are comprised of individuals who are either much worse off or much better off psychologically than population-based samples. This may partially explain the equivocal findings of disease-specific studies. A fourth methodological problem with many studies of pediatric conditions is reliance on unvalidated instruments or one method of measurement. Use of multiple methods of assessment will allow researchers to evaluate the extent to which measures are method-specific or converge in their assessments. Fifth, few studies have examined the long-term impact of pediatric chronic disease. Currently, we know little about whether the psychosocial impact of chronic disease is stable or varies depending on the developmental issues the child is facing or other factors in the child's life. Further, we know little about the influence of age or developmental level on psychosocial morbidity. Sixth, studies need to carefully control for sociodemographic and medical variables that may influence psychosocial morbidity. Seventh, much of the research has focused on psychopathology. Social competence is an equally important factor to evaluate, particularly since mortality is less of an issue than in the past. In general, our assessments of social competence are not as sophisticated as our assessments of psychopathology. New techniques, including observational studies of parent–child or peer–child interaction, may be very valuable to assess social competencies.

In sum, while there is a tremendous amount of individual variation in adjustment to pediatric chronic illness, children with chronic conditions do appear to be about twice as likely as healthy children to show some form of psychosocial impairment. These impairments are more likely to appear as internalizing symptoms rather than problems with peer relationships, self-esteem, or academic difficulties. Children with neurological or sensory impairments appear particularly vulnerable to adjustment problems.

MODELS OF CHILDREN'S ADAPTATION TO CHRONIC ILLNESS

Several general and disease-specific conceptual models delineating factors related to the adjustment of children with chronic illness were developed in the 1980s and early 1990s (Fiese & Sameroff, 1989; Hanson, 1992; Jessop & Stein, 1983; Stein & Jessop, 1982; Thompson, 1985; Wallander, Varni, Babani, Banis, & Wilcox, 1989; Wertlieb, Jacobson, & Hauser, 1990). These models paralleled trends in the literature on children's adjustment to stress, and were developed in part as a response to the failure to find large differences in adjustment between chronically ill children and controls.

Jessop and Stein (1983) argue that to understand the meaning of a disease in the lives of patients and their families, a noncategorical approach to chronic childhood illness is needed. In this approach, common features of chronic illnesses and individuals' reactions to them are emphasized, rather than the unique features of any one disease. Noncategorical measures such as the functional status of the child and the amount of burden the illness places on the family are suggested for use in this type of an approach. Thus, Stein, Jessop, and their colleagues include children who have different chronic diseases in their studies and examine the relations between noncategorical measures and adjustment. In addition to theoretical reasons, Jessop and Stein note that this approach is needed to generate the sample sizes necessary to perform sophisticated data analyses. In support of their view, Stein and Jessop (1989) present data from one institutional and one population-based study that demonstrate that diagnostic groupings are not very useful in examining correlates of illness. In their analyses, there was more variation within diagnostic groups than between diagnostic groups.

In a related vein, Thompson (1985) and Wallander et al. (1989) have advocated transactional approaches for studying chronic illnesses. In their models, child adjustment is determined by several sets of factors, including disease parameters (e.g., severity, functional impairment), demographic variables, family functioning or family resources, intrapersonal factors (e.g., temperament, competence, locus of control), and the child's coping processes. Thompson emphasizes maternal coping processes and adjustment to a greater extent than Wallander and colleagues. Hanson (1992) and Wertlieb et al. (1990) have developed models specific to the adjustment of children with diabetes, which are conceptually similar to those of Thompson (1985) and Wallander et al. (1989).

Kliewer, Sandler, and Wolchik (1994) have developed a transactional model of parent and family influences on coping processes in children that can be applied to families with a chronically ill child. Kliewer et al. (1994) suggest that parents influence their children's threat appraisals and coping efforts through three processes, which then influence psychological adjustment. Parents coach their children to react emotionally and to use particular coping strategies when faced with problems, model their own emotional responses and coping efforts in response to stress, and create a home environment that either invites open communication and cohesion or stifles them.

Transactional approaches lend themselves to address the question of why some children with a particular disease function well and others with the same disease function poorly. This approach may still be disease-specific, but it allows clinicians and researchers to identify children who are most in need of intervention. Transactional models such as those developed by Wallander et al. (1989) and Kliewer et al. (1994) are also useful when children with differing chronic conditions are "pooled" into one study. For example, in these studies, dimensions of family functioning that apply across conditions may be examined. The models suggested by Wallander et al. and Kliewer et al. are compatible with the noncategorical approach advocated by Stein and Jessop (1989). However, Wallander et al. and Kliewer et al. emphasize coping processes to a greater extent than do Stein and Jessop.

The disease-specific and the noncategorical approaches can contribute to our understanding of the effects of chronic illness. The disease-specific approach investigates mechanisms by which children develop specific problems to a common condition and identifies families that are most negatively impacted. The noncategorical approach studies common processes across diseases that threaten children's well-being. The key question for both approaches focuses on the mechanisms involved in the development of problems and the identification of high-risk groups. In the next section, I will review representative literature on the relations between coping and adjustment and on the influence of social environmental variables on coping and adjustment in chronically ill children and adolescents.

Relations between Coping Processes and Adjustment

Coping processes refer to both how a child *appraises* or evaluates a situation (e.g., is it threatening?) and the efforts he or she uses to manage the associated affect or to solve the problem. Sandler and coauthors (Chapter 1, this volume) provide an overview of ways in which coping has been conceptualized. One key distinction is between problem-focused coping, which aims to address the source of the distress, and emotion-focused coping, which aims to manage affect related to the stressful situation (Lazarus & Folkman, 1984). Weisz's (Weisz, Rothbaum, & Blackburn, 1984) distinction between primary- and secondary-control coping is similar to Lazarus and Folkman's conceptualization. Other distinctions that are made are between active and avoidant coping (Ayers, Sandler, West, & Roosa, 1996) and between behavioral and cognitive coping efforts (Moos & Billings, 1982). Pediatric researchers have often developed their own coping measures, perhaps because measures used in the developmental and clinical literatures were not valid or meaningful for children with chronic illnesses or were too lengthy to be used in pediatric settings.

A number of recent studies with diverse groups of chronically ill children have demonstrated links between children's coping behavior and psychological adjustment. For example, in a study of 64 children with diabetes, Band and Weisz (1990) found that coping was significantly related to medical adjustment for older, but not younger, children. Additionally, coping style was uniquely predictive of parent-rated sociobehavioral adjustment and conduct problems in older children but not younger children. In all cases, greater levels of primary-control coping (which is conceptually similar to problem-focused coping) was associated with more favorable adjustment.

Delamater and colleagues have examined the contribution of coping to the adjustment of children with insulin-dependent diabetes mellitus (IDDM) in several studies. Delamater, Smith, Lankester, and Santiago (1988) found that several diabetes-specific coping measures were significantly associated with worse metabolic control in a study of 47 adolescents with IDDM. Higher scores on self-blame, keeps to self, and wishful thinking were related to worse control. Grey, Cameron, and Thurber (1991) replicated this effect in their investigation of 103 children with diabetes. Children who used avoidant coping were more depressed and more likely to have problems with metabolic control. In contrast, Hanson, Cigrang, et al. (1989) found that avoidant coping was unrelated to metabolic control in 135 youth with IDDM, but was significantly related to lower regimen compliance. In one of the few longitudinal studies in this area, Jacobson, Hauser, Lavori, and Wolfsdorf (1990) found that coping (conceptualized in terms of defense level, adaptive strength, and locus of control) assessed at the start of the study predicted adherence to the diabetic regimen over a 4-year period.

In a study of 50 children with sickle-cell disease, Thompson, Gil, Burbach, Keith, and Kinney (1993) found that children's strategies for coping with pain explained an additional 21% of the variation in child-reported behavior symptoms after accounting for number of illness complications, pain frequency, type of sickle cell disease (SCD), SES, sex, and age. Specifically, negative thinking by children (e.g., catastrophizing) was associated with greater levels of behavior problems. In another study with 39 children with sickle-cell disease, Lewis and Kliewer (1996) demonstrated that active coping was negatively linked to self-reported anxiety and health care utilization, while avoidant coping was positively related to anxiety. Coping strategies moderated, but did not mediate, links between self-rated hopefulness and anxiety. When active, support, or distraction coping was high, hope was negatively related to anxiety. These relations held after controlling for sociodemographic variables and disease severity.

Ebata and Moos (1991) investigated the relation between coping and adjustment in adolescents, including 45 adolescents with rheumatic disease. In regression analyses predicting psychological well-being, distress, and behavior problems, age, gender, and group membership were controlled. Severity and challenge appraisals were entered as predictors, followed by coping variables. Overall, adolescents who use more approach coping, such as positive reappraisal and problem-solving and less avoidance coping, were more psychologically healthy.

In sum, the majority of the evidence suggests that coping that is more problem focused is related to better adjustment while avoidant coping and coping that focuses on the self (e.g., self-blame) are related to poorer adjustment. These relations hold across different types of chronic illness and a variety of indicators of adjustment, including both physiological and psychological measures. Little is known, however, about the specific situations in which active coping is the most adaptive or avoidant coping the most harmful. It may be that the adaptive nature of coping efforts depends in part on the stage of the disease, the medical demands placed on the child and the family, and the prognosis.

Relations between Environmental Variables and Coping and Adjustment

The majority of existing empirical work has examined relations between environmental influences and adaptation; less is known about the relations between environmental influences and coping. Environmental influence variables include qualities of the family environment, such as the level of cohesion, conflict, organization, expressiveness, or adaptability; social support from family or friends; the adaptation of other family members, particularly mothers; beliefs and coping strategies of parents; and impact of the illness on the family.

Several studies have focused on qualities of the family environment. Hanson and colleagues have conducted a number of studies examining environmental influences on the adjustment of youth with IDDM. Hanson's comprehensive model delineating factors associated with adjustment in children with IDDM and a summary of her programmatic research may be found in Hanson (1992). In a study of 95 youth, Hanson, DeGuire, Schinkel, Henggeler, and Burghen (1992) found that high levels of family flexibility and low levels of illness-specific nonsupport were related to dietary adherence. High family affection and low illness-specific support were associated with psychosocial adaption. Family factors did not successfully predict metabolic control or illness-specific psychosocial adjustment. Other studies (Hanson, Henggeler, Harris, Burghen, & Moore, 1989) found that flexible family relations, high family cohesion, and high marital satisfaction were significantly related to good metabolic control, but these effects were most evident for those with the shortest IDDM duration.

Hanson, Cigrang, et al. (1989) also examined relations between the family environment and coping efforts of 135 adolescents with IDDM. They found that lower family cohesion was related to higher ventilation and avoidant coping, after controlling for age and stress. Additionally, there was a family adaptability × IDDM duration interaction. For adolescents with a long duration of IDDM, family rigidity was associated with avoidant coping.

In a study of 46 children with IDDM, Wertlieb, Hauser, and Jacobson (1986) found that family conflict was positively related and family organization was negatively related to psychological adjustment problems. Family environment was also associated with adherence in a longitudinal study of 52 children with diabetes (Hauser, Jacobson, Lavori, & Wolfsdorf, 1990). Long-term (4-year) adherence was most strongly predicted by higher family conflict. Parental and child perceptions of cohesion predicted improvement in adherence and overall higher adherence.

Weist, Finney, Barnard, Davis, and Ollendick (1993) used an empirical approach to determine psychosocial variables related to optimal metabolic control of diabetes in 56 children and their families. Children were classified as either in optimal or nonoptimal control of diabetes, then were compared on measures of behavioral symptoms, competence, coping, family environment, health locus of control, and diabetes knowledge and care. Children in the optimal control category had parents who reported their families as more controlling compared with children in the nonoptimal control category.

The main and stress-buffering effects of quality of the family environment on the psychological adjustment of 53 adolescents with spina bifida were investigated by Murch and Cohen (1989). Self-reports of anxiety, depression, and self-esteem were obtained. Family conflict and control were positively related to depression and anxiety and negatively related to self-esteem. Cohesion and depression were negatively related, and expressiveness, cohesion, and independence were positively related to self-esteem. In terms of interactions with life stress, family conflict and control buffered the stress-adjustment relation, while a high level of independence exacerbated the effects of life stress.

Several studies have included multiple groups of chronically ill youngsters. Wallander et al. (1989) examined the relations between family resources and parent reports of psychological adjustment in 153 children with either juvenile diabetes, juvenile rheumatoid arthritis, chronic obesity, spina bifida, or cerebral palsy. After controlling for maternal education and family income, family resources explained significant amounts of variance in child adjustment. In particular, more conflict was related to more externalizing problems and cohesion and conflict were positively related to social competence, while control was negatively related to competence.

As part of a study of 187 healthy and chronically ill children, Perrin,

Ayoub, and Willett (1993) evaluated the effects of the family environment on a composite index of child adjustment. Adjustment ratings from parents, children, and teachers were obtained and analyzed separately. After controlling for SES, verbal intelligence, age, and gender, family environment was significantly related to child adjustment for all three reporters.

Family environment also predicted parent-rated adjustment in a sample of 60 children who were either healthy or had asthma or diabetes (Hamlett, Pellegrini, & Katz, 1992). Family cohesion and conflict were significantly related to externalizing symptoms after controlling for disease type, although the direction of effects was not reported. Adequacy of maternal support predicted internalizing symptoms.

Walker, Van Slyke and Newbrough (1992) examined associations between child management problems, maternal caretaking burden, family problems, and child adjustment. Family problems, which included limits on family opportunities, family disharmony, financial stress, and maternal concerns, specifically feeling a personal burden for the child, were positively related to child adjustment problems.

Finally, Kliewer and Lewis (1995) tested three models of family influence on the coping processes of 39 children and adolescents with sickle-cell disease. After controlling for relevant demographic and disease parameters, active coping was positively related to living in a more cohesive family environment, and hope (conceptualized as a generalized cognitive appraisal) was associated with receiving active coping suggestions from parents.

The majority of studies on environmental influences on children's coping and adjustment to chronic illness have assessed dimensions of the family environment. As the above review indicates, family cohesion, affection, flexibility, and expressiveness in particular are associated with good psychological and physical adjustment and with active coping. Conversely, family conflict is associated with poor psychological and physical adjustment. These relations hold even after controlling for relevant disease parameters. Most of the empirical work has taken a "main effects" approach when exploring associations between environmental variables and adjustment. A limited number of studies have examined features of the social environment as either a moderator or mediator in predicting adjustment.

In addition to the family environment, maternal functioning and general family functioning have been studied. Studying the psychological adjustment of 45 children with cystic fibrosis, Thompson, Gustafson, Hamlett, and Spock (1992) found that maternal anxiety was positively related to children's internalizing and externalizing symptoms, after controlling for disease severity, SES, and the child's age and gender.

Kager and Holden (1992) examined the direct and moderating influences of family and individual variables on the adjustment of 64 children and adolescents with IDDM. Maternal reports of the helpfulness of coping behaviors in managing her child's illness was negatively related to a child's general self-worth, suggesting that mothers' attempts to manage stress are more helpful when their children are less competent.

General family dysfunction was related to self-reported depressive symptomatology and parent-reported behavioral and emotional symptoms in a sample of 44 children with cystic fibrosis (Pumariega, Pearson, & Seilheimer, 1993). However, the authors only report zero-order correlations between variables of interest, so it is unclear if these environmental indicators explain additional variation in adjustment beyond that explained by control variables.

The contribution of environmental factors to the physical (Ross et al., 1993) and psychological (Daltroy et al., 1992) adjustment of youth with juvenile rheumatoid arthritis has also been studied. Using data from a 28-day pain diary, Ross et al. found that child distress, maternal distress, and family disharmony were associated with self-reported pain after controlling for disease characteristics. In a study with 102 children with juvenile rheumatoid arthritis, Daltroy et al. found that social competence was predicted by age, disease duration and severity, maternal physical health, and maternal employment status. Mothers who enjoyed good or excellent physical health and worked part-time rated their children as being more socially competent relative to less healthy mothers who were employed full-time.

The contribution of maternal, paternal, and adolescent ratings of parent–teen relationships to the social and physical adjustment of 115 adolescents with diabetes was examined by Wysocki (1993). Regression analyses revealed that ratings of skill deficits/overt conflict by all three respondent groups were associated with poorer social and physical adjustment.

In addition to diabetes, support has been identified as important in the adjustment of children with cancer. Varni, Katz, Colegrove, and Dolgin (1994) studied the effects of perceived support from classmates, parents, teachers and friends on the psychological adjustment of 30 children recently diagnosed with cancer. After controlling for age and gender, classmate support was associated with better self- and other-rated adjustment. Kazak and Meadows (1989) used a short-term (6 months) longitudinal design to study the adjustment, family adaptability, and social support of 35 adolescents who survived childhood cancer. Perceived social acceptance was positively associated with satisfaction with emotional support and family adaptability. Perceived scholastic competence was also related to family adaptability.

In sum, studies focused on maternal adjustment, general family dysfunction or disharmony, and level of support have revealed that better physical and psychological adjustment is associated with higher levels of maternal functioning, family harmony, and perceptions of support. Additional research is needed to specify the processes by which social environmental factors influence children's physical and psychological well-being. In the following section, developmental issues faced by chronically ill youth will be discussed, with attention to the specific ways in which chronic illnesses might interfere with these adaptive tasks.

ADAPTIVE TASKS AND DEVELOPMENTAL ISSUES

As Garrison and McQuiston (1989) note, chronically ill children face the same developmental tasks and challenges as healthy children. Infants and toddlers need to develop (1) a sense of self that is differentiated from the environment (Piaget, 1952), (2) a basic trust of others (Erikson, 1963), and (3) a sense of autonomy (Erikson, 1963). In childhood, developmental tasks include expanding self-understanding, learning more about how society works, developing behavioral standards, and managing behavior. These tasks are related to what Erikson calls the crisis of industry versus inferiority. Learning to be productive—to master and complete tasks—leads to a sense of competence. Also important during middle childhood is connection with peers. It is at this stage in the life span that individuals begin to shift investment toward the peer group, and friendships with peers become more salient (Hartup, 1989). During adolescence, developing a sense of identity that is unique and important (Erikson, 1968) is central. According to Erikson, this may be achieved by deciding on a career or by developing intimate relationships with others. Intimate, romantic relationships are important to adolescents and involve incorporating one's sexuality into notions about the self. The task of identity development is connected with the task of autonomy development. Adolescents need to assert themselves and expand relationships with others outside the family. However, as Grotevant and Cooper (1986) argue, retaining an emotional connection with parents, rather than becoming emotionally disengaged from them, is healthy.

Chronic illness may interfere with these developmental tasks in multiple ways. A sense of basic trust, which develops from consistent, predictable experiences (Boyce, Jensen, James, & Peacock, 1983; Erikson, 1963), may be compromised due to frequent hospitalizations that require separations from parents and by painful medical procedures. Children with sickle-cell disease, cystic fibrosis, or cancer are particularly likely to experience these challenges to development.

The push toward autonomy in toddlers is exercised through manipulation and exploration of objects in the physical world. The sense of independence develops as toddlers have opportunities to do things for themselves. When young children are very ill or their mobility is restrained by medical procedures, they have fewer opportunities to explore the environment and exercise independent behavior. Concern for their ill children's well-being may also make parents overprotective, thus fostering dependent, rather than independent behavior (Cerreto & Travis, 1984). Children with conditions whose symptoms may be exacerbated by physical activity (e.g., cystic fibrosis, asthma, sickle-cell disease, arthritis, hemophilia) may be most at risk for poor autonomy development.

Developing a healthy notion of self, good peer relationships, and sense of competence may be challenged by the constraints of living with a chronic illness, particularly if a child's social interactions are limited (Garrison & McQuiston, 1989). Chronic illnesses that result in decreased school attendance or limited participation in play or sports activities or that require adherence to medical routines or treatments that make the child seem "different" all present coping challenges.

Identity and autonomy development present adaptive challenges to the chronically ill adolescent. Chronically ill adolescents who are slow to mature physically, as is the case with adolescents with sickle-cell disease or cystic fibrosis, may have a poor body image (McCracken, 1984). As is the case with healthy youth, concerns about physical appearance can affect the development of intimate, romantic relationships. Behavioral autonomy is also difficult, particularly for adolescents whose medical regimens are complicated and require parental involvement. Additionally, medical regimens that involve daily insulin injections, urine or blood testing, chest therapy, blood transfusions, or assorted medications make it difficult for the adolescent to perceive him- or herself as similar to peers. Concomitant with concerns about peer relations and a desire to become more independent is the emergence of adolescent egocentrism. Egocentric thinking during adolescence often results in increased risk taking, primarily because adolescents underestimate potential harm associated with risky behavior. For the chronically ill adolescent, risk taking can have life-threatening implications, particularly if it involves nonparticipation in the prescribed medical regimen or experimentation with substances that interact with medication (Garrison & McQuiston, 1989; McAnarney, 1985).

Finally, because of their enhanced cognitive ability to consider the future, chronically ill adolescents face issues of morbidity and mortality in ways that children do not. In fact, Koocher (1984) suggests that it is the uncertainty about the duration and outcome of the illness that is the most distressing to chronically ill youth. It is difficult for chronically ill adolescents to think about career options or long-term relationships if they are uncertain if they will be alive or well enough to participate in these activities.

It is difficult to know what specific features of a chronic illness make it stressful and challenging for children. Unfortunately, there are sparse data on this issue. Some work has addressed stress from the parents' perspective (e.g., Quittner, DiGirolamo, Michel, & Eigen, 1992), but less is known about the dimensions of illness that children identify as challenging. The most stressful components of chronic illnesses most likely vary across individuals, across particular illnesses, and within individuals over time. Anecdotal evidence suggests that young cancer patients may be primarily concerned about how their illness affects their family. They may worry about the emotional strain of the disease on parents and siblings. This may be true for children with other chronic illnesses as well. For early adolescents, clinical observations suggest that concerns about being normal may predominate, and adolescents may become very self-conscious about appearance.

Jessop and Stein (1985) have noted that uncertainty about the course of a disease is very psychologically unsettling and is associated with greater psychological disturbance on the part of the mother and greater perceived impact of the illness on the family. Koocher (1984) also has suggested that the lack of predictability may be the most stressful for some children, particularly for those with illnesses that have moderate survival rates. Alternatively, a high level of functional impairment or visibility could be what is most distressing. However, data from Jessop and Stein (1985) suggest that visibility is less consequential than uncertainty. Further, children with conditions that were not visible had more negative consequences relative to children with visible conditions.

Understanding the adaptive challenges that chronically ill children face and the impact of the social environment on coping and adjustment is a necessary first step toward the design and testing of interventions for children and their families. Although conceptual models of relations between environmental resources, children's coping processes, and children's adjustment to chronic illness exist, most studies have tested only portions of a larger conceptual model. Large sample sizes and longitudinal designs are needed to adequately test complex models of adjustment, particularly those that specify moderated or mediated effects. Models of adjustment that are well-defined prior to the design of interventions have the greatest opportunity for advancing our understanding of how to effectively assist chronically ill youth. The following section examines interventions designed to facilitate adjustment to chronic illness. Interventions that target children's psychosocial adjustment as a primary or secondary outcome are reviewed. Interventions that are (1) designed to affect the health care system broadly (e.g., Jessop & Stein, 1994), (2) focused only on physical health outcomes, (3) aimed primarily at parents, or (4) focused specifically on painful medical procedures or injury prevention are not covered.

INTERVENTIONS TO FACILITATE ADJUSTMENT TO CHRONIC ILLNESS

In an editorial introduction to a special issue on interventions in pediatric psychology, LaGreca and Varni (1993) note that only 9.1% of the research articles published in the *Journal of Pediatric Psychology* from 1988 to 1992 dealt with efforts to improve the status or functioning of the child, parent, or family; an additional 3.8% dealt with the prevention of problems or disorders. LaGreca and Varni note that the paucity of published research documenting the empirical effects of treatment is likely due to the difficulty of conducting these types of studies, relative to other research endeavors. It is clear that interventions with chronically ill children and families are occurring, though these programs may not be evaluated. In this section, I will describe the general targets and modes of intervention with chronically ill youth, and then review recent empirical work.

As Johnson (1988) notes, interventions with chronically ill children have focused on management of the illness, coping with the disease, and effects on the family. Interventions focused on coping with the illness are concerned with assessment and treatment of psychological reactions, stress resistance and vulnerability, and procedure-specific psychological responses. Interventions targeting effects on the family have been concerned with impacts on the functioning of parents and siblings, as well as how the disease changes relationships within the family system. However, most interventions with chronically ill youth are aimed at management of the illness; coping efficacy and effects on the family are secondary considerations. Additionally, most interventions with chronically ill youth are disease specific. This is probably the case because management issues tend to be unique to disease type, or at least are perceived that way by health care providers. Garrison and McQuiston (1989) comment that programs may be delivered in a prevention mode (health education and preparation for anticipated symptoms or procedures), an intervention mode (treatment after significant problems develop), or a case-monitoring mode (follow-up programs for children defined at risk). Stein, Jessop, and Ireys (1988) provide a slightly different perspective, noting that their intervention work has used one of three general approaches: enhancing coordination and continuity of the health care system, enhancing social support for children and families, and enhancing cognitive competence, usually via education.

Researchers have typically drawn on established theory and/or empirical literature to design their intervention programs, or in some cases have used a needs assessment approach (e.g., Mason, Olson, Myers, Huszti, & Kenning, 1992; Wilson, Mitchell, Rolnick, & Fish, 1993). Interventions that have been evaluated have drawn heavily from prior theoretical and empirical work on the adjustment of youth with specific chronic illnesses.

A number of interventions have been conducted with adolescents with diabetes, motivated in part by the difficulty of maintaining metabolic control during this developmental period. Satin, LaGreca, Zigo, and Skyler (1989) were the first to report on the outcome of a family-oriented group intervention for these adolescents. Their intervention is based on evidence that adolescents who come from conflicted or dysfunctional families typically display behavioral or psychosocial adjustment problems (Wertlieb et al., 1986), as well as difficulties with metabolic control. Although Satin et al. do not specify mediators in their intervention, in addition to metabolic status, adolescents were evaluated on perceptions of themselves and parents completed measures of their perceptions of children and families with diabetes, their adolescent's self-care, and the family environment. Satin et al. randomly assigned 32 families to either a multifamily group (MF), a multifamily plus parent simulation of diabetes group (MF + S), or a wait-list control group (C). The two treatment conditions were 6 weeks long and were family oriented. Relative to controls, adolescents in the MF + S group improved their metabolic control, and adolescents in both intervention groups had more positive perceptions of a "teenager with diabetes" at posttreatment. There were no group differences on the parent perception or family environment variables. Thus, it is clear that changes in parental attitudes or in family environment did not account for improvements in metabolic control. Satin et al. note that while it is unclear what factors accounted for the improvements in metabolic control, there was indirect evidence suggesting that behavioral changes in diabetic management were prevalent in the families with the most improvements.

In contrast to the family intervention conducted by Satin et al., Boardway, Delamater, Tomakowsky, and Gutai (1993) evaluated the effects of a stress management training program for adolescents with diabetes. The program was built in part on the evidence that stress is associated with both maladaptive coping and poor metabolic control. Thus, it was reasoned that by lowering stress, adaptive coping and metabolic control could be improved. Nineteen patients were randomly assigned to either the stress management group or a standard outpatient treatment. The stress management program consisted of ten sessions over 3 months and three additional sessions over 3 months. A 3-month follow-up without treatment was conducted. The stress management program was conducted in a group format, and focused on accurate assessment behaviors, coping skills, assertiveness training, and dietary and insulin administration skills. Results indicated that diabetes-specific stress (a measure of the "hassles" associated with being a diabetic teenager) decreased significantly for adolescents in the stress management group, but metabolic control, general life-stress events, regimen adherence, coping styles, and self-efficacy about diabetes did not differ across groups at posttest or follow-up. Thus, the intervention affected change in the hypothesized mediator, but did not improve other variables in the model, including metabolic control.

The psychosocial functioning of children newly diagnosed with cancer was the focus of an intervention by Varni, Katz, Colegrove, and Dolgin (1993). This multisite intervention was based on data demonstrating the stress-buffering effects of social support on adjustment in children with chronic physical disorders, data linking social skills to the development of social support, and knowledge that children with problematic peer relationships are at risk for long-term adjustment problems. Varni et al. reasoned that if children's social competence could be improved, they would attract more support from peers and teachers and demonstrate fewer adjustment problems. Sixty-four children were randomly assigned to either a social skills training group or a school reintegration standard treatment group. Children completed measures of depressive symptoms, anxiety, self-esteem, and perceived social support. Parents rated their child's adjustment and social competence. At the 9-month follow-up, children who received the social skills training showed significant increases in classmate and teacher support relative to their pretreatment levels (but not lower depression or anxiety, or higher esteem). Parents reported decreases in problem behavior and increases in social competence for this group. These changes were not observed in the standard treatment group. Unfortunately, measures of competence on the skills taught in the intervention were not reported; thus, it is unclear whether changes in these social skills accounted for the observed effects.

Sanders, Shepherd, Cleghorn, and Woolford (1994) compared a cognitive–behavioral family intervention for children with recurrent abdominal pain to standard pediatric care. Their intervention was designed to specifically test the hypotheses that the family intervention would result in improvements in children's active coping and maternal caregiving, and these behavior changes would in turn lead to reduced pain for the children and less interference of the pain in the child's daily activities. Forty-four children were randomly assigned to the treatment conditions. Measures of maternal caregiving, children's coping, child adjustment, treatment expectancies, relapse, and diary and observational measures of pain were collected at pretreatment, posttreatment, and 6- and 12-month follow-ups. Results indicated that children in both conditions had significant improvements in pain intensity and pain behavior. However, children in the cognitive–behavioral treatment had lower levels of long-term relapse, higher rates of complete elimination of pain, and lower rates of pain interfering with their daily activities. Regression analyses indicated that change in pain from pre- to posttreatment was predicted by children's active coping and maternal caregiving. However, all participants were included in these analyses (even those who did not receive training in coping), and treatment group was not controlled in the analyses. Thus, though it appears that the hypothesized mediators affected the pain outcomes, it is unclear whether the intervention influenced coping or caregiving. It may be that the small sample size of the treatment groups precluded these analyses.

Silver, Coupey, and Bauman (1992) used a 3-month peer counseling training intervention to attempt to improve the well-being of 32 inner-city adolescents, half of whom were chronically ill. The intervention was based on the premise that adolescents who participate in training and service programs show increased personal growth, greater self-acceptance and confidence, and better social interaction. Fourteen youths who completed the training and were invited to become counselors showed improved ego development and fewer psychiatric symptoms relative to a comparison sample of adolescents who did not receive training and to adolescents who received the training but were not invited to become counselors or who declined counseling jobs. Silver et al. suggest that psychological readiness influences which adolescents will benefit from this type of intervention.

Some studies have attempted to influence hypothesized mediators of physical health, but have not directly assessed health outcomes. For example, Kubly and McClellan (1984) evaluated the effects of self-care instruction on asthmatic children. Twenty-eight families were randomly assigned to either a self-care group or a knowledge-only control group. Families in the self-care group were instructed in breathing exercises, self-medication, and knowledge of asthma. Children completed a health locus of control scale (assessing responsibility) and parents and children completed a self-care activity questionnaire before and after the intervention. Results indicated that at posttreatment children in the treatment group had greater increases in their health locus of control scores, but did not differ from controls on measures of self-care. It appears as though this intervention affected children's perceptions of responsibility for their health. However, relations between health locus of control and self-care and pulmonary function were not reported; thus, it is unclear whether heightened responsibility will lead to increased self-care and/or better pulmonary outcomes.

The above studies were all focused on changing children's physical symptoms of and adjustment to chronic illness or changing the mediators thought to affect those outcomes. Most of these studies approach intervention with strong empirical justification, but they fail to adequately specify or test the mediators they propose are responsible for changes in physical or psychological functioning. Models that include moderators, such as examining the impact of age or developmental level on the efficacy of the intervention, are even more rare. Lack of follow-up beyond 12 months is also problematic. Small sample size is the biggest barrier to testing intervention models in a sophisticated way. LaGreca and Varni (1993) offer some creative solutions to this problem, including conducting multicenter studies, using crossover designs, or studying the effects of within-group parameters to a greater extent.

SUMMARY AND FUTURE DIRECTIONS

A significant percentage of children have chronic illnesses. Fewer of these children are dying than in the past; as a consequence, attention has shifted from dealing with mortality to understanding and preventing psychosocial morbidity. The best available data indicate that while there is tremendous variability in response to chronic illness, these children are about twice as likely to develop some form of psychiatric disturbance relative to healthy peers. Disturbances are most likely to occur in the area of internalizing symptoms and to children with diseases characterized by neurological or sensory impairments. What is less clear is the long-term impact of having a chronic illness, whether the impact of a disease varies by the developmental issues a child is facing, and whether subtle effects on socioemotional functioning not detected by global measures of pathology or competence exist. We also know almost nothing about the specific features of having a chronic illness that make it stressful for youth and the specific adaptive challenges these children face at different points in their development. Answers to these questions would help in identifying the groups of chronically ill children most in need of intervention.

Over the past decade, a number of fairly sophisticated models of children's adaptation to chronic illness have been developed. In general, the empirical literature has not kept pace with the amount of theorizing. Despite this deficit, knowledge about factors that affect children's adjustment is accumulating. First, children's coping strategies are related to their adjustment, with problem-focused coping strategies generally associated with better adjustment, while avoidant and self-focused strategies are related to poorer adjustment. These associations are fairly robust and apply to physiological and psychological outcomes. Second, family cohesion, flexibility, and warmth are associated with active coping and with good psychological and physical adjustment; families high on conflict and dysfunction have children who are less well adjusted. Problems with maternal adjustment are also associated with poor child outcomes. With few exceptions, these findings are of the "main effects" variety, and provide little information about ways in which risk or protective factors interact. Current data also do not address the mechanisms of family influence (e.g., why do cohesive families have children who are better adjusted?) or provide information about how situational demands might interact with coping to influence adjustment. Additionally, we know little about the broader contextual influences (neighborhood, media, culture) on the coping processes of children with chronic illness. This information is necessary, since conceptual models and interventions increasingly adopt a stress and coping framework.

At this point, there is limited empirical work on interventions for chronically ill youth. Prior to the design of effective interventions, further generative research using population-based samples that examines moderators and mediators of adjustment needs to be conducted. Programmatic research that follows from carefully conceived models of adaptation and solid generative studies will be the most successful in advancing our understanding of adjustment to chronic illness and in shaping our efforts to improve the lives of children with these conditions.

ACKNOWLEDGMENT
I thank Susan Pinson and K. Heather Wood for their assistance in gathering reference material.

REFERENCES

Allen, K. D., Warzak, W. J., Greger, N. G., Bernotas, T. D., & Huseman, C. A. (1993). Psychosocial adjustment of children with isolated growth hormone deficiency. *Children's Health Care, 22,* 61–72.

American Cancer Society. (1995). *Cancer facts and figures.* New York: American Cancer Society.

Ayers, T. S., Sandler, I. N., West, S. G., & Roosa, M. (1996). A dispositional and situational assessment of children's coping: Testing alternative models of coping. *Journal of Personality, 64,* 923–958.

Band, E. B., & Weisz, J. (1990). Developmental differences in primary and secondary control coping and adjustment to juvenile diabetes. *Journal of Clinical Child Psychology, 19,* 150–158.

Billings, A. G., Moos, R. H., Miller, J. J., & Gottlieb, J. E. (1987). Psychosocial adaptation in juvenile rheumatic disease: A controlled evaluation. *Health Psychology, 6,* 343–359.

Boardway, R. H., Delamater, A. M., Tomakowsky, J., & Gutai, J. P. (1993). Stress management training for adolescents with diabetes. *Journal of Pediatric Psychology, 18,* 29–45.

Boyce, W. T., Jensen, E. W., James, S. A., & Peacock, J. L. (1983). The family routines inventory: Theoretical origins. *Social Science and Medicine, 17,* 193–200.

Breslau, N. (1985). Psychiatric disorder in children with physical disabilities. *Journal of the Academy of Child Psychiatry, 24,* 87–94.

Brown, R. T., Armstrong, F. D., & Eckman, J. R. (1993). Neurocognitive aspects of pediatric sickle cell disease. *Journal of Learning Disabilities, 26,* 33–45.

Brown, R. T., & Madan-Swain, A. (1993). Cognitive, neuropsychological, and academic sequelae in children with leukemia. *Journal of Learning Disabilities, 26,* 74–90.

Butler, R. W., & Copeland, D. R. (1993). Neuropsychological effects of central nervous system prophylactic treatment in childhood leukemia: Methodological considerations. *Journal of Pediatric Psychology, 18,* 319–338.

Cadman, D., Boyle, M., Szatmari, P., & Offord, D. R. (1987). Chronic illness, disability, and mental and social well-being: Findings of the Ontario Child Health Study. *Pediatrics, 79,* 805–813.

Celano, M. P., & Geller, R. J. (1993). Learning, school performance, and children with asthma: How much at risk? *Journal of Learning Disabilities, 26,* 23–32.

Cerreto, M. C., & Travis, L. B. (1984). Implications of psychological and family factors in the treatment of diabetes. *Pediatric Clinics of North America, 31,* 698–710.

Cousens, P., Waters, B., Said, J., & Stevens, M. (1988). Cognitive effects of cranial irradiation in leukemia: A survey and meta-analysis. *Journal of Child Psychology and Psychiatry, 29,* 839–852.

Daltroy, L. H., Larson, M. G., Eaton, H. M., Partridge, A. J., Pless, I. B., Rogers, M. P., & Liang, M. H. (1992). Psychosocial adjustment in juvenile arthritis. *Journal of Pediatric Psychology, 17,* 277–289.

Delamater, A. M. (1992). Stress, coping, and metabolic control among youngsters with diabetes. In A. M. LaGreca, L. J. Siegel, J. L. Wallander, & C. E. Walker (Eds.), *Stress and coping in child health* (pp. 191–211). New York: Guilford.

Delamater, A. M., Smith, J. A., Lankester, L., & Santiago, J. V. (1988). *Relationship of coping responses to metabolic control in diabetic adolescents.* Paper presented at the First Florida Conference on Child Health Psychology, Gainesville.

Drotar, D., & Bush, M. (1985). Mental health issues and services. In N. Hobbs & J. M. Perrin (Eds.), *Issues in the care of children with chronic illness* (pp. 514–550). San Francisco: Jossey-Bass.

Ebata, A. T., & Moos, R. H. (1991). Coping and adjustment in distressed and healthy adolescents. *Journal of Applied Developmental Psychology, 12,* 33–54.

Eiser, C. (1990). Psychological effects of chronic disease. *Journal of Child Psychology and Psychiatry, 31,* 85–98.

Eiser, C. (1994). Making sense of chronic disease: The 11th Jack Tizard Memorial Lecture. *Journal of Child Psychology and Psychiatry and Allied Disciplines, 35,* 1373–1389.

Erikson, E. H. (1963). *Childhood and society* (2nd ed.). New York: Norton.

Erikson, E. H. (1968). *Identity: Youth and crisis.* New York: Norton.

Fiese, B. H., & Sameroff, A. J. (1989). Family context in pediatric psychology. *Journal of Pediatric Psychology, 14,* 293–314.

Garralda, M. E., Jameson, R. A., Reynolds, J. M., & Postlethwaite, R. J. (1988). Psychiatric adjustment in children with chronic renal failure. *Journal of Child Psychology and Psychiatry, 29,* 79–90.

Garrison, W. T., & McQuiston, S. (1989). *Chronic illness during childhood and adolescence. Psychological aspects* (Developmental Clinical Psychology and Psychiatry, Vol. 19). Newbury Park, CA: Sage.

Glasgow, R. E., & Anderson, B. J. (1995). Future directions for research on pediatric chronic disease management: Lessons from diabetes. *Journal of Pediatric Psychology, 20,* 389–402.

Gortmaker, S. L., & Sappenfield, W. (1984). Chronic childhood disorders: Prevalence and impact. *Pediatric Clinics of North America, 31,* 3–18.

Grey, M., Cameron, E., & Thurber, F. W. (1991). Coping and adaptation in children with diabetes. *Nursing Research, 40,* 144–149.

Grotevant, H., & Cooper, C. (1986). Individuation in family relationships: A perspective on individual differences in the development of role-taking skill in adolescence. *Human Development, 29,* 82–100.

Hamlett, K. W., Pellegrini, D. S., & Katz, K. S. (1992). Childhood chronic illness as a family stressor. *Journal of Pediatric Psychology, 17,* 33–47.

Hanson, C. L. (1992). Developing systemic models of the adaptation of youths with diabetes. In A. M. LaGreca, L. J. Siegel, J. L. Wallander, & C. E. Walker (Eds.), *Stress and coping in child health* (pp. 212–241). New York: Guilford.

Hanson, C. L., Cigrang, J. A., Harris, M. A., Carle, D. L., Relyea, G., & Burghen, G. A. (1989). Coping styles in youths with insulin-dependent diabetes mellitus. *Journal of Consulting and Clinical Psychology, 57,* 644–651.

Hanson, C. L., DeGuire, M. J., Schinkel, A. M., Henggeler, S. W., & Burghen, G. A. (1992). Comparing social learning and family systems correlates of adaptation in youths with IDDM. *Journal of Pediatric Psychology, 17,* 555–572.

Hanson, C. L., Henggeler, S. W., Harris, M. A., Burghen, G. A., & Moore, M. (1989). Family system variables and the health status of adolescents with IDDM. *Health Psychology, 8,* 239–253.

Hartup, W. W. (1989). Social relationships and their developmental significance. *American Psychologist, 44,* 120–126.

Hauser, S. T., Jacobson, A. M., Lavori, P., & Wolfsdorf, J. I. (1990). Adherence among children and adolescents with insulin-dependent diabetes mellitus over a four-year longitudinal follow-up: II. Immediate and long-term linkages with the family milieu. *Journal of Pediatric Psychology, 15,* 527–542.

Hauser, S. T., Jacobson, A. M., Wertlieb, D., Weiss-Perry, B., Follansbee, D., Wolfsdorf, J. I., Herskowitz, R. D., Houlihan, J., & Rajapark, D. C. (1986). Children with recently diagnosed diabetes: Interactions with their families. *Health Psychology, 5,* 273–296.

Hauser, S. T., Pollets, D., Turner, B., Jacobson, A., Powers, S., & Noam, G. (1979). Ego development and self-esteem in diabetic adolescents. *Diabetes Care, 2,* 465–471.

Jacobson, A. M., Hauser, S. T., Lavori, P., & Wolfsdorf, J. (1990). Adherence among children and adolescents with insulin-dependent diabetes mellitus over a four-year longitudinal follow-up: I. The influence of patient coping and adjustment. *Journal of Pediatric Psychology, 15,* 511–526.

Jessop, D. J., & Stein, R. E. (1983). A noncategorical approach to psychosocial research. *Journal of Psychosocial Oncology, 1,* 61–64.

Jessop, D. J., & Stein, R. E. (1985). Uncertainty and its relation to the psychological and social correlates of chronic illness in children. *Social Science and Medicine, 20,* 993–999.

Jessop, D. J., & Stein, R. E. (1994). Providing comprehensive health care to children with chronic illness. *Pediatrics, 93,* 602–607.

Johnson, S. B. (1988). Psychological aspects of childhood diabetes. *Journal of Child Psychology and Psychiatry, 29,* 729–738.

Kager, V. A., & Holden, E. W. (1992). Preliminary investigation of the direct and moderating effects of family and individual variables on the adjustment of children and adolescents with diabetes. *Journal of Pediatric Psychology, 17,* 491–502.

Kaplan, S. L., Busner, J., Weinhold, C., & Lenon, P. (1987). Depressive symptoms in children and adolescents with cancer: A longitudinal study. *Journal of the American Academy of Child and Adolescent Psychiatry, 26,* 782–787.

Kashani, J. H., Koenig, P., Shepperd, J. A., Wilfley, D., & Morris, D. A. (1988). Psychopathology and self-concept in asthmatic children. *Journal of Pediatric Psychology, 13,* 509–520.

Kazak, A. E., & Meadows, A. T. (1989). Families of young adolescents who have survived cancer: Social–emotional adjustment, adaptability, and social support. *Journal of Pediatric Psychology, 14,* 175–191.

Kliewer, W., & Lewis, H. (1995). Family influences on coping processes in children and adolescents with sickle cell disease. *Journal of Pediatric Psychology, 20,* 511–525.

Kliewer, W., Sandler, I. N., & Wolchik, S. (1994). Family socialization of threat appraisal and coping: Coaching, modeling, and family context. In K. Hurrelmann & F. Festmann (Eds.), *Social networks and social support in childhood and adolescence* (pp. 271–291). Berlin: Walter de Gruyter.

Koocher, G. P. (1984). Terminal care and survivorship in pediatric chronic illness. *Clinical Psychology Review, 4,* 571–583.

Koocher, G. G. P., & O'Malley, J. E. (1981). *The Damocles syndrome: Psychological consequences of surviving childhood cancer.* New York: McGraw-Hill.

Korsch, B. M., & Fine, R. (1985). Chronic kidney disease. In N. Hobbs & J. M. Perrin (Eds.), *Issues in the care of children with chronic illness* (pp. 282–298). San Francisco: Jossey-Bass.

Kubly, L. S., & McClellan, M. S. (1984). Effects of self-care instruction on asthmatic children. *Issues in Comprehensive Pediatric Nursing, 7,* 121–130.

LaGreca, A. M., & Varni, J. W. (1993). Editorial: Interventions in pediatric psychology: A look toward the future. *Journal of Pediatric Psychology, 18,* 667–679.

Lavigne, J. V., & Faier-Routman, J. (1992). Psychological adjustment to pediatric physical disorders: A meta-analytic review. *Journal of Pediatric Psychology, 18,* 133–157.

Lazarus, R. S., & Folkman, S. (1984). *Stress, appraisal, and coping.* New York: Springer.

Lemanek, K. L., Moore, S. L., Gresham, F. M., Williamson, D. A., & Kelley, M. L. (1986). Psychological adjustment of children with sickle cell anemia. *Journal of Pediatric Psychology, 11,* 397–426.

Lewis, H., & Kliewer, W. (1996). Hope, coping, and psychological and physical adjustment among children with sickle cell disease: Tests of mediator and moderator models. *Journal of Pediatric Psychology, 21,* 25–41.

Mason, P. J., Olson, R. A., Myers, J. G., Huszti, H. C., & Kenning, M. (1992). AIDS and hemophilia: Implications for interventions with families. In M. C. Roberts & J. L. Wallander (Eds.), *Family issues in pediatric psychology* (pp. 95–109). Hillsdale, NJ: Erlbaum.

McAnarney, E. R. (1985). Social maturation. A challenge for handicapped and chronically ill adolescents. *Journal of Adolescent Health Care, 6,* 90–101.

McCracken, M. J. (1984). Cystic fibrosis in adolescence. In R. Blum (Ed.), *Chronic illness and disabilities in childhood and adolescence* (pp. 397–427). New York: Grune & Stratton.

Moos, R. H., & Billings, A. G. (1982). Conceptualizing and measuring coping resources and processes. In L. Goldberger & S. Breznitz (Eds.), *Handbook of stress: Theoretical and clinical aspects* (pp. 212–230). New York: Free Press.

Mrazek, D., Anderson, I., & Strunk, R. (1985). Disturbed emotional development of severely asthmatic pre-school children. In J. E. Stevenson (Ed.), *Recent research in developmental psychopathology* (pp. 81–93). Oxford: Pergamon.

Mulhern, R. K., Carpentieri, S., Shema, S., Stone, P., & Fairclough, D. (1993). Factors associated with social and behavioral problems among children recently diagnosed with brain tumor. *Journal of Pediatric Psychology, 18,* 339–350.

Murch, R. L., & Cohen, L. H. (1989). Relationships among life stress, perceived family environment, and the psychological distress of spina bifida adolescents. *Journal of Pediatric Psychology, 14,* 193–214.

Newacheck, P. A., & Stoddard, J. J. (1994). Prevalence and impact of multiple childhood chronic illnesses. *Journal of Pediatrics, 124,* 40–48.

Newacheck, P. A., & Taylor, W. R. (1992). Childhood chronic illness: Prevalence, severity, and impact. *American Journal of Public Health, 82,* 364–371.

Noll, R. B., Bukowski, W. M., Davies, W. H., Koontz, K., & Kulkarni, R. (1993). Adjustment in the peer system of adolescents with cancer: A two-year study. *Journal of Pediatric Psychology, 18,* 351–364.

Noll, R. B., Ris, M. D., Davies, W. H., Bukowski, W. M., & Koontz, K. (1992). Social interactions between children with cancer or sickle cell disease and their peers: Teacher ratings. *Journal of Developmental and Behavioral Pediatrics, 13,* 187–193.

Perrin, E. C., Ayoub, C. C., & Willett, J. B. (1993). In the eyes of the beholder: Family and maternal influences on perceptions of adjustment of children with a chronic illness. *Developmental and Behavioral Pediatrics, 14,* 94–105.

Piaget, J. (1952). *The origins of intelligence in children*. New York: International Universities Press.

Pumariega, A. J., Pearson, D. A., & Seilheimer, D. K. (1993). Family and childhood adjustment in cystic fibrosis. *Journal of Child and Family Studies, 2,* 109–118.

Quittner, A. L., DiGirolamo, A. M., Michel, M., & Eigen, H. (1992). Parental response to cystic fibrosis: A contextual analysis of the diagnosis phase. *Journal of Pediatric Psychology, 17,* 683–704.

Ross, C. K., Lavigne, J. V., Hayford, J. R., Berry, S. L., Sinacore, J. M., & Pachman, L. M. (1993). Psychological factors affecting reported pain in juvenile rheumatoid arthritis. *Journal of Pediatric Psychology, 18,* 561–573.

Rovet, J. F., Ehrlich, R. M., Czuchta, D., & Akler, M. (1993). Psychoeducational characteristics of children and adolescents with insulin-dependent diabetes mellitus. *Journal of Learning Disabilities, 26,* 7–22.

Sanders, M. R., Shepherd, R. W., Cleghorn, G., & Woolford, H. (1994). The treatment of recurrent abdominal pain in children: A controlled comparison of cognitive–behavioral family intervention and standard pediatric care. *Journal of Consulting and Clinical Psychology, 62,* 306–314.

Satin, W., LaGreca, A. M., Zigo, M. Z., & Skyler, J. S. (1989). Diabetes in adolescence: Effects of multifamily group intervention and parent simulation of diabetes. *Journal of Pediatric Psychology, 14,* 259–275.

Silver, E. J., Coupey, S. M., & Bauman, L. J. (1992). Effects of a peer counseling training intervention on psychological functioning of adolescents. *Journal of Adolescent Research, 7,* 110–128.

Stein, R. E., & Jessop, D. J. (1982). A noncategorical approach to chronic childhood illness. *Public Health Reports, 97,* 354–362.

Stein, R. E., & Jessop, D. J. (1989). What diagnosis does not tell: The case for a noncategorical approach to chronic illness in childhood. *Social Science and Medicine, 29,* 769–778.

Stein, R. E., Jessop, D. J., & Ireys, H. T. (1988). Prevention of emotional problems in children with chronic illness and their families. In L. A. Bond & B. M. Wagner (Eds.), *Families in transition: Primary prevention programs that work* (pp. 286–308). Newbury Park, CA: Sage.

Sullivan, B. J. (1978). Self-esteem and depression in adolescent diabetic girls. *Diabetes Care, 1,* 18–22.

Tew, B., & Laurence, K. (1985). Possible personality problems among 10-year old spina bifida children. *Child: Care, Health, and Development, 11,* 375–390.

Thompson, R. J., Jr. (1985). Coping with the stress of chronic illness. In A. N. O'Quinn (Ed.), *Management of chronic disorders of childhood* (pp. 11–41). Boston: G. K. Hall.

Thompson, R. J., Gil, K. M., Burbach, D. J., Keith, B. R., & Kinney, T. R. (1993). Role of child and maternal processes in the psychological adjustment of children with sickle cell disease. *Journal of Consulting and Clinical Psychology, 61,* 468–474.

Thompson, R. J., Gustafson, K. E., Hamlett, K. W., & Spock, A. (1992). Psychological adjustment of children with cystic fibrosis: The role of child cognitive processes and maternal adjustment. *Journal of Pediatric Psychology, 17,* 741–755.

Thompson, R. J., Hodges, K., & Hamlett, K. W. (1990). A matched comparison of adjustment in children with cystic fibrosis and psychiatrically referred and nonreferred children. *Journal of Pediatric Psychology, 15,* 745–759.

Ungerer, J., Horgan, B., Chaitow, J., & Champion, J. B. (1988). Psychosocial functioning in children and young adults with juvenile arthritis. *Journal of Pediatrics, 81,* 195–202.

Varni, J. W., Katz, E. R., Colegrove, R., Jr., & Dolgin, M. (1993). The impact of social skills training on the adjustment of children with newly diagnosed cancer. *Journal of Pediatric Psychology, 18,* 751–767.

Varni, J. W., Katz, E. R., Colegrove, R., & Dolgin, M. (1994). Perceived social support and adjustment of children with newly diagnosed cancer. *Developmental and Behavioral Pediatrics, 15,* 20–26.

Walker, L. S., Van Slyke, D. A., & Newbrough, J. R. (1992). Family resources and stress: A comparison of families of children with cystic fibrosis, diabetes, and mental retardation. *Journal of Pediatric Psychology, 17,* 327–343.

Wallander, J. L., Varni, J. W., Babani, L. V., Banis, H. T., & Wilcox, K. T. (1989). Family resources as resistance factors for psychological maladjustment in chronically ill and handicapped children. *Journal of Pediatric Psychology, 14,* 157–173.

Weist, M. D., Finney, J. W., Barnard, M. U., Davis, C. D., & Ollendick, T. H. (1993). Empirical selection of psychosocial treatment targets for children and adolescents with diabetes. *Journal of Pediatric Psychology, 18*, 11–28.

Weisz, J. R., Rothbaum, F. M., & Blackburn, T. C. (1984). Standing out and standing in: The psychology of control in American and Japan. *American Psychologist, 39*, 955–969.

Wertlieb, D., Hauser, S. T., & Jacobson, A. M. (1986). Adaptation to diabetes: Behavior symptoms and family context. *Journal of Pediatric Psychology, 11*, 463–479.

Wertlieb, D. L., Jacobson, A. M., & Hauser, S. T. (1990). The child with diabetes: A developmental stress and coping perspective. In P. T. Costa, Jr. & G. R. VandenBos (Eds.), *Psychological aspects of serious illness: Chronic conditions, fatal diseases, and clinical care* (pp. 65–101). Washington, DC: American Psychological Association.

Wilson, S. R., Mitchell, J. H., Rolnick, S., & Fish, L. (1993). Effective and ineffective management behaviors of parents of infants and young children with asthma. *Journal of Pediatric Psychology, 18*, 63–81.

Worshel, F. F., Nolan, B. F., Willson, V. L., Purser, J. S., Copeland, D. R., & Pfefferbaum, B. (1988). Assessment of depression in children with cancer. *Journal of Pediatric Psychology, 13*, 101–112.

Wysocki, T. (1993). Associations among teen–parent relationships, metabolic control, and adjustment to diabetes in adolescents. *Journal of Pediatric Psychology, 18*, 441–452.

11

The Nexus of Culture and Sensory Loss
Coping with Deafness

MARK T. GREENBERG, LILIANA J. LENGUA,
and ROSEMARY CALDERON

What is it like to be a small child,
In a school, in a room void of sound—
With a teacher who talks and talks and talks;
And then when she does come around to you,
She expects you to know what she's said?
You have to be deaf to understand.

What is it like to be curious,
To thirst for knowledge you can call your own,
With an inner desire that's set on fire—
And you ask a brother, sister, or friend
Who looks in answer and says, "Never Mind"?

You have to be deaf to understand.
What is it like to comprehend
Some nimble fingers that paint the scene,
And make you smile and feel serene,
With the "spoken word" of the moving hand
That makes you part of the word at large?

You have to be deaf to understand.
What is it like to "hear" a hand?
Yes, you have to be deaf to understand.
[excerpts taken from poem by Willard Madsen,
professor of journalism, Gallaudet]

The development and adaptation of deaf children and their families is an area of study that is fascinating and complex. Having a significant hearing loss may have radically different consequences for the child and his or her family, de-

MARK T. GREENBERG • Human Development and Family Studies, Penn State University, University Park, Pennsylvania 16802.   LILIANA J. LENGUA • Department of Psychology, University of Washington, Seattle, Washington 98195.   ROSEMARY CALDERON • Department of Psychiatry, Children's Hospital Medical Center (CHMC), Seattle, Washington 98195.

Handbook of Children's Coping: Linking Theory and Intervention, edited by Wolchik and Sandler. Plenum Press, New York, 1997.

pending on such factors as the hearing status of the child's parents, the etiology of deafness, the age at which deafness occurred, the type of communication approach(es) adopted by the family, the type of schooling that is selected, and the amount and nature of contact that both the deaf child and his or her parents have with other deaf children and adults. All of these factors (and more) will influence how the child and family perceive deafness and its social, educational, and vocational consequences.

As a group, deaf children and adolescents are at risk for a number of adverse outcomes. These include low academic achievement, delays in some cognitive and social–cognitive processes, as well as higher rates of social maladaptation and psychological distress and disorder (Greenberg & Kusche, 1989; Marschark, 1993). However, not all deaf children develop adjustment problems, and the impact of deafness is mediated and moderated by several factors, including the quality of family environment, parental adaptation to deafness, family coping, the nature of school and community resources (including the deaf community), as well as the child's own characteristics and transactions with his or her ecology. Given this, it is important to identify factors that play a role in children's adaptive adjustment to deafness, and individual and family coping may be one such variable.

In this chapter, we present a conceptualization of coping that we have applied to deaf children and their families. In doing so, we inform the reader of the unique issues faced by deaf children, discuss the risks and stresses faced by deaf children and their families, and discuss what is currently known from empirical research regarding factors that influence outcomes in this population. We will first discuss contextual and cultural issues that impact the deaf child and his or her family. We then review research on social–cognition and personality research in deaf children and youth. Given this background, we then propose a conceptual model of coping as it fits within a larger process model for understanding factors that influence the development of deaf children and youth. Finally, we review two studies that examine aspects of our overall model. The first study investigates how parental stresses and coping resources affect family and child development in middle childhood. The second study reviews a school-based prevention program intended to improve the coping and adjustment of deaf children.

CONTEXTUAL ISSUES IN DEAFNESS

There have been a number of studies investigating children's coping with physical disabilities or chronic illnesses (see Chapter 10, this volume), and coping with deafness shares some similarities with these other areas. For example, as discussed by Kliewer (Chapter 10, this volume), most research in coping with chronic illness or disabilities note that families of these children experience more stressors and the children themselves are faced with more daily challenges or hassles relative to normative populations. Also, there is evidence that the psychological adjustment of these children is related to appraisals of disability- or illness-specific stressors and the types of coping strategies (active/approach vs. avoidant) they use. Thus, on the face of it, one might think that substituting "deafness" for other disability terms would make little difference in terms of children's coping and adaptation; however, this is not the case. This is because deafness can be defined not only by its sensory/medical consequences (degree of hearing loss, sound reception) or its educational/functional consequences, but also from a sociological or cultural perspective. For the reader to understand what this means, it will be necessary to begin by pointing out four distinctive features of deafness.

Deaf Culture

The fact that many deaf persons communicate with each other manually and are believed to have done so for all of recorded history has a profound influence on the lives of deaf persons. Although the topic has been hotly debated as to whether deafness is a "defined" culture, the fact that it has its own language and communicative style is an essential fact (Gannon, 1981; Padden & Humphries, 1988). Although only recently legitimized by linguistics (Baker & Cokely, 1980), native sign languages (in the case of the United States, American Sign Language) have been the glue for cultural ties and intergenerational transmission of culture for deaf people throughout the world.

Furthermore, not only language but a variety of other factors help to define deaf culture and identity. A few exemplars will suffice.* First, the great majority of deaf persons marry and/or live with other deaf persons during adult life (Schein & Delk, 1974). Second, there are numerous organizations of deaf persons in America and throughout the world that uniquely connect deaf persons for political, athletic, and cultural affairs (Gannon, 1981; Garretson, 1994; Nash & Nash, 1981; Schein, 1989). Third, for over 100 years in America, deaf persons have had their own university that has undergone significant cultural transformations from a institution directed by hearing persons for deaf people to one that is directed and advised primarily by deaf persons (Erting, 1994; Gannon, 1993).

Intergenerational Discontinuity of Deafness

Given the richness of deaf culture, one might expect significant cross-generational, familial continuity; however, this is not the case. Of the estimated 65,000 profoundly deaf children in America (Schildroth & Hotto, 1993), over 90% of deaf children are born to hearing parents. Further, most deaf parents bear hearing children. Although there are numerous forms of deafness that are genetic, there are few forms that result from dominant genes, and relatively rarely do two deaf persons marry who carry the same recessive genes. Although studies show that for as many as 50% of children the specific reason for deafness is unknown (Marschark, 1993), the great majority of causes of deafness are

---

*There are variety of other defining features of deaf culture. The interested reader is referred to following sources (Erting, 1994; Padden & Humphries, 1988; Schein, 1989).

due to factors that occur in the prenatal or perinatal period, or in early child-hood. Thus, one dilemma faced by a majority of deaf children is that they are likely to become part of (consciously adopt) a clearly defined minority culture in which there are no other members in their family. This "recognition" that deaf children of hearing parents are like "minority" children, who will belong to their own culture and have their own language, has broad implications for both child and parental coping. In their family of origin, they have no other minority members to show them that culture and language. Further, to be a successful member of society and gain the full access to its richness and oppor-tunities, they will need to learn to live at least to some extent in both worlds: that of the hearing and that of the deaf (Kannapell, 1994).

Deafness and Schooling

For over two centuries, deaf persons have been educated in unique school facilities in which language and culture are transmitted. Regardless of whether native sign language and culture were promoted, tolerated, or banned, the residential school provided the ecology for the cultural socialization of younger deaf children by older deaf children and adults. Deaf children who had little understanding of their deafness except that they wore hearing aids and had difficulty speaking, when placed in a residential school were introduced to a world that provided them with a unique and valued identity, one that could not be bestowed by their hearing parents. Thus, a great deal more than traditional educational subjects was attained at these schools. Of equal value was a sense of belonging and identity born of a new-found language and cultural history; with these new tools, a revised perception of "hearing" culture and how it might be circumvented and/or accommodated was gained.

Recent Changes in the Schooling of Deaf Children: Familial Impact

Given the centrality of both the family and school for the development of deaf children, a review of recent changes in the relations between families and schools is necessary. During the past two to three decades, there have been dramatic shifts in the nature of schooling for deaf children. These shifts have led to new and more important roles for parents in the educational develop-ment and social–emotional adjustment of their children, and thus, highlight the importance of the family's coping/adjustment to deafness. Three major shifts in educational policy have altered placement. The first is the "revolu-tion" in deaf education that led to the use of some form of manual communica-tion as a central component of schooling. In some cases, this has led to signifi-cant improvements in family communication. As a result, parents have become more involved with their child and his or her education. As parents feel more competent to communicate, and as local schools offer programs that utilize Total Communication (in one of its many forms),* there have been less com-

---

*Total Communication is a philosophy that all possible modes of communication should be incor-porated into the education of deaf children. It has been actualized in a variety of forms that invariably include a form of manual communication in addition to speech and auditory training.

pelling reasons for sending children to distant locations to be educated (e.g., residential schools).

The second change in policy in America is the result of the enactment of Public Law 94-142. This law authorized local school districts (regardless of the number of deaf and hearing-impaired children in their catchment area) to develop local plans for educating deaf and other disabled children. Regardless of the heterogeneity in the "quality" of these plans and the controversial nature of defining "the least restrictive environment" for deaf children, the effects of this law have been to place more responsibility on the local schools and families. Finally, Public Law 99-457, enacted in 1986, mandates that family members should be the central focus of plans for early intervention.

Increasing numbers of children are now being educated in neighborhood schools and are remaining at home rather than residing in state residential schools (Moores, Cerney & Garcia, 1990). Thus, there has been a significant decrease in residential school enrollment for deaf children. A comparison of school attendance for 1974 (pre-PL 94-142) and 1984 revealed that during that 10-year period, public residential school enrollment declined by 18.3% and private residential school enrollment declined by 69%, whereas public day classes increased by 30%. In addition to a decline in public residential school enrollment, 40% of those attending a residential program are now day students, commuting to school from home (Moores, 1987). In the most recent report (Schildroth & Hotto, 1993), residential school attendance declined an additional 6%. Approximately 70% of deaf children now attend local public schools. For most elementary school-aged children, the deaf school institution and staff are no longer the child's "home and family." Deaf children remain in the "hearing community" and are residing with their hearing families much longer, and fewer deaf children are being introduced into the "deaf community" through the cross-generational process of attending a residential state educational institution (Mowry, 1994).

Appraisal and Identity: Defining Deafness

A central notion in coping research is that the nature of one's appraisal of an event will have significant consequences for the process of coping. For this reason, deafness presents an extraordinarily interesting case because there are multiple levels at which appraisal and attribution will affect social–interpersonal processes. First, how both the child and parent appraise deafness itself will have important developmental consequences for how environments (both academic and interpersonal) are selected, what stressors will be faced, and what culturally based solutions will be offered and accepted. Thus, the study of coping in both the deaf child and her or his family needs to include consideration of cultural issues (minority status, minority language, bilingualism), as well as medical and functional features of a loss of sensory capacity.*

---

*It is important for the reader to note that we intentionally chose not to use either the words "handicap" or "disabled," since they both imply a deficiency. There are many deaf people who do not appraise themselves in this way; they only acknowledge a single sensory loss (Padden & Humphries, 1988).

At every turn in the study of deaf persons and their families, one is met with alternative worldviews that alter the meaning of deafness. There is no better venue to comprehend this than in its very definition. *Deafness, hearing-impaired,* and *hard-of-hearing* are hotly debated terms that in part are influenced by whether one is taking a medical, psychological, or cultural perspective (Marschark, 1993; Padden & Humphries, 1988). The medical definition of deafness is based on measurement of audiological function. Those individuals with 70 and above decibel loss (severe or profound losses) are generally considered deaf because their hearing loss, even when strongly amplified, in many cases does not permit them to understand speech (Meadow-Orlans, 1987). Medically related professionals often use the term *hearing-impaired* interchangeably with the term *deaf,* or characterize an individual as hard-of-hearing depending on the specifics of the audiogram (degree of hearing loss in the speech range). The psychological perspective focuses more on the functional significance of the hearing loss, that is, to what degree does it impact day-to-day functioning. Thus, the term *deaf* is more likely to be used when a person cannot rely exclusively on speech and is likely to use a manual mode of communication. In contrast, the terms *hearing-impaired* and *hard-of-hearing* are more often used with a child who benefits from auditory stimulation and relies on sound and speech for communication, independent of their extent of hearing loss.

The cultural perspective is symbolized by the use of the word, *Deaf,* with an upper case "D." It indicates a particular group of deaf people who share a common language and culture. They hold a set of beliefs about themselves and their connection to the larger society. This definition distinguishes these "Deaf" people from other persons with hearing losses of various levels who "live in the hearing culture" and do not identify themselves with "Deaf culture." The latter group also includes some persons who have progressive hearing losses or are late deafened (Woodward, 1972). Those who identify themselves as Deaf do not refer to themselves as hearing-impaired or hard-of-hearing, although they may have only a moderate hearing impairment from an audiological standpoint. These worldviews of hearing loss often clash, and they present a confusing set of alternative models of defining deafness.

There are two further aspects of "definitional identity" that may affect appraisal and coping. First, these definitions may come from outside of the family (professionals), the family's own labeling, or the self-declared identity of the deaf child. Second, there is often a temporally ordered, "developmental" sequence that becomes part of the adaptation process itself. The infant or young child's hearing loss is most often initially defined from a medical perspective; that is, medical tests are performed to determine the level of hearing loss, and parents are provided a set of numbers that characterize that loss. The physicians and audiologists may use these numbers to determine a specific cutoff point in deciding whether to refer a child for intervention, as well as in deciding what label to use in describing this sensory loss. In contrast, hearing parents, and most teachers and other professionals working with the child, generally adopt a psychological or functional perspective toward the hearing loss and how it may impact that child's learning, behavior, and relationships. Last, as the child grows into adolescence and young adulthood, his or her hearing loss or deafness takes on cultural connotations related to the individual's identity formation and lifestyle choices (Carty, 1994; Stone & Stirling, 1994). Thus, regardless of the nature of the sensory loss, one young adult may identify himself as hearing-impaired, handicapped, and/or as missing a needed sensory capacity, while another person may identify herself as Deaf, and that deafness provides identity through involvement with other Deaf persons. Thus, the individual's self-definition may play an important role in how his or her deafness is experienced, how the individual appraises and copes with daily events or hassles, and ultimately the individual's psychological adjustment.

The definitional complexity faced by the deaf child and his or her family is significant and has been faced also by researchers in deafness. Because of the need for a defining feature of deafness, most research has grouped children by their degree of hearing impairment. In most instances, in this chapter we will refer to children with medically and psychologically defined deafness, i.e., those children with hearing losses of greater than 70 decibels (severe to profound deficits) and whose hearing impairment significantly impacts their development and social interactions.

Personality Development, Social Competence, and Maladjustment in Deaf Children

Early studies in the "psychology of deafness" led to a stereotypic characterization in which deaf children and adults generally were seen as impulsive, immature, and egocentric in their social orientations. However, these characterizations were likely due to a combination of factors, including generalizing from clinical populations, the use of inappropriate assessment measures, and the inability of examiners to use the deaf person's best modes of communication (Greenberg & Kusche, 1989). It is now obvious that deaf persons vary widely in their characteristics, personalities, motives, and interests. Thus, the notion of a "deaf personality" has been invalidated. However, because many deaf children (and adults) share developmental experiences that are less than optimal, including early and continued communicative deprivation, difficulties in their families of origin, less than adequate educational experiences, and continuing social stigma and prejudice, a significant portion of deaf persons show developmental misintegrations of language, cognition, and affect (see Greenberg & Kusche, 1993).

Social Cognition

Many deaf children show delays in numerous subdomains of the construct of social–cognition. Although there are wide individual differences among deaf children, and there are many who do not show any delays, compared to hearing children they do show significant deficits as a group in such areas as impulse control (Harris, 1978), empathy development (Bachara, Raphael, & Phelan, 1980), role-taking ability (Kusche & Greenberg, 1983), the ability to interpret facial expressions (Odom, Blanton, & Laukhuf, 1973; Pietzrak, 1981; Sugarman, 1969), social-problem solving (Coady, 1984; Luckner & McNeil, 1994), social attributions (Kusche, Garfield, & Greenberg, 1983), and moral development (DeCaro & Emerton, 1978). In addition, deaf children often experience important gaps in understanding social interactions in the hearing world, in part due to sensory loss and its attendant deprivation of incidental learning (Marschark, 1993). Both Meadow (1980) and Greenberg and Kusche (1989) have provided extensive reviews of this literature.

Personality

A variety of studies have found that, compared to hearing adolescents, deaf adolescents have more external locus of control (Blanton & Nunnally, 1964; Bodner & Johns, 1976; Dowaliby, Burke, & McKee, 1983), lower self-esteem (Garrison, Emerton, & Layne, 1978), and greater learned helplessness (McCrone, 1979). Because few measures of personality have been effectively translated into sign language, there has been a paucity of recent research on this topic.

While comparisons between hearing and deaf children illustrate the need to improve the social and cognitive conditions of deaf children, they unfortunately focus on a deficit model approach to deafness (Carver & Doe, 1989). In contrast, a focus on the assets and conditions that promote healthy social and cognitive outcomes is essential for the development of preventive interventions.

Childhood Psychiatric Disorder

At present, there are a disproportionately high number of deaf children with adjustment problems, as well as serious mental health problems (Hindley, Hill, McGuigan, & Kitson, 1994; Meadow & Trybus, 1979). According to Meadow and Trybus's (1979) review, the prevalence of moderate and severe emotional disorders in this population has been reported to range from 8% in a survey of 44,000 children (Jensema & Trybus, 1975) to 20 to 30% in smaller, clinical–experimental investigations (Freeman, Malkin, & Hastings, 1975; Meadow, 1980; Schlesinger & Meadow, 1972; Vernon, 1969). It appears that the types of problems found with deaf children are similar to those of hearing children (Hindley et al., 1994; Hirshoren & Schaittjer, 1979). However, some studies have found additional deaf-specific factors that include problems in communication and isolation (Reivich & Rothrock, 1972).

Summary

In spite of significant improvements throughout the world in the education of deaf children, there is little question that many deaf children experience communicative and social deprivation that affect both cognitive and social development. As a result, there is an unusually high incidence of deaf children who experience communicative delays, and these, in turn, may lead to both delays in social–cognitive skills and psychosocial disorders that range from poor peer relationships to more serious behavioral and emotional difficulties. Although some conditions that cause deafness (genetic, prenatal, and postnatal) may also present risk factors for social adjustment and disorder, there is little reason to believe that the general population of deaf persons are at significantly greater risk for such disorders solely due to their sensory loss.*

Utilizing a Stress and Coping Model for Conceptualizing the Influence of Deafness

There are a number of rationales for why we have found a stress and coping model useful in understanding the effects of deafness. These are enumerated below.

Major Life Stresses Unique to Deaf Children and Families

Similar to hearing individuals and families, deaf children and youth experience major life stressors that may be very debilitating, e.g., deaths of family members, illness, divorce, and so forth. Deaf persons also experience a number of unique life stressors that concern consolidation of their identity at critical times, e.g., at family separation and entrance to a residential school, upon peer rejection in mainstream school contexts, or at a variety of other possible times that are unique to each person.

For the hearing parent of a deaf child, there are also unique challenges that are best characterized as "role strain" (Pearlin & Schooler, 1978). That is, parenting a deaf child could best be considered a potentially chronic stressor (Calderon & Greenberg, 1993; Quittner, Glueckauf, & Jackson, 1990) that presents a series of developmental, educational, and sometimes medical challenges. There are a number of reasons for this chronic stress. First, from a phenomenological perspective, most parents report that having a deaf child is a difficult adjustment (Greenberg, 1983; Gregory, 1976; Schlesinger & Meadow, 1972). Second, communication is quite difficult to establish; this is true even if it is also sometimes fun and creative (Meadow-Orlans, 1990). Third, because of these communication issues, parents often feel like they are placed in the role of the teacher instead of the parent. Fourth, deaf children are reported by their parents to be more difficult to manage, especially in the preschool years, because communication is visual and it is more difficult to get their attention. Parents of hearing children are used to using auditory means of maintaining contact (e.g., calling out a last warning or suggestion as children run out the door). Fifth, parents are likely to be learning about a new culture and language. Last, there are always new hurdles for parents to cope with, such as new skills and techniques to enhance the child's development, numerous additional meetings to attend with professionals and parents, ensuring that programs for their child are adequate, and being an advocate for deaf children and deafness. Parents often report that these stresses significantly affect their marriage and relationships with extended family and friends. Quittner et al. (1990) reported that hearing parents of deaf preschoolers reported significantly higher parenting stress, more limited social support networks, and higher emotional distress

---

*A clear exception to this statement is a significant portion of the deaf population who were deafened from rubella during the early 1960s. Rubella not only led to deafness in some cases, but also a mosaic of other disorders that affected the central nervous system, including mental retardation, motor difficulties, and so forth.

than parents of hearing children. They did not examine the effects of these family stressors on the functioning of the deaf children. Interestingly, there has not been a systematic investigation of stresses experienced by families with deaf children nor is there a measure of family stress specific to this experience.

The Experience of Daily Hassles

Many deaf persons are likely to experience more daily, small hassles (minor life stressors) relative to hearing individuals. These are often related to such issues as language and communication differences or deficits, the experience of stigma or prejudice from the hearing culture, and experiences of isolation. How the individual appraises these stressors is a function of such complex factors as cognitive level and understanding, communicative level and competence to map experiences, socialization experience, beliefs about the world (e.g., perceived control), and present psychological state (e.g., morale). The deaf individuals' appraisals of the nature of these daily hassles may have a strong impact on how they choose to cope with the stressors and on their adaptation. For example, communication differences can be viewed as a challenge to express ideas or needs, which might elicit creative problem-solving strategies, or as a threat to being understood or having ones' needs met, which might elicit self-defeating thoughts or avoidance of social contact. Thus, the appraisal of hassles as a challenge may lead to better adaptation, whereas the appraisal of threat may lead to ineffective coping and adjustment problems (Quitnner et al., 1990).

Although there is no empirically based literature on coping with the daily hassles of communication, stigma, and prejudice that accompany the "deaf experience," there are a number of deaf persons who have written eloquent descriptions of the everyday experience of being deaf (Bienvenu, 1994; Bragg, 1989; Heppner, 1992; Jacobs, 1989; Kisor, 1990). In a fascinating project on coping in young deaf adults, Foster (1987) examined the stresses faced by deaf college graduates in the employment context and the different ways that they cope with the issues of communication and isolation with their co-workers. For the student of coping, these are invaluable resources for understanding the experience of deaf adults.

Considerations of Severity and Pathology

While the experience of major and minor life stressors is one reason that a stress and coping model is applicable, there are at least three other rationales for this approach. First, most psychological problems of deaf persons are not major psychoses. Although there is no evidence of elevated rates of schizophrenia (Rainier & Altshuler, 1971), it is believed that a higher proportion of deaf persons experience depression, hopelessness, and other difficulties that would be conceptualized in *Diagnostic and Statistical Manual of Mental Disorders,* 4th ed. (American Psychiatric Association, 1994) (DSM-IV) terms as "adjustment reactions." There has been almost no investigation of the epidemiology of psychiatric disorders in the general deaf population, and while it has been suggested that there are higher rates of addictive behavior disorders, there is little empirical evidence.

Second, within the literature on mental health and deafness, the "pathological model" has reigned supreme and has contained the underlying assumption that deaf persons' personalities are damaged, i.e., that the problem/illness commonly resides solely in the individual rather than the person–environment ecology (Levine, 1981). By utilizing a coping model, ecological and communicative considerations are more clearly conceptualized as a component of both the etiology and the treatment of most psychological problems.

A further reason for adopting a coping model is related to our current knowledge of family functioning with deafness. Research prior to the mid-- 1980s usually adopted a stress–pathology model in which hearing impairment was a stressor or deficit from which pathology was the likely outcome. In most studies, families with deaf children were compared to those with hearing children to demonstrate the negative effects of deafness. This literature is univariate, subject to numerous methodological shortcomings, and absent of theory. Further, the findings did not support a stress–pathology perspective (Calderon & Greenberg, 1993). Instead, the findings indicated a wide range of family and child functioning, with some parents and children at high risk for poor adaptation and some functioning adaptively. Thus, rather than viewing deaf children and their parents as a homogeneous group, it is more useful to determine what differences characterize families and children with differential outcomes. Such an analysis of individual differences needs to be integrated with an examination of how other ecologies (extended family, school, peers, community) transactionally impact the family (Friedrich, Greenberg, & Crnic, 1986).

The Process of Stress and Coping

There are a variety of models that attempt to explain the stress and coping process (Caplan, 1981; Goldberger & Brenitz, 1982; Lazarus, 1966; Pearlin, Lieberman, Menaghan, & Mullan, 1981; Seyle, 1976). Although these models differ on particular points, this process can be summarized in three steps. First, one experiences a stress or stressor (e.g., an external event, thought, emotion). Second, one appraises the meaning and significance of the event. Given a "stressful" appraisal, the individual attempts to mediate or reduce the stress through coping behaviors that are intended to minimize its impact. Finally, if one is "unsuccessful" in coping effectively, psychiatric or medical symptoms or negative changes in interpersonal relationships are likely to occur.

The Mutual Relation of Appraisal and Coping

Appraisal and coping mutually and reciprocally influence one another. Thus, while they can be divided for heuristic purposes, the question of causal direction is like "the chicken and the egg." The coping strategies an individual employs are likely to be influenced by how the individual appraises the stressor (Cohen & Lazarus, 1979). Likewise, the effectiveness of one's coping will influence whether an event is appraised as stressful, benign, or challenging. For example, unsuccessful coping attempts may lead an individual to view stressors with hopelessness or helplessness.

The model we have adopted (and adapted) is primarily drawn from the work of Richard Lazarus and colleagues (Folkman, Schaefer, & Lazarus, 1980; Lazarus & Folkman, 1984). This is a very general model of stress and coping that can be applied to a variety of contexts, and it is especially useful for understanding deaf children and their families. Coping can be defined as attempts to manage (master, tolerate, reduce, minimize) environmental and internal demands, and the conflicts between them, that tax or exceed one's resources (Lazarus & Launier, 1978). It can occur prior to, during, or after a stress or group of stressors. Coping is generally considered to be a state, not a trait. That is, it is a continual, transactional process that is often situation specific (Wrubel, Benner, & Lazarus, 1981).

Lazarus and Launier (1978) have characterized two main types of coping. The first—action-oriented responses (problem-focused strategies)—attempts to change the environmental situation that the individual feels is responsible for the threat or stress. That is, action-oriented coping focuses on the "troubled" person–environment relationship. Examples of action-oriented coping are removing oneself from the stress context, gaining more information, decision making, communicating one's feelings, and interpersonal problem solving (Lazarus & Folkman, 1984).

The second broad type—intrapsychic or palliative forms of coping (emotion-focused strategies)—seeks to modulate or regulate the internal emotional reaction to stress or threat. Examples include cognitive restructuring or redefinition of the situation, minimization, selective focus on positive aspects of the situation, avoidance, utilizing defense mechanisms, and using biofeedback to regulate reactions to stress. Emotion-focused strategies are utilized to alter, suppress, or defend against uncomfortable feelings that are experienced (either consciously or unconsciously) as stressful.

Most often, people use a combination of both active and palliative forms of coping. They often work together, i.e., reducing one's emotional stress may lead to better work performance, which may in turn further reduce one's distress. However, they may also inhibit one another, i.e., denial of the diagnosis of deafness (avoidance) may lead to serious delays in intervention (active/ approach). In addition, the effectiveness of a coping strategy may depend on the match or fit of the strategy with the stressor (Compas, 1987). With low-controllability situations, palliative strategies may be preferable, whereas with controllable situations, action-oriented strategies may be optimal.

Coping Resources

Folkman, Schaefer, and Lazarus (1980) view coping resources as moderators of stress and have delineated four types of coping resources that are thought to interact with the effects of stress as appraised within the individual's cognitive–phenomenological framework (Lazarus & Folkman, 1984). They have categorized the domains of coping resources as (1) problem-solving skills (e.g., seek and analyze information, generate solutions, consider consequences); (2) social networks (e.g., support from and satisfaction with spouse, friends, extended family, neighbors); (3) utilitarian resources (e.g., income, professional services, education); and (4) general and specific beliefs (e.g., self-efficacy, internal locus of control, religiosity, spirituality).* It is important to note that the resources described above are not mutually exclusive; indeed, there is notable overlap. For example, early intervention (a utilitarian resource) also provides social support. Similarly, problem-solving ability is likely to be related to self-efficacy (a general belief). The presence and perception of adequate skills, social support, and utilitarian resources may reduce the stress or threat perceived in an event, increase one's efficacy expectations, and determine the coping strategies employed.

COPING AND CHILDHOOD DEAFNESS: A MODEL

As may now be apparent, characterizing the factors influencing the coping of deaf children and their families is complex. There is the individual's and family's need to cope with the diagnosis of hearing loss or impairment, the stressors introduced into the family, decisions regarding methods of communication and type of schooling, and the daily hassles that present themselves to the family as well as the deaf child. As a result of this complexity, it is important to consider not only the deaf child's coping efforts, but also the coping approach of the child's family, as well as the role of educational and community resources.

Figure 1 presents a working model of major factors affecting family and child adjustment in hearing families with a deaf child. According to this model, child social and academic adjustment is a direct function of both parental adjustment and quality of parenting, as well as the child's affective, behavioral, and cognitive–linguistic skills (ABC skills; see a later section in this chapter for further elaboration of the ABCD model). Further, both parent adjustment/quality and child ABC skills are mediated by coping resources as specified in Lazarus and Folkman's model (i.e., problem-solving skills, social support, use of utilitarian resources, and general and specific beliefs). Thus, parents who carefully thinking through problems, engage a community of supportive and knowledgeable persons, utilize effective personal and community resources, and believe that their decisions are critical to their child's development are likely to have children who show better adjustment. Further, for hearing parents, early, positive contact with a variety of deaf adults is hypothesized to create healthy parental appraisals of the meaning of their child's deafness, which, in turn, facilitates their use of other coping resources including the effective acquisition of sign language for both themselves and their child and understanding the "cultural gap" often faced by deaf children as they develop their identity (Carver, 1988; Freeman, Boese, & Carbin, 1981; Hill, 1993; Stone, & Stirling, 1994). Similarly, we hypothesize that positive contact between the deaf child and the deaf community assists in the construction of a healthy identity, which, especially during adolescence, impacts ABC skills and

*Folkman et al. consider a fifth resource domain of health–energy–morale. We consider this domain to be best viewed as an outcome or likely mediating result of the other coping resources. However, it is acknowledged that this factor will also reciprocally influence the utilization of other coping resources.

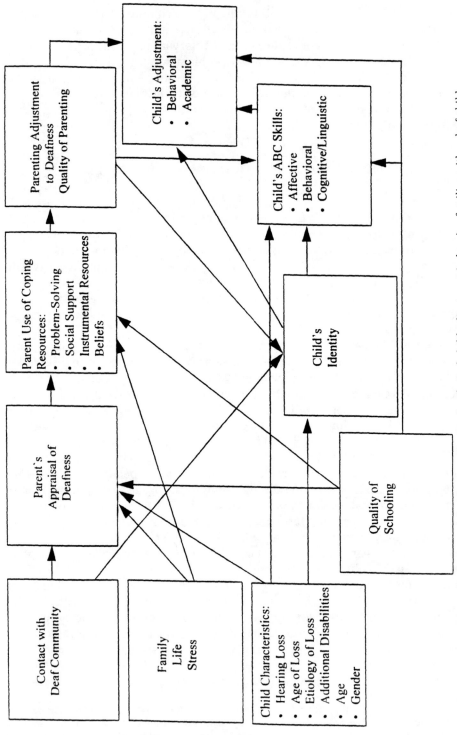

Figure 1. Working model of factors affecting family and child adjustment in hearing families with a deaf child.

adjustment (Bet-Chava, 1993). Obtaining quality schooling for the deaf child that combines a challenging educational program with contact with a deaf peer group is also believed to impact parental appraisal and coping, child ABC skills, and ultimate child adjustment. Finally, those variables listed at the left of Fig. 1 may operate as moderators of these processes. Thus, degree of general negative life stress (e.g., family instability, family violence, unemployment, frequent family relocations) as well as characteristics of the deaf child (degree of hearing loss, etiology of hearing loss, age at hearing loss, additional disabilities, age, and gender) may lead to different processes and outcomes for both the child and family.

Few of the complex relations specified in Fig. 1 have been substantiated by empirical research; most of these hypothesized connections are drawn from the results of fragmented empirical findings and the wisdom of many persons working in the field of childhood deafness. In the remaining sections of this chapter, we review two projects that have attempted to investigate portions of this overall model.

Family Coping and Child Outcome

Parent and Child Psychological Outcomes

Although a great deal has been written about the needs of families with deaf children (Lederberg, 1993; Luterman, 1987) and a variety of models of the developmental processes of family life have been proposed, there has been little quality research on the *multivariate* nature of family coping with deafness. The field has been plagued by inadequate, univariate conceptualizations of family influence (Calderon & Greenberg, 1993). However, there are clear indications that parent problem-solving skills, social supports, and beliefs about deafness all play significant roles in the parents' own adjustment, as well as that of their children (see below, as well as Calderon & Greenberg, 1997, for a review of this literature).

In our own laboratory, we have conducted a series of studies examining the role of coping resources in the development of hearing families with deaf children. These projects began with a study indicating the powerful effect of early intervention programs for families of young deaf children. The study included a quasi-experimental posttest design and compared 12 families who had received a model intervention to 12 families who had received existing community services. Within the intervention program studied, parents received utilitarian resources (access to professionals, teaching instructional techniques, sign language classes, seminars on deafness) and access to a social network that included hearing parents as well as deaf adults. As a result, parents demonstrated differences in attitudes, beliefs, and knowledge regarding deafness (Greenberg, 1983; Greenberg, Calderon, & Kusche, 1984). It appears that the provision of social support may be especially important during the months and years just after diagnosis (Lederberg & Mobley, 1990; MacTurk, Meadow-Orlans, Koester, & Spencer, 1993; Meadow-Orlans, 1990, 1994; Meadow-Orlans & Steinberg, 1993).

More recently, we have extensively studied a sample of 36 families and their school-aged children and investigated part of the coping model described above (Calderon, 1988). The majority of the families were Caucasian, middle-class, and married. All participating families used a total communication approach with their deaf child, and all the children were living at home and attending self-contained classrooms for deaf children in public schools. Children's mean age was about 10 years old and aided hearing loss was a 62-decibel loss (severe); unaided losses were usually in the profound range.

Through a home interview and questionnaires, we assessed the four domains of coping resources, parents' current level of adjustment to having a deaf child, the current level of personal and family life adjustment, the negative impact of current life experiences, and the perceived emotional well-being of their child. Maternal problem-solving skills were assessed with a standardized task that provided dilemmas common to families with deaf children (e.g., finding baby-sitters, locating the most appropriate school, obtaining additional services). Social support assessed relations within the family, extended family, community, and in relation to professionals. Beliefs were assessed in the domains of parenting locus of control and religiosity. Children also were rated by their teachers on emotional and social adjustment.

Two types of parental outcomes were examined: their general personal adjustment and their specific adjustment to their deaf child. These outcomes were related to parental coping resources and current negative life stress, as well as the child's hearing loss and age. Thus, in relation to our overall model (Fig. 1), this study examined how child characteristics, family life stress, and parental coping resources affected parental adjustment. Child adjustment was then examined as a result of parents' adjustment, current negative life stress, parent coping resources, child hearing loss, and age.

Utilizing a hierarchical multiple regression model in which child age, hearing loss, and current life stress were first entered as covariates, results indicated that negative life stress and social support were significantly related to maternal personal adjustment, whereas only social support predicted specific maternal adjustment to her deaf child. In addition, higher maternal marital satisfaction was also strongly associated with both maternal outcomes. Utilitarian resources (socioeconomic status, knowledge of deafness), maternal problem-solving skills, and maternal beliefs did not predict additional variance in maternal adjustment outcomes.

Similar to maternal adjustment, overall paternal personal adjustment was related to general life stress, paternal locus of control, and intimate social support (marital satisfaction). In contrast to that of mothers, no significant relationships were present between any paternal coping resources and father's specific adjustment to his deaf child.

With regard to child outcome, as measured by teacher ratings of children's behavior, child's age and maternal problem-solving skills were the most salient predictors. Maternal problem solving not only demonstrated a direct relationship to teacher ratings, but also demonstrated a buffering role in relation to age. Older children with mothers who showed better problem-solving skills were rated by teachers as more adaptive than were older children with mothers demonstrating lower problem-solving skills. Maternal belief in chance also showed an interaction with age. For older children, mothers who believed in chance as a reason for child improvement had children who were rated as more poorly adjusted. Thus, although maternal problem-solving ability was not significantly related to their *own* adaptation, it clearly showed importance for child outcome. These results also suggest that coping resources may differently impact outcomes for different persons and at different phases of development.

While specific coping resources were related to child outcome, both maternal and paternal overall personal adjustment were highly related to teacher assessment of child functioning. The relationship between parent personal adjustment and teacher-rated adjustment demonstrates a connection between the child's home and school environments. Children raised in a home environment with more positive familial interactions might be expected to have higher self-esteem, fewer behavior problems, and more resources for coping with their own appraised stressors.

Parental Resources and Child Skills and Achievement

In a related study using the same sample and family data, we investigated how family stress and coping were related to the deaf children's social–cognitive development and academic achievement (Calderon, Greenberg, & Kusche, 1991). The children were assessed with an extensive battery of academic–cognitive, social–cognitive, and neuropsychological measures. Using hierarchical regression, findings indicated that maternal problem-solving skills showed a significant contribution to the child's emotional understanding, reading achievement, and child's social problem-solving skills. Furthermore, high maternal belief in chance was negatively related to the child's social problem-solving skills. Utilitarian resources (socioeconomic status, parental sophistication regarding their child's education and communication needs) were positively correlated with child's reading achievement. Finally, mothers who indicated more positive maternal adjustment specific to their deaf child had children who showed lower impulsivity, greater cognitive flexibility, and higher social understanding. General maternal personal adjustment was not strongly related to the various child outcomes.

In summary, we found that maternal coping resources were related to both general maternal adjustment, as well as directly to the child's functioning as assessed by the parents, the teachers, and our own direct child testing. Applying the Folkman et al. model, we found that each of the four domains of coping resources showed a significant impact on either the parent's adjustment (social support, beliefs), the child's adjustment (problem solving and beliefs), or the child's cognitive and social–cognitive skills (problem solving, beliefs, utilitarian resources). In addition, the resources that had the most influence on child outcome (i.e., problem-solving skills and understanding of communication and education needs) are factors that are not innate but are potentially modifiable, and thus provide a hopeful perspective on how research on coping can help to influence the targets of intervention and intervention strategies. Although this study is useful in illustrating the use of a coping model using independent reports of child outcome, it has significant limitations, and thus requires replication. Its limitations include small sample size (and thus low power to detect effects), unrepresentative composition (all children using total communication, living in an urban location, and attending local schools), and the fact that aspects of the overall coping model (quality of contact with the deaf community, parent appraisal of the meaning of deafness, quality of schooling) were not investigated.

Although the presence of a hearing impairment is different from many other stressors because of its chronicity, the application of Folkman et al.'s (1980) stress and coping model to the broader social system of the family shows promise as a step toward a better understanding and explanation of differential outcome in families with a hearing-impaired child. Aside from providing a unifying approach in understanding the disparate variables examined in previous studies, this model suggests that deafness, itself, does not lead to maladaptive outcomes. Instead, family stress and parental use of coping resources strongly impact parent and child adjustment. It also encourages the consideration of coping resources in the larger ecological contexts of the individual, family, peer groups, and societal institutions.

Children's Coping

Deaf children are often hindered by their delays in communicative development and social–cognitive skills when they face a number of important challenges. One of the challenges facing most deaf individuals is coming to terms with their deafness and construing it in a way that will lead to more positive adaptation. This is likely to entail actively confronting their deafness, rather than avoidance or repression of its implications, and forming cognitive interpretations that facilitate a positive identity and worldview. This challenge is likely to be of most importance in later childhood and adolescence. A second challenge for deaf youth is meeting the demands presented by daily hassles in a way that allows them to have positive interactions with others and to negotiate the hearing world. To meet these challenges and to show healthy social adjustment and relations with both deaf and hearing peers and adults, effective integration of affective, cognitive, and behavioral skills is essential. This is likely to require active problem solving, effective utilization of support systems, and cognitive strategies that enhance one's beliefs about control and efficacy. However, given the previously documented delays in emotional understanding, difficulties in understanding social interactions, and deficits in problem-solving skills, some deaf children are ill-equipped to cope adequately. This highlights the need for preventive intervention with school-aged deaf children. However, at present there are almost no empirically evaluated school or community-based preventive interventions for school-aged children (see Greenberg, in press).

Promoting Social Competence in Deaf Children: The PATHS Curriculum

In 1982, we began a series of studies on the use of a school-based curriculum, PATHS (promoting alternative thinking strategies), that was designed to improve the social competence and reduce the behavioral difficulties of deaf children (Kusche & Greenberg, 1995). The curriculum is grounded in a theory of development and change: the ABCD (affective–behavioral–cognitive–

dynamic) model, which places primacy on the dynamic developmental integration of affect and emotion language, manifest behavior, cognitive understanding and expectancies, and linguistic and communicative skills for understanding social competence and clinical disorder. Basic to this model is the premise that the child's coping, as reflected in behavior and internal regulation, is a function of her or his emotional awareness, affective–cognitive control, and social–cognitive understanding. Further, the child's coping ability is conceptualized as a function of (1) constitutional factors, (2) the degree of sensitivity and nurturance in the environment, (3) the degree of trauma the child has experienced, and (4) the quality of cognitive and linguistic stimulation that is present.*

Implicit in this developmental model is the idea that during the maturation process, some components of emotional development precede later forms of cognition. As a result, in early development, affect is an important precursor of other modes of thinking, and subsequently must be integrated with other developmental functions for optimal maturation. Findings in the neurobiology of emotional and brain development provide support for this model (Fox & Davidson, 1984; Harris, 1986; Heilman & Satz, 1983; Luria, 1980).

Based on the ABCD model, the overall objective of the PATHS curriculum was to teach deaf children effective interpersonal problem-solving skills. To do so, there were four constituent goals. The first goal was to assist children to learn to "stop and think," a response that facilitates the development and use of verbal thought. Second, we provided children with enriched linguistic experiences and dialoguing to help mediate their understanding of self and others. Third, we provided a variety of experiences in which the children learned to integrate emotional understanding with cognitive and linguistic skills to analyze and solve problems. The children were taught that feelings are signals that communicate useful information. If people learn to attend to what their feelings are telling them, the information can be beneficially utilized in making decisions about what to do next. Fourth, we encouraged the generalization of self-control, emotional understanding, and problem-solving to other social contexts, including the remainder of the classroom day, playgrounds, lunchroom, and other peer-related contexts.

Although the goal of PATHS was to teach deaf children how to resolve interpersonal problems, we have found that there are at least three major (and a variety of minor) skills that are necessary prerequisites for effective problem solving. From a developmental standpoint, these are critical skills for effective coping. The first is adequate communication skills. The ability to recognize a problem, generate alternatives, and consider their consequences all rely heavily on the reflective use of language.

The second skill is the ability to label and understand one's emotions. Poor identification of one's feelings and those of others' will often lead to the wrong solutions. In our work, we have found that deaf children are clearly delayed and impoverished in their linguistic differentiation of emotions (Kusche et al., 1983). For example, the children often showed fusion of concepts such as feeling disappointed and angry, or angry and jealous, or ashamed and shy. We

*See Greenberg and Kusche (1993) for a complete description of the ABCD model.

believe that an accurate and rich semantic framework of emotions is critical for healthy adjustment (Pine, 1985) and successful problem solving. In addition, being able to communicate one's feeling to others is often a very effective coping solution.

The third prerequisite is taking another's point of view. If one is either not able to, does not remember to, or cannot accurately take the point of view of another person in a problem situation, one is often likely to generate selfish, unsatisfactory solutions. We have found that deaf children are cognizant of the difference between their perspective and another's, but are often delayed in the ability to correctly infer the other's view (Kusche & Greenberg, 1983). Thus, our work indicated that communication, affective awareness, and perspective taking all play central roles in effective coping.

Participants and Design

The intervention sample included 70 severely and profoundly deaf children who were involved in 3 consecutive years of longitudinal data collection. The children ranged in ages from 6 to 13 years. All of the children had hearing parents and attended self-contained classrooms in local school that utilized total communication (operationalized as the simultaneous use of signs and speech). All of the children had an unaided hearing loss of at least a 70 decibel (better ear); the average loss was 92 decibel. The design included the random assignment of classrooms to Intervention and wait-list control status: assignment occurred after pretesting. The PATHS curriculum consisted of a 60-lesson manual that was used daily in the classroom for 20–30 minutes over a period of 6 months. The teachers and their assistants received 3 days of training prior to the school year and then received weekly observations, group supervision, and individual consultations. During the second year, the children in the wait-list control group (and new children who entered the classrooms) received a revised version of the curriculum that had been expanded to include approximately 15 more lessons. At each assessment time (pretest, posttest, follow-up), a variety of measures were utilized to assess social problem solving, emotional understanding, academic achievement, and teacher and parent ratings of behavioral adaptation.

The Intervention

The PATHS curriculum is a daily classroom program designed to improve self-control, emotional understanding, and social problem-solving skills. During the past 10 years it has undergone major revisions; however, the research discussed here concerns its original version (see Greenberg & Kusche, 1993, for further information).

There were three units in the versions of the PATHS curriculum that were used in our original research with deaf children. The first, titled the Turtle Unit, focused on the development of self-control and problem identification. Training in self-control is a necessary first step in problem solving, and the unit primarily consisted of an adaptation of the Turtle Technique (Schneider & Robin, 1978). This technique consists of a series of structured lessons accompanied by a reinforcement program that is individually tailored by each class-room teacher. Through a series of lessons the children were told a metaphorical story about a young turtle who has both interpersonal and academic difficulties that arise through "not stopping to think," and these problems are manifest in aggressive behavior. With the assistance of a "wise old turtle," the young turtle learns to solve his or her problems through developing self-control. These lessons present a relaxed and indirect procedure for teaching self-control and practice in role-playing. Thus, the children learn that they can control/inhibit their negative behavior by using a cue procedure, e.g., going inside their shells, when they feel angry, upset, or otherwise distressed. The Turtle Technique was taught/rehearsed during the 30-minute per day curriculum time and was then generalized throughout the day through the use of a reinforcement system selected by the teacher. The self-control or "Turtle" section of the curriculum comprised the first 12 lessons.

The second section, the Feelings Unit, consisted of teaching emotional and interpersonal understanding. This section contained approximately 25 lessons and continued for approximately 15 weeks. The lessons covered approximately 30 different affective states and were taught in a developmental hierarchy beginning with basic emotions (happy, sad, angry, etc.) and later introducing more complex emotional states (jealousy, guilt, pride). As the ability to label emotional states is a central focus of the ABCD model, major emphasis was placed on encouraging such labeling as a precursor for effective self-control and optimal problem resolution. Further, the children were also taught cues for recognizing their own feelings and the recognition of emotions in others, affective self-monitoring techniques, training in attributions that link causes and emotions, perspective-taking skills in how and why to consider another's point of view, empathic realization of how one's behavior can affect other people, and information regarding how the behavior of others can affect oneself. These lessons included group discussions, role-playing skits, art activities, stories, and educational games.

The third section of the curriculum taught interpersonal cognitive problem solving. The section contained approximately 20 lessons and required 10–15 weeks. The skills in the preceding domains were considered prerequisites for learning "formal" interpersonal problem solving. However, from the beginning of the Turtle Unit, children were implicitly taught problem solving and teachers were actively dialoguing with the children as problems arose.

Following the conceptual model developed by D'Zurilla and Goldfried (1971), Shure and Spivack (1978), and Weissberg, Gesten, Liebenstein, Doherty-Schmid, and Hutton (1980), the problem-solving model covered the topics of (1) problem identification, (2) goal selection, (3) generation of alternatives, (4) consideration of consequences, (5) choosing a plan, and (6) trying again if the initial plan was unsuccessful. In addition, our model emphasized both stopping and calming down as the initial step and identifying the feelings of participants in the problem (added between steps 1 and 2 above).

Following from the ABCD model, it is important to note that the curriculum focused on the integration of behavioral, affective, cognitive, and social–cognitive skills. These included teaching behavioral aspects of self-control and using language/representation to help children become more aware on a moment-to-moment basis of their internal affective signals. In addition, the curriculum promoted practice of the pedagogical aspects of problem solving, as well as generalization for using problem solving in real-life contexts during the school day. In terms of the Folkman et al. model, the PATHS curriculum focuses primarily on improving problem-solving skills and altering attributions (beliefs) that should lead to improved relationships (social support) with both adults and peers.

Results

The results, assessed using analysis of covariance (with the pretest scores used as covariates), generally indicated significant improvements for children receiving the PATHS curriculum (see Greenberg & Kusche, 1993, for an extended discussion of measures and results). Results of social problem-solving interviews indicated significant improvements in role-taking, expectancy of outcome, and means–end problem-solving skills. Intervention children also generated a significantly higher percentage of prosocial solutions and a lower percentage of both neutral and negative solutions. Similar improvements were found on both emotional recognition and the reading of emotion labels. In addition, intervention children showed a significant increase in reading achievement on the Stanford Achievement Test, and those intervention children above age 9 showed a significant higher score on the Wechsler Intelligence Scale for Children—Revised Mazes subtest compared to controls. Teacher ratings indicated significant improvements in emotional adjustment and frustration tolerance. These improvements in both behavior and social–cognition were large in magnitude 1 month after intervention (overall effect size of 1.1 SD across all measures) and were maintained up to 2 years postintervention. Further, very similar findings were found for an independent replication sample (the wait-list control group plus new students). Thus, teaching self-control, emotional understanding, and problem-solving skills led to changes in these skills themselves, as well as to improved behavior.

To partially examine our model of change and assess mediation of effects, prepost change scores were computed for each outcome measure within the intervention group. Correlations were then computed between change in the hypothesized mediators and change in the adjustment variables. The results of this analysis provided support for the theoretical model and can be summarized as follows: (1) increases in emotional understanding and role-taking ability were significantly related to changes in problem-solving skills: (2) increases in role-taking skills were related to teacher ratings of improvement in emotional adjustment and reduction in behavior problems; (3) increases in problem-solving skills were related to large increases in teacher ratings of emotional adjustment; and (4) increases in the generation of prosocial alternatives to peer dilemmas were related to increases in overall social competence and decreases in school-related behavior problems (see Greenberg & Kusche, 1993, for details).

We have found that a coping model helps to reconceptualize some of the difficulties shown by some deaf children as deficits in problem-solving skills. Rather than defects in their personality structure, these deficits may be seen as deficits in social, cognitive, and communicative skills. The PATHS curriculum was successful in altering social–cognitive and affective skills, as well as behavior. In addition, a change score analysis indicated that increases in affective–cognitive understanding appear to be related to behavioral improvements. We believe that the direction of "causal" effects is likely to go from social–cognitive integrations to behavior.

Although curricular-based interventions appear promising for improving the social competence of deaf children, it is clear that such intervention needs to be teacher-based and sustained across grades. This is indicated by results of short-term, experimental demonstrations. For example, Regan (1981) utilized a shortened nine-session version of a well-known self-control training program with a small sample of children and found no effects on behavioral impulsivity.

Although PATHS began as a specific curriculum for deaf children to be conducted within a school year, over the past decade it has been considerably expanded to a multiyear model. Recently, we have reported findings showing significant effects with hearing children (both regular and special needs children) on emotional understanding and behavioral adaptation (Greenberg, Kusche, Cook & Quamma, 1995; Kusche & Greenberg, 1991). The curriculum now contains approximately 120 lessons and is used over a 2- to 3-year period on a regular basis in the classroom (Kusche & Greenberg, 1995).

Further Issues and Future Directions

In this chapter, we have presented an overall model of coping in families with deaf children and reviewed research examining the role of family coping resources, the child's communicative development, and the impact of preventive intervention in promoting healthy adaptation in deaf children. Although there has been some research on coping and adaptation in deaf children and their families, this area has been understudied. Given our model, there are a number of directions we suggest for future research.

Measurement

Given the unique circumstances of deaf children and their families, it is notable that there has been a dearth of measures developed, or appropriately modified from other populations, to assess the unique circumstances, stresses, and coping resources of families and children (Meadow-Orlans, 1990). To study coping and adaptation, it is necessary for measurement to capture the ecology and phenomenological context of the participants. This includes not only better measures of specific, unique stresses associated with parenting a deaf child (cf. Quittner et al., 1990), but also measures of the understanding and utilization of resources: for example, parents adaptation to deafness, sophistication regarding educational and cultural aspects of deafness, problem solving of deafness-specific dilemmas, their contact with and utilization of deaf persons at different periods in the child's development, and so forth. Similarly, in studying the coping of deaf children, there is a need for a measure(s) of the specific hassles experienced by deaf children of different ages in different educational contexts (mainstream vs. deaf-only classrooms, day vs. residential school environments). Further, there is a need to develop measures of coping style that can be used for deaf children (probably utilizing videotape signing as the preferred modality). It is likely that both quantitative and qualitative research will contribute important pieces to the completion of these measurement needs, with the use of deaf children and their hearing parents as informants who can help guide the research. As with the study of the stresses experienced by deaf adults, personal accounts of the coping processes of parents are very instructive (Spradley & Spradley, 1978).

Tests of Theoretical Models

Also in the future, comprehensive tests of ecological models are needed. We have presented a theoretical model for the factors and processes that influence development in deaf children. Research in our laboratory has produced evidence in support of parts of the model, but further research is needed to test the complex interrelations among the multiple factors that are likely to influence deaf children's developmental outcomes.

A second aspect of theory testing that would further our understanding are tests of the processes of coping themselves. There are three directions we suggest. First, we need to investigate the differences in coping processes between families and children who make different types of appraisals. The second direction is to examine different styles of coping (e.g., approach vs. avoidance) and how these relate to adaptation. Finally, it would be useful to examine how coping styles may show "goodness of fit" to specific situations. For example, do families who utilize emotion-focused coping with uncontrollable events, i.e., diagnosis of deafness, and problem-solving coping with controllable events show better adaptation than families who show patterns with less "fit?" An important component of testing such a goodness of fit is to first develop measures of parents' conceptions of the controllability of events. These are important steps in proceeding on the path of a more state-based, contextualized study of coping processes.

Developmental Issues in Adolescence: The Influence of Interpersonal Relations

A third direction for future research is greater attention to developmental issues, and, in particular, to issues related to adolescent development. With the advent of adolescence, the effects of both identity development and social networks are likely to play an increasingly important role in the adaptation of deaf children (Carty, 1994; Carver, 1988). Although the development of a healthy identity is likely in part to result from factors discussed above (e.g., family, individual, and ecological–educational factors), new developmental forces complicate the picture.

There are two types of social relations that have a powerful influence on adolescent competence and risk: (1) the quality of intimate attachments (Armsden & Greenberg, 1987), and (2) membership in social groups/networks that provide support. Intimate attachments are defined by the affective quality of feelings of intimacy, solidarity, and trust (Bowlby, 1982), including the extent to which an individual can draw on others for support at a true level of involvement and concern in times of need. In young deaf children, we have reported that the quality of the child–parent attachment is related to the quality of communication (Greenberg & Marvin, 1979). There has been no research on the nature or effect of parent–deaf child attachments in middle childhood or adolescence and little study of the peer relations of deaf children (see Lederberg, 1993, for review). However, during adolescence, peers may take on a more powerful role in providing intimate support.

In contrast to intimate attachments, the social network or group might include a variety of individuals, including relatively close friends, members of one's extended family, co-workers or classmates, neighbors, casual acquaintances, and members of organizations or groups in which the adolescent actively participates. This "less intimate social support" can be a powerful influence on mental health and coping ability. Both intimate attachments and/or one's social group can be invaluable resources for coping with stress by providing a variety of functions, including emotional support, information, advice, feelings of solidarity, and actual physical or financial assistance. As more deaf children are educated in mainstream settings, and thus have fewer early and adolescent experiences with deaf adults, the nature and function of the deaf adolescent's social network may be of particular importance for the following three reasons. First, a social network provides a sense of connection or feeling of belonging to *some* type of "community." For a deaf person it could be either the "deaf" world or the "hearing" world or both. However, given that most deaf children grow up as a "minority" with few or no role models to help them establish their identity, the feeling of belonging is both quite important and in some cases difficult for the individual to establish (Reagan, 1990). The second function that certain types of social support may provide is to control the meaning of events. That is, events that an individual may appraise as very stressful or problematic may be reappraised as natural and not "crazy." Through the network interactions, the individual comes to realize that "I'm not the only one who has this problem." This function is dependent on the individual having access to other individuals that share similar issues, identities, and concerns. In the area of deafness, such groups have been effectively utilized for hearing parents and for deaf children. However, there has been little or no use of such groups for deaf adolescents living in hearing families, especially in mainstream settings.

The third and related function of such network groups is to open up new channels of information for the individual, and thus provide the individual with more coping options, e.g., different alternative solutions to problems. Individuals who are isolated or have "deficient" social networks are likely to be less able to deal adequately with stress for the variety of reasons mentioned above. Traditionally, the deaf adolescent's network developed through attendance at a residential school, as well as through special summer camp experiences, and participation in athletic, activity-based and fraternal networks involving other deaf adolescent and adults. As enrollment at residential schools has dramatically declined, deaf adolescents are at greater risk (especially in rural areas), since they may not have access to social networks where they feel they belong and that can help to "normalize" the experience of being "an outsider in a hearing world." The role of contact with the deaf community (adults, older peers, and a deaf peer group) has been understudied. As we hypothesize that social support from deaf persons may impact both the child and youth's self-identity and as a result affect their adjustment, the study of the influence of social networks, especially those with other deaf persons, is warranted.

With the exception of two studies (Charlson, Strong, & Gold, 1992; Mertens, 1989), there has been little exploration of how school placement, social support networks, or intimate relations affect adaptation in adolescents who are deaf. Both studies indicated that deaf teens educated solely in mainstream settings were more likely to be academically challenged, yet socially isolated and lonely. Since adolescence is believed to be a time of significant risk, as well as a critical time for the formation of identity, such information is essential for the development of effective programs to strengthen identity and adaptation (Cohen, 1991). In this regard, there is a need to pay special attention to the potential role of deaf adults in affecting these developmental processes (Hill, 1993).

Brubaker (1994) has suggested the utility of applying the model of acculturative stress (Berry, 1989) for understanding the different modes by which deaf adults adjust to their cultural minority status (i.e., assimilation, integration, separation, and marginalization). Such models of individual differences may yield valuable information regarding how one's self-definition (i.e., Deaf vs. hard of hearing) and other factors, such as type of schooling, relate to one's attitude in interacting with the dominant hearing culture. A similar model might be applied to deaf youth to understand how attitudes toward the dominant hearing culture affect their style of coping as well as their postsecondary and employment decisions.

CONCLUSIONS

The study of stress, coping, and adaptation in families with deaf children and in the children themselves is of great interest for two reasons. First, it provides a population that shares issues related to disability with those related to culture in a unique manner. Second, the study of deaf children provides an extremely interesting population in which to study resiliency and risk. Finally, there is a significant need for improvements in both universal and targeted prevention for families and children; research on coping should be a critical step in the design of the next generation of intervention strategies.

REFERENCES

American Psychiatric Association. (1994). *Diagnostic and statistical manual of mental disorders* (4th ed.). Washington, DC: Author.

Armsden, G. C., & Greenberg, M. T. (1987). The inventory of parent and peer attachments: Individual differences and their relationship to well-being in adolescence. *Journal of Youth and Adolescence, 16,* 427–454.

Bachara, G. H., Raphael, J., & Phelan, W. J., III. (1980). Empathy development in deaf preadolescents. *American Annals of the Deaf, 125,* 38–41.

Baker, C., & Cokely, D. (Eds.). (1980). *Sign language and the deaf community*. Silver Spring, MD: National Association of the Deaf.

Berry, J. W. (1989). Psychology of acculturation. In J. Berman (Ed.), *Nebraska symposium on motivation* (Vol. 37, pp. 201–234). Lincoln: University of Nebraska Press.

Bet-Chava, Y. (1993). Antecedents of self-esteem in deaf people: A meta-analytic review. *Rehabilitation Psychology, 38,* 221–234.

Bienvenu, M. J. (1994). Reflections of deaf culture in deaf humor. In C. J. Erting (Ed.), *The deaf way: Perspectives from the International Conference on Deaf Culture* (pp. 16–22). Washington, DC: Gallaudet University Press.

Blanton, R. L., & Nunnally, J. C. (1964). Semantic habits and cognitive style processes in the deaf. *Journal of Abnormal and Social Psychology, 68,* 397–402.

Bodner, B., & Johns, J. (1976). *A study of locus of control and hearing-impaired students.* Paper presented at the A. G. Bell Association for the Deaf, Boston.

Bowlby, J. (1982). *Attachment and loss. Vol. 1: Attachment* (2nd ed.). New York: Basic Books (Original work published 1969).

Bragg, B. (1989). *Lessons in laughter: The autobiography of a deaf actor.* Washington, DC: Gallaudet University Press.

Brubaker, R. G. (1994). Acculturative stress: A useful framework form understanding the experience of deaf Americans. *Journal of the American Deafness and Rehabilitation Association, 28,* 1–15.

Calderon, R. (1988). Stress and coping in hearing families with deaf children: A model of factors affecting adjustment. *Dissertation Abstracts International, 49, 8B.* (University Microfilms No. 8820402).

Calderon, R., & Greenberg, M. T. (1993). Considerations in the adaptation of families with school-aged deaf children. In M. Marschark & M. D. Clark (Eds.), *Psychological perspectives on deafness* (pp. 27–48). Hillsdale, NJ: Erlbaum.

Calderon, R., & Greenberg, M. T. (1997). The effectiveness of early intervention for children with hearing impairments. In M. J. Guralnick (Ed.), *The effectiveness of early intervention: Second generation research* (pp. 455–482). Baltimore, MD: Paul H. Brooks.

Calderon, R., Greenberg, M. T., & Kusche, C. (1991). The influence of family coping on the cognitive and social skills of deaf children. In D. Martin (Ed.), *Advances in cognition, education, and deafness* (pp. 195–200). Washington, DC: Gallaudet University Press.

Caplan, G. (1981). Mastery of stress: Psychosocial aspects. *The American Journal of Psychiatry, 138,* 413–420.

Carty, B. (1994). The development of deaf identity. In C. J. Erting (Ed.), *The deaf way: Perspectives from the International Conference on Deaf Culture* (pp. 40–43). Washington, DC: Gallaudet University Press.

Carver, R. J. (1988). Social factors in the development of the deaf child. *Canadian Journal of the Deaf, 2,* 81–92.

Carver, R. J., & Doe, T. M. (1989). Rehabilitation or oppression? Options for the humanization of the deaf. *Canadian Journal of the Deaf, 3,* 87–99.

Charlson, E., Strong, M., & Gold, R. (1992). How successful deaf teenagers experience and cope with isolation. *American Annals of the Deaf, 137,* 261–270.

Coady, E. A. (1984). *Social problem solving skills and school related social competency of elementary age deaf students: A descriptive study.* Unpublished doctoral dissertation, University of Washington, Seattle, WA.

Cohen, F. E., & Lazarus, R. S. (1979). Coping with the stress of illness. In G. C. Stone, F. Cohen, & N. E. Adler (Eds.), *Psychological stress and psychopathology* (pp. 124–148). New York: McGraw-Hill.

Cohen, O. P. (1991). At-risk deaf adolescents. *The Volta Review, 93,* 57–72.

Compas, B. E. (1987). Coping with stress during childhood and adolescence. *Psychological Bulletin, 101,* 393–403.

DeCaro, P., & Emerton, R. G. (1978). *A cognitive–developmental investigation of moral reasoning in a deaf population.* Paper Series, Department of Research and Development, National Technical Institute for the Deaf.

Dowaliby, F. J., Burke, N. E., & McKee, B. G. (1983). A comparison of hearing-impaired and normally hearing students on locus of control, people orientation, and study habits and attitudes. *American Annals of the Deaf, 128,* 53–59.

D'Zurilla, T. J., & Goldfried, M. R. (1971). Problem solving and behavior modification. *Journal of Abnormal Psychology, 78,* 107–126.

Erting, C. J. (Ed.). (1994). *The deaf way: Perspectives from the International Conference on Deaf Culture.* Washington, DC: Gallaudet University Press.

Folkman, S., Schaefer, C., & Lazarus, R. S. (1980). Cognitive processes as mediators of stress and coping. In V. Hamilton & D. M. Warburton (Eds.), *Human stress and cognition* (pp. 210–248). London: Wiley.

Foster, S. B. (1987). Employment experiences of deaf college graduates: An interview study. *Journal of the American Deafness and Rehabilitation Association, 21,* 1–15.

Fox, N. A., & Davidson, R. J. (Eds.). (1984). *The psychobiology of affective development.* Hillsdale, NJ: Erlbaum.

Freeman, R., Boese, R., & Carbin, C. (1981). *Can't your deaf child hear?* Baltimore: University Park Press.

Freeman, R. D., Malkin, S. F., & Hastings, J. O. (1975). Psycho-social problems of deaf children and their families: A comparative study. *American Annals of the Deaf, 120,* 391–405.

Friedrich, W. A., Greenberg, M. T., & Crnic, K. A. (1986). Empirical studies of handicapped children and their families: Measurement issues and conceptual framework. In S. Landesman-Dwyer & P. Vietze (Eds.), *Research on the impact of residential settings on mentally retarded persons* (pp. 229–249). Baltimore: University Park Press.

Gannon, J. R. (1981). *Deaf heritage: A narrative history of deaf America.* Silver Spring, MD: National Association of the Deaf.

Gannon, J. R. (1993). *The week the world heard Gallaudet.* Washington, DC: Gallaudet University Press.

Garretson, M. D. (Ed.). (1994). *Deafness: life and culture.* Silver Spring, MD: National Association of the Deaf.

Garrison, W. M., Emerton, R. G., & Layne, C. A. (1978). *Self-concept and social interaction in a deaf population.* Rochester, NY: National Training Institute for the Deaf.

Goldberger, L., & Brenitz, S. (Eds.). (1982). *Handbook of stress: Theoretical and clinical aspects.* New York: Free Press.

Greenberg, M. T. (1983). Family stress and child competence: The effects of early intervention for families with deaf infants. *American Annals of the Deaf, 128,* 407–417.

Greenberg, M. T. (in press). Educational interventions: Prevention and promotion of competence. In P. Hindley & N. Kitson (Eds.), *Mental health and deafness.* London: Whurr Publications.

Greenberg, M., Calderon, R., & Kusche, C. (1984). Early intervention using simultaneous communication with deaf infants: The effect on communication development. *Child Development, 55,* 607–616.

Greenberg, M., & Kusche, C. (1989). Cognitive, personal and social development of deaf children and adolescents. In M. C. Wang, M. C. Reynolds, & H. J. Walberg (Eds.), *Handbook of special education: Research and practice* (pp. 484–526). Oxford, England: Pergamon Press.

Greenberg, M. T., & Kusche, C. A. (1993). *Promoting social and emotional development in deaf children: The PATHS project.* Seattle: University of Washington Press.

Greenberg, M. T., Kusche, C. A., Cook, E. T., & Quamma, J. P. (1995). Promoting emotional competence in school-aged deaf children: The effects of the PATHS curriculum. *Development and Psychopathology, 7,* 117–136.

Greenberg, M. T., & Marvin, R. S. (1979). Attachment patterns in profoundly deaf preschool children. *Merrill-Palmer Quarterly, 25,* 265–279.

Gregory, S. (1976). *The deaf child and his family.* New York: John Wiley.

Hamilton, V. (1982). Cognition and stress: An information processing model. In L. Goldberger & S. Brenitz (Eds.), *Handbook of stress: Theoretical and clinical aspects* (pp. 41–71). New York: Free Press.

Harris, J. E. (1986). *Clinical neuroscience.* New York: Human Sciences Press.

Harris, R. I. (1978). The relationship of impulse control to parent hearing status, manual communication, and academic achievement in deaf children. *American Annals of the Deaf, 123,* 52–67.

Heilman, K. M., & Satz, P. (Eds.). (1983). *Neuropsychology of Human Emotion.* New York: Guilford Press.

Heppner, C. M. (1992). *Seeds of disquiet: One deaf woman's experience.* Washington, DC: Gallaudet University Press.

Hill, P. (1993). The need for deaf adult role models in early intervention programs for deaf children. *ACEHI Journal, 19,* 14–20.

Hindley, P. A., Hill, P. D., McGuigan, S., & Kitson, N. (1994). Psychiatric disorder in deaf and hearing-impaired children and young people: A prevalence study. *Journal of Child Psychology and Psychiatry, 35,* 917–934.

Hirshoren, A., & Schaittjer, C. J. (1979). Dimensions of problem behavior in deaf children. *Journal of Abnormal Child Psychology, 7,* 221–228.

Jacobs, L. M. (1989). *A deaf adult speaks out* (3rd ed.). Washington, DC: Gallaudet University Press.

Jensema, C. J., & Trybus, R. (1975). *Reported emotional/behavioral problems among hearing impaired children in special educational programs: United States 1972–1973.* Series R, Number 1, Washington, DC: Office of Demographic Studies, Gallaudet College.

Kannapell, B. (1994). Deaf identity: An American perspective. In C. J. Erting (Ed.), *The deaf way: Perspectives from the International Conference on Deaf Culture* (pp. 44–48). Washington, DC: Gallaudet University Press.

Kisor, H. (1990). *What's that pig outdoors? A memoir of deafness.* New York: Hill & Wang.

Kusche, C. A., Garfield, T. S., & Greenberg, M. T. (1983). The understanding of emotional and social attributions in deaf adolescents. *Journal of Clinical Child Psychology, 12,* 153–160.

Kusche, C. A., & Greenberg, M. T. (1983). The development of evaluative understanding and role-taking in deaf and hearing children. *Child Development, 54,* 141–147.

Kusche, C. A., & Greenberg, M. T. (1991). *Improving classroom behavior and emotional understanding in special needs children: The effects of the PATHS curriculum.* Paper presented at the Society for Research in Child Development, Seattle, WA.

Kusche, C. A., & Greenberg, M. T. (1995). *The PATHS curriculum.* Seattle, WA: Developmental Research & Programs.

Lazarus, R. S. (1966). *Psychological stress and the coping process.* New York: McGraw-Hill, 1966.

Lazarus, R. S., & Folkman, S. (1984). *Stress, appraisal and coping.* New York: Springer.

Lazarus, R. S., & Launier, R. (1978). Stress-related transactions between person and environment. In L. A. Pervin & M. Lewis (Ed.), *Perspectives in interactional psychology* (pp. 44–72). New York: Plenum Press.

Lederberg, A. (1993). The impact of deafness on mother-child and peer relationships. In M. Marschark & M. D. Clark (Eds.), *Psychological perspectives on deafness* (pp. 93–122). Hillsdale, NJ: Erlbaum.

Lederberg, A. R., & Mobley, C. E. (1990). The effect of hearing impairment on the quality of attachment and mother–toddler interaction. *Child Development, 61,* 1596–1604.

Levine, E. S. (1981). *The ecology of early deafness.* New York: Columbia University Press.

Luckner, J. L., & McNeill, J. H. (1994). Performance of a group of deaf and hard-of-hearing students and a comparison group of hearing students on a series of problem-solving tasks. *American Annals of the Deaf, 139,* 371–377.

Luria, A. R. (1980). *Higher cortical functions in man.* New York: Basic Books.

Luterman, D. (1987). *Deafness in the family.* Boston: Little, Brown.

MacTurk, R. H., Meadow-Orlans, K. P., Koester, L. S., & Spencer, P. E. (1993). Social support, motivation, language, and interaction: A longitudinal study of mothers and deaf infants. *American Annals of the Deaf, 138,* 19–25.

Marschark, M. (1993). *Psychological development of deaf children.* New York: Oxford University Press.

McCrone, W. (1979). Learned helplessness and level of underachievement among deaf adolescents. *Psychology in the Schools, 16,* 430–434.

Meadow, K. P. (1980). *Deafness and child development.* Berkeley: University of California Press.

Meadow, K. P., & Trybus, R. J. (1979). Behavioral and emotional problems of deaf children: An overview. In L. J. Bradford & W. G. Hardy (Eds.), *Hearing and hearing impairment* (pp. 91–111). New York: Grune & Stratton.

Meadow-Orlans, K. P. (1987). An analysis of the effectiveness of early intervention programs for hearing-impaired children. In M. J. Guralnick & F. C. Bennett (Eds.), *The effectiveness of early intervention for at-risk children* (pp. 325–362). New York: Academic Press.

Meadow-Orlans, K. P. (1990). The impact of child hearing loss on the family. In D. F. Moores & K. P.

Meadow-Orlans (Eds.), *Educational and developmental aspects of deafness* (pp. 321–338). Washington, DC: Gallaudet University Press.

Meadow-Orlans, K. P. (1994). Stress, support, and deafness: Perceptions of infants' mothers and fathers. *Journal of Early Intervention, 18,* 91–102.

Meadow-Orlans, K. P., & Steinberg, A. G. (1993). Effects of infant hearing loss and maternal support on mother–infant interactions at 18 months. *Journal of Applied Developmental Psychology, 14,* 407–426.

Mertens, D. M. (1989). Social experiences of hearing impaired high school youth. *American Annals of the Deaf, 134,* 15–19.

Moores, D. F. (1987). *Educating the deaf: Psychology, principles, and practices* (3rd ed.). Boston: Houghton Mifflin Company.

Moores, D. F., Cerney, B., & Garcia, M. (1990). School placement and least restrictive environment. In D. F. Moores & K. P. Meadow-Orlans (Eds.), *Educational and developmental aspects of deafness* (pp. 115–136). Washington, DC: Gallaudet University Press.

Mowry, R. L. (1994). What deaf high school students tell us about their social networks. In C. J. Erting (Ed.), *The deaf way: Perspectives from the International Conference on Deaf Culture* (pp. 642–649). Washington, DC: Gallaudet University Press.

Nash, J. E., & Nash, A. (1981). *Deafness in society.* Lexington, MA: Lexington.

Odom, P. B., Blanton, R. L., & Laukhuf, C. (1973). Facial expressions and interpretation of emotion-arousing situations in deaf and hearing children. *Journal of Abnormal Child Psychology, 1,* 139–151.

Padden, C., & Humphries, T. (1988). *Deaf in America: Voices from a culture.* Cambridge, MA: Harvard University Press.

Pearlin, L., & Schooler, C. (1978). The structure of coping. *Journal of Health and Social Behavior, 30,* 241–256.

Pearlin, L. I., Lieberman, M. A., Menaghan, E. G., & Mullan, J. T. (1981). The stress process. *Journal of Health and Social Behavior, 22,* 337–356.

Pietzrak, W. (1981). Perception of the emotions of others by deaf school children. *Defektologiya, 4,* 37–92.

Pine, F. (1985). *Developmental theory and clinical process.* New Haven, CT: Yale University Press.

Quittner, A. L., Glueckauf, R. L., & Jackson, D. N. (1990). Chronic parenting stress: Moderating versus mediating effects of social support. *Journal of Personality and Social Psychology, 59,* 1266–1278.

Rainier, J. D., & Altshuler, K. Z. (1971). A psychiatric program for the deaf: Experience and implications. *American Journal of Psychiatry, 127,* 1527–1532.

Reagan, T. (1990). Cultural consideration in the education of deaf children. In D. F. Moores & K. P. Meadow-Orlans (Eds.), *Educational and developmental aspects of deafness* (pp. 73–84). Washington, DC: Gallaudet University Press.

Regan, J. J. (1981). *An attempt to modify cognitive impulsivity in deaf children: Self-instruction versus problem-solving strategies.* Unpublished doctoral dissertation, University of Toronto.

Reivich, R. S., & Rothrock, I. A. (1972). Behavior problems of deaf children and adolescents: A factor-analytic study. *Journal of Speech and Hearing Research, 15,* 93–104.

Schein, J., & Delk, M. (1974). *The deaf population of the US.* Washington, DC: Gallaudet University Press.

Schein, J. D. (1989). *At home among strangers.* Washington, DC: Gallaudet University Press.

Schildroth, A. N., & Hotto, S. A. (1993). Annual survey of hearing-impaired children and youth: 1991–1992 school year. *American Annals of the Deaf, 138,* 163–171.

Schlesinger, H. S., & Meadow, K. (1972). *Sound and sign.* Berkeley: University of California Press.

Schneider, M., & Robin, A. (1978). *Manual for the Turtle Technique.* Unpublished manual, Department of Psychology, State University of New York at Stony Brook.

Selyle, H. (1976). *The stress of life.* New York: McGraw-Hill.

Shure, M. B., & Spivak, G. (1978). *Problem-solving techniques in childrearing.* San Francisco: Jossey Bass.

Spradley, T. S., & Spradley, J. P. (1978). *Deaf like me.* New York: Random House.

Stone, R., & Stirling, L. O. (1994). Developing and defining an identity: Deaf children of deaf and hearing parents. In C. J. Erting (Ed.), *The deaf way: Perspectives from the International Conference on Deaf Culture* (pp. 49–53). Washington, DC: Gallaudet University Press.

Sugarman, I. R. (1969). *The perception of facial expressions of affect by deaf and nondeaf high school students*. Unpublished doctoral dissertation, Columbia University, New York.

Vernon, M. (1969). Sociological and psychological factors associated with hearing loss. *Journal of Speech and Hearing Research, 12,* 541–563.

Weissberg, R. P., Gesten, E. L., Liebenstein, N. L., Doherty-Schmid, K. D., & Hutton, H. (1980). *The Rochester Social Problem Solving (SPS) Program*. Rochester, NY: University of Rochester Press.

Woodward, J. (1972). Implications for sociolinguistics research among the deaf. *Sign Language Studies, 1,* 1–7.

Wrubel, J., Benner, P., & Lazarus, R. S. (1981). Social competence from the perspective of stress and coping. In J. M. Wine & M. Smye (Eds.), *Social competence* (pp. 44–77). New York: Guilford Press.

12

Children's Coping with Stressful Medical Procedures

LIZETTE PETERSON, KRISTA K. OLIVER, and LISA SALDANA

Childhood is a time in which children are cared for and protected by their parents. Medical procedures involving children thus provide a paradoxical situation for children and their families. Nowhere else in their experience are children subjected to a planned event that is frightening and often painful, while the parents look on passively or even assist in restraining the children. This same paradox of adult presence without protection, which presents such a challenge to children and their families, allows a unique opportunity for the investigation of how children cope with anxiety-provoking and painful experiences. Because most elective medical procedures are planned in advance, children and their families' responses to a procedure can and have been meticulously explored through observation, interview, self-report, parent ratings, and physiological assessment (Peterson, 1984).

Investigations of children's and families' responses to medical procedures may yield data relevant to children's reactions to other situations involving fear and tissue damage that cannot be as readily observed, such as the more ubiquitous event of minor childhood injury (Peterson & Starr, 1994). Such investigations of emotion-focused coping, which characterize adaptive responding to medical procedures, may also provide an interesting contrast to other forms of stress such as school failure, where instrumental or action-based coping to change the situation may be most adaptive (Band & Weisz, 1988). Thus, because of the predictability, relatively high degree of threat, and sharp temporal focus, the study of children's coping with medical procedures may serve as the

LIZETTE PETERSON, KRISTA K. OLIVER, and LISA SALDANA • Department of Psychology, University of Missouri at Columbia, Columbia, Missouri 65211.
Handbook of Children's Coping: Linking Theory and Intervention, edited by Wolchik and Sandler. Plenum Press, New York, 1997.

ideal laboratory for understanding how children cope with frightening events that must be endured rather than altered.

Research on children's reactions to medical procedures has grown from a few dozen studies conducted prior to the late 1960s to a literature of hundreds of investigations. The field has encompassed a variety of medical procedures, ranging from threatening but nonpainful procedures such as cast removal (Johnson, Kirchoff, & Endress, 1975) to brief procedures that involve short duration and mild intensity of pain such as injections (e.g., Powers, Blount, Bachanas, Cotter, & Swan, 1993) and venipunctures (e.g., Manne et al., 1992), to highly threatening procedures such as cardiac catheterization (e.g., Cassell, 1965) and to extremely painful procedures such as burn debridement (Elliott & Olson, 1983) and bone marrow aspirations (Jay & Elliott, 1990). Procedures could be organized by temporal parameters (very brief vs. lengthy), degree of pain (cast removal is painless, burn debridement is excruciating), or goal of the procedure (diagnostic vs. treatment). Instead, researchers have tended to group procedures together if the medical procedures involve psychological threat in the form of potential tissue damage or pain and require children to submit to the procedure cooperatively, to alter their natural behavioral inclinations to fight or flee, and to manage their subjective cognitive and emotional response to the procedure. Nearly all of these procedures involve needles or other sharp tools, they are episodic (i.e., have a clearly marked beginning and end), and they are more easily performed on a cooperative child. Such procedures have been the focus of the bulk of research on preparation for medical procedures.

THE POPULATION TO BE SERVED

All but the most underprivileged children in the United States undergo routine immunization injections as part of well-child care (Peterson & Oliver, 1994). Diagnostic tests such as finger pricks and venipunctures are very common procedures for children as well. Each year, 5 million children undergo some kind of diagnostic or treatment-oriented medical procedure (Bush, Melamed, Sheras, & Greenbaum, 1986). Thus, the question of coping with medical procedures is relevant to a very large population of children. This population includes healthy children who either receive preventive preparation in case a later medical procedure takes place (e.g., Elkins & Roberts, 1985) or who undergo a planned medical procedure that is an anomaly in a life otherwise typical of any child in the community (e.g., Peterson & Toler, 1986). However, much of the literature has focused on children who require medical procedures for chronic and sometimes life-threatening illness (e.g., Smith, Ackerson, & Blotcky, 1989), and thus researchers are beginning to recognize the importance of and explicitly target features such as the different effects of prior medical experience (described later in this chapter) that will influence children's response to procedural stressors.

Rather than attempting a comprehensive overview of this burgeoning area, in this chapter we will offer examples that characterize past and current findings on children's and their families' responses to medical procedures. Some of the classic work in the field has great present-day relevance and, as will be seen in the next section, some of this older work can serve to inform us concerning the potential negative effects of the child's isolation from family and from meaningful information that characterized past pediatric practices.

We will first consider the past and current influence of medical procedures on children's short- and long-term adaptation. In general, younger children tend to be more distressed by medical procedures than older children; we will explore the reasons for this finding. We will then give an overview of a coping model frequently applied to stressful medical procedures and will emphasize the importance of clearly articulating the phase of coping (from appraising the stressor, to encountering the stressor, to recovering from the stressor; see transactional model of coping, Lazarus & Lanier, 1978) under investigation.

There are many different processes that influence children's responses to stressful procedures. Two in particular have received extensive attention in recent years. The role of the child's characteristic methods of coping and the influence of parental presence versus absence provide good representations of the richness and complexity of current study of the internal (coping style) and ecological (parent support) processes that may influence a child's response to a medical procedure.

Despite recent emphasis on descriptive models, there has also been considerable progress made in designing preventive interventions to reduce the stress of undergoing a medical procedure; thus, current preventive preparation strategies will be overviewed next. Finally, possible directions for future descriptive, intervention-oriented, and theoretical work will be considered.

ADAPTATION FOLLOWING MEDICAL PROCEDURES

Historical Perspective

The early literature on children's reactions to medical procedures tended to describe global responses to the entire hospitalization experience. The descriptions painted a dark, frightening picture, reporting increases in both externalizing behaviors such as anger, aggression, and irritability (e.g., Jensen, 1955), and internalizing problems such as panic and crying (e.g., Prugh, Staub, Sands, Kirschbaum, & Lenihan, 1953). Some researchers described regressive responses to hospitalization such as an increase in separation anxiety, behavioral disturbances such as eating problems and sleep disruption, and both insomnia and nightmares following hospitalization (e.g., Jackson, Winkley, Faust, & Cermack, 1952). The early descriptive reports were sufficiently distressing that some clinicians indicated a concern that children might suffer lasting negative effects, both in terms of specific fears of medical procedures and general problems in personality development (e.g., Chapman, Loeb, & Gibbons, 1956). Then, Douglas (1975) published a compelling documentation of problematic effects seen in adults as a result of their hospitalization as children 20 years earlier. He followed British children who had been hospitalized prior to age 5 and a nonhospitalized comparison group of children. In early adulthood, he examined several measures of adjustment including behavioral disturbances, learning disabilities, and unemployment. Each of these measures showed worse adjustment in adulthood in the group previously hospitalized as children. This well-regarded study raised serious concerns about potential long-term effects of early hospitalization.

Changes in Pediatric Hospitalization

Although early reports indicated immediate and lasting negative effects following medical procedures, the typical pediatric hospitalization experience has changed dramatically in practically every way since those early reports. One of the biggest changes has been in sustained parental support during hospitalization. There is some controversy concerning whether parents should be present during the actual medical procedures, which will be discussed later in this chapter, but there is no doubt that in the vast majority of cases, parental presence is extremely beneficial to the child in a medical setting (see reviews by Melamed, 1993; Peterson, Mori, & Carter, 1985). Early studies documented that children had fewer emotional and behavioral disturbances and recovered more rapidly if their parent remained with them during hospitalization (Brain & Maclay, 1968). A shift from being allowed to visit once a week to full rooming-in privileges had occurred for most hospitals by the mid-1970s (Hardgrove, 1980), and some physicians made emphatic statements at that time suggesting that no child should be treated in a hospital that did not allow the parent to remain with the child (e.g., Gabriel, 1977). Thus, one major change has been that most hospitals now encourage parental contact with the child throughout hospitalization. Indeed, parents who did not take advantage of such opportunities reported that the overnight separation from their child was more stressful to the child than postoperative pain, vomiting, or bleeding (Peterson & Shigetomi, 1982).

A second major environmental change was made in the organization of pediatric wards and nursing practices. Contrary to past surgical procedures, it is now unusual for a child to be placed on an adult ward. Furthermore, rather than the generic white and sterile hospital environment of the 1960s, many children now are comforted by illustrations on the walls, footprints on the ceiling that lead back to the ward after surgery, and nurses specially trained to deal with children (e.g., Wilson, 1982). Pediatric psychologists have assisted in teaching the on-line nursing staff behavioral techniques to deal with common child management difficulties, such as bedtime problems (e.g., Rapoff, Christophersen, & Rapoff, 1982), and nurses, in turn, work to encourage parental involvement in caregiving (Roskies, Mongeon, & Gagnon-Lefebre, 1978).

The types of medical procedures performed on children today have also changed. For example, some surgeries such as routine tonsillectomies are no longer recommended, and over 40% of all surgeries are now performed as ambulatory or same-day surgery, involving being admitted early in the morning and returning home the same day (Polister, 1988). This allows children to remain in a comforting, familiar environment right up to the time of the surgery and then return to it during recovery.

Finally, as a later section of this chapter will document, preventive preparation for medical procedures takes place more routinely now. Thus, enhanced familial support, a child-friendly hospital environment, changes in surgical procedures, and better psychological preparation for medical procedures all have improved children's reactions to hospitalization and to medical procedures.

This is not to say that children do not experience clear distress during frightening or painful procedures. Most researchers report a gamut of immediate negative reactions, ranging from verbal expression of fear and discomfort and nonverbal indictors such as moaning, whimpering, and crying, to resistant behaviors such as kicking, pushing, or hitting (e.g., Faust, Olson, & Rodriguez, 1991; Lumley, Abeles, Melamed, Pistone, & Johnson, 1990; Peterson, Schultheis, Ridley-Johnson, Miller, & Tracy, 1984). However, most studies examining effects as much as 1 year following surgery find no evidence of negative carryover from procedures such as minor elective surgeries (e.g., Peterson & Shigetomi, 1982). Although no direct negative effects from minor surgery experiences have been reported following current hospital practices, research does suggest that the ability to cope with general life stresses early in life tends to produce better coping with problems later in childhood (Cicchetti & Schneider-Rosen, 1986). Although no long-term data exist, it seems logical that early feelings of self-efficacy in medical settings may be formed in these early encounters, and that such feelings may contribute to better coping later on. Thus, in addition to warranting intervention because of children's immediate and sometimes overwhelming distress, children's coping effectively with medical procedures is deserving of concern, study, and intervention because of its potential impact on future response to medical situations and on the child's general sense of self-efficacy.

As noted earlier, because childhood is a time when children are typically cared for and protected by adults, invasive medical procedures in which an adult deliberately causes a child to experience fear or pain are often difficult for the child to comprehend. This is particularly true for very young children, as will be seen in the following section, who are just beginning to build a sense of coping efficacy.

DEVELOPMENTAL ISSUES

Components of Coping and Development

The developmental implications for children's coping with medical procedures are profound. Children are accustomed to someone else serving as the coping agent. This adult coping agent typically adjusts the environment and his or her own responding to fit the child's temperament and stages of arousal (Field, 1985). When the caregiver fails to provide such coping, the child may feel abandoned. With age, children assume more responsibility for dealing with their own emotions, although adults continue in their protective role to some extent until late adolescence (Peterson, 1989).

In addition to mere lack of experience in coping, young children lack some of the prerequisites for effective coping. Their limited cognitive abilities make it difficult for them to interpret parameters of the procedure such as duration or intensity. Thus, for small children, visually salient procedures involving very brief but intense discomfort such as venipunctures and injections are particularly distressing (Eland & Anderson, 1977; Poster, 1983). Preschool-aged children are also more likely to harbor frightening misconceptions, such as the notion that all one's blood could leak out during a venipuncture (Sheridan, 1975). Harbeck and Peterson (1992) found that preschool children's thinking about pain was qualitatively different from that of older children. Unlike older children, preschool children do not have a clear idea of what pain is like; they do not understand why procedures hurt or how pain might be helpful or beneficial. Furthermore, they often lack a memory for past painful procedures, which may make an upcoming procedure more unfamiliar and confusing.

Verbally based techniques such as self-instruction and visually based techniques such as distraction and imagery depend on linguistic and visual–spatial skills that may be poorly developed in preschool children. Relaxing one's muscles requires experience and an ability to voluntarily direct action, which may be limited in younger children. Thus, preschool age children seem set up to cope especially poorly with medical procedures.

Not only are preschool age children less prepared to cope well, they respond less well to information-based preparations overall (Vernon & Thompson, 1993). However, Rasnake and Linscheid (1989) demonstrated that matching level of preprocedure information to preschool children's conceptual abilities resulted in lowered observer-rated distress during proctoscopy in comparison to children receiving standardized information or developmentally advanced information. Thus, understanding how to adjust preparation based on the child's developmental level seems an important challenge for preparation research.

Assessing Age Effects: A Surprising Absence of Results

As we have noted earlier (Peterson, 1989), despite the clear belief on the part of pediatric psychologists that developmental influences are of paramount importance in understanding children within medical settings, this research area has typically not examined age as a primary variable. There may be a variety of reasons for this. First, there has been a small but steady stream of results (samples of which are reported below) that have universally shown that where age effects exist, they are in the predictable direction of younger children coping more poorly than older children. Thus, age effects may no longer be of primary interest to some scientists, since their effects seem well known.

Second, research on response to medical procedures is extremely difficult to conduct and has tended to be underfunded. Sample size has been a primary concern for this area. Thus, investigators have often restricted samples to homogeneous age groups, matched groups for age, or covaried age effects out, some explicitly labeling age as a "nuisance" variable (Faust et al., 1991) rather than regarding age as a primary independent variable. Finally, some types of research have been limited to children 7 years of age and older who could provide interview and self-report data and who are most likely to understand and benefit from preparation. Thus, although in the United States, preschool children tend to be the age group most frequently admitted to a hospital (Azarnoff & Woody, 1981), the unique methods of coping they use and their developmental response to preparation have received little research attention.

Studies that have explored age effects have reported that in comparison to elementary school age children, preschool children recall prior procedures less well (Harbeck & Peterson, 1992), remember less of the preparation information they have been given (Melamed, Robbins, & Fernandez, 1982), are less likely to ask questions (Pidgeon, 1981) and to seek out information effectively (Peterson & Toler, 1986), and tend to comprehend medically relevant information less well (Simeonsson, Buckley, & Munson, 1979). Their coping strategies (coping strategies will be considered in more detail in the next section) tend to show more avoidance (Miller, Roussi, Caputo, & Kruus, 1995), more action- and less emotion-focused coping (Band & Weisz, 1988), and less usage of cognitive coping strategies (Brown, O'Keefe, Sanders, & Baker, 1986; Olson, Johnson, Powers, Pope, & Klein, 1993). All of these findings tend to predict less adaptive coping.

Preschool children's evidently lower level of positive coping skills appear to yield more problematic reactions to medical procedures. Preschool children report more distress during medical exams (Weisz, McCabe, & Dennig, 1994) and show higher levels of observable distress (Peterson & Shigetomi, 1981; Peterson, Schultheis, et al., 1984) and lower levels of cooperation during invasive procedures such as blood tests (Peterson & Toler, 1986). They cry and scream more (Manne, Bakeman, Jacobsen, & Redd, 1993), evidence generally higher levels of behavioral distress during medical procedures (Bachanas & Roberts, 1995), and show more postoperative problems such as coughing and choking (Peterson & Toler, 1986). Given that preschool children seem more poorly prepared to cope with medical procedures and evidence more problematic responses to them, one important avenue for future research will be methods to promote the early development of effective coping strategies and ways of amplifying skills in preschool age children.

PROCESSES INFLUENCING CHILDREN'S COPING

A Developmental Model of Coping

As if it were not complex enough to map the developmental changes in children's cognitive, linguistic, visual–spatial, and support-eliciting abilities that may be relevant to coping, the current literature suggests that these changes are best superimposed on a model of coping that focuses on at least three definitive episodes or stages of a threatening stimulus (see Lazarus & Lanier, 1978, for complete explication). First, the child experiences the *antici-pation/preparation* phase. During this phase, the child learns that a medical procedure must occur and is provided with various details about the procedure. The next phase is labeled *encounter;* during encounter the child must actually contact the medical procedure. During the final phase, *recovery,* the child must return to a preprocedure existence. There has been no published research directly focused on assisting in the recovery phase, and thus all the research reviewed in the next section focuses either on anticipation/preparation or encounter coping.

One source of great confusion is the belief that coping with the stressor occurs only during encounter. In reality, each of the phases involves a stressor (anticipation/preparation = learning of the procedure; encounter = the medical event; recovery = challenge to return to normal), the need for coping, and an outcome for that phase. Another source of confusion occurs when the child's coping response to the stressor (what the child does to limit his or her distress) is confused with the outcome of coping. For example, reduced crying might erroneously be labeled as a successful coping response rather than being correctly regarded as the outcome of successful coping. Other researches have used the term "coping response" only to signify a coping response with a positive outcome, whereas most researchers use the term to signify any coping attempt, regardless of its success.

Some researchers have reviewed the literature without considering whether a given study focused on coping within the anticipation/preparation phase (e.g., an active, information-seeking approach to the stressor of planning a medical procedure) or coping within the encounter phase (e.g., anxiously asking questions to delay a procedure). Such reviewers have concluded that there is little consistency in conclusions about what constitutes effective coping across studies. It is essential for the reader and the clinician to understand that adaptive coping responses a child may make during anticipation/preparation are likely to bear no resemblance to the adaptive coping during encounter. Manne et al. (1993) clearly demonstrated that techniques such as information seeking or self-assertion were not stable across phases of coping.

It would seem more logical to expect that a technique might have differing degrees of success depending on phase. For example, as will be seen below, information seeking results in positive outcomes during anticipation/preparation but negative outcomes during encounter. Further, the desired outcome in one phase is not necessarily the desired outcome in the next phase. Reduced arousal in encounter, for example, does not necessarily come from reduced arousal in the anticipation/preparation phase. In fact, one study suggested that increased arousal at the end of the anticipation/preparation phase may indicate successfully engaged anticipation/preparation coping, which in turn indicates a readiness to successfully deal with and produce lower arousal in encounter (Melamed, 1982). With these caveats as a beginning, we will now sample some of the exciting recent conceptualizations of how children cope with medical procedures.

Coping Research Base

Coping Models Based on Anticipation/Preparation Phase Responses

There have been a variety of different approaches to measuring how children cope with anticipation/preparation, but most have focused on the extent to which the child actively seeks out and takes in versus avoids information during the anticipation/preparation phase, the phase in which the child is preparing for but not yet in encounter with the medical procedure. In an early study focused on anticipation/preparation coping, Siegel (1981) reported that hospitalized children who sought out information about medical procedures could accurately report such information-seeking behavior in a structured interview. Such children were observed during encounter to be less anxious, more cooperative, and more tolerant of pain than children who avoided information during anticipation/preparation.

Our laboratory (Peterson & Toler, 1986) utilized Siegel's interview strategy to categorize children as information seeking versus information avoiding and found, as Siegel had, that children who reported gathering information actually knew more about their upcoming hospital procedure and initiated discussion prior to their blood test and anesthesia induction than children who avoided information. Information-seeking children were also less distressed than information-avoiding children after the encounter phase blood test and postsurgery period.

LaMontagne (1984, 1987) labeled the coping dimensions she studied "active" versus "avoidant," and found that active coping during the anticipation/preparation phase was associated with an internal locus of control. Using LaMontagne's interview, Thompson (1994) measured information-seeking or information-limiting styles of coping with anticipation/preparation. She found that individuals with a strong information-seeking *or* a strong information-avoiding strategy of coping tended to be less anxious than children who used combined strategies of receiving information. Although this may seem puzzling, recall that none of the studies using the LaMontagne interview measured actual response to the medical procedure in encounter. Thus, high information seekers may have lower self-reported anxiety because they feel prepared for encounter and individuals low in information avoidance may have low anxiety because they have remained unaware of the stressor to come. These latter individuals would not be predicted to remain low anxious during encounter by the other studies reviewed in this section.

There have been other ways of innovatively measuring the extent to which children will welcome versus block information during anticipation/preparation. For example, Knight et al. (1979) gave both an interview and a Rorschach interpretation at the same time that information about surgery was given to the child. Knight and colleagues categorized children as open to information (coping with intellectualization or mixed defenses) or defending (coping with denial, displacement, or projection) and found the former group to have lower anxiety during encounter (as indexed by urine cortisol) and better nurses' ratings of ward adjustment.

Burstein and Meichenbaum (1979) observed children in three distinct settings. First, prior to hospitalization, they recorded in a free play situation whether children played with either medically relevant toys (information seeking) or nonrelevant toys (information avoiding). Then, they used a self-report questionnaire to explore defensiveness in the children. Finally, these children were asked to report on how anxious they were on a hospital ward during recovery from a surgical procedure. Data across the three time periods were related. Children who played with the medically relevant toys gave less defensive answers on the questionnaire. More importantly, these children reported less anxiety while hospitalized following surgery.

Hubert, Jay, Saltoun, and Hayes (1988) used trained observers to assess children during the anticipation/preparation phase's formal participant modeling preparation program. They found that children who were observed to avoid information during the anticipation/preparation program were later observed to be more likely to act out during encounter with the bone marrow aspiration procedure. Such children also had higher observed distress on the hospital ward.

The findings of this literature are quite consistent; children who cope by seeking out information during anticipation/preparation tend to perform more adaptively than children who avoid information. This consistency stands in contrast to much of the adult literature on the related concept of sensitization–repression. As we have argued elsewhere (Schultheis, Peterson, & Selby, 1987), the adult literature typically describes sensitizers as high in anxiety and worry. Also labeled "vigilants" and "monitors," these individuals seem to bring a negative cognitive structure to appraisal that does not seem to fit the information-seeking children described here. Miller et al. (1995) make this point extremely well in one of the best applications of this conceptual framework to children. They showed children who cope by monitoring (worrying about the threat) to be more anxious, especially if they also try to avoid information. High monitors who do not avoid information, in contrast, have the lowest anxiety ratings. Thus, our strong recommendation would be that the literature on information seeking should not be confused with the larger "sensitizer" or "monitor" literature, or with any of the studies in the next section that examine information seeking during encounter rather than anticipation/preparation. Information seeking during anticipation/preparation serves a very different function than it does during encounter, as will be seen in the next section.

As a final intriguing note, the literature on children's information processing frequently uses memory for stressful medical procedures as an index of the degree to which threat disrupts ability to understand and recall information. Recent findings in that area suggest that children who (through either disposition or experimenter intervention) are experiencing high efficacy for control over the coming stressor actually process threatening cues better than neutral cues, whereas the reverse is true for children with a low sense of control (Cortez & Bugental, 1995). Thus, it may not be the tendency to approach per se, but it may be the child's sense of coping efficacy that influences information seeking in anticipation/preparation. That is, children who feel better equipped to cope with stress may be more open to accepting information about potentially frightening aspects of the procedure. This is an exciting concept to explore in future research.

Coping Models Based on Encounter Phase Responses

Smith and her colleagues (Smith et al., 1989; Smith Ackerson, Blotcky, & Berkow, 1990) utilized Siegel's (1981) interview but altered it to ask about how the child responded to the medical procedure itself. Their categorization of "information seeking" included behaviors such as positive self-statements, and "information avoiding" included such coping strategies as imagery, distraction, and relaxation; clearly, these categories were not the same coping styles referred to by the literature just reviewed on information avoiding in anticipation/preparation. Smith et al. (1990) failed to find any age effects on coping and also failed to find coping style to be related to fearfulness, reports of pain, or behavioral observations of distress.

Peterson, Harbeck, Chaney, Farmer, and Thomas (1990) similarly adapted

Siegel's interview to ask about both anticipation/preparation and encounter coping. However, rather than using the information-seeking versus information-avoiding labels that are relevant to anticipation/preparation, we regarded encounter coping as having two dimensions: Proactive versus reactive and stimulus approach versus stimulus blocking. Thus, examples of proactive/stimulus blocking would include techniques such as distraction, imagery, relaxation, and self-instruction. A proactive/stimulus approach would be to think about the sensation as not being painful (e.g., My arm is made of plastic, it is numb). Reactive reactions tended to involve worry about how to escape (stimulus blocking) or being uncooperative (stimulus approach). We found that self-reported information seeking in anticipation/preparation predicted proactive coping during the encounter phase.

Other investigators have categorized encounter responses into similar categories. For example, Brown et al. (1986) and Olson et al. (1993) labeled responses that were similar to the proactive techniques just described as "coping" (positive self-talk, relaxation, thought stopping) and categorized responses that were similar to the reactive coping responses described above as "catastrophizing" (focus on negative affect, escape or avoidance). The rate of encounter cognitive coping increased in both studies with age and in Brown et al. was negatively related to anxiety.

Other researchers have described the different potential goals of coping rather than focusing tightly on the goal of relieving subjective distress. As was discussed earlier, Band and Weisz (1988) examined 6-, 9-, and 12-year-old's coping to six different life situations (e.g., separation, school failure, and medical stress). They described a coping dichotomy of primary coping (similar to problem-focused coping, in which coping is "aimed at influencing objective conditions or events," p. 247) and secondary coping (similar to emotion-focused coping, in which the goal of coping is "maximizing one's goodness of fit with conditions as they are," p. 247), along with a category called relinquished control, which was used only 3.5% of the time. Thus, children tended to report doing something rather than nothing in response to the situations. The school failure seemed to call for more primary coping, while medical stress was more often responded to with secondary coping. Overall, with increasing age, children seemed to move away from primary to secondary coping. This was particularly true with medical procedures.

Weisz et al. (1994) replicated this developmental finding with children with leukemia who were faced with a series of painful medical procedures. Children who utilized more secondary coping had better general adjustment (lower Child Behavior Checklist scores, indicating less psychopathology), rated themselves as less distressed, and showed less distress on behavioral observations.

Summary

The studies reviewed in the last two sections provide a representative sample of the studies that have evolved categorical systems for children's coping with anticipation and with encounter, and have gathered descriptive data on the child's coping, in isolation from other environmental variables. This research demonstrates the orderliness of the majority of these data and reveals that proactive emotion-focused coping during encounter is associated with improved behavioral outcomes for children. In contrast, primary or instrumental coping, particularly when it is reactive rather than proactive, is associated with a lack of cooperation, negative emotional responses, and behavioral acting out.

It is unfortunate that so little work has looked at responding across phases. Because coping is typically a response directed toward a specific task (either preparation for, encounter with, or recovery from a stressor), it is essential for researchers to more clearly recognize the phase of responding under investigation. Ultimately, research that can follow children through their attempts at preparation during anticipation to assess how these attempts have allowed them to succeed or fail at coping during encounter may be the most valuable in planning interventions. Finally, very little research has been addressed toward the recovery phase. It may be that a sense of self-efficacy or awareness of one's potential for coping is best realized during the recovery phase. This remains for future research to investigate, however.

The next section reports on studies that have combined parental response categorization with categorizing children's coping responding. As will be seen, these studies are plagued more with both conceptual and methodological difficulties than the previous studies, and firm conclusions regarding these studies are much more difficult to identify. Because of the preliminary nature of this area, it will be merely overviewed before the larger section describing the role of parental presence and other family factors will be considered.

Parental Factors in Coping

Dyadic Interaction Studies

One of the earliest and best attempts to measure dyadic interaction patterns was reported by Bush et al. (1986). They observed 4- to 10-year-old children and their parents as they entered the examining room and ceased when the physician entered the room. Thus, it is unclear if this interaction is more appropriately viewed as occurring within anticipation/preparation or encounter. It appears to be more like the encounter situations reported in the past literature, but clearly constitutes a borderline case. Four classes of child outcome behavior were reported (prosocial, distress, attachment, and exploration) and six distinct forms of parental behaviors were observed (distraction, reassurance, ignoring, informing, agitation, and restraining). There were many interesting relationships observed, but we will focus here on child distress as the most relevant child variable to treatment. Not surprisingly, maternal agitation was linked to increased child distress and parental distraction to decreased child distress. Surprisingly, maternal reassurance was also linked to increased child distress. The authors noted that reassurance occurred more often with younger children and may have been elicited by children's distress rather than causing it.

Lumley et al. (1990) examined the interaction of maternal coping style with child temperament during encounter with anesthesia induction. Maternal coping style was characterized as high or low on two dimensions. The dimensions were obtained by identifying six categories of coping (distraction from medical topics, informing about medical topics, restraining, ignoring, reassuring, and agitation) and then combining the categories empirically rather than conceptually, using factor analysis to create a distraction–information cluster (formed with distraction, informing, and restraining) and emotional noninvolvement cluster (with ignoring, reassuring, and agitation). Four- to ten-year-old children's temperament was categorized as either withdrawing or approaching, using the Parent Temperament Questionnaire.

Lumley et al. (1990) found that the distraction–informing style of the parent interacted with the withdrawal–approaching temperament of the child. Specifically, children with a withdrawal temperament were highly distressed during anesthesia induction if their mothers were low distracting and high informing. However, children with an approach temperament had low distress during induction if their mothers were low distracting and high informing. In contrast, children with a withdrawal temperament had low distress if their mothers were high distracting and low informing, whereas this maternal pattern resulted in high distress among children with an approach temperament. However, this interaction was found on only one of a number of dependent variables, and thus should be regarded as suggestive rather than definitive.

Manne et al. (1992) similarly videotaped 43 adult–child dyads during encounter with a medical procedure. In this case, the procedure was encounter with a painful, brief medical procedure (venipuncture). Three child behaviors (cope, momentary distress, and cry/scream) and six parental behaviors (explain, distract, command to cope, give control to child, praise, and criticize/threaten) were observed. These authors used a sequential analysis to examine how the dyad members influenced each other. For example, child distress and crying were followed by increased explaining and decreased distraction by the adult. In turn, adult explaining was unlikely to be followed by child coping, and adult distraction diminished the chance the child would cry. It is difficult, if not impossible, to demonstrate causal relationships with such analyses. We are left wondering if parents' explaining leads children to be distressed and to fail to cope or if parents tend to explain if their child's coping falters and distress increases. These authors argue, however, that following explaining, greater-than-expected increases of child distress did not occur, but following child distress, greater-than-expected increases of explaining did occur. Thus, it seems more likely that distress causes explaining rather than vice versa, if there exists a causal relationship at all. In addition, it is unclear whether the child would fare better or worse if parents ceased explaining.

Frank, Blount, Smith, Manimala, and Martin (1995) described an award-winning masters thesis that utilized a sequential analysis strategy. This article began by reviewing a series of similar studies by Blount and his colleagues that focused on a variety of parent and child behaviors. These studies generally described three specific adult variables: coping promoting (including nonprocedural talk, humor, coping command), distress promoting (including reassurance, criticism, apology, giving control to the child, and empathy), and adult neutral behavior (including praise and commands to child). These causally labeled variables represent the combined scores for the conceptually dissimilar variables they include; the groupings were determined by correlations between these variables on earlier sequential analysis. Thus, variables that had been followed by child distress were labeled "distress promoting," despite the fact that (as was just seen in the Manne et al., 1992) a parent behavior that precedes child distress need not be causally related to it. In any case, the combined group of variables labeled "parental distress promoting" did predict a significant portion of the variance of child distress behavior in the Frank et al. (1995) study.

In addition to allowing more description of dyadic interaction (which is certainly of interest from a developmentalist's perspective), the primary purposes of describing naturalistic sequences of child and parent behavior is presumably to discover potential causal relationships that could serve to steer recommendations about more effective parent–child coping interactions. Because of the correlational nature of the data, it is difficult for such a study to do more than hypothesis build. It remains for an experimental intervention study to actively test the causal effects of parental coping responses suggested by the above studies. It is not clear why naturally occurring parental coping responses would be preferable to manipulate than those interventions (reviewed in the second-to-the-last section in this chapter) that have been used successfully in the past to create effective parental coping assistance. In any case, this area of research faces a number of challenges in the coming years before clear contributions to clinical intervention strategies are likely to be realized.

It is not surprising that such complicated sequences of parent–child behavior present difficulties in interpretation. As will be seen in the next section, even the mere presence or absence of parents during a procedure has led to conflicting results.

Parental Presence

As was noted in the introduction to this chapter there is no question concerning the positive influence of parental presence during the general period of hospitalization (Peterson et al., 1985). Early studies documented the positive influence of parental presence both for children's general hospitalization experience (Brain & Maclay, 1968) and for children undergoing specific stressful procedures such as anesthesia induction (Vernon, Foley, & Shulman, 1967) or a tooth filling (Frankl, Shiere, & Fogels, 1962). However, not all professionals have welcomed parental presence during medical procedures. For example, surveys of dentists (Roder, Lewis, & Law, 1961) and literature reviews (Gershen, 1976) have commented on the historical strong preference of dentists for parental absence.

More recently, some research has suggested that in certain circumscribed situations, parental presence may be related to more, rather than less, distress in children. We have previously noted that those medical procedures that involve highly visual, high-intensity, low-duration sensations such as injections, finger pricks, and venipunctures seem to present particular challenges to young children. Shaw and Routh (1982) observed 1.5- to 5-year-old children receiving an injection. Gross, Stern, Levin, Dale, and Wojnilower (1983) viewed 4- to 10-year-olds experiencing a venipuncture, and Gonzalez et al. (1989) rated children ages 3 to 5 who were receiving an injection. All three studies found that children were more distressed in the parent-present than in the parent-absent condition. Gross et al. suggested that children with parents present were not necessarily subjectively more anxious, but were acting distressed to elicit intervention and comfort from the mother, thus demonstrating a higher level of observable cues in her presence than in her absence.

Alternatively, some mothers may have been actively behaving in a way that caused their children to be more anxious. Historically, many health care workers have noted that some parents model fearful reactions to medical procedures, both verbally and with nonverbal cues such as facial signs of fear and covering their eyes (Venham, 1973). Fishman, Cook, Hammock, Gregory, and Thomas (1989) reported data consistent with this premise. They found children with fearful mothers displayed greater distress when the mother was present, whereas children of low-fear mothers were more distressed when their mothers were absent. Melamed (1993) similarly noted that maternal trait anxiety was associated with maternal agitation and ineffective distraction during an injection. Thus, maternal cuing of child distress behavior may in part be responsible for some increases in distress seen when the mother is present during a high-intensity, short-duration procedure.

It thus seems important to develop ways of decreasing such maternal anxiety. Jay and Elliott (1990) recently described a preparation program not for the children but for the parents, which used cognitive restructuring and relaxation to lower the parent's anxiety, and found less observable distress in the parents as a result. Programs that give parents a specific role such as that of coping coach also show diminished parental anxiety (Peterson & Shigetomi, 1981). Further, given that such studies (reviewed below) have shown that when parents are effective coping coaches for their children, both adult and child anxiety is reduced, it would seem likely that the potential negative effects of parental presence during invasive diagnostic procedures might be avoided if the parents were not only less anxious but also appropriately trained to deal effectively with their children's distress. The next section documents the use of parental training as one of the strong current directions in planning prevention interventions for children undergoing stressful medical procedures.

PREVENTIVE INTERVENTION

Preparation for medical procedures has historically been one of the earliest and best-researched areas in pediatric psychology (see reviews by Peterson & Harbeck, 1988; Siegel, 1976). There was early agreement that children profited from receiving accurate information (Prugh & Jordon, 1975). Later studies argued that in addition to simple information, children needed assistance in effectively dealing with procedures that evoked fear and pain. Four research traditions arose to offer such assistance: stress point preparation, modeling, hypnosis/distraction coaching, and coping training/stress inoculation. Each of these traditions will be described, and some examples of those studies with the most rigorous methodology and the best empirical evidence of their success will be considered. These studies used different outcome variables (from physiological to observed distress to subject reports of anxiety) and because of the nature of preparation, relied on randomized, posttest-only designs and typically small samples of only 10 to 20 children in any one treatment condition. They often measured different points during the hospital experience; most focused on both pre- and postsurgery measures. Most treatments lasted half an hour or less and were applied by nurses or paraprofessionals. Their common ground is that all of these techniques were determined to have beneficial preparation effects on children's later response to medical procedures.

Stress Point Preparation

A "stress point" was defined in this area as any one of a number of discrete, temporally limited stressors likely to occur during the child's hospital experience. Common stress points for a pediatric surgery stay might include admission, blood test, preoperative injection, separation from parents, and anesthesia induction. Wolfer and Visintainer (1975) assigned one nurse to be with the parent and the child directly before each stress point to inform and answer questions about and to support coping with each of the stressors. Children receiving these treatments appeared less distressed and experienced more rapid recoveries from surgery (e.g., taking fluids and ambulating sooner) in comparison with children receiving only routine care. Such special nursing care was shown by several investigators to reduce both parental and child anxiety (Ferguson, 1979; Skipper & Leonard, 1968; Skipper, Leonard, & Rhymes, 1968).

Models

Cassell (1965) utilized a puppet model to describe not only procedures but potential reactions children might have to a cardiac catheterization. Children receiving this procedure were not only less distressed during the procedure but were also more willing to return to the hospital for another visit. Melamed and Siegel (1975) published the first of a series of studies showing that a film of a peer model ("Ethan") experiencing hospitalization and surgery was an effective method of decreasing both observed distress and self-reported anxiety. They suggested that such a film offered both a desensitization experience and a model of appropriate responding; it was a clearly effective preparation vehicle. Melamed's group went on to describe many of the effective parameters of filmed modeling, including variables such as age and time (elementary school age children benefited from preparation more temporally removed from the event, whereas preschool age children needed more proximal treatment) (Melamed, Meyer, Gee, & Soule, 1976). They also documented the diminished effectiveness of modeling with children who had previously experienced surgery (Melamed, Dearborn, & Harmecz, 1983) or who were experiencing same-day surgery (Faust & Melamed, 1984).

Subsequent research offered replication of the positive effects of modeling and still more variations on the theme. Peterson, Schultheis, et al. (1984) demonstrated that a local (homemade) modeling film and a live puppet show were equally effective as Melamed and Siegel's "Ethan" film, and all three modeling programs resulted in lower distress and lower self-reported fear in comparison to a control group. Peterson, Schultheis et al. (1984) showed that a hospital tour and exposure to medical instruments in the absence of a modeling component failed to provide the preventive benefits in reduced observable distress and self-reported anxiety seen from a modeling preparation. Pinto and Hollandsworth (1989) used a modeling film either with or without the parents present. Children who viewed the film showed a more positive response on every variable measured, from physiologically indexed anxiety in the form of the palmar sweat to observer-rated anxiety and self-reported fear. Parents who viewed the film were also less anxious than parents who did not view it. Interestingly, parents who did not view the film but whose child did were less anxious than parents of control-group children. Pinto and Hollandsworth (1989) also added a unique and important dimension to their study by demonstrating that prepared children actually required fewer medications and less time in the hospital, saving the hospital money and demonstrating the cost-effectiveness of intervention.

Hypnosis and Distraction

Stress point preparation and modeling programs were effective tools in preparing children for an entire hospital experience. However, for medical procedures that involved a more focused, threatening, and painful stressor, such as bone marrow aspiration or burn debridement, different techniques were required. Hypnosis was one of the earliest techniques employed (LaBaw, Holton, Tewell, & Eccles, 1975). Zeltzer and LeBaron (1982) used both clinician-coached techniques (such as distraction) and hypnosis to reduce pain in child cancer patients, ages 6–17, who were undergoing bone marrow aspirations and lumbar punctures. The hypnosis was made up of "intense imaginal involvement" in which the child's attention was engaged in novel and exciting imaginary situations. Both kinds of techniques reduced pain, but hypnosis was more effective in reducing anxiety. More recent studies have replicated these findings (e.g., Kuttner, Bowman, & Teasdale, 1988), have described different applications depending on the developmental level of the child (e.g., Kuttner, 1989), and have offered case examples for highly challenging situations such as emergency room interventions (Kohen, 1986).

Elliott and Olson (1983) used relaxation plus deep breathing, attention distraction, and rewards to assist pediatric burn patients in coping. Kelley, Jarvie, Middlebrook, McNeer, and Drabman (1984) similarly used both cartoon viewing as distraction and small rewards for inhibiting distress cues to assist two children undergoing hydrotherapy treatment. Jay, Elliott, Ozolins, and Olson (1983) successfully treated ten highly distressed pediatric cancer patients using modeling, positive imagery, reinforcement for lying still, and deep breathing. Finally, Dahlquist, Gil, Armstrong, Ginsberg, and Jones (1985) had a clinical psychologist or graduate student coach three children in cue controlled relaxation, controlled breathing, pleasant imagery, and positive self-talk during chemotherapy venipunctures and found that the children and medical staff (but not parents) rated child distress as greatly diminished.

These multicomponent, behavioral preparation programs have much in common with the coping/stress inoculation procedures in the next section. They are placed here because the primary instigator of the technique, like the hypnosis studies, is the clinician. Elliott and Olson (1983) actually attempted to remove from the room the pediatric psychologist who coached the child during the medical procedures and found that the children no longer benefited from the techniques. In contrast with this need to retain the clinician–coach, for the studies in the next section, there was no clinician present to serve as a coach. Thus, for the coping/stress inoculation techniques, the parent–child team or the child him- or herself was the therapeutic agent.

Coping/Stress Inoculation

One of the difficulties of the literature on children's coping with medical procedures is the use of the single word "coping" paired with multiple meanings. Not only is "coping" used to signify behaviors the child and parent emit to attempt to deal effectively with a stressor (sometimes the label means *only* the effective responses and sometimes all responses), but in this context it also means the behaviors the children are taught to use to deal with the stressors in the encounter phase.

One direction for studies using coping skill instruction or stress inoculation was the involvement of parents as legitimate treatment agents. Peterson and Shigetomi (1981) asked whether modeling, coping training, or the combination of both delivered to mother–child dyads might be most successful in reducing child distress. Using the parents as coping coaches, we found that the coping skills training, including deep breathing, relaxation, self-instruction, and imagery in combination with the "Ethan" modeling film, was most effective when children were faced with highly stressful procedures such as the venipuncture and the preoperative injection. Children who received the coping technology tended to drink, eat, and void sooner after surgery and their parents felt less anxious and more effective.

Zastowny, Kirschenbaum, and Meng (1986) did not use a model contrast group, but they did similarly use parents as coping coaches. They taught parents generally about dealing with stress and about stress inoculation techniques (preparation, confrontation, coping with feelings, and self-reinforcement), and they trained parents to cue their children in deep breathing and distraction. Children whose parents received such training were more cooperative, especially during stressful procedures such as the preoperative injection, and were rated as better adjusted following surgery. Trained parents also reported that they themselves experienced less anxiety.

For mothers of preschool children experiencing a cardiac catheterization, stress management training was also found to be the most effective preparation by Campbell et al. (1992), who contrasted such preparation with education, supportive psychotherapy, all three active techniques together, and a no-treatment control group. Children whose mothers were in the stress management groups were observed to be less distressed and more cooperative during both the venipuncture and the catheterization procedure, in comparison to children whose parents received other preparations. In addition, stress management group children were rated by their mothers as having a more favorable post-hospital adjustment than the other children.

Siegel and Peterson (1980, 1981) similarly tried to pose the "which is the more effective preparation" question for preschool children by contrasting the use of sensory information (an adult allowed children to hear auditory cues, small olfactory cues, and provided a positive but accurate sensory description of the procedure) and coping skills training (the adult provided the same training packages as used in Peterson & Shigetomi, 1981) with nonspecific support (the adult read the children a story from "Winnie the Pooh"). The children were experiencing their first tooth filling, which occurred in the absence of their parents, because this low-income preschool sample had their dental work completed while in day care. Sensory information and coping were equally effective, and both resulted in increased behavioral cooperation and decreased observable distress when compared with the nonspecific support intervention.

The tendency in these original coping skills preparation programs to involve the parents when possible and to combine techniques seemed to presage the current strategies being tested. The area seems to be moving toward programs that combine several empirically validated techniques in an effort to create the most effective technology possible. Examples of such programs can be seen in the next section.

Composite Techniques

One of the early interpretations of the effectiveness of modeling preparations was the concept that the model suggested coping skills for children to imitate. Klingman, Melamed, Cuthbert, and Hermecz (1984) noted that participant modeling (where the child is encouraged and given time to imitate the model) was more effective in preparing children for medical procedures than symbolic modeling (where the child simply observes the model). When Faust et al. (1991) began preparing children for same-day surgery, they recognized that a simple modeling preparation used in the past had been ineffective with same-day surgery patients, presumably because there was too little time for the children to assimilate the information in the film (Faust & Melamed, 1984). Faust et al. (1991) elected to combine coping skills training with modeling. Through a slide-and-tape presentation, they trained 4- to 10-year-old children alone or with their parents to engage in deep breathing and imagery, using a child model. Children who had received the participant modeling treatment, regardless of whether their mothers were present or not, showed fewer distressed behaviors postsurgery than the control children.

Manne et al. (1990) described an ingenious method to afford children control over their breathing and distraction during brief invasive procedures such as venipunctures. They used a party blower and asked parents to coach their children to control the party blowers' expansion by blowing it very slowly, while the parent counted. This simple technique was very successful in reducing children's uncooperative and distressed behavior. Blount et al. (1992) later replicated these findings.

Similarly, Powers et al. (1993) used parents as coaches for distraction, use of party blowers, and counting techniques with their 3- to 5-year-old children who were to experience painful injections and venipuncture for intravenous treatment. This study was able to examine maintenance of such treatment over time. Parent coping-promoting behaviors did decrease over time but always remained above baseline. Children continued to intermittently use the techniques, but periodically failed to use the coping behaviors, with subsequent intermittent behavioral distress. The need for more extensive training or booster sessions with a clinician–coach may be indicated, but even if such intervention were required, this would remain a very cost effective treatment.

Summary

As this section of the chapter indicates, there have been a variety of approaches to preparation for medical procedures, and each of the techniques reviewed here has been found to be effective in reducing children's observable or self-reported distress. A logical question is, if all of these techniques offer some degree of effectiveness, which is the most effective? Hospital administrators would want to go further and play degree of success in reducing distress off against cost of the preparation. Unfortunately, this literature is singularly unenlightening concerning comparative effectiveness and cost. These studies examined many different medical procedures with children of different ages and medical histories, using different outcome measures taken at different times during the medical procedure. The multicomponent procedures rarely utilized a component analysis, and it was rare that investigators examined long-term effects of the procedures. The few comparative studies offered mixed conclusions. For example, Peterson and Shigetomi (1981) found modeling plus coping to be more successful than modeling alone in reducing observed and subjective reported distress, but only for dependent variables involving high levels of immediate stress (e.g., venipuncture, presurgery injection). A year after they received intervention, one third of the parents receiving coping (but not modeling) reported that the treatment continued to influence their children's behavior. In the absence of explicit within-study comparisons, differences in subjects, medical procedures, preparation types, and outcome variables make cross-study comparisons highly suspect. One important avenue for future research is to cease proving that new techniques are effective and to begin to explore which methods of preparation are the most effective.

Establishing comparative effectiveness is only one of the challenges that awaits this area in the future. As will be seen in the final section of this chapter, the challenge of widespread implementation, continued involvement of the family, the conceptual justification of descriptive work, and renewed sensitivity to individual differences such as developmental level and characteristic coping style all remain for future research in this expanding area.

FUTURE RESEARCH CHALLENGES

Implementation

Peterson and Ridley-Johnson (1980), in a good news/bad news report, noted that although their survey of pediatric hospitals revealed that most hospitals did have presurgical preparation programs, most of these programs involved didactic presentations and hospital tours, which have been found by research reviewed in this chapter to be inferior preparation vehicles. Recently, a similar survey by O'Byrne, Peterson, and Saldana (in press) revealed mild improvements, with half of the pediatric hospitals in this country reporting use of modeling films for child surgery patients and training children in relaxation and coping prior to fingerpricks, oncology procedures, cardiac catheterization, and surgery. However, hospital administrators, pediatric surgeons, and the nursing staff, who make decisions at various levels concerning preparation, receive their information from in-service presentations, workshops, word of mouth, and occasionally from medical journals. According to this survey, only 28% read psychology journals such as *Journal of Consulting and Clinical Psychology, Behavior Therapy, Health Psychology,* and *Journal of Pediatric Psychology,* the repositories of the majority of the studies just reviewed. It is a common lament in clinical psychology that researchers are not effective politicians in arranging the adoption of our techniques.

Studying dissemination is a challenge not often undertaken by the coping literature. Most attempts have been surveys like those cited above, which merely report the level of success or failure in introducing research findings into practice. O'Byrne et al. (in press) attempted to go beyond merely describing implementation levels, to exploring those characteristics of the agent responsible for designing preparation programs that might predict whether that agent would select techniques suggested by the research literature as more effective. The agent's professional degree (BA, RN/MS, PhD/MD), length of time in current hospital position, source of information (workshops, media, nursing journals, psychology journals), past evaluation of the program, and knowledge of coping techniques were used as predictors, with the criterion to be predicted a numerical index of the extent to which the technique was suggested as effective by the literature. Only two of these variables successfully predicted the type of procedures used to prepare children in pediatric hospitals for fingerpricks and venipunctures. Specifically, use of research journals and greater knowledge of coping techniques predicted more effective techniques being used. However, none of these factors significantly predicted selection of preparation techniques for oncology procedures, special procedures, or surgeries. Intensive study, perhaps using open-ended survey questions or interviews, of the process by which techniques are selected may be necessary prior to interventions to improve implementation of research findings. We do not even know at present whether research findings are ever accessed by decision makers, whether the results are available but are not compelling, or whether the results are compelling but the technology is viewed as too expensive or too innovative for adoption in hospitals that tend to be fiscally very conservative.

In addition to understanding how the process naturalistically takes place, experimental endeavors could be undertaken to assess the pathways for enhanced dissemination of research results. If research results focused not only on effectiveness in terms of improved psychosocial functioning, but also underlined patient satisfaction, reduced medication and length of hospital stay, and relative ease of administration, they might be more readily adopted. It also would be of interest whether it is more important for the information to contact physicians (who "own" the child patients and dictate many aspects of their care), hospital administrators (who allocate funds and staff for preparation and who are alert to public relations issues and cost savings), or nursing staff and child life workers (who actually operate the programs).

Other areas of psychology have documented grass roots efforts that culminate in citizens demanding legal changes to support requirements such as safety belts (e.g., Fawcett, Seekins, & Jason, 1987). If those systems such as the American Academy of Pediatrics and the American Association for Care of Children in Hospitals that have taken political stands recommending that parents accompany their hospitalized children and that children receive preparation for surgery could be induced to recommend changing from techniques with no empirical supporting data to those techniques shown by research to be effective, large-scale changes might result. The technology exists to mount such a campaign; following its success in a research report would be invaluable.

Family Involvement

Thus far, the literature has demonstrated that separation from the parent is an unnecessary stressor and that for the most part parental presence is a valuable aid. Additional study is needed of those immediate, invasive procedures in which parental presence may be problematic. There are many hypotheses concerning why children may be more distressed in their parents' presence. A pragmatic solution would seem to be the examination of whether parental presence is a positive or negative feature if the parent is an effective coping coach. The current literature involving parents indicates that not only are children less distressed with a parent coping coach, but the parent is less distressed and feels more competent as well.

There is a small literature on siblings of chronically ill children and some anecdotal reports regarding siblings of pediatric surgery patients. Now that nearly half of surgery patients and most child cancer patients are with their families until the hour of the procedure and back again before night, the study of the impact of family dynamics for children undergoing medical procedures seems overdue. There are a myriad of questions that might be asked. Is it beneficial for the hospitalized child to receive support from siblings? Is it good for the siblings? Should the same parent remain with the hospitalized child or is it helpful to alternate parent support? Is prolonged separation of the parents to afford caregiving to the hospitalized child detrimental to the marriage? Are two parents at the hospital better than one? What is the cost to the homebound siblings? How does the family's need for mutual support shift with length of hospitalization or with the child's developmental level? These are only a small sample of the research questions that would enrich this area.

Questionable Value of Current Descriptive Study of Dyadic Interactions

Areas within psychology go through cycles in which, on one hand, observational studies describe human reactions and observed patterns of reactions are used to generate conceptual models, and, on the other hand, experimental studies operate from a given conceptual model and yield cause-and-effect solutions. It is a good argument to suggest that before effective prevention programs can be mounted, solid descriptive work is needed to create a theoretical basis for subsequent intervention (Chassin, Presson, & Sherman, 1985). However, the extent to which the observational studies exploring parent cues to child coping are yielding a conceptual basis different from that which already exists is dubious. None of these studies has revealed any new techniques that could be taught to parents and their children. None revealed mechanisms for coping that were unknown before. For example, one of the best descriptive findings that can be applied from this literature is that when parents make a request for the child to cope, the child is more likely to cope. Now that some studies have revealed no new technologies, the extensive time and effort of such a study might be better directed to improving existing interventions.

Individual Differences

Once effective technology is available, clinicians can afford the luxury of asking "which treatment from which clinician will work best with which child in which situation?" As was noted earlier, age is widely acknowledged as a very important determinant of coping, but studies have not yet focused on which techniques work best with which age children. Effective techniques need to be found for very young children in particular. Similarly, previous procedural experience and disease stage are important subject variables deserving of study. Finally, it is clear that different medical procedures may demand different prevention techniques. It would be helpful if there was more multicomponent preparation with follow-up to ascertain what tools families actually use in which situations and how effective these strategies are.

Phases of the Stressor

Early in this chapter, we argued for a developmental model of coping that would take into account differences in anticipation/preparation, encounter, and recovery phases. There is the presumption that interventions in the first phase influence the second and third phases, but most studies do not provide appropriate measures of each phase. Consider how such research might intersect with the study of individual coping styles, or with parental coaching of coping, or both. Does knowing how a child typically approaches anticipation/preparation or how the parent usually coaches during anticipation/preparation allow us to select an optimal intervention technique to reduce distress in anticipation/preparation? Further, is low distress in anticipation/preparation necessarily related to low distress during encounter? For most programs, reduced distress in encounter rather than anticipation/preparation is typically the goal. We have also presumed that effective coping in encounter improves coping in recovery and the child's long-term sense of self-efficacy in medical situations. Empirical validation of these presumptions seems vital. Ultimately, the most valuable research will be that which must take place to ensure optimal long-term consequences.

CONCLUSIONS

We began this chapter by suggesting that children's encounters with medical procedures were an ideal arena within which to study children's coping with stress and pain. The volume of knowledge that exists in this area is merely overviewed in this chapter. It seems likely that children's responses to many other stressful situations that involve enduring rather than changing the situation could be assisted with such knowledge. It is unclear whether children's feelings of high or low self-efficacy in this arena influence other areas of their coping, but this seems likely. This current volume and other areas where research on children's coping is brought together seem to be important steps to unite the fields of knowledge on children's coping in order to enrich and enhance our understanding of each.

REFERENCES

Azarnoff, P., & Woody, R. D. (1981). Preparation of children for hospitalization in acute care hospitals in the United States. *Pediatrics, 68,* 361–368.

Bachanas, P. J., & Roberts, M. C. (1995). Factors affecting children's attitudes toward health care and responses to stressful medical procedures. *Journal of Pediatric Psychology, 20,* 261–275.

Band, E. B., & Weisz, J. R. (1988). How to feel better when it feels bad: Children's perspectives on coping with every day stress. *Developmental Psychology, 24,* 247–253.

Blount, R. L., Bachanas, P. J., Powers, S. W., Cotter, M. C., Franklin, A., Chaplin, W., Mayfield, J., Henderson, M., & Blount, S. D. (1992). Training children to cope and parents to coach them during routine immunizations: Effects on child, parent, and staff behaviors. *Behavior Therapy, 23,* 689–705.

Brain, D., J., & Maclay, I. (1968). Controlled study of mothers and children in hospital. *British Medical Journal, 1,* 278–280.

Brown, J. M., O'Keefe, J., Sanders, S. H., & Baker, B. (1986). Developmental changes in children's cognitions to stressful and painful situations. *Journal of Pediatric Psychology, 11,* 343–357.

Burstein, S., & Meichenbaum, D. (1979). The work of worrying in children undergoing surgery. *Journal of Abnormal Child Psychology, 7,* 121–132.

Bush, J. P., Melamed, B. G., Sheras, P. L., & Greenbaum, P. E. (1986). Mother–child patterns of coping with anticipatory medical stress. *Health Psychology, 5,* 137–157.

Campbell, L. A., Kirkpatrick, S. E., Berry, C. C., Penn, N. E., Waldman, J. D., & Mathewson, J. W. (1992). Psychological preparation of mothers of preschool children undergoing cardiac catheterization. *Psychology and Health, 7,* 175–185.

Cassell, S. (1965). Effects of brief puppet therapy upon the emotional responses of children undergoing cardiac catheterization. *Journal of Consulting and Clinical Psychology, 29,* 1–8.

Chapman, A. H., Loeb, D. G., & Gibbons, M. J. (1956). Psychiatric aspects of hospitalizing children. *Archives of Pediatrics, 73,* 77–88.

Chassin, L. A., Presson, C. C., & Sherman, S. J. (1985). Stepping backwards in order to step forward: An acquisition-oriented approach to primary prevention. *Journal of Consulting and Clinical Psychology, 53,* 612–622.

Cicchetti, D., & Schneider-Rosen, K. (1986). An organizational approach to childhood depression. In M. Rutter, C. E. Izard, & P. B. Read (Eds.), *Depression in young people: Clinical and developmental perspectives* (pp. 71–134). New York: Guilford Press.

Cortez, V. L., & Bugental, D. B. (1995). Priming of perceived control in young children as a buffer against fear-inducing events. *Child Development, 66,* 687–696.

Dahlquist, L. M., Gil, K. M., Armstrong, D., Ginsberg, A., & Jones, B. (1985). Behavioral management of children's distress during chemotherapy. *Journal of Behavior Therapy and Experimental Psychiatry, 16,* 325–329.

Douglas, J.W.B. (1975). Early hospital admission and later disturbances of behaviour and learning. *Developmental Medicine and Child Neurology, 17,* 456–480.

Eland, J. M., & Anderson, J. E. (1977). The experience of pain in children. In A. Jacox (Ed.), *Pain: A source book for nurses and other professionals* (pp. 453–473). Boston: Little, Brown.

Elkins, P. D., & Roberts, M. C. (1985). Reducing medical fears in a general population of children: A comparison of three audiovisual modeling procedures. *Journal of Pediatric Psychology, 10,* 65–75.

Elliott, C. H., & Olson, R. A. (1983). The management of children's behavioral distress in response to painful medical treatment for burn injuries. *Behaviour Research and Therapy, 21,* 675–683.

Faust, J., & Melamed, B. G. (1984). Influence of arousal, previous experience, and age on surgery preparation of same-day surgery and in-hospital patients. *Journal of Consulting and Clinical Psychology, 52,* 359–365.

Faust, J., Olson, R., & Rodriguez, H. (1991). Same-day surgery preparation: Reduction of pediatric patient arousal and distress through participant modeling. *Journal of Consulting and Clinical Psychology, 59,* 475–478.

Fawcett, S. B., Seekins, A., & Jason, L. A. (1987). Policy research and child passenger safety legislation: A case study and experimental evaluation. *Journal of Social Issues, 43*(2), 133–148.

Ferguson, B. F. (1979). Preparing young children for hospitalization: A comparison of two methods. *Pediatrics, 64,* 656–664.

Field, T. M. (1985). Attachment as psycho-biological attunement: Being on the same wavelength. In M. Reite & T. Field (Eds.), *Psychobiology of attachment and separation* (pp. 90–118). New York: Academic Press.

Fishman, B. E., Cook, E. W., Hammock, S. J., Gregory, B. R., & Thomas, J. P. (1989, April). *Familial transmission of fear: Effects of maternal anxiety and presence on children's response to dental treatment.* Paper presented at the Florida Conference on Child Health Psychology, Gainesville, FL.

Frank, N. C., Blount, R. L., Smith, A. J., Manimala, M. R., & Martin, J. K. (1995). Parent and staff behavior, previous child medical experience, and maternal anxiety as they relate to child procedural distress and coping. *Journal of Pediatric Psychology, 20,* 277–289.

Frankl, S. N., Shiere, F. R., & Fogels, H. R. (1962). Should the parent remain with the child in the dental operatory? *Journal of Dentistry for Children, 29,* 150–163.

Gabriel, H. P. (1977). A practical approach to preparing children for dermatologic surgery. *Journal of Dermatological Surgery and Oncology, 3,* 523–526.

Gershen, J. A. (1976). Maternal influence on the behavior patterns of children in the dental situation. *Journal of Dentistry for Children, 43,* 28–32.

Gonzalez, J. C., Routh, D. K., Saab, P. G., Armstrong, F. D., Shifman, L., Gueria, E., & Fawcett, N. (1989). Effect of parent presence on children's reactions to injections: Behavioral, physiological, and subjective aspects. *Journal of Pediatric Psychology, 14,* 449–462.

Gross, A. M., Stern, R. M., Levin, R. B., Dale, J., & Wojnilower, P. A. (1983). The effect of mother–child separation on the behavior of children experiencing a diagnostic medical procedure. *Journal of Consulting and Clinical Psychology, 51,* 783–785.

Harbeck, C., & Peterson, L. (1992). Elephants dancing in my head: A developmental approach to children's concepts of specific pains. *Child Development, 63,* 138–149.

Hardgrove, C. B. (1980). Helping parents on the pediatric ward: A report on a survey of hospitals with "living-in" programs. *Pediatrician, 9,* 220–223.

Hubert, N. C., Jay, S. M., Saltoun, M., & Hayes, M. (1988). Approach/avoidance and distress in children undergoing preparation for painful medical procedures. *Journal of Clinical Child Psychology, 17,* 194–202.

Jackson, K., Winkley, R., Faust, O. A., & Cermack, E. (1952). The problem of emotional trauma in the hospital treatment of children. *Journal of the American Medical Association, 149,* 1536–1538.

Jay, S. M., & Elliott, C. H. (1990). A stressful inoculation program for parents whose children are undergoing painful medical procedures. *Journal of Consulting and Clinical Psychology, 58,* 799–804.

Jay, S. M., Elliott, C. H., Ozolins, M., & Olson, R. (1983). *Behavioral management of children's distress during painful medical procedures.* Unpublished manuscript.

Jensen, R. A. (1955). The hospitalized child: Round table. *American Journal of Orthopsychiatry, 25,* 293–318.

Johnson, J. E., Kirchoff, K. T., & Endress, M. P. (1975). Altering children's distress behavior during orthopedic case removal. *Nursing Research, 24,* 404–410.

Kelley, M. L., Jarvie, G. J., Middlebrook, J. L., McNeer, M. F., & Drabman, R. S. (1984). Decreasing burned children's pain behavior: Impacting the trauma of hydrotherapy. *Journal of Applied Behavior Analysis, 17*, 147–158.

Klingman, A., Melamed, B. G., Cuthbert, M. I., & Hermecz, D. A. (1984). Effects of participant modeling on information acquisition and skill utilization. *Journal of Consulting and Clinical Psychology, 52*, 414–422.

Knight, R. B., Atkins, A., Eagle, C., Evans, N., Finkelstein, J. W., Fukushima, D., Katz, J., & Weiner, H. (1979). Psychological stress, ego-defense, and cortisol production in children hospitalized for elective surgery. *Psychosomatic Medicine, 41*, 40–49.

Kohen, D. (1986). Applications of relaxation/mental imagery (self-hypnosis) in pediatric emergencies. *The International Journal of Clinical and Experimental Hypnosis, 34*, 283–294.

Kuttner, L. (1989). Management of young children's acute pain and anxiety during invasive medical procedures. *Pediatrician, 16*, 39–44.

Kuttner, L., Bowman, M., & Teasdale, M. (1988). Psychological treatment of distress, pain, and anxiety for young children with cancer. *Developmental and Behavioral Pediatrics, 9*, 374–381.

LaBaw, W., Holton, C., Tewell, K., & Eccles, D. (1975). The use of self-hypnosis by children with cancer. *The American Journal of Clinical Hypnosis, 17*, 233–238.

LaMontagne, L. L. (1984). Children's locus of control beliefs as predictors of preoperative coping behavior. *Nursing Research, 32*, 76–79, 85.

LaMontagne, L. L. (1987). Children's preoperative coping: Replication and extension. *Nursing Research, 36*, 163–167.

Lazarus, R. S., & Lanier, R. (1978). Stress-related transactions between person and environment. In L. A. Pervin & M. Lewis (Eds.), *Perspectives in interactional psychology* (pp. 287–327). New York: Plenum Press.

Lumley, M. A., Abeles, L. A., Melamed, B. G., Pistone, L. M., & Johnson, J. H. (1990). Coping outcomes in children undergoing stressful medical procedures: The role of child–environment variables. *Behavioral Assessment, 12*, 223–238.

Manne, S. L., Bakeman, R., Jacobsen, P., Gorfinkle, K., Bernstein, D., & Redd, W. (1992). Adult–child interaction during invasive medical procedures. *Health Psychology, 11*, 241–249.

Manne, S. L., Bakeman, R., Jacobsen, P., & Redd, W. H. (1993). Children's coping during invasive medical procedures. *Behavior Therapy, 24*, 143–158.

Manne, S. L., Redd, W. H., Jacobsen, P. B., Gorfinkle, K., Shorr, O., & Rapkin, B. (1990). Behavioral intervention to reduce child and parent distress during venipuncture. *Journal of Consulting and Clinical Psychology, 58*, 565–572.

Melamed, B. (1982). Reduction of medical fears: An information processing analysis. In J. Boulougouris (Ed.), *Learning theory approaches to psychiatry* (pp. 205–218). New York: Wiley-Interscience.

Melamed, B. G. (1993). Putting the family back in the child. *Behaviour Research and Therapy, 31*, 239–247.

Melamed, B. G., Dearborn, M. I., & Hermecz, D. A. (1983). Necessary considerations for surgery preparation: Age and previous experience. *Psychosomatic Medicine, 45*, 517–525.

Melamed, B. G., Meyer, R., Gee, C., & Soule, L. (1976). The influence of time and type of preparation on children's adjustment to hospitalization. *Journal of Pediatric Psychology, 1*, 31–37.

Melamed, B. G., Robbins, R. L., & Fernandez, J. (1982). Factors to be considered in psychological preparation for surgery. In D. Routh & M. Wolraich (Eds.), *Advances in developmental and behavioral pediatrics* (pp. 51–72). New York: JAI.

Melamed, B. G., & Siegel, L. J. (1975). Reduction of anxiety in children facing hospitalization and surgery by use of filmed modeling. *Journal of Consulting and Clinical Psychology, 43*, 511–521.

Miller, S. M., Roussi, P., Caputo, G. C., & Kruus, L. (1995). Patterns of children's coping with an aversive dental treatment. *Health Psychology, 14*, 236–246.

O'Byrne K., Peterson, L., & Saldana, L. (in press). *Predicting the selection of effective prehospital preparation programs: Pediatric hospital response to survey.* Health Psychology.

Olson, A. L., Johnson, S. G., Powers, L. E., Pope, J. B., & Klein, R. B. (1993). Cognitive coping strategies of children with chronic illness. *Developmental and Behavioral Pediatrics, 14*, 217–223.

Peterson, L. (1984). A brief methodological comment on possible inaccuracies induced by multimodal measurement analysis and reporting. *Journal of Behavior Medicine, 7*, 307–313.

Peterson, L. (1989). Coping by children undergoing stressful medical procedures: Some conceptual, methodological, and therapeutic issues. *Journal of Consulting and Clinical Psychology, 57,* 380–387.

Peterson, L., & Harbeck, C. (1988). *The pediatric psychologist: Issues in professional development and practice.* Champaign, IL: Research Press.

Peterson, L., Harbeck, C., Chaney, J., Farmer, J., & Thomas, A. M. (1990). Children's coping with medical procedures: A conceptual overview and integration. *Behavioral Assessment, 12,* 197–212.

Peterson, L., Mori, L., & Carter, P. (1985). The role of the family in children's responses to stressful medical procedures. *Journal of Clinical Child Psychology, 14,* 98–104.

Peterson, L., & Oliver, K. K. (1994). Prevention of injuries and diseases. In M. C. Roberts (Ed.), *Handbook of pediatric psychology* (pp. 185–199). New York: Guilford Press.

Peterson, L., & Ridley-Johnson, R. (1980). Pediatric hospital response to surgery on prehospital preparation for children. *Journal of Pediatric Psychology, 5,* 1–7.

Peterson, L., Ridley-Johnson, R., Tracy, K., & Mullins, L. L. (1984). Developing cost-effective presurgical preparation: A comparative analysis. *Journal of Pediatric Psychology, 9,* 274–296.

Peterson, L., Schultheis, K., Ridley-Johnson, R., Miller, D. V., & Tracy, K. C. (1984). Comparison of three modeling procedures on the presurgical and postsurgical reactions of children. *Behavior Therapy, 15,* 197–203.

Peterson, L., & Shigetomi, C. (1981). The use of coping techniques to minimize anxiety in hospitalized children. *Behavior Therapy, 12,* 1–14.

Peterson, L., & Shigetomi, C. (1982). One-year follow-up of elective surgery child patients perceiving preoperative preparation. *Journal of Pediatric Psychology, 7,* 43–48.

Peterson, L., & Starr, L. (1994, April). *Coping with medical procedures and injury: Issues in children coping with medical procedures.* Paper presented at the 15th Annual Scientific Session of the Society of Behavioral Medicine, Boston, MA.

Peterson, L., & Toler, S. M. (1986). An information seeking disposition in child surgery patients: Some preliminary evidence. *Health Psychology, 5,* 343–358.

Pidgeon, V. (1981). Children's concepts of illness: Implications for health teaching. *Maternal–Child Nursing Journal, 14,* 23–35.

Pinto, R. P., & Hollandsworth, J. G. (1989). Using video tape modeling to prepare children psychologically for surgery: Influence of parents and costs versus benefits of providing preparation services. *Health Psychology, 8,* 79–95.

Polister, P. (1988). Ambulatory surgery: Some issues and considerations. *American College of Surgery Bulletin, 73,* 26–29.

Poster, E. C., (1983). Stress immunization: Techniques to help children cope with hospitalization. *Maternal–Child Nursing Journal, 12,* 119–134.

Powers, S. W., Blount, R. L., Bachanas, P. L., Cotter, M. W., & Swan, S. C. (1993). Helping preschool leukemia patients and their parents cope during injections. *Journal of Pediatric Psychology, 18,* 681–695.

Prugh, D. G., & Jordon, K. (1975). Physical illness or injury: The hospital as a source of emotional disturbances in child and family. In I. N. Berlin (Ed.), *Advocacy for children in mental health* (pp. 208–249). New York: Brunner/Mazel.

Prugh, D. G., Staub, E. M., Sands, H. H., Kirschbaum, R. M., & Lenihan, E. A. (1953). A study of the emotional reactions of children and families to hospitalization and illness. *American Journal of Orthopsychiatry, 23,* 70–106.

Rapoff, M. A., Christophersen, E. R., & Rapoff, K. E. (1982). The management of common childhood bedtime problems by pediatric nurse practitioners. *Journal of Pediatric Psychology, 7,* 179–196.

Rasnake, L. K., & Linscheid, T. R. (1989). Anxiety reduction in children receiving medical care: Developmental considerations. *Journal of Developmental and Behavioral Pediatrics, 10,* 169–175.

Roder, R. E., Lewis, T. M., & Law, D. B. (1961). Physiological responses of dentists to the presence of the parent in the operatory. *Journal of Dentistry for Children, 28,* 263–270.

Roskies, E., Mongeon, M., & Gagnon-Lefebre, B. (1978). Increasing participation in the hospitalization of young children. *Medical Care, 16,* 765–777.

Schultheis, K., Peterson, L., & Selby, V. (1987). Preparation for stressful medical procedures and person x treatment interactions. *Clinical Psychology Review, 7,* 329–352.

Shaw, E. G., & Routh, D. K. (1982). Effects of mother presence on children's reaction to adverse procedures. *Journal of Pediatric Psychology, 7,* 33–42.

Sheridan, M. S. (1975). Talk time for hospitalized children. *Social Work, 20,* 40–44.

Siegel, L. J. (1976). Preparation of children of hospitalization: A selected review of the research literature. *Journal of Pediatric Psychology, 1,* 26–30.

Siegel, L. J. (1981, April). *Naturalistic study of coping strategies in children facing medical procedures.* Paper presented at the meeting of the Southeastern Psychological Association, Atlanta, GA.

Siegel, L. J., & Peterson, L. (1980). Stress reduction in young dental patients through coping skills and sensory information. *Journal of Consulting and Clinical Psychology, 48,* 785–787.

Siegel, L. J., & Peterson, L. (1981). Maintenance effects of coping skills and sensory information on young children's response to repeated dental procedures. *Behavior Therapy, 12,* 530–535.

Simeonsson, R. J., Buckley, L., & Munson, L. (1979). Conceptions of illness causality in hospitalized children. *Journal of Pediatric Psychology, 4,* 77–84.

Skipper, J. K., & Leonard, R. C. (1968). Children, stress, and hospitalization: A field experiment. *Journal of Health and Social Behavior, 9,* 275–287.

Skipper, J. K., Leonard, R. C., & Rhymes, J. (1968). Child hospitalization and social interaction: An experimental study of mothers' feelings of stress, adaptation, and satisfaction. *Medical Care, 6,* 496–506.

Smith, K. E., Ackerson, J. P., & Blotcky, A. D. (1989). Reducing distress during invasive medical procedures: Relating behavioral interventions to preferred coping style in pediatric cancer patients. *Journal of Pediatric Psychology, 14,* 405–419.

Smith, K. E., Ackerson, J. P., Blotcky, A. D., & Berkow, R. (1990). Preferred coping styles of pediatric cancer patients during invasive medical procedures. *Journal of Psychosocial Oncology, 8,* 59–70.

Thompson, M. L. (1994). Information-seeking coping and anxiety in school-age children anticipating surgery. *Children's Health Care, 23,* 87–97.

Venham, L. L. (1973). *The effect of the mother's presence on the child's response to a stressful situation.* Unpublished manuscript. University of Connecticut, Storrs.

Vernon, D.T.A., Foley, J. M., & Shulman, J. L. (1967). Effect of mother–child separation and birth order on young children's responses to two potentially stressful experiences. *Journal of Personality and Social Psychology, 5,* 162–174.

Vernon, D.T.A., & Thompson, R. H. (1993). Research on the effect of experimental interventions on children's behavior after hospitalization: A review and synthesis. *Journal of Developmental and Behavioral Pediatrics, 14,* 36–44.

Weisz, J. R., McCabe, M. A., & Dennig, M. D. (1994). Primary and secondary control among children undergoing medical procedures: Adjustment as a function of coping style. *Journal of Consulting and Clinical Psychology, 62,* 324–332.

Wilson, A. M. (1982). A familiar face. *Anaesthesia, 37,* 1225.

Wolfer, J. A., & Visintainer, M. A. (1975). Pediatric surgery patients' and parents' stress responses and adjustment. *Nursing Research, 24,* 244–255.

Zastowny, T. R., Kirschenbaum, D. S., & Meng, A. L. (1986). Coping skills training for children: Effect on distress before, during, and after hospitalization for surgery. *Health Psychology, 5,* 231–247.

Zeltzer, L., & LeBaron, S. (1982). Hypnosis and nonhypnotic techniques for reduction of pain and anxiety during painful procedures in children and adolescents with cancer. *Journal of Pediatrics, 101,* 1032–1035.

13

Children and Families Coping with Disaster

CONWAY F. SAYLOR, RONALD BELTER, and SHERRI J. STOKES

A unique environment in which to capture the effects of stress and coping in children is the aftermath of disaster. At a basic level the disaster environment provides an opportunity to learn how essentially well-adjusted children and families cope with the short- and long-term effects of a sudden, unanticipated, monumental set of stressors. At an applied level, there is a compelling and widespread need for supportive interventions throughout the stages of the disaster and its aftermath if psychological sequelae are to be minimized. The purposes of this chapter are: to define disaster as it pertains to children and families; to examine the nature of stressors associated with various types of disasters; to highlight key findings from the growing literature on disaster's impact on children; to review recent literature pertaining specifically to stress and coping by children in disasters; and to introduce intervention techniques that have been developed to minimize the ill effects of disasters on their young victims.

It is impossible to address these issues in a single chapter without excluding relevant and important studies, theories, and populations. The chapter title refers to children and families because the research in this area supports a strong relationship between the coping and adjustment of children and that of their parents or other family members. It is arguable that the most important step in treating the child disaster victim is to see that the parents' needs are being met. In fact, the analogy has been made to adults in an airplane crisis placing the oxygen mask over their own faces before trying to assist their

CONWAY F. SAYLOR • Department of Psychology, The Citadel, Charleston, South Carolina 29409. RONALD BELTER • Department of Psychology, University of West Florida, Pensacola, Florida 32514. SHERRI J. STOKES • New Hope Treatment Center, Charleston, South Carolina 29483.

Handbook of Children's Coping: Linking Theory and Intervention, edited by Wolchik and Sandler. Plenum Press, New York, 1997.

children with their masks (American Academy of Pediatrics, 1995). Furthermore, most assessment and interventions with children postdisaster involve the members of family systems as well as broader systems such as school or community networks. The well-developed literature on adults' stress and coping and disasters, while directly relevant, is beyond the scope of this chapter, but is nicely reviewed elsewhere (e.g., Austin, 1992; Freedy & Hobfall, 1995; Freedy, Kilpatrick, & Resnick, 1993).

The focus on children does not limit our coverage of data specific to elementary school-aged children or toddlers and preschoolers. However, it does reflect the fact that the disaster literature, still in its early development, tends to group wide age ranges in its outcome studies. For economy, the term *children* will be used in this chapter to refer to youngsters from birth to 18 years. However, the importance of examining all findings in the context of diverse cognitive and psychosocial developmental stages cannot be overemphasized.

Finally, *disaster* is a broad term that can include acts of nature such as hurricanes, earthquakes, floods, and fires; man-made disasters such as bombings, shootings, war, or hostage-taking; and technology-related disasters such as transportation accidents, nuclear accidents, and bridge or building collapses. Thorough reviews of each type of disaster can be found elsewhere (Saylor, 1993). Because there has been a recent surge of writing in the area of childrens' reactions to natural disasters and because this area encompasses most of the pertinent issues in coping with such a stress, the literature on natural disasters will be reviewed in greater depth in this chapter. However, the reader should bear in mind that the findings and experiences of natural disaster victims may be similar to those noted in other types of disasters or personal trauma as well.

DEFINING DISASTER

While the definition of disaster can vary from source to source, there is generally a consensus that, unlike other forms of trauma, a disaster is a public event that directly impacts on multiple individuals and families. It is a relatively sudden event that is out of the range of ordinary experience and is so severe in its destructive impact that no one, regardless of premorbid function or experiences, could be expected to be unaffected by it (Saylor, 1993; Vogel & Vernberg, 1993). Some definitions also specify that a disaster is an event with a discreet beginning and end. However, a growing literature on longer-term outcomes indicates that the aftermath may be a more important element of the impact than the initial visible event itself (e.g., McFarlane, 1987; Swenson et al., 1996) and suggests that we may be unable to say exactly where the endpoint of a disaster lies. A catastrophic or near-catastrophic disaster is one that may kill, injure, or displace many thousands of people, and disrupt the business and services of entire communities (American Red Cross, 1991).

As Vernberg and Vogel (1993) note, there are several stages to the disaster process, each with different characteristics in terms of stress and intervention. In the predisaster preparation phase, personnel are trained and networked and plans are established so that communities are as prepared as possible to assist children and families in the event of any kind of disaster. The disaster impact phase begins when the actual natural or man-made disaster strikes and continues until the nature and scope of the disaster are first assessed and communicated to those affected. Within 24 hours, victims and their families are considered to be entering the short-term adaptation phase, in which initial debriefing and crisis intervention will take place. The long-term adaptation phase is the period beyond 3 months postdisaster impact, a period that may extend for some children and families for months, years, or even a lifetime. The issues, the personnel needs, the nature of the stresses, the systems most relevant to intervention, and the interventions themselves change across these phases, creating a need for fluid and coordinated efforts on behalf of child disaster victims (American Academy of Pediatrics, 1995; Vernberg & Vogel, 1993).

EPIDEMIOLOGY

There have been no epidemiological studies to date that enable us to gauge the numbers of children who will be exposed to and/or experience symptoms subsequent to a disaster in their lifetimes. Even in geographic regions known to have been impacted by disasters, it can only be ascertained how many children were screened or in other ways identified as "contacts" in officially declared disaster zones. This kind of reporting could be not so much a reflection of the numbers of children affected, but rather a reflection of the amount or scope of funding for the organization reporting these contacts. Hurricane Andrew (1990) was the most severe hurricane ever to strike the mainland of the United States. In the aftermath of Hurricane Hugo (1989), the federal government was relatively prompt and thorough in its response to this disaster, including the funding of a statewide counseling initiative. In their final report to the federal government, in 1994, the state of Florida reported that 14,948 children had been included in "crisis counseling cases," with 398 children being among those referred for "additional services." While not shedding light on disaster exposure in the general population, these figures underscore the importance of developing this area of clinical investigation. There are hundreds of large federal disaster areas officially declared each year. If this many children or more can be directly affected in one state in a single disaster, then disaster exposure is worthy of consideration as a potential childhood trauma for significant numbers of children.

STRESSORS ASSOCIATED WITH DISASTER

The hallmark of disasters is that they immediately plunge the child and family into situations in which they are exposed to multiple stressors, acute and chronic, which may all influence adjustment and may all need to be addressed with diverse and multifaceted intervention techniques. The interrelated and in some cases self-perpetuating stresses experienced by disaster victims bear examination at several levels. First, at a conceptual level, the stresses tend to have several important characteristics: they differ and evolve across disaster stages; they are measurable in both "objective" and "subjective" terms; they may come from "inside" or "outside" the child; they may be experienced more prominently at one level (e.g., affective, cognitive, or behavioral) than another; and, finally, the behavioral and emotional reactions to one set of stressors may themselves become the next set of stressors. At a pragmatic level, typical patterns of different types of disasters may change the nature of the stress experienced. Examples of characteristics that shape the impact of a disaster include whether it is predictable versus unpredictable, sudden versus gradual, catastrophic versus relatively small in scope, occurring locally versus in another community, brief or prolonged in duration, and has someone versus no one to blame.

The complex interaction of these conceptual and pragmatic factors can be illustrated by considering the experience of children who go through a hurricane. Indeed, the stressors change with the stage. At the disaster impact stage, stresses include the harrowing 24 hours of awaiting and surviving the storm's arrival: the sounds and sights of destruction, the fears for their own and others' safety, the sight of their familiar worlds changed forever. In the short- and long-term aftermath, there are new challenges to cope with such as distress in the family as financial burdens mount; insurance adjustor and contractor worries; changes in school, child care, or parent work routines; and parental distress. Each of these stressors is quantifiable in objective terms (e.g., how much damage the home sustained, how many more hours the parents are emotionally or physically absent from the child due to demands of rebuilding) and in subjective terms (e.g., how severe and disturbing the child and family perceive their losses and life changes to be). Stresses may come from "inside" the child in terms of new fears of wind and storms that impede adaptive function, or from "outside" in terms of recreation facilities that are destroyed, friends who are displaced, and routines that are more difficult due to damage to roads, schools, and day care facilities. The reactions to the initial trauma, the hurricane, may themselves become additional stressors. For example, sleep disturbance due to nightmares may result in sleep deprivation and related behavioral difficulties, or separation anxiety induced by the experience may interfere with successful return to important school and childcare routines.

In Table 1, examples of the stresses children experience in a natural disaster are presented in ways that highlight both disaster stage and component or source of stress (environmental, affective, cognitive, behavioral). In most cases, stress impacts, is interpreted, and is reacted to in several of these modes simultaneously and interactively. However, as a precursor to examining impact of disaster-related stress and interventions for children experiencing this stress, it is important to separate them out.

As mentioned, the stresses of disaster can be categorized pragmatically as well as conceptually. Table 2 provides examples of disasters that vary on key dimensions thought to correlate with the nature and extent of disaster impact (Saylor, 1993). This list is illustrative, not comprehensive, and omits various disasters that may have mixed characteristics or be ambiguous in these dimensions. The relationship between these characteristics and disaster is not always straightforward and bears further investigation. For example, if a disaster is predictable, there are more opportunities to prepare and even protect children

Table 1. Examples of Possible Hurricane-Related Stressors by Source and Stage

Source	Stressor	Example
Disaster impact stage		
Environment	Sight, sound, smells of disaster occurring	Child hears wind roaring, feels house shake
Cognitive	Concept and appraisal of situation including perceived life threat or imminent injury	Child sees flood filling his living room and decides he or she is about to drown
Affective	Arousal related to terrifying situation	Child panics at the "explosive" sound of a tree coming through the roof
Behavioral	Uncomfortable or extraordinary actions	Child crouches in bathtub with siblings as parent tries to protect him or her from storm
Short-term adaptation stage		
Environmental	Sights and sounds of widespread injury	Child sees rescue workers, property destruction, or bodies and debris being removed from nearby homes
Cognitive	Initial realization of losses and destruction	Child processes that his or her home has been demolished and a neighbor is missing, perhaps dead
Affective	Anger, anxiety, shock, denial, despair	Child grieves for lost loved ones, as well as loss of "secure community"
Behavioral	Sleep and appetite disturbance, with related behavior problems	Child refuses to sleep alone, is more demanding, and regresses in days and weeks following hurricane
Long-term adaptation stage		
Environmental	Extended stresses of rebuilding, recovering, and returning to routines	Child as still not returned to his or her home or original school 6–9 months after hurricane
Cognitive	Reflection on disaster, including attributions and blame	Child is preoccupied with thoughts of how he or she might have saved his or her friend whose family was killed
Affective	Later stages of grief, self-perpetuating anxiety related to cues of disaster	Child becomes anxious during storms, and becomes agitated as news reports of seasonal hurricanes are broadcast
Behavioral	Avoidance, acting out, ritualistic behaviors associated with preparing for or avoiding similar disaster	Child repeatedly packs up toys and replays "evacuation"; child refuses to be in a room with windows during even a milder storm

from direct exposure to the trauma. There should also be fewer human casualties and fewer children who witness death or fear for their lives during disaster impact. In that regard, unpredictable disaster may be associated with more severe stress than predictable. The flip side is that adults and children who have had opportunities to prepare and still are in the impact zone for

Table 2. Examples of Disasters Which Vary on Key Dimensions
of Stressors

Dimensions	
Predictable	**Unpredictable**
Hurricanes	Earthquakes
Flooding	Transportation disasters
War	Random shootings, bombs
Larger group affected	**Smaller group affected**
Earthquakes	Lightning strikes
Hurricanes	Tornadoes
Nuclear accidents	Shootings/hostages
Gradual	**Sudden**
Flooding	Earthquake
Some fires	Explosion
Brief impact	**Prolonged impact**
Earthquakes	War
Lightning/tornadoes	Flooding
Transportation accident	Nuclear accidents
Home/community	**Elsewhere/isolated**
Natural disasters	Boat, train, or plane crash
Terrorism in country	in another part of country
Floods	or world
Earthquake	
Someone to blame	**No one to blame**
Shooting, bombings	Earthquakes
Transportation disasters	Hurricanes
Building/dam collapses	Mudslides

whatever reasons may be more burdened by the trauma and loss incurred. For example, a family that did not try to evacuate a flood zone until it was too late and lost a parent in the raging water might experience greater long-term adjustment difficulties than a family that lost a parent in a plane crash for which there was no way to anticipate the danger.

Researchers who have studied transportation accidents have reported that stress may be heightened by being isolated and away from one's support systems (Yule, 1993). For example, a child from New York who survives a plane crash over Iowa might be without family and community support for days or even weeks, particularly if he is too injured to return home. After the July 1996 crash of TWA Flight 800, tempers flared as families waited in hotel rooms in New York away from community support for the opportunity to identify their children's remains. While data are not yet available from this disaster, earlier studies would predict that this experience might disrupt and perhaps prolong the grief and adaptation process for the parents, siblings, and close friends of the young crash victims.

Nearly all these key characteristics have a flip side. In large-scale disasters in one's own community, there are fewer healthy, unscathed persons from the local trusted community available to serve as resources. For example, after Hurricane Hugo, a large percent of the professionals in the medical and mental health communities were trying to serve the short- and long-term needs of the families in their community while recovering from severe losses in their own households. Collaborative programs (Red Cross, FEMA) described later in this chapter are countering this factor, but data are lacking in whether or not and how people outside of the "trauma membrane" (Rozenski et al., 1993) can contribute to stress reduction for young disaster victims. In a smaller disaster, there may be more resources immediately available, but affected families may feel forgotten or alone in their stress, coping, and grief soon after the initial coverage diminishes.

A final point to be noted about children's experiences of the stresses accompanying disaster is that exposure to these stresses can be either "direct" or "indirect." In the Oklahoma City bombing of 1995, direct exposure victims might be the children who were personally on the premises when the blast occurred, who were injured, and/or saw others injured and killed. No less affected would be children who were not physically present, but who lost parents and other loved ones in the same horrific moment. Children in Oklahoma City and nationwide almost certainly received indirect exposure through the in-depth, graphic media coverage of all aspects of the explosion and rescue efforts, as well as by witnessing their own families' fears and grief after the incident.

The impact of media coverage on direct disaster victims has recently raised an issue (Libow, 1992), as have the psychological and ethical implications of creating an enormous population of indirectly exposed children, through media exposure and/or exploitation of disaster (Sugar, 1988). To date there have been few empirical studies of indirect exposure to disaster on children. One bit of data in support of indirect exposure is evidence that children express distress and have symptoms of anxiety and depression at a higher rate when their parents or other immediate family members are in combat or imprisoned during wars (for review, see Swenson & Klingman, 1993). This, however, is not the same as distress in youngsters whose sole exposure is through the media. It has been speculated that children who are exposed by television to the grizzly aftermath of a disaster in which children are killed (such as the bombing in Oklahoma City or the TWA 800 crash) might be more likely to fear or imagine that they might perish in this way. Research needs to be conducted to provide an empirical basis on which to guide ethical media coverage.

IMPACT OF DISASTERS

In spite of the complex nature of the stress associated with disaster, it has been possible to document trends in the kinds of reactions noted in children who experience a disaster, as well as to identify risk factors that are associated with more severe symptom presentation. The trends from recent literature will be noted in this section, with emphasis on the natural disaster literature.

Types of Reactions

The earliest studies of child reactions to disaster appeared in the 1950s and 1960s, and relied on subjective clinical appraisal of victims. More recent studies have employed more sophisticated designs using standardized measures with both the child and the child's parents. These studies indicate that children experience a wide range of emotional and behavioral reactions to disasters (Belter & Shannon, 1993; Vogel & Vernberg, 1993). For example, in storm-related disasters, a higher frequency and severity of postdisaster fear of storms has been reported in exposed children (Dollinger, O'Donnell, & Staley, 1984; Milne, 1977; Swenson et al., 1996). Symptoms of sleep disturbance (Dollinger, 1986; Junn, Guerin, & Rushbrook, 1990; Sullivan, Saylor, & Foster, 1991), increased dependency (Block, Silber, & Perry, 1956; Guerin, Junn, & Rushbrook, 1991), decreased school performance (Gleser, Green, & Winget, 1981; Milne, 1977; Shannon, Lonigan, Finch, & Taylor, 1994), regressive enuresis (Durkin, Khan, Davidson, Zaman, & Stein, 1993), and other somatic complaints (McFarlane, Policansky, & Irwin, 1987; Nader, Pynoos, Fairbanks, & Frederick, 1990; Schwarz & Kowalski, 1991), have also been noted as common short and long-term responses in children.

Since the first appearance of posttraumatic stress disorder (PTSD) in the *Diagnostic and Statistical Manual of Mental Disorders,* 3rd edition, revised (DSM-III-R) (American Psychiatric Association, 1980), studies of children and disasters have documented the presence of PTSD symptoms in a significant proportion of child disaster victims (Vogel & Vernberg, 1993). In addition to the first criterion of exposure to a traumatic event, the three main symptom cluster criteria required for the diagnosis remain essentially unchanged in the DSM-IV (American Psychiatric Association, 1994). These three essential features of PTSD are: persistent reexperiencing of the trauma, persistent avoidance of trauma-related stimuli and/or numbing of general responsiveness, and persistent increased arousal. The DSM-IV has introduced a new diagnostic category—Acute Stress Disorder—similar to PTSD with the exception of more prominent dissociative features and a time frame within the first 4 weeks following the traumatic event. Given that this is a new diagnostic category, the prevalence of acute stress disorder in child disaster victims is unknown and should become a focus of future research. In clinical practice, the diagnosis of PTSD usually entails a subjective appraisal of the child by means of interview with the child and a well-informed caretaker such as a parent or teacher. The use of objective measures to systematically collect data to be applied to standard diagnostic criteria is the exception rather than the rule in clinical practice. Such scientific rigor is becoming more common in recent research efforts to assess PTSD in child disaster victims, but there is still considerable variability (Vogel & Vernberg, 1993). Thus, the reliability and validity of methods employed to assess PTSD varies and should be carefully examined when reviewing the literature.

Recent studies have indicated that the postdisaster PTSD symptoms most frequently reported in children are from the reexperiencing cluster, with relatively fewer symptoms from the other two clusters of avoidance/numbing and hyperarousal (La Greca, Silverman, Vernberg, & Prinstein, 1996; Schwarz & Kowalski, 1991; Vernberg, La Greca, Silverman, & Prinstein, 1996). These studies also indicate that although the prevalence of general PTSD symptoms is high in a large percentage of the children studied, a relatively smaller yet substantial percentage meet full criteria for the diagnosis of PTSD. Vernberg et al. (1996) reported that 14% of their sample of 3rd to 5th grade children had few or no PTSD symptoms related to their experience of Hurricane Andrew, 3 months after the hurricane. The remainder of the sample consisted of 55% reporting very severe symptoms, 25% severe, 26% moderate, and 30% mild symptoms of PTSD. In a longitudinal follow-up study of these same children, LaGreca et al. (1996) identified 39% of the sample who met full diagnostic criteria for PTSD at the 3-month interval, 24% at the 7-month interval, and 18% at the 10-month interval. Thus, while PTSD symptoms were reported by the majority of the sample, a smaller yet substantial percentage of these subjects met the complete diagnostic criteria for the diagnosis of PTSD, based on a child self-report measure. While this prevalence diminished over time, 18% of the sample still met diagnostic criteria 10 months after exposure to the hurricane.

Shannon et al. (1994) assessed PTSD symptoms in a large sample (n = 5657) of school children aged 9 to 19 years, 3 months after experiencing Hurricane Hugo. In this sample, reexperiencing symptoms of PTSD were reported by 51.3% of the preadolescents, 21.1% of the early adolescents, and 16.2% of the late adolescents. Numbing and avoidance symptoms were reported by 15.5% of preadolescents, 10.3% of early adolescents, and 8.7% of late adolescents. Finally, symptoms of hyperarousal were reported by 59.9% of preadolescents, 35.6% of early adolescents, and 23.1 of late adolescents. Despite this high prevalence of PTSD symptoms in the sample, only 5.42% of the sample met all three diagnostic criteria for PTSD using the same self-report measure employed in the Hurricane Andrew studies. The difference in prevalence of PTSD between these two samples is most likely due to the difference in the severity of exposure to these two hurricane disasters in the samples. The issue of extent of exposure to trauma is one of several relevant factors that have been described in the literature as risk factors, to be discussed in the next section.

Risk Factors

Various characteristics of the child, family, and disaster have been studied as potential factors that might exacerbate or insulate the child from the impact of a traumatic experience such as a disaster. Studies of gender differences in child reactions to disasters have yielded somewhat mixed results. A large number of studies have reported greater frequency or severity of a variety of problems in girls (Burke, Moccia, Borus, & Burns, 1986; Green et al., 1991; Lonigan, Shannon, Finch, Daugherty, & Taylor, 1991; Lonigan et al., 1994; Seroka, Knapp, Knight, Siemon, & Starbuck, 1986; Yule, 1993). A few studies have found higher levels of anxiety (Burke, Borus, Burns, Milstein, & Beasley, 1982) and acting out (Gillis, 1991; Gleser et al., 1981) in boys. Still other studies have reported no gender differences (Block et al., 1956; Dollinger, 1986; Milne, 1977). The inconsistency of findings related to gender differences reflects problems in methodology related to small sample sizes, subjective measures, and inconsistently defined diagnostic criteria characteristic of earlier research studies. More recent studies with more rigorous methodology have suggested that gender differences may interact with other factors to influence the type of symptoms displayed by child victims. For example, Shannon et al. (1994) found the girls in their sample reported symptoms related to emotional reactions and processing, while the boys reported more cognitive and behavioral symptoms.

There are only limited reports of ethnic or racial differences in the literature. For example, Shannon et al. (1994) found higher levels of varied symptoms and specific PTSD symptoms in African-American subjects, even when controlling for severity of exposure. By contrast, Vernberg et al. (1996) found no ethnic group differences in their sample, when they accounted for level of exposure. Thus, it is unclear how ethnic and racial characteristics, either alone or in interaction with other factors, affect reactions to disaster.

Studies of age differences have also yielded mixed results. Many studies have employed samples limited to a narrow age range, thus precluding consideration of age differences. However, among those studies with samples spanning a broad age range, the findings suggest that younger children have higher rates of some symptoms such as fears, enuresis, and dependency, while older children have higher rates of other symptoms such as depression, anxiety, and PTSD (Block et al., 1956; Gleser et al., 1981; Green et al., 1991; Milne, 1977; Seroka et al., 1986). Other studies have reported a higher frequency and severity of PTSD symptoms in younger children, compared to older children (Lonigan et al., 1994; Shannon et al., 1994). It would appear that, in general, younger children are at greater risk for symptoms that are typically more prevalent in their age range in the general population (e.g., regressive, dependent behavior), while older children and adolescents are more likely to present with symptoms that are consistent with their developmentally higher cognitive and affective functioning (e.g., anxiety, depression).

The extent to which the child's premorbid functioning affects his or her reaction to a disaster is difficult to determine, given the need to retrospectively identify predisaster conditions. Yet, some studies have found that premorbid problems such as a preexisting psychiatric condition or anxiety are associated with postdisaster symptoms (Earls, Smith, Reich, & Jung, 1988; Lonigan et al., 1994). Other studies indicated that premorbid factors were not related to severity of symptoms (Dollinger, 1986; Pynoos et al., 1987). Studies of premorbid factors are necessarily limited by the availability of good predisaster data on target samples. The unpredictability of disasters precludes prospective data collection and leaves researchers dependent on the discovery of preexisting data or on retrospective recall of subjects about predisaster issues. There are inherent problems with both types of data, which limit the conclusions one can draw regarding predisaster factors. Thus, although it appears to be conceptually relevant as a risk factor, the extent to which specific aspects of predisaster functioning represent a risk factor is not clear and requires further study.

There have been a limited number of studies that have indicated that the impact of a disaster on the child's parents is also a relevant factor for the child's reaction. These studies have found a positive relationship between parental symptoms and maladjustment, and the severity of the child's reactions to the disaster (Block et al., 1956; Earls et al., 1988; Green et al., 1991; McFarlane et al., 1987; McFarlane, 1988). However, most of these studies employed parent report for assessing both parent and child symptoms, and thus the correlations between parent and child symptoms may represent shared method variance.

Only the Earls et al. (1988) study employed both parent and child report of symptoms on a structured diagnostic interview. Thus, the association between parent symptoms and child symptoms is not clear. Further research is needed to assess the extent to which the type and severity of the child's symptoms can be expected to vary relative to the extent to which the parents have difficulty coping.

An obvious risk factor that has clear support in the literature is the severity of exposure to the trauma. In numerous studies, degree of exposure to the trauma through physical proximity, perceived threat to life, loss of or separation from family members, displacement from home, personal injury or damage to property, witnessing injury to others or damage to property, and so forth is clearly associated with the severity of the child's reaction (Vernberg et al., 1996; Vogel & Vernberg, 1993). The more directly exposed to the trauma and the more severe the impact of damage and disruption of life, the greater the negative psychological impact on the child. While an objective assessment of exposure to trauma is important, the child's subjective appraisal and personal experience of the trauma seem more likely to be the critical factors in determining risk for negative psychological impact.

In summary, negative psychological reactions to natural disasters are quite prevalent in children and adolescents of all ages. This is manifested in a wide range of symptoms, with the most prevalent and severe presentation consisting of symptoms of PTSD. Although the severity of symptoms seems not to vary significantly or consistently by age, gender, or racial/ethnic background, the type of symptom tends to vary somewhat by age and gender. It also appears that the child's predisaster functioning, parental and family postdisaster functioning, and the child's perceived severity of exposure to trauma are important factors that affect the child's reaction to the disaster.

The research on the impact of disasters on children has become increasingly more sophisticated. More recent studies have employed larger samples and objective, multimethod approaches to data collection compared to the early studies that employed interview measures, poorly defined diagnostic criteria, and generally small samples. More recent studies have also relied more heavily on child self-report measures in addition to or in lieu of parent report measures. Previous research has revealed significant discrepancies between parent report and self-report measures of a variety of internal states (Achenbach, McConaughy, & Howell, 1987; Kazdin, Esveldt-Dawson, Unis, & Rancurello, 1983; Kazdin, French, Unis, & Esveldt-Dawson, 1983; McConaughy, 1993; Phares, Compas, & Howell, 1989). It is generally accepted that children tend to be more reliable informants in regard to variables that may not be readily expressed to or observed by their parents. In particular, under circumstances of a disaster that affects the entire family, parents who are themselves significantly affected may not be well informed about their childrens' subjective perception of and reaction to the disaster experience (Belter, Finch, Foster, & Imm, 1995). The observed tendency is for parents to underestimate and underreport the level of distress and symptoms experienced by their children. Further research on risk factors should continue to emphasize child self-report, integrating data obtained from multiple sources postdisaster, as well as available data related to predisaster factors.

COPING AND SUPPORT RESOURCES

Compas and Epping (1993) present a very good overview of the process of coping in children, emphasizing developmental issues and family influences on coping. They note that coping efforts of children vary not only by developmental level of the child, but also over the course of time as the situational demands of the disaster change to present new challenges for coping. They also emphasize that an individual child's coping with a disaster occurs in a social context and is influenced to a large degree by the circumstances of the family and other important social systems in which the child functions (e.g., school, neighborhood, peer groups). These circumstances will determine whether those social systems offer resources to facilitate effective coping or barriers to impede effective coping. As a result, assessment of coping efforts should focus not only on individual coping skills but also on the various social systems that impact the effective application of those skills.

Compared with the research on the impact of disasters on children, the research on children's use of coping and support resources in response to a natural disaster is rather limited. There is some evidence that with young children, behavior that qualifies as a PTSD symptom may represent a developmentally appropriate coping strategy. For example, reenactment play that has been reported in children (Block et al., 1956; Saylor, Swenson, & Powell, 1992) can be regarded as an effort to gain mastery and to work through or discharge emotion related to the trauma. Saylor et al. (1992) collected anecdotes that parents of preschoolers reported in the year following Hurricane Hugo. None of the children in the sample had been treated by psychiatric professionals (by parent report), but all had been between the ages of 2 and 4 when Hugo struck their homes and community. Parents reported hurricane-related play such as packing up toys to "evacuate" and play-acting the "boarding up" of a playhouse over and over again. Other children reportedly anthropomorphized "Hugo" to be a character that they could successfully fight off with their toy swords and guns. Still others reenacted the hurricane scene with food (e.g., Hugo "blowing down" broccoli stalk "trees" at the dinner table; cookie bear "roofers" working on a gingerbread house) or drawings. There were no data to document the impact of these spontaneous behaviors, other than parent report that their children seemed soothed or reassured once the games were completed, particularly those whose themes included mastery or "fending off" the disaster. Research is needed to document the nature and impact of spontaneous play and other "intuitive" coping techniques used by resilient children following disasters.

In an initial study of coping strategies employed by children following a Hurricane Hugo, Dunn (1991) found a positive relationship between number and severity of PTSD symptoms and total number of coping strategies employed. A measure of children's coping strategies, the Kidcope (Spirito et al., 1988), was employed to assess use of both positive and negative coping strategies. A factor analysis yielded two primary factors: (1) adaptive coping, comprised of distraction, cognitive restructuring, problem solving, social support, and emotional calming; and (2) maladaptive coping, comprised of self-criticism, emotional escalation, blaming others, and social withdrawal. In this sample, the children reported using a significantly greater number of positive or adaptive strategies than negative or maladaptive strategies. However, greater use of both positive and negative strategies was related to higher levels of PTSD symptoms. The perceived effectiveness of the strategies was not related to PTSD symptoms.

Vernberg et al. (1996) employed a similar distinction of positive and negative coping strategies in their study of children who endured Hurricane Andrew. They obtained results consistent with Dunn's (1991) study, with children who reported higher levels of PTSD symptoms also reporting using higher levels of both types of coping. These findings indicate that children with higher levels of PTSD were responding to the higher demands of the disaster situation with increased coping efforts. However, the use of negative coping strategies was a stronger predictor of PTSD symptoms than was the use of positive strategies.

Finally, in a longitudinal extension of the above study, La Greca et al. (1996) found that the use of negative coping strategies also predicted PTSD symptoms over time. At the 7-month postdisaster interval, three coping strategies labeled positive coping, blame/anger, and social withdrawal were associated with higher levels of PTSD symptoms in this sample. At the 10-month interval, only one coping strategy—blame/anger—was associated with higher PTSD symptoms. This is the only study done to date that has prospectively supported different outcomes for different coping strategies used by children following a natural disaster.

With regard to support resources, Vernberg et al. (1996) and La Greca et al. (1996) reported that access to a range of supportive resources (e.g., family, teachers, peers) was a significant predictor of PTSD symptoms. Children with access to good supportive resources reported lower levels of PTSD symptoms. These findings emphasize the importance of different sources of support to facilitate coping with the varied stressors of a natural disaster within the different systems with which the child interacts. Over time, children who reported high levels of support in the early postdisaster period reported fewer PTSD symptoms at 7 and 10 months after the hurricane.

The limited research on coping and support indicates that children tend to employ a wide range of both positive and negative coping strategies and that the higher the level of stress reaction, the greater the coping effort or number of strategies employed. Limited data suggest that the use of negative strategies predicts higher levels of PTSD symptoms over time. However, further research on outcome of coping efforts is needed. Ready access to a wide range of supportive resources appears to facilitate effective coping, and thus reduce the risk for prolonged presence of symptoms.

Before intelligent approaches to intervention and its evaluation can be undertaken, much more research is needed regarding the coping employed by children and adolescents following disaster. The few studies cited here suggest that some children may spontaneously employ developmentally appropriate coping to recover from disaster. Others may be able to learn more adaptive coping techniques from family, school, or mental health professionals.

Research should be conducted along several paths: What are the coping strategies spontaneously employed by youngsters exhibiting the fewest problems postdisaster? Can models of coping with other child abuse or chronic illness be applied to the disaster area? In what ways do the stress and coping of disaster victims differ from those of youngsters coping with other trauma? How do developmental and cultural factors influence the type of coping and its effectiveness? At the present time, the model proposed by Vernberg et al. (1996) is the most comprehensive framework for understanding variations in emergence and longevity of symptoms of distress in children following a disaster. The extent or severity of exposure to the traumatic event interacts with characteristics of the child (e.g., age, gender, ethnicity), in the context of social support available to the child, which can promote or impede effective coping with the disaster. The literature generally supports the notion that the child directly exposed to a severely stressful traumatic event, who has few resources for social support and employs negative coping strategies, is at highest risk for severe and prolonged symptoms. Thus, efforts to prevent or reduce the severity and longevity of symptoms would focus on preventive efforts to reduce the extent of exposure, secondary efforts to develop social support resources, and tertiary efforts to build and employ more effective coping strategies.

In the next section, approaches to intervention with children and families after disaster will be reviewed. While the influence of related literatures (e.g., treating PTSD in adults, coping with a child's chronic illness) is evident in the design of these interventions, it is important to note that clinicians have generally been thrust into the disaster environment to intervene as best they could with an incomplete datebase to underlie their work.

INTERVENTION FOLLOWING DISASTER

There has been a host of interventions suggested for children and families following disasters. On the positive side, many have been constructed based on the empirical data described above about what the impact might be and which children might be at greatest risk (e.g., Galante & Foa, 1986; Klingman, 1993; LaGreca, Vernberg, Silverman, Vogel, & Prinstein, 1994). Other intervention strategies have been drawn from more well-developed models whose efficacy has been demonstrated with adults after traumatic experiences or with children experiencing trauma other than disaster (e.g., Freedy & Hobfall, 1995). Unfortunately, there is almost no research documenting the effectiveness of any intervention techniques with children after disaster.

Vernberg (1996) chaired a symposium at the American Psychological Association that featured some of the first controlled studies of interventions with children after a disaster. In this symposium, Gurwitch, Messenbaugh, Leftwich, Corrigan, and Pfefferbaum (1996) discussed obstacles to implementation and preliminary findings from projects designed to identify and intervene with children stressed by the bombing in Oklahoma City. A project was proposed for preschool-aged (6 months to 5 years) children and their parents directly exposed to the bombing as it affected their YMCA day care. The well-designed study involved in-depth screening of both parents and children, followed by random assignment of interested participants to one of two interventions: parent support group only or parent support group in conjunction with a parallel child group. Both groups proposed to have specific goals related to reduction of PTSD symptoms and milder adjustment problems. A second project proposed for elementary school children in the Oklahoma City area targeted a larger population using a similar model. While empirically sound and clinically promising, both projects suffered from lack of support and cooperation among agencies, a lack of understanding of or commitment to the projects by potential referral sources, and a resulting shortage of participants. This report highlighted the wide discrepancy between our growing knowledge and expertise in the disaster area and our success at implementing recommended interventions in an environment where they can be properly received and evaluated.

In the same symposium, McDermott (1996) reported on intervention delivered to Australian school children aged 6 to 18 following a major bushfire in which an entire forest perished, 86 houses were destroyed, and one elementary school was razed. Following routing, 6-month screening, and debriefing in the affected schools, McDermott and his colleagues assessed and intervened with children using a guided workbook. Although there was no significant differences on the overall Impact of Event Scale (IES) score between children randomly assigned to treatment versus control group, the authors noted treatment group reductions on the IES avoidance subscale and positive parent and teacher ratings regarding the intervention. McDermott (1996) further noted the relationships between exposure and symptom presentation discussed earlier in this chapter and highlighted the fact that all participants showed high distress. McDermott, like Gurwitch et al. (1996), noted reluctance by many parents for their children to be participants in any intervention and/or reassessment, particularly more than 1 year postdisaster.

The most promising findings based on a controlled intervention trial were reported by Chemtob and Hamada (1996), who intervened with Hawaiian school children following a major hurricane. In combination, the three studies in the Vernburg (1996) symposium represent the state of the art at this time for designing interventions that involve parents, schools, and professionals in collaboration, for involving replicable workbook and manualized treatment package, and for attempting to implement interventions in an environment where they can be evaluated. In the next decade, screening and controlled, longitudinally evaluated interventions should be the highest priority for clinical research initiatives in the children and disaster area.

In the next section, intervention models that might lend themselves to empirical scrutiny are referenced, along with "model" programs which have been described and/or implemented, but not necessarily evaluated, in recent disasters. The organization of this section again highlights the importance of separately considering the issues and needs associated with each of the different disaster stages.

Disaster Models

In sampling the most current and promising interventions, it is again helpful to consider the context of disaster stage. Moreover, it is important to consider intervention in the context of the systems surrounding the child: family, peers, school systems, and communities. Scott (1994) describes a model developed by the National Organization for Victim Assistance (NOVA) that captures the change in intervention focus over stages. In this model, children are assisted with immediate needs for safety and security in the impact stage, then are helped to ventilate and validate in the short term, while predicting and preparing for the extended adjustment period to follow in the long-term adjustment phase.

Applying this model to a tornado, children in the safety and security stage would be moved to the safest location, such as a storm-proof shelter or a location under heavy furniture, and comforted as much as possible by nearby adults as the twister's immediate impact is felt. In the ventilate and validate stage, children might be encouraged to join in school- or community-based debriefing and group counseling sessions to hear that they are not alone, that their feelings are common in this situation, and that they will have help and support in their recovery. Some children even at this early stage will be able to openly express their feelings of terror or resentment that the adults could not keep the disaster from striking. Others will need more time to process their own experiences and may find it intrusive to be asked to "share" in the early stages of adjustment. The predicting and preparing stage may last months or even years as youngsters cope with what has happened and prepare themselves for the now real possibility that they might experience an unpredictable twister again.

Most interventions described for individual children and families have focused on the short- and long-term adaptation phases. School and community interventions, while seeking to identify those in need of more intensive follow-up, tend to be more active in support, networking, and broad screening during the earlier stages of disaster impact and short-term adaptation. It is important to note that few psychosocial interventions can be successfully implemented before the immediate needs of safety and survival are addressed (Saylor, 1993). Thus, any interventions taking place in the first 24 hours need to be focused on basic tasks of information gathering or dissemination and support of personnel involved in rescue efforts (Vernberg & Vogel, 1993). In this section, promising models for intervention in key systems and stages will be highlighted.

No intervention should proceed without good assessment of the risk factors and symptoms discussed in the previous section. Review of relevant assessment techniques is beyond the scope of this chapter, but issues and potential measurement techniques are elaborated elsewhere (American Academy of Pediatrics, 1995; Finch & Daugherty, 1993; Frederick, 1985; LaGreca et al., 1994; Saylor, Swenson, Stokes, Wertlieb, & Casto, 1994). Adequate assessment not only has implications for cost-effective identification of intervention candidates, but also is a prerequisite for the kind of intervention outcome research that is sorely needed in the disaster area.

The most important intervention of all is predisaster planning and training. In the final section of this chapter, we will feature exciting efforts that network and train potential intervention providers (Carll, 1994; Yeast, 1994). This planning, training, networking, prevention model is in fact the direction of the future, as multiple agencies and disciplines mobilize around the concept that the best time to intervene in disasters is before they ever occur.

Intervention Immediately after Impact

Immediately following a catastrophe, efforts are primarily geared toward those needing emergency medical care and restoring safety. The task of restoring safety is a complicated one involving an individual's physical as well as psychological or emotional safety (Pynoos & Nader, 1988). Debriefing is necessary by professionals in order to provide accurate information regarding the specifics of the disaster, location/reunification of children or family members, deaths that have occurred, and available resources. Debriefing can only be done if an effective method of communicating with one another is employed immediately following the disaster (American Academy of Pediatrics, 1995; Mitchell, 1993; Shelby, 1994; Vernberg & Vogel, 1993).

Short-Term Interventions

Following the initial upheaval after a disaster, children and families make attempts to restoring some type of normalcy in the midst of destruction. Interventions during this period must be carefully assessed and implemented, since an individual's or family's long-term adjustment is, at some level, determined by the effectiveness of immediate coping efforts.

As stated earlier, restoring a sense of normalcy is extremely important to children and adults following a disaster. Children spend most of their day in a classroom; thus, it makes sense to return to their most comfortable setting as soon as possible. Klingman (1993) offers a model of intervention that is implemented using the school system as social support. A second model that describes in detail aspects of prevention and intervention utilizing the school setting is that of Nader and Pynoos (1993). Empirically based concrete resources for intervening with children in elementary schools are now in a manual that provides professionals with easily accessible information (LaGreca et al., 1994). These resources and models share a common focus on the use of the school's own administrative staff as supports, the importance of implementing in-school screening and treatment teams, the recognition of potential for teacher support and influence on children, the promotion of parent support groups, the importance of rituals/services for losses, and the transition to proper mental health services outside the school system as severe or persistent needs are identified.

Typically following a disaster, mental health centers serve a secondary prevention role. Assistance with coping and problem solving in the midst of crises may be sought at clinics where there are trained professionals; but more often, the clinics will sit empty while outreach takes place in the community. Although the role and function of mental health systems may vary with the nature of the crisis, it is important that trained mental health professionals be available for rapid outreach intervention. Outreach programs are more effective than traditional mental health services offered at a single location (Joyner & Swenson, 1993).

Other systems that can be instrumental in providing assessment and short-term interventions to children and families are the inpatient and outpatient pediatric services. The American Academy of Pediatrics has made a priority of providing education and information about psychosocial needs of children and families after a disaster. Waeckerle (1994) described the vitality of medical professionals' involvement in planning and responses to disasters in communities.

Long-Term Interventions

Those needing longer-term interventions are primarily those children exhibiting PTSD symptomatology. Although each child experiences trauma differently, there are several common principles that can be used in treating traumatized children: helping the child reexperience the trauma in treatment; early intervention; and involvement of caretakers and other significant adults in treatment (Gillis, 1993). Specific intervention techniques, such as flooding, that are useful in treatment of PTSD in children have been documented by Saigh (1989). Children and adolescents exhibiting symptoms of PTSD may benefit from individual therapy using a psychodynamic approach (Terr, 1989). Other approaches such as cognitive–behavioral therapies have also been demonstrated to be effective (Yule, 1993). Group and family therapies have been used as adjunct interventions with children and adolescents presenting with symptoms months to years postdisaster (Gillis, 1993).

FUTURE DIRECTIONS: PREDISASTER PLANNING AND TRAINING

As is the case with studies of intervention with child disaster victims, the literature evaluating prevention is sparse. However, a strong theoretical and empirical base underlies several promising collaborative initiatives to truly institute prevention programs. Primary prevention models specific to children and disasters have been proposed (e.g., Pynoos & Nader, 1988; Vernberg & Vogel, 1993), and in combination with broader models of community preparation (e.g., Waeckerle, 1994) provide a sound course for future initiation. The characteristic of disasters as sudden and unanticipated makes it necessary to train and prepare when the disaster itself is abstract. Today we are in the predisaster stage of tomorrow's disaster.

The term "primary prevention" refers to efforts to prevent a disorder or adverse reaction to a disaster before it occurs. Such efforts would take place during the predisaster preparation phase in the model proposed by Vernberg and Vogel (1993). Primary prevention focused on the child and family in this phase would consist of community education programs to prepare citizens for a disaster, such as hurricane-preparedness programs. Such programs focus on educating the general public about the potential dangers of a potential disaster and the steps to take in advance to minimize the adverse effects of the disaster. Such steps would include identifying evacuation routes from a hurricane, seeking safe shelter in a tornado, stockpiling water and other supplies, and so forth. We are not aware of any formal efforts to study the efficacy of such primary prevention programs in preventing the adverse psychological impact of disasters on children. One research focus should be on the extent to which the general public is influenced by these primary prevention efforts and actually follow through with advance planning and preparation.

There has been tremendous progress since 1989 in another important aspect of primary prevention: training and networking professionals to respond effectively to the needs of children and families after disasters. The American Academy of Pediatrics (1995), in collaboration with the Federal Emergency Management Association, sponsored a multidisciplinary task force to develop a handbook for pediatricians to quickly prepare them to mobilize on behalf of children in a disaster. The guide was disseminated to every American Academy of Pediatrics' member in the Oklahoma City area within days of the 1995 bombing, and is readily available for predisaster training and preparation.

Psychologists have organized model collaborative programs that involve the kind of training, networking, and interagency collaboration required to make intervention effective in the predisaster phase. The American Psychological Association and American Counseling Association have established a formal partnership with the American Red Cross to coordinate training of mental health volunteers in a 2-day program that includes a component on children (Yeast, 1994). Another predisaster preparation phase effort consists of a National Disaster Relief Network coordinated by the American Psychological Association, with the cooperation of various state psychological associations (Carll, 1994). Both initiatives target adults, with some mention of children.

In an important recent development, the American Psychological Association council approved a motion for a select task force to draft a guide specific to intervention issues with children involved in disaster. In 1996–1997, the product of this task force should add a significant resource to disaster-related prevention and intervention initiatives. With a trained interdisciplinary network in place ahead of time, a quick and effective response by volunteer psychologists (and other professionals) should be facilitated in the disaster impact and short-term adaptation phases of the next natural and technological disasters. As yet, formal evaluation of the efficacy of these efforts in minimizing adverse reactions in children has not systematically occurred. Such research is needed to establish the specific aspects of preventive intervention that are effective and how they can be enhanced in a cost-effective disaster relief effort. It seems clear, however, that in large-scale disasters that affect large numbers of people, coordination of intervention resources by various community organizations is critical in meeting the challenges of a crisis that grossly overwhelms the community's resources.

CONCLUSIONS

Disasters present a unique set of stressors to children and families. While the precise nature and severity of the stress varies with the type of disaster and systems impacted, researchers have identified characteristics that place children at increased risk for posttraumatic stress symptoms. Recent research has also begun to document patterns of support and coping that may be linked to successful recovery from disaster. Promising intervention procedures have been introduced for the individual child disaster victim as well as the family, school, and community. Collaboration across disciplines and agencies has already yielded more sound intervention possibilities, and additional procedures are currently being mapped out by experts in the field. Continued collaboration is needed in all stages of disaster preparation and intervention if children's psychological needs are to be effectively met. Additional research is needed in all aspects of children affected by disasters, but especially in the implementation and evaluation of empirically based intervention programs.

REFERENCES

Achenbach, T. M., McConaughy, S. M., & Howell, C. T. (1987). Child/adolescent behavioral and emotional problems: Implications of cross informant correlations for situational specificity. *Psychological Bulletin, 101*(2), 213–232.

American Academy of Pediatrics. (1995). *Psychosocial issues for children and families in disasters: A guide for the primary care physician.* Oak Grove Village, IL: American Academy of Pediatrics Press.

American Psychiatric Association. (1980). *Diagnostic and statistical manual of mental disorders* (3rd ed.). Washington, DC: Author.

American Psychiatric Association. (1994). *Diagnostic and statistical manual of mental disorders* (4th ed.). Washington, DC: Author.

American Red Cross. (1991). *Disaster services regulations and procedures.* Washington, DC: American Red Cross.

Austin, L. S. (1992). *Responding to disaster: A guide for mental health professionals.* Washington DC: American Psychiatric Association Press.

Belter, R., & Shannon, M. (1993). Impact of natural disasters on children and families. In C. F. Saylor, (Ed.), *Children and disasters* (pp. 85–104). New York: Plenum Press.

Belter, R. W., Finch, A. J., Jr., Foster, K. Y., & Imm, P. S. (1995). Disconcordance between parent and child reports: What does it mean? Paper presented at the Southeastern Psychological Association annual conference, Savannah, GA.

Block, D., Silber, E., & Perry, S. (1956). Some factors in the emotional reaction of children to disaster. *American Journal of Psychiatry, 113,* 416–422.

Burke, J., Borus, J., Burns, B., Millstein, & Beasley, M. (1982). Change in children's behavior after a natural disaster. *American Journal of Psychiatry, 139,* 1010–1014.

Burke, J. D., Moccia, P., Borus, J. F., & Burns, B. J. (1986). Emotional distress in fifth-grade children ten months after a natural disaster. *Journal of the American Academy of Child Psychiatry, 25,* 536–541.

Carll, E. K. (1994). Disaster intervention with children and families: National and state initiatives. *Children, Youth, and Family Services Quarterly, 17*(3), 21–23.

Chemtob, C. M., & Hamada, R. S. (1996). Maile Project: A controlled treatment with hurricane-traumatized children. Paper presented at the American Psychological Association Meeting, Toronto, CA.

Compas, B., & Epping, J. (1993). Stress and coping in children and families: Implications for children coping with disaster. In C. F. Saylor (Ed.). *Children and disasters* (pp. 11–28). New York: Plenum Press.

Dollinger, S. J. (1986). The measurement of children's sleep disturbances and somatic complaints following a disaster. *Child Psychiatry and Human Development, 16,* 148–153.

Dollinger, S. J., O'Donnell, J. P., & Staley, A. A. (1984). Lightning-strike disaster: Effects on children's fears and worries. *Journal of Consulting and Clinical Psychology, 52,* 1028–1038.

Dunn, S. E. (1991). *The impact of a catastrophic natural disaster on children: PTSD symptomatology and coping strategies.* Unpublished manuscript.

Durkin, M., Khan, N., Davidson, L., Zaman, S., & Stein (1993). The effects of a natural disaster on child behavior: Evidence for posttraumatic stress. *American Journal of Public Health, 83*(11), 1549–1553.

Earls, F., Smith, E., Reich, W., & Jung, K. G. (1988). Investigating psychopathological consequences of a disaster in children: A pilot study incorporating a structured diagnostic interview. *Journal of the American Academy of Child and Adolescent Psychiatry, 27,* 90–95.

Finch, A. J., & Daugherty, T. K. (1993). Issues in the assessment of posttraumatic stress disorder in children. In C. F. Saylor (Ed.) *Children and disasters* (pp. 45–66). New York: Plenum Press.

Frederick, C. J. (1985). Children traumatized by catastrophic situations. In S. Eth and R. S. Pynoos (Eds.), *Posttraumatic stress disorders in children* (pp. 73–99). Washington, DC: American Psychiatric Press.

Freedy, J. R., & Hobfall, S. E. (1995). *Traumatic stress: From theory to practice.* New York: Plenum Press.

Freedy, J., Kilpatrick, D., & Resnick, H. (1993). Natural disasters and mental health: Theory, assessment, and intervention. *Journal of Social Behavior and Personality, 8*(3), 49–103.

Galante, R., & Foa, D. (1986). An epidemiological study of psychic trauma and treatment effectiveness for children after a natural disaster. *Journal of the American Academy of Child Psychiatry, 25,* 357–363.

Gillis, H. M. (1991, August). Children's responses and symptomatology following the Stockton, California school-yard shooting. In R. Belter (Chair), *Short- and long-term effects of trauma in children and adolescents.* Symposium conducted at the meeting of the American Psychological Association, San Francisco.

Green, B. L., Korol, M., Grace, M. C., Vary, M. G., Leonard, A. C., Gleser, G. C., & Smitson-Cohen, S. (1991). Children and disaster: Gender and parental effects on PTSD symptoms. *Journal of the American Academy of Child and Adolescent Psychiatry, 30,* 945–951.

Gillis, H. (1993). Individual and small-group psychotherapy for children involved in trauma and disaster. In C. F. Saylor (Ed.) *Children and disasters* (pp. 165–186). New York: Plenum Press.

Gleser, G. C., Green, B. L., & Winget, C. (1981). *Prolonged psychosocial effects of disaster: A study of Buffalo Creek.* New York: Academic Press.

Guerin, D. W., Junn, E., & Rushbrook, S. (1991). Preschoolers' reactions to the 1989 Bay Area earthquake as assessed by parent report on the Child Behavior Checklist. In J. M. Vogel (Chair), *Children's response to natural disasters: The aftermath of Hurricane Hugo and the 1989 Bay Area earthquake.* Symposium conducted at the biennial meeting of the Society for Research in Child Development, Seattle.

Gurwitch, R., Messenbaugh, A., Leftwich, M., Corrigan, S., & Pfefferbaum, B. (1996). *Brief intervention with children following the Oklahoma City bombing.* Paper presented at the American Psychological Association Meeting, Toronto, CA.

Joyner, C., & Swenson, C. (1993). Community-level intervention after a disaster. In C. F. Saylor (Ed.), *Children and disasters* (pp. 211–229). New York: Plenum Press.

Junn, E. N., Guerin, D. W., & Rushbrook, S. (1990). *Children's reactions to earthquake disaster.* Paper presented at the annual convention of the American Psychological Association, Boston.

Kazdin, A. E., Esveldt-Dawson, K., Unis, A. S., & Rancurello, M. D. (1983). Child and parent evaluations of depression and aggression in psychiatric inpatient children. *Journal of Abnormal Child Psychology, 11,* 401–413.

Kazdin, A. E., French, N. H., Unis, A. S., & Esveldt-Dawson, K. (1983). Assessment of childhood depression: Correspondence of child and parent ratings. *Journal of the American Academy of Child Psychiatry, 22,* 157–164.

Klingman, A. (1993). School-based intervention following a disaster. In C. F. Saylor (Ed.). *Children & disasters* (pp. 187–210). New York: Plenum Press.

LaGreca, A., Silverman, W., Vernberg, E., & Prinstein, M. (1996). Symptoms of posttraumatic stress in children after Hurricane Andrew: A prospective study. *Journal of Consulting and Clinical Psychology, 64*(4), 712–713.

LaGreca, A., Vernberg, E., Silverman, W., Vogel, A., & Prinstein, M. (1994). *Helping children prepare for and cope with natural disasters: A manual for professionals working with elementary school children.* Miami, Florida: Bell Foundation South.

Libow, J. (1992). Traumatized children and the news media: Clinical considerations. *American Journal of Orthopsychiatry, 62*(3), 379–386.

Lonigan, C. J., Shannon, M. P., Finch, A. J., Jr., Daugherty, T. K., & Taylor, C. M. (1991). Children's reactions to a natural disaster: Symptom severity and degree of exposure. *Advances in Behaviour Research Therapy, 13*(3), 135–154.

Lonigan, C. J., Shannon, M. P., Taylor, C. M., Finch, A. J., & Sallee, F. R. (1994). Children exposed to disaster: Risk factors for the development of post-traumatic symptomatology. *Journal of the American Academy of Child and Adolescent Psychiatry, 33*(1), 94–105.

McConaughy, S. H. (1993). Advances in empirically based assessment of children's behavioral and emotional problems. *School Psychology Review, 22*(2), 285–307.

McDermott, B. (1996). *Sutherland Bushfire Trauma Project: A randomized controlled treatment trial.* Paper presented at the American Psychological Association Meeting, Toronto, CA.

McFarlane, A. C. (1987). Post-traumatic phenomena in a longitudinal study of children following a natural disaster. *Journal of the American Academy of Child Psychiatry, 29,* 677–690.

McFarlane, A. C. (1988). Recent life events and psychiatric disorder in children: The interaction with preceding extreme adversity. *Journal of Child Psychology and Psychiatry, 29,* 677–690.

McFarlane, A. C., Policansky, S. K., & Irwin, C. (1987). A longitudinal study of the psychological morbidity in children due to a natural disaster. *Psychological Medicine, 17,* 727–738.

Milne, G. (1977). Cyclone Tracy: II. The effects on Darwin children. *Australian Psychologist, 12*(1), 55–62.

Mitchell, J. T. (1993). *Critical incidents stress debriefing: An operations manual.* Ellicott City, MD: Chevron Publishing.

Nader, K., & Pynoos, R. (1993). School disaster: Planning and initial interventions. *Journal of Social Behavior and Personality, 8*(5), 299–230.

Nader, K., Pynoos, R., Fairbanks, L., & Frederick, C. (1990). Children's PTSD symptoms one year after a sniper attack at their school. *American Journal of Psychiatry, 147,* 1526–1530.

Phares, V., Compas, B., & Howell, D. C. (1989). Perspectives on child behavior problems: Comparisons of children's self-reports with parent and teacher reports. *Psychological Assessment: A Journal of Consulting and Clinical Psychology, 1*(1), 68–71.

Pynoos, R. S., & Nader, K. (1988). Psychological first aid and treatment approach to children exposed to community violence: Research implications *Journal of Traumatic Stress, 1,* 445–473.

Pynoos, R., & Nader, K. (1993). Issues in the treatment of posttraumatic stress disorder in children and adolescents in J. Wilson & B. Raphael (Eds.), *The international handbook of traumatic stress syndromes* (pp. 535–539). New York: Plenum Press.

Pynoos, R. S., Frederick, C., Nader, K., Arroyo, W., Steinberg, A., Eth, S., Nunez, F., & Fairbanks, L. (1987). Life threat and posttraumatic stress in school-age children. *Archives of General Psychiatry, 44,* 1057–1063.

Rozensky, R., Sloan, I., Schwarz, E., & Kowalski, J. (1993). Psychological responses of children to shootings and hostage situations. In C. F. Saylor (Ed.). *Children and disasters* (pp. 123–136). New York: Plenum Press.

Saigh, P. A. (1989). The use of *in vitro* flooding in the treatment of traumatized adolescents. *Journal of Behavior and Developmental Pediatrics, 10,* 17–21.

Saylor, C. F. (1993). *Children and disasters.* New York: Plenum Press.

Saylor, C. F., Swenson, C. C., & Powell, P. (1992). Hurricane Hugo blows down the broccoli: Preschoolers' post-disaster play and adjustment. *Child Psychiatry and Human Development, 22*(3), 139–149.

Saylor, C., Swenson, C., Stokes, S., Wertlieb, D., & Casto, Y. (1994). The Pediatric Emotional Distress Scale (PEDS): A brief screening measure for child trauma victims. Presented at the American Psychological Association Meeting. Los Angeles, CA.

Schwarz, E. D., & Kowalski, J. M. (1991). Malignant memories: Posttraumatic stress disorder in children and adults following a school shooting. *Journal of the American Academy of Child and Adolescent Psychiatry, 30*(6), 936–944.

Scott, R. (1994). Dealing with the aftermath of a crisis, trauma, and disaster: An overview of intervention strategies for children. *Children, Youth, and Family Services Quarterly, 17*(3), 6–9.

Seroka, C. M., Knapp, C., Knight, S., Siemon, C. R., & Starbuck, S. (1986). A comprehensive program for postdisaster counseling. *Social Casework: The Journal of Contemporary Social Work, 67,* 37–44.

Shannon, M. P., Lonigan, C. J., Finch, A. J., & Taylor, C. M. (1994). Children exposed to disaster: I. Epidemiology of profiles. *Journal of the American Academy of Child Psychiatry, 33* 80–93.

Shelby, J. (1994). Psychological intervention with children in disaster relief shelters. *Children, Youth, and Family Services Quarterly, 17*(3), 14–18.

Spirito, A., Stark, L., & Williams, C. (1988). Development of a brief coping checklist for use with pediatric populations. *Journal of Pediatric Psychology, 13,* 389–407.

Sugar, M. (1988). A preschooler in a disaster. *American Journal of Psychotherapy, 42,* 619–629.

Sullivan, M. A., Saylor, C. F., & Foster, K. Y. (1991). Post hurricane adjustment of preschoolers and their families. *Advances in Behaviour Research and Therapy, 13*(3), 163–171.

Swenson, C., & Klingman, A. (1993). Children and war. In C. F. Saylor (Ed.). *Children and disasters* (pp. 137–164). New York: Plenum Press.

Swenson, C., Saylor, C., Powell, P., Stokes, S., Foster, K., & Belter, R. (1996). Mothers' ratings of children's adjustment 14 months following a hurricane. *Orthopsychiatry, 66*(1), 122–130.

Terr, L. (1989). Treating psychic trauma in children: A preliminary discussion. *Journal of Traumatic Stress, 2,* 2–20.

Vernberg, E. (1996). *Issues and advances in evaluating postdisaster interventions.* Paper presented at the American Psychological Association meeting, Toronto, Canada.

Vernberg, E., La Greca, A., Silverman, W., & Prinstein, M. (1996). Prediction of posttraumatic stress symptoms in children after Hurricane Andrew. *Journal of Abnormal Psychology, 105,* 237–248.

Vernberg, E., & Vogel, S. (1993). Interventions with children after disasters. *Journal of Clinical Child Psychology 22*(4), 485–498.

Vogel, S., & Vernberg, E. (1993). Children's psychological responses to disasters. *Journal of Clinical Child Psychology, 22*(4), 464–484.

Waeckerle, J. F. (1994). Disaster medicine: Challenges for today. *Annals of Emergency Medicine, 23*(4), 715–718.

Yeast, C. (1994). APA disaster response network: Psychological response to survivors of traumatic events. *Children, Youth, and Family Services Quarterly, 17*(3), 19–20.

Yule, W. (1993). Technology-related disasters. In C. F. Saylor (Ed.). *Children and disasters* (pp. 105–122). New York: Plenum Press.

IV

Social Environmental Stressors

14

Children's Coping in the Academic Domain

ELLEN A. SKINNER and JAMES G. WELLBORN

Each child who fails to learn is a personal tragedy and a social loss. Children with inadequate education are more likely to become adults who are unemployed, on welfare, imprisoned, or who bear children out of wedlock. A nation whose future depends upon a smaller pool of future workers is undermined by each child who fails to acquire essential knowledge and skills.

National Commission on Children, 1993

School failure is expensive—to American society, to families, and to individual children. According to some estimates, the national rate of school dropout hovers between 25 and 30% (United States Department of Education, 1985). Its distribution across geography, race, and ethnic groups ranges from essentially zero in some predominantly Caucasian suburban school districts to over 60% for African-American inner-city children (Hamack, 1986; Levin, 1986). Over 700,000 young people drop out of school each year (Dryfoos, 1990). Adolescents who leave before completing a high school degree are more likely to face unemployment and to earn significantly lower incomes (Rumberger, 1987). In addition, they are more likely to participate in a host of socially undesirable activities, including drug and alcohol use, gang activity, teenage pregnancy, and delinquent acts (Fad & Ryser, 1993).

Costs at the individual level are more difficult to reckon with statistics, but they are easy to imagine. Leaving school changes an individual's life trajectory, including not only their career path and financial status, but also the kind of

ELLEN A. SKINNER • Department of Psychology, Portland State University, Portland, Oregon 97207. JAMES G. WELLBORN • Tennessee Christian Medical Center, Madison, Tennessee 37221.

Handbook of Children's Coping: Linking Theory and Intervention, edited by Wolchik and Sandler. Plenum Press, New York, 1997.

person they will marry, the number and timing of their children, and even the kind of parenting they will provide (Dryfoos, 1990; Rutter, 1989). Children who remain in school, but do not do well, have more distressing interpersonal interactions with parents and teachers, do not have as many friends, and think less of their scholastic competence and abilities (Dweck & Elliott, 1983; Marge & Waters, 1988). These difficulties, which are detectable as soon as children begin formal education but seem to become relatively stable starting as early as third grade (Stipek, Recchia, & McClintic, 1992), can interfere with development in related areas, including cognition, motivation, and social functioning.

Discussions of the factors that influence scholastic success and school completion reflect the growing recognition that students' academic participation and performance are multiply determined by cultural factors, such as the uneven distribution of resources and changing demands on the labor force; by sociological factors, such as the goals and strategies of educational institutions; by the climates provided by specific schools, families, and neighborhoods; and by the individual personalities, abilities, and motivations of students and their teachers, parents, and peers. Each of these factors has its ideological and disciplinary proponents, and each leads to different implications about the targets of educational reform designed to optimize student learning and school completion (Rush & Vitale, 1994).

A relatively recent addition to these discussions, as a key factor that may influence student success and satisfaction in school, has been the concept of academic coping, or how children interpret and react to academic challenges, setbacks, and difficulties. Why has the notion of coping in schools not been considered more fully up to now? First, there is the general trend in the literature on educational reform away from the consideration of individual child factors (such as intelligence or motivation) as explanations for student outcomes and toward a consideration of more global and systemic factors. Second, from the perspective of the literatures on coping, schools have not typically been considered to be major stressors in children's lives. Traditionally, children have been considered to "cope" only with nonnormative and potentially traumatic events, such as divorce, parental illness, or medical treatments (Garmezy, 1983; Rutter, 1983). However, the recent analysis of "common stressors" has opened the way for the study of how children cope with everyday problems, such as those encountered in school (Causey & Dubow, 1992). With this shift, researchers have begun to consider the variety of issues children face at school (Dickey & Henderson, 1989), children's understanding of the nature of these stressors, such as their controllability (Causey & Dubow, 1992; Compas, Banez, Malcarne, & Worsham, 1991), and how children attempt to cope with these events through behaviors such as direct action, problem solving, support seeking, distraction, distancing, or acceptance (Causey & Dubow, 1992; Dickey & Henderson, 1989; Ebata & Moos, 1989; Tero & Connell, 1984; Work, Levinson, & Hightower, 1987).

Despite the recent recognition of its potential importance, the research on academic coping per se is small, compared both to the literatures on other factors that influence children's school performance and to the literatures on how children cope with other stressors. Only a handful of scales exist that directly assess children's domain specific coping in schools, and several of these are unpublished. The scales that do exist are still in the validation stage, and no consensus has been reached about the core categories of academic coping, about the most effective types of coping in schools, or about the mechanisms by which such coping may be expected to affect its outcomes. Despite the fact that school performance has been considered to be an indicator of positive adjustment in intervention studies that target coping with other stresses (e.g., divorce) (Alpert-Gillis, Pedro-Carroll, & Cowen, 1989), few intervention studies to date have had academic coping as their direct target.

Although research on academic coping per se is limited, several other lines of research can be considered relevant because they examine certain reactions children may show to problems and failures in school (Compas, 1987). Work on mastery versus helplessness (Dweck, 1991; Dweck & Wortman, 1982; Harter, 1978) has examined in detail children's emotional, behavioral, and motivational reactions to failure and noncontingency in academic settings. Work on autonomy and self-determination (Deci & Ryan, 1985; Grolnick & Ryan, 1989; Ryan, 1982) has investigated children's reactions to external pressures, coercion, and extrinsically motivating tasks, and has studied their effects on behavioral engagement and intrinsic motivation for learning. And, work on help seeking in the classroom (Nelson-LeGall, 1985; special section, 1990) has analyzed the individual and interpersonal factors that make children more (or less) likely to go to teachers when they encounter difficulties with academic material.

Taken together, these theories and research represent a great deal of knowledge about children's perspectives and reactions to stressors in school. The purpose of this chapter is to draw these together, using a framework of coping to organize and integrate this work. Focusing on these processes through the lens of coping emphasizes core questions in these diverse literatures, such as the nature of stress and the consequences of different patterns of responses, and allows these questions to be answered, not only on their own terms, but also in relation to each other. A more comprehensive approach also allows for more informed speculation about intervention. The analysis of factors that facilitate and impede coping, in both children themselves and in their close relationships with teachers and parents, can suggest routes toward optimizing children's coping in school.

COPING AS AN ORGANIZING FRAMEWORK

Despite the apparent heterogeneity of the literatures on children's responses to problems in school, it may be surprising to discover that, at a very general level, they share a set of core assumptions about the factors that shape these processes. First, they assume that experiences of stress involve not just the objective features of the (in this case) academic environment, but also include the interactions of the individual child with that social and physical context, as well as the child's own interpretations of those interactions. In the coping literatures, this assumption is represented in definitions of stress that focus on person–context relations and in analyses of reactions to stress that begin with processes of cognitive appraisal (e.g., Lazarus & Folkman, 1984). In the other literatures, this assumption is represented by a focus on the self and the role of self-perceptions (e.g., self-esteem) and interpretations of the environment (e.g., influences of powerful others) in shaping children's reactions to problems, such as whether they will seek help (Nelson-LeGall, 1985).

Second, all these approaches assume that a major task consists of describing the different patterns of action children show in response to academic difficulties and explaining the factors that contribute to these individual differences. In the coping literature, the goal has been to answer this question "extensively," that is, to identify a broad range of different reactions (such as distancing or externalizing) and then to trace their antecedents backward, for example, in children's personality (Kliewer, 1991). In the self-perception literatures, the approach has been more "intensive," attempting to start with one set of self-system processes (e.g., self-determination) and then to describe in detail the patterns of action that result when this self-system is challenged or threatened (Deci & Ryan, 1985).

Third, all approaches have emphasized that patterns of action have both short- and long-term consequences for children. Short-term consequences (often referred to as "effectiveness" in the coping literature) describe the effects of the pattern of action or coping on the resolution of the current interaction. For example, in a disciplinary encounter, an aggressive student response is likely to result in further sanctions from the teacher. Or, a helpless response to initial failure is likely to interrupt successful problem solving. Furthermore, these short-term consequences can also have long-ranging effects, for example, resulting in more subsequent stressful interactions with teachers and learning activities, and eventually even preventing children from developing the cognitive and motivational resources they need to succeed in school.

These three themes are represented in the general conceptualization of the coping process used in this chapter. According to this perspective, children's encounters with stress have an impact on their views of themselves and the world, which in turn have a direct influence on their coping and patterns of action in those stressful situations. These actions, in turn, influence the outcomes of stressful encounters, which feed back upon the context and feed forward into the child's own development.

This general view of the coping process is used to organize the sections of this chapter. First, we consider the nature of stress in the academic context. Then we review definitions, dimensions, and categories of coping used to describe children's responses to stress in school. Third, we examine the correlates or outcomes of different patterns of coping. We conclude with suggestions for optimizing children's coping in the classroom. Throughout, our own work within a motivational framework will be used in an attempt to tie together these issues (for more detail, see Skinner & Wellborn, 1994).

STRESS IN ACADEMIC CONTEXTS

Children's own reports validate the notion that schools can be stressful places for students. If children are asked to name the most upsetting event of the last month (Spirito, Stark, Grace, & Stamoulis, 1991) or to describe things that happened that made them feel bad (Compas, Malcarne, & Fondacaro,

1988), events from school are consistently among the three most common problems they name (with family and peer relations usually the other two). When asked specifically to describe what bothers them at school, children as young as kindergarten are able to report their experience of multiple stressors. In a study in which 141 kindergarten through second grade children were asked about what worried or upset them in school, they most often mentioned schoolwork (26.8%), peer relationships (21%), personal injury or loss (17.3%), and loss of personal comfort (14.7%); they also mentioned discipline (6.9%), relations with teachers (6.3%), and family events (6.3%) (Dickey & Henderson, 1989). Adolescents were also able to report the multiple stressors they experience in school, including worry about examination results and study pressures, problems with the classroom environment (such as noise or crowding), issues with school authority, the difficulty of self-management, and challenges in accepting the self and relating to peers (Fanshawe & Burnett, 1991).

A closer examination of their specific answers reveals that children report being bothered by a multitude of big and small events: bad grades on tests and homework, anxiety about not doing well in the future, not understanding material presented in class, not knowing the answer if asked by the teacher, following the rules and threats of punishment for infractions, and concern that the teacher does not like them. These lines of research clearly support the notion that school can have costs for children (Ingraham, 1985). However, they are not very informative about *why* these experiences should be stressful or about the theoretical dimensions that underlie these experiences.

A Motivational Perspective on Stress in Schools

In answering questions about why certain school experiences threaten or challenge children, motivational theories rely on the concept of "psychological needs." The model of motivation used here posits three basic innate psychological needs: relatedness, competence, and autonomy (Connell, 1990; Connell & Wellborn, 1991; Deci & Ryan, 1985). These three needs are challenged or supported by opportunities provided by the social context. According to this perspective, school contexts are stressful to the extent that they challenge or threaten children's basic fundamental human needs.

If the model assumes that all children come with needs for relatedness, competence, and autonomy, however, how can it be useful in explaining individual differences in children's reactions to common school experiences? All children will sometimes fail in their attempts to solve problems or to understand material presented in class. All children must follow school rules, which by their nature are often constraining. All children will sometimes be overlooked by teachers. Why are these experiences stressful for some children, whereas they are not noticed or are even seen as challenges by other children? According to the motivational perspective, one answer lies in individual differences in children's self-system processes.

Consistent with many self theories (Harter, 1983), the motivational model posits that children actively construct beliefs or internal representations of themselves, the social context, and interactions between the two. We refer to these belief sets as *self-system processes* or organized constructions about the self in relation to the social context. These are based on an individual child's history of interactions with the social and physical environments and are shaped by the cognitive and social processes that help interpret these interactions. Consistent with the notion of fundamental needs, we posit that children's self-system processes are organized around relatedness, competence, and autonomy (Connell & Wellborn, 1991). To understand these issues completely, it is necessary to explain the nature of the innate psychological needs postulated, the kinds of experiences that can impinge on them, and the individual vulnerabilities that make these experiences stressful.

Competence, Chaos, and Control

The need with which most researchers in the academic domain are familiar is children's need for competence. Competence or effectance refers to the need to experience oneself as effective in interactions with the social and physical environment (White, 1959). Although sometimes not mentioned explicitly, the assumption of this need underlies explanations of many theories of control, causal attributions, helplessness, and self-efficacy (Skinner, 1995).

Children's needs for competence can be challenged or threatened by social contexts that are characterized by chaos. Chaotic contexts are noncontingent, inconsistent, random, arbitrary, discriminatory, or unfair; they also include social contextual situations in which information is lacking about how to produce desired effects, such as when the rationales for rules are not explained, when children are asked to attempt activities that are too difficult for them, when strategies for producing outcomes are not well-specified, when practice and opportunities for independent attempts are not sufficient, or when guidance and feedback for strategy implementation are not provided.

The self-system processes connected to the need for competence have been studied by researchers interested in perceived control (for reviews, see Bandura, 1977, 1986, 1989; Dweck, 1991; Folkman, 1984; Schunk, 1984; Seligman, 1975; Skinner, 1995, 1996; Weiner, 1979, 1985, 1986; Weiss, 1986). In general, these belief sets refer to convictions about the capacity of the self to enact effective strategies and about the responsiveness of the environment to one's efforts. Situations that are highly chaotic or children who are pessimistic with respect to their own competence are hypothesized to produce interpretations of setbacks and failures as evidence of incompetence and as forecasting long-term difficulty. In general, children with self-system vulnerabilities react to academic difficulties with appraisals that reflect an overly generalized negative view (1) of the self (which we label "self-derogation") and (2) of the possibility of the context being responsive to the child's needs (which we label "catastrophizing"). In the coping literature, these are referred to as primary appraisals and they contribute to the initial distress children experience in reaction to negative events.

In the specific case of competence, we have found that children with low perceived control, when imagining school problems ("When something bad happens to me in school, like not doing well on a test or not being able to answer an important question in class . . ."), are more likely to endorse items reflecting self-derogation of competence (e.g., "I feel like the dumbest person in the world" or "I feel totally stupid") and catastrophizing about the impossibility of future control (e.g., "I worry that I won't do well on anything" or "I worry that I'll never learn how to do it") (Edge & Skinner, 1997; Skinner, 1993).

Based in part on these appraisals, children with low perceived control tend to react to even relatively mild instances of failure or resistance (such as not being able to think of an answer right away) with confusion and panic. In contrast, children with high perceived control do not react with extreme distress to academic failures and setbacks. They seem to focus instead on overcoming these obstacles with goal-directed concentrated action (for reviews, see Dweck & Elliott, 1983; Skinner, 1995).

Autonomy, Coercion, and Self-Determination

Also familiar to many researchers in the academic domain is children's need for autonomy. Autonomy or self-determination refers to the need to experience oneself as the origin of one's actions, to perceive oneself as free to choose one's own goals and course of action (for reviews, see deCharms, 1968; Deci & Ryan, 1985). Again, although not always explicitly acknowledged, this need can provide one explanation for why certain experiences in school, such as graded performance or competition, can be stressful: Because they can undermine children's autonomy (Ames & Ames, 1984, 1985; Ryan & Grolnick, 1986). The general term used to describe interactions that can undermine autonomy is *coercion*. These refer to interactions in which children are pressured, for example, by rules or rewards, to behave in certain ways or to express certain feelings; it may refer to a lack of autonomy support or to direct attempts to pressure, constrain, or force children to accept certain goals or courses of action.

Children's perceptions about the extent to which they are free to show the goals and course of action of their choice have been studied by researchers interested in self-determination, autonomy orientations, goal orientations, or self-regulatory styles (Ames & Ames, 1984, 1985; Deci & Ryan, 1985; Dweck & Leggett, 1988; Ryan & Connell, 1989). In general, these belief systems refer to children's internalized reasons for engaging in behaviors that may or may not be intrinsically interesting (such as homework or tests).

Situations that are highly coercive or children with low autonomy produce interpretations of difficult interactions that emphasize their pressured quality. For example, we found that the lower a child's self-determined autonomy orientation, the more likely he or she was to appraise challenging situations (e.g., "When something bad happens to me in school, like not doing well on a test or not being able to answer an important question in class) with self-derogation ("I feel like it's all my fault" or "I feel like I'm to blame") and catastrophizing ("It really spoils the subject for me" or "I don't care about that subject any more") (Edge & Skinner, 1997; Skinner, 1993).

Children with orientations that are nonautonomous can react to even mild resistance with high distress or frustration and are unable to prevent themselves from responding in underregulated ways (e.g., rebellion) or can pressure themselves to respond in overregulated ways (e.g., perseveration), both of which are nonautonomous. In contrast, when children are autonomous in their orientations for engaging in learning activities, they react to obstacles and setbacks with little distress and, instead, with interest and flexibility, interpreting environmental feedback as information that can be used to guide performance and not as pressure to act in some specific manner.

Relatedness, Neglect, and Internal Working Models

The third need, although long recognized as paramount in family settings, has only recently come to the attention of researchers interested in children's school experiences; it is children's need for relatedness. Relatedness or belongingness refers to the need to experience oneself as lovable and loving, as a valued member of a group or community (Ainsworth, 1979, 1989). This need may contribute to explanations of why attachments to teachers and peers as well as feelings of community within schools may predict children's participation and learning in those settings (Lynch & Cicchetti, 1992).

Social interactions that undermine a child's need for relatedness can be summarized in the construct of neglect. In the school context, neglect refers to the absence of involvement, such as when children are ignored or overlooked by teachers, or when teachers fail to communicate their regard and affection for children, or when teachers or the school climate in general are cold, distant, and uncaring, or even hostile and rejecting of children. Parents may also show neglect, if they express no interest in their children's school work or experiences.

The self-system processes of relatedness have been conceptualized by attachment researchers as internal working models of attachment figures (Bretherton, 1985; Cassidy, 1988; Crittendon, 1990; Lynch & Cicchetti, 1992) and relational schemes (Baldwin, 1992). In general, these refer to children's convictions about their own lovability or intrinsic worth, and their expectations that social partners can be trusted to be warm and available in times of need. We have found that children with insecure internal working models tend to report that they react to challenges (e.g., "When something bad happens to me in school, like not doing well on a test or not being able to answer an important question in class") with more self-derogation ("I feel like nobody will like me" or "I feel like nobody will have anything to do with me") and catastrophizing (e.g., "I feel like I let everybody down" or "I feel like I didn't come through for people") (Edge & Skinner, 1997; Skinner, 1993).

Children with maladaptive beliefs about relatedness, for example, who doubt their own value or who view social partners as likely to be dangerous, react to even mildly stressful events with anxiety and expectations for severe social consequences. Hence, they would be more likely to conceal problems or avoid social contacts. In contrast, children with adaptive self-system processes in this area react to potential threats to relatedness, such as neglect or being overlooked by a teacher, with little distress and with active attempts to reestablish contact.

Self as a Source of Distress and as an Intrapersonal Resource

In sum, a motivational theory suggests that one source of individual differences in children's coping arises as a function of their appraisals of potentially stressful events as threatening or impinging on their basic needs. Children's self-system processes of relatedness, competence, and autonomy should influence whether a failure or setback in school is viewed by a child simply as a source of information about where more work and help are needed or, instead, as an indication of sweeping incompetence, with shameful and anxiety-provoking interpersonal consequences. This analysis of the role of the self in coping allows for the a priori identification of children who are likely to respond to difficulties in school with distress. And it explains why some children are so overwhelmed by daily hassles in school: Because these setbacks feed directly into existing self-system vulnerabilities. An overview of this model is presented in Fig. 1.

These self-systems may also be a route by which parents, even though physically absent from the school setting, can make their presence felt (e.g., Connell & Wellborn, 1991; Grolnick & Slowiaczek, 1994; Wellborn, 1996; Yoder, 1996). Children bring their history of interactions with parents around issues of relatedness, competence, and autonomy with them to the classroom in the form of their self-system processes. For example, maladaptive relatedness beliefs formed in neglectful interactions with parents may make children fearful of their teachers' reactions to their failures, and so may lead them to conceal their difficulties from teachers. In a parallel vein, children's low perceived control, based on interactions with noncontingent parents, may lead children to assume that there is nothing they can do to overcome initial failures to understand academic material. Or, children's highly reactive autonomy orientation based on coercive interactions with parents may provoke them to react obstinately to even the mildest rule enforcement from teachers.

WAYS OF COPING IN SCHOOL

How do children respond to the challenges and threats provided by their everyday school experiences? What are the different ways children can cope with stressors in the academic domain? Although this issue is central to any conceptualization of coping in school, no current theory claims to be comprehensive in its answer. Theories and measures derived from a coping perspective suggest a variety of possible responses to classroom stresses. Theories derived from self-perception perspectives tend to focus in more detail on one or two patterns of responses. Each of these perspectives will be reviewed briefly, followed by a presentation of the motivational perspective which tries to integrate both.

Coping Perspective

Despite disagreement about the precise definition of coping itself, consensus seems to exist about some general parameters of children's coping (Compas, 1987). First, children can cope, not only through behavioral acts, but also with emotional and cognitive responses. Second, coping includes not just responses that are effective in ameliorating stress, but also attempts that do not succeed. And third, instead of being considered as a traitlike "style," coping in most situations can be thought of as a profile of activities that may vary depending

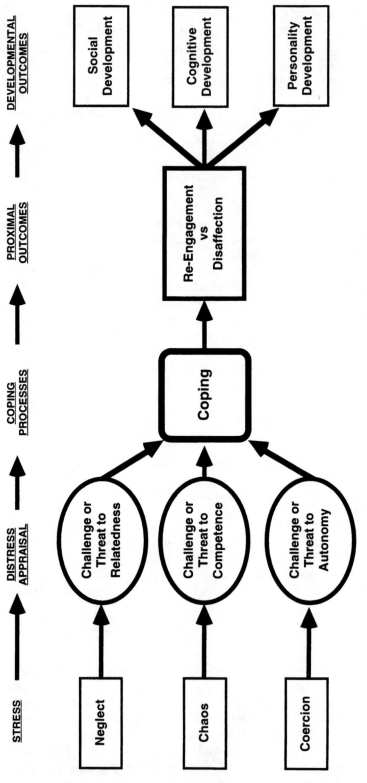

Figure 1. A simple model of the coping process. (Adapted from Skinner & Wellborn, 1994.)

on the kind of stressor, its domain, and the point in time during the coping process (see Lazarus & Folkman, 1984, for a discussion of these issues in adults).

Theorists have sometimes found it useful to think in terms of overarching dimensions. Two different perspectives, both adapted from the adult literature, have tended to guide thinking in this area. The first distinguishes coping that is problem focused, or aimed at solving the problem that created the stress, from coping that is emotion focused, or aimed at reducing the emotional distress created by the problem (Compas et al., 1988; Lazarus & Folkman, 1984; for a review of assessments based on this distinction, see Knapp, Stark, Kurkjian, & Spirito, 1991). The second main perspective distinguishes kinds of coping that bring the child into more contact with the stressful situation from coping that removes the child from the interaction, using such terms as approach versus avoidance (Roth & Cohen, 1986), blunting versus monitoring (Miller & Green, 1990), or repression versus sensitization (Ebata & Moos, 1991; see Skinner et al., 1997 for a review).

Most coping theories and measures of coping, building on these general distinctions, have looked at a variety of coping "strategies" or ways of coping. Only a few of these theories and measures have been designed explicitly to tap children's responses to problems and setbacks in the academic domain. They are listed in Table 1. The general formats of most of these scales include "stems," which describe the stressful academic situation, and "items," which describe children's coping responses. In addition, some scales are formatted like checklists, in which children are asked to imagine a problem they are having in school and then to check off from the list of coping items those that they used in response to that problem. Others include domain-specific stems (such as, "Think of a time something bad happened in school") and children are asked to rate different coping responses, usually on a scale of 1 to 4 or 1 to 5. To derive coping categories, theorists usually start with a range of possible responses and then used factor analyses to discover sets of items which may tap one "way" or category of coping.*

As can be seen in Table 1, the resulting categories are heterogeneous, ranging from very general syndromes, such as internalizing and externalizing behavior, to relatively specific responses, such as problem solving, distraction, or resignation. In addition, the number and kinds of categories differ from measure to measure. However, some commonalties can be discerned. All category systems refer to a cluster of reactions involving "planful problem solving." Categories in this cluster include problem solving itself, as well as cognitive decision making, self-reliance, direct action, and logical analysis. A second cluster common to many approaches involves seeking contact with others, including seeking problem-focused support and guidance and seeking social support or emotional reassurance.

A third cluster involves avoiding contact with the stressful situation,

*Other operationalizations have been used as more indirect indicators of coping, such as the use of mastery or self-image questionnaires (Klebanov & Brooks-Gunn, 1992), DSM-III-R global assessment of functioning (Plante, Goldfarb, & Wadley, 1993), or combinations of achievement motivation and anxiety (Wade, 1981). Although they may be related to children's adaptation to school, these "inferred" strategies do not directly map onto notions of coping categories, and so are not discussed in this section.

Table 1. Categories of Coping on Assessments That Include Children's
Academic Coping

Author(s)	Ways of coping	
Ayers et al. (1989)	Cognitive decision making	Direct problem solving
	Problem-focused support	Positive cognitive restructuring
	Seeking understanding	Emotion-focused support
	Expressing feelings	Physical release of emotion
	Distracting actions	Avoidant actions
	Cognitive avoidance	Problem behavior
	Lack of coping	
Band & Weisz (1988)	Direct problem solving	Social/spiritual support
	Problem-focused crying	Emotion-focused crying
	Problem-focused aggression	Emotion-focused aggression
	Problem-solved avoidance	Cognitive avoidance
	Pure cognition	
	Doing nothing	
Brown, O'Keefe,	Coping strategies	Catastrophizing cognitions
Sanders, & Baker	Positive self-talk	Focus on negative/pain
(1986)	Attention diversion	Escape/avoidance
	Relaxation, deep breathing	Fear of unlikely consequence
	Thought stopping	Fear of response of other
	Task orientation	Self-denigration, self-blame
	Talking with someone else	Anxious anticipation
	Problem solving	Worry/rumination
Causey & Dubow	Approach	
(1992)	Social support, problem solving/self-reliance	
	Avoidance	
	Distancing, internalizing, externalizing	
Coleman (1992)	Confrontative coping	Distancing
	Self-controlling	Seeking social support
	Accepting responsibility	Escape avoidance
	Planful problem solving	Positive reappraisal
	Helplessness	
Compas, Malcarne, &	Problem-focused coping	
Fondacaro	Emotion-focused coping	
(1988)		
Dickie & Henderson	Direct action	Distraction
(1989)	Social support	Acceptance/resignation
	Redefinition	Catharsis/venting
	Relaxation/fun activity	
Ebata & Moos (1989)	Approach	
	Positive reappraisal, logical analysis, guidance/support, problem solving	
	Avoidance	
	Cognitive avoidance, resigned acceptance, alternative rewards, emotional discharge	
Fad & Ryser (1993)	Copes appropriately when insulted	
	Copes acceptably when bossed	

Table 1. (*Continued*)

Author(s)	Ways of coping
	Able to express anger appropriately Can handle being lied to Avoid arguments when provoked Copes in acceptable way if someone takes something belonging to him/her Copes with being blamed unfairly

Fagen (1984)	Changing self when frustrated
	  Modify goals, try new paths to goal, identify positives in self, accept limitations
	Changing environment when frustrated
	  Encounter external source of frustration, seek help/assistance

Fanshawe & Burnett (1991)	Negative avoidance Anger Family communication Positive avoidance
Horowitz, Boardman, & Redlener (1994)	Social support/ventilating feelings Optimistic appraisal and change Distancing
Lepore & Kliewer (1989) (from Kliewer, 1991)	Monitoring Blunting
Rush & Vitale (1994)	Difficulty accepting adult authority Unable to solve conflicts without negative verbal or physical confrontation Disciplinary action is not serving as a deterrent Unable to make and keep friends in his or her age group Unable to cope with new situations
Spirito, Stark, Grace, & Stamoulis (1991)	Distraction Social withdrawal Wishful thinking Self-criticism Blaming others Problem solving Emotional regulation Cognitive restructuring Social support Resignation

Tero & Connell (1984); Mellor-Crummey et al., (1989)	Positive coping
	  Problem-focused strategies
	  Placing positive values on negative events
	Defensive coping
	  Projection
	  Denial
	Anxiety amplification

Timberlake, Barnett, & Plionis (1993)	Use of words to eradicate difference Use of activity to camouflage differences Use of actions to encapsulate difference

Work, Levinson, & Hightower (1987)	Approach
	  Seeking social support, self-reliance
	Avoidance
	  Distancing, wishful thinking

through means such as distracting or avoidant action, cognitive avoidance, distancing, escape, denial, social withdrawal, or wishful thinking. A fourth cluster involves uncontrolled emotional discharge, including responses such as venting, physical release of emotion, externalizing behaviors, aggression, confrontation, and blaming others. A final cluster includes "not coping," that is, doing nothing, becoming helpless, resigned, and accepting failure. This is sometimes accompanied by anxiety and self-blame. Less frequently mentioned are more cognitive strategies, such as cognitive re-structuring, positive reappraisal, optimism, accepting responsibility, redefinition, and active attempts to modify goals, accept limitations, or identify the positive in the self.*

Self-Perception Perspective on Reactions to Stress

The literature on self-perceptions shows more consensus about the kinds of reactions to problems and setbacks promoted by different views of the self. However, the range of reactions described is correspondingly more narrow. For each self-perception studied, only a handful of "coping categories" are considered relevant.

According to the attachment perspective, the self-systems associated with relatedness predict reactions to stressful events (such as separation or novelty) that involve going to trusted others for aid or comfort (Ainsworth, 1979, 1989). Extrapolating this work to the academic domain, the prediction would be that children with a warm and trusting relationship with teachers and parents would be more likely to turn to them in times of distress or need, such as when they are having academic difficulties. The research that directly addresses help seeking in the academic domain (Nelson-LeGall, 1985; Newman, 1990) suggests that other self-perceptions may be involved in addition to self-esteem, such as perceived competence, but it reinforces the notion that one important response to difficulties in school is to seek help from the teacher.

In the literatures on perceived control, two reactions to difficulties or failure have been characterized as "mastery oriented" versus "helplessness" (Dweck, 1991; Seligman, 1975). A helpless response to setbacks includes passivity, confusion, anxiety, self-recrimination, withdrawal, and attempts to escape from the situation. In contrast, a mastery-oriented response includes

---

*A continuing question in this area has been the validity of children's reports of their own coping responses (e.g., Weisz, 1993). Occasionally, researchers have tried to examine whether children's self-reports of their coping responses in school are related to the reports of their coping provided by peers (Causey & Debow, 1992) or teachers (Connell & Illardi, 1987). Although some positive correlations have been found, especially with more observable behavioral coping response categories (such as externalizing behavior or seeking social support) (Causey & Debow, 1992), the correspondence, especially for more intrapsychic coping (such as denial or anxiety amplification), is modest at best. This low correspondence may suggest caution about the use of children's own self-reports of coping or it may suggest that many of the coping responses of interest to researchers are not directly accessible to outside observers. Following a year-long observational study, in which we attempted to capture different types of coping through videotapes in the classroom, we have concluded that both the expression and display rules of the classroom context make many forms of academic coping unavailable to observers, even though our interviews and questionnaires confirmed that these same coping processes are very salient to the children who are experiencing them.

boosting concentration, narrowing the focus of attention, strategy generation and testing, and augmented effort and persistence. These responses have been produced in academic situations in the laboratory and have also been observed in classrooms, from kindergarten to college.

In the work on autonomy, two nonautonomous reactions to environmental pressures have been suggested: rebellion and conformity (Deci & Ryan, 1985). Conformity is considered nonautonomous because it consists of simply submitting to external pressure. Perhaps surprisingly, rebellion is also considered nonautonomous because it consists of doing the opposite of what is requested, and so is still controlled by external forces. Autonomous responses to external (or internal) constraints can include either going along with them or not, but doing so in a way that is choiceful, intentional, voluntary, willing, flexible, free of tension, and fully committed.

A Motivational Perspective on Patterns of Coping

The goal of the motivational conceptualization of coping was to formulate a definition of coping that was motivationally based and yet "developmentally friendly," that is, appropriate to work with children as well as adults. We define coping as action regulation in the face of psychological stress (Skinner & Wellborn, 1994). Action is the critical outcome of motivational processes (Wellborn, 1991) and consists of behavior, emotion, and orientation (or outlook). Hence, coping refers to the ways children (and people more generally) mobilize, manage, energize, guide, channel, and direct their behavior, emotion, and orientation in stressful circumstances, or how they fail to do so. We consider this definition to be developmentally friendly, because it assumes that how action regulation is accomplished not only differs between individuals but also changes with age and developmental level. Specifically, this definition links the coping concept with the rich literatures on the development of children's regulation of behavior (Kopp, 1982), attention (Mischel & Mischel, 1983), and emotion (Fox, 1994; Chapter 2, this volume).

In generating a list of ways children could cope, we wanted a set of dimensions of coping that could be derived from the coping definition and could in turn be used to generate a set of categories that would be reasonably comprehensive, encompassing categories used by both coping and self-perception theories, and also be flexibly applicable across domains and age groups (see Skinner & Wellborn, 1994).

Dimensions of Coping

To form a matrix of kinds of coping, we crossed the three objects of regulation (behavior, emotion, and orientation) with the three sources of psychological stress (neglect, chaos, and coercion). To these core dimensions, we hypothesized that one additional dimension would be added as children became able to differentiate self from context in their self-system processes. We expected that in their appraisals of the stressful situation, children would come to target, as the source of the distress, either the self or the context or both. The matrix of coping dimensions is presented in Fig. 2. We have filled in the 36 general

COPING RESPONSES

COPING REACTIONS	APPRAISALS		Regulation of Behavior	Regulation of Emotion	Regulation of Orientation
RELATEDNESS					
SELF	CHALLENGE	"I will love."	Cooperate ("I work on it with somebody I like.")	Appreciate ("I'm glad my teacher is there.")	Support ("I think of all the people I can go to.")
SELF	THREAT	"I am alone."	Delegation ("I try to get someone to do it for me.")	Self-pity ("I feel sorry for myself.")	Abandonment ("No one even cares.")
CONTEXT	CHALLENGE	"I will reduce neglect."	Contact-seeking ("I talk with the teacher about it.")	Comfort-seeking ("I talk to someone who will cheer me up.")	Help-seeking ("I think about how to get help next time if I need it.")
CONTEXT	THREAT	"The world is cold."	Concealment ("I try to keep anybody from finding out about it.")	Detachment ("I say 'Who cares what anybody thinks.")	Isolation ("I stay away from people.")
COMPETENCE					
SELF	CHALLENGE	"I will learn."	Strategize ("I try to think of different ways to do it.")	Resolve ("I tell myself 'You can do it.")	Repair ("It makes me want to try even harder.")
SELF	THREAT	"I am helpless."	Confusion ("I get all confused.")	Self-doubt ("I tell myself 'You can't do this.'")	Discouragement ("I just don't want to do any more.")
CONTEXT	CHALLENGE	"I will reduce chaos."	Information-seeking ("I try to find out more about it.")	Optimism ("I can usually get it right in the end.")	Prevention ("I try to figure out how to do better next time.")
CONTEXT	THREAT	"The world is unpredictable."	Escape ("I try to get out of it.")	Pessimism ("I'll probably miss it.")	Procrastination ("I put off working on it.")
AUTONOMY					
SELF	CHALLENGE	"I will decide."	Flexibility ("I skip it and come back to it later.")	Accept Responsibility ("I think about the part I may have played.")	Reevaluation ("I decide whether I want to do anything about it.")
SELF	THREAT	"I don't know what I want."	Perseveration ("I go over the problem again and again and again.")	Self-blame ("I blame myself for not working hard enough.")	Obsession ("I can't stop thinking about it.")
CONTEXT	CHALLENGE	"I will reduce coercion."	Negotiation ("I go along with it for now.")	Blamelessness ("I say 'These things happen.")	Rededication ("I think about how this may be useful to me later on.")
CONTEXT	THREAT	"The world is hostile."	Aggression ("I'd just like to rip it to shreds.")	Projection ("I say the test was not fair.")	Devaluation ("I say 'Who needs school anyway.")

Figure 2. Categories of coping.

categories of coping that we believe correspond to the combinations of dimensions.

Development and Domain of Coping

Fortunately or unfortunately, the exact categories that fill the matrix will probably differ depending on the developmental level of individuals and the contextual constraints of the domain of the stressor. For example, in reports of their coping with everyday stressors in school and friendship (Skinner, Altman, & Sherwood, 1991a), younger children (age 7) showed more evidence of actively regulating their behaviors than their emotions (for parallel developmental differences, see also Band & Weisz, 1988; Compas et al., 1988), and even older children (age 10) did not often spontaneously report regulation of their orientations or outlooks.

Furthermore, children's coping responses were constrained by the power structures, norms, and rules of the classroom (Skinner et al., 1991a). With friends, children were able to show aggression or to simply avoid peers with whom they had difficulties. However, in school, children cannot easily aggress against their teachers; they can only be "oppositional." They cannot easily avoid taking tests or escape from school; therefore, they can only express this option through procrastination or mental escape (see also Band & Weisz, 1988; Causey & Dubow, 1992; Compas et al., 1988; Spirito et al., 1991; Stark, Spirito, Williams, & Guevremont, 1989; Wellborn, Mellor-Crummey, Connell, & Skinner, 1990, for domain differences in coping).

Categories of Academic Coping

We attempted to capture the variety of ways children can cope in school through a self-report questionnaire of the 36 categories of coping (Skinner & Wellborn, 1992). It was based on open-ended interviews with children about their responses to problems and difficulties they had actually experienced in school (Skinner, Altman, & Sherwood, 1991b). We based the items on the general categories, then adapted them to the academic domain and to the developmental level of school-aged children, using children's own words from the open-ended interviews to describe the coping responses whenever possible (see Skinner et al., 1991a). The analysis of these scales is underway, including their psychometric properties as well as their interrelationships to each other and to short- and long-term coping consequences. For example, the competence ways of coping show high internal consistencies and factor structures consistent with the matrix (Edge & Skinner, 1997). However, the complete structure of this matrix remains to be tested.

The different coping categories can, as is typical for coping research, be considered separately. However, given the structure of the matrix (see Fig. 2), they can also be grouped into complexes of behavior, emotion, and orientation, corresponding to the rows of the matrix. For example, a helpless pattern of coping can be found in the row corresponding to competence, self, and threat; this combination of confused behavioral regulation, self-doubt, and discouragement would be expected to co-occur when children do not believe that they are competent to overcome academic failures and setbacks. As another example, an externalizing coping combination can be found in the row corresponding to autonomy, context, and threat; behavioral aggression, projection (blaming others), and devaluation would be expected to co-occur in children who rebel against the coercion of school activities. Hence, each row can be considered a complex of action (behavior, emotion, and orientation) in response to psychological stress.

Implications of a Motivational Model of Coping Categories

This more comprehensive way of thinking about coping may add to the literatures on coping and on self-perceptions, at both the specific and the general levels. Specifically, this dimensionalization suggests several differentiations that may be useful to work on help seeking, perceived control, and autonomy. For help seeking, it suggests that the opposite of help seeking may not simply be passivity, it may be "concealment"; that is, children may actively try to prevent adults from discovering that they need assistance. The different categories in the matrix are also consistent with suggestions in the literature that it may be important to distinguish different kinds of contact seeking with adults (Nelson-LeGall, 1985). We have differentiated contact seeking in general from going to the teacher for comfort or for help. We have also distinguished help seeking (going to the teacher for instrumental aid needed to complete the task oneself) from attempts to get someone else to do the work (termed "delegation").

To the research on perceived control, this dimensionalization adds the notion that helplessness due to perceived incompetence may manifest itself differently than helplessness due to perceived noncontingency. A combination of confusion–self-doubt–discouragement is distinguished from an escape pattern, which includes active attempts to leave the situation, pessimism, and avoidance or procrastination. In a similar vein, this dimensionalization recognizes a characterization of two nonautonomous responses to threats to autonomy: one often referred to as internalizing behavior (perseveration, self-blame, and obsession) and the other as externalizing behavior (aggression, projection, and devaluation).

At the specific level, this dimensionalization also may add something to coping theories: a wider range of positive coping. Most lists of coping categories have only one or two positive modes (usually centered around problem solving and support seeking), whereas they include a much larger variety of negative modes (see Table 1 for examples in the academic domain). The current dimensionalization maintains a one-to-one correspondence between positive and negative modes, and specifically suggests that information seeking, flexible experimentation, cooperation, contact seeking, and negotiation be added to positive ways of coping. The dimensionalization also dispels the impression that behavioral or problem-focused coping is homogeneously positive, whereas emotion-focused coping is usually maladaptive. An equal number of positive and negative behavior and emotion regulation responses are included. Finally, this dimensionalization also explicitly adds an orientation or outlook component to coping. This aspect of coping may become increasingly important as children approach adolescence (Fanshawe & Burnett, 1991).

At the most general level, the motivational dimensionalization implies that many different perspectives can be considered as different facets of coping. It suggests that the different categories of coping may be best considered in relation to each other. For example, it becomes clear that high perceived control is not sufficient to produce optimal coping. Children also need to feel autonomous and related if they are to remain flexible in their responding and to go to adults when they need additional help. And it suggests that whether help seeking has positive or negative consequences may depend on its effects on other forms of coping, for example, whether help seeking interferes with strategizing (e.g., as "delegation") or is used to supplement more independent forms of coping.

It also suggests that a deeper set of dimensions than approach versus avoidance may be needed to detect when different ways of coping will be adaptive or maladaptive. Following the regulation literature (for a review, see Chapter 2, this volume), we suggest that coping will be adaptive to the extent that it is organized (vs. disorganized), flexible (vs. rigid), and benign (vs. punitive). Hence, two ways of "approach coping," such as strategizing versus perseverance, may be shown to be differentially adaptive, because the former is flexible whereas the latter rigid. Or two forms of "avoidance coping," such as escape versus reevaluation, may be differentially adaptive, because the former is disorganized whereas the latter is organized. Finally, two modes of emotion regulation, such as accepting responsibility versus self-blame, may differ in adaptiveness, because the former is benign whereas the latter is punitive.

OUTCOMES IN ACADEMIC COPING

What are the outcomes of children's coping in the academic domain? What are the costs and benefits that can accrue to children based on the way they respond to problems in school? The few studies that pertain to these questions are summarized in Table 2. They are of two types. One set of studies describes the correlates of different ways of coping; the second set examines the differences between preselected groups on their profiles of coping.

Table 2. Outcomes and Correlates of Coping in the Academic Domain

Author	Subjects	Coping and outcome
Causey & Dubow (1992)	4th to 6th grades	Problem solving was positively correlated with perceived control, self-esteem, academic performance. Social support was positively correlated with perceived control. Internalizing was positively correlated with perceived control and anxiety. Externalizing was negatively correlated with perceived control, self-esteem, and academic performance.

(continued)

Table 2. (*Continued*)

Author	Subjects	Coping and outcome
Coleman (1992)	$N = 42M$ 21 gifted IQ LD 21 average IQ LD 6th–9th grade	Gift/LD reported more planful problem solving coping than Avg/LD Avg/LD reported more distancing, escape/avoid, and helplessness coping than gift/LD. No differences between gift/LD and avg/LD in confrontive, self-control, social support, accepting responsibility, and positive reappraisal coping. No differences between gift/LD and avg/LD in total number of coping categories employed.
Connell & Illardi (1987)	$N = 121$	Denial coping and anxiety amplification coping were negatively correlated with teacher reports of cognitive competence and self-esteem. Positive, denial, and anxiety amplification coping are negatively correlated with academic achievement.
Fad & Ryser (1993)	$N = 96$	Academically successful students were rated by teachers as having better coping skills than were academically unsuccessful students.
Illardi & Bridges (1988)	$N = 55$ M; 57 F 4th–6th grade	Subjects did not differ on anxiety amplification or projection. Males who underrate their competence used more denial coping compared to teacher report. Males who overrate their competence used more positive coping compared to teacher report.
Klebanov & Brooks-Gunn (1992)	$N = 126$ F	"Mastery and coping" were significantly related to English and math grades in middle school and to math grades 4 years later.
Mantzicopoulos (1990)	$N = 54$ M; 66 F 4th–6th grade	Academic coping style did not differentiate subjects on behavioral conduct. Subjects with positive coping styles had significantly higher social acceptance and global self-worth scores compared to subjects with defensive or self-blame coping styles. Subjects with positive coping styles had higher scores on scholastic competence than subjects with self-blame coping styles. Subjects with a positive coping style had higher scores on academic achievement tests than subjects with defensive and self-blame coping styles.
Plante & Goldfarb (1993)	$N = 61$ M; 39 F	Coping was positively correlated with verbal/comprehension factor, perceptual/organizational factor, and the freedom from distractibility factor on the WISC-R intelligence test. Coping was significantly correlated with reading achievement, math achievement, and written language scores. Main effects for coping were reported for scores on

Table 2. (*Continued*)

Author	Subjects	Coping and outcome
		the performance factor and the freedom from distractibility factor. An interaction effect for stress and coping was also reported for scores on the achievement test with poor copers who are stressed scoring lower on the Reading measure.
Wade (1981)	$N = 475$ M; 481 F 4th grade	Approach coping subjects performed better on English, math, and reading achievement tests compared to avoidance coping subjects.

For some coping categories, these studies present a consistent picture. First, coping responses that fall into the cluster of "planful problem solving" were generally positive; they were connected with higher perceived control, self-esteem, self-worth, school grades, and achievement test performance. Second, helpless responses (such as confusion and avoidance) and externalizing behaviors (such as venting or aggression) both seemed maladaptive; they were negatively correlated with this same set of variables.

The picture was less clear for social support-seeking and internalizing behaviors (such as anxiety and self-blame). In some studies, support seeking was unrelated to academic outcomes; in others it was positively related, for example, to perceived control. This may reflect a general problem in the literature on academic help seeking (Nelson-LeGall, 1985): Children with low academic competence tend to need help more frequently (producing a negative relation between frequency of help-seeking behavior and academic competence), but children with high academic self-confidence are more likely to actually seek help on the infrequent occasions when they need it (producing a positive relation between help seeking and performance).

The work on internalizing responses to problems in school is likewise unclear. Although it has been found that anxious and self-blaming responses to failure can hinder performance, nevertheless, internalizing responses are sometimes positively linked with academic competence and performance, perhaps because they may reflect the desire to do well in school, generally considered a positive force in performance. When Wade (1981) separated high anxious subjects into those with high versus low achievement motivation, she indeed discovered that subjects who were highly anxious but also highly motivated showed higher levels of attainment (in English, math, and reading) than correspondingly high anxious subjects whose achievement motivation was low. Wade (1981) speculates that these groups may differ on whether they use their anxiety to fuel increased work on difficult subject material (an approach strategy) or to guide escape responses (an avoidance strategy).

Critique of Research

As suggested repeatedly by researchers in this area, studies of the correlates of coping generally suffer from several shortcomings. First and foremost is a general issue, critical to the evaluation of research on the short- and long-term outcomes of different ways of coping: the distinction between ways of coping and consequences of coping. In some studies, externalizing behavior is used as a coping category (sometimes labeled "venting" or "emotional discharge") and in some studies it is an outcome of interest. The same holds for internalizing behaviors, in which self-blame and anxiety have been used as both coping responses and outcomes. And, in our own work, when "strategizing" (attempting to think of alternative solutions for a problem) is the coping response, it seems not too surprising that continued engagement is the short-term outcome.

Empirical solutions to this problem seem straightforward. Researchers should minimize overlap between measures of coping categories and consequences within a study. Or, as we have in our studies, researchers can use higher levels of abstraction (not tied to a single coping response and consequence) and consider the use of alternative reporters (e.g., children for coping and teachers for engagement). Nevertheless, the conceptual solution is not so clear. What criteria should be used to determine whether a set of emotions or behaviors is a coping response or a coping outcome? Fuller discussion of this issue should be useful.

A second important issue is that almost all studies examining "outcomes" of coping are cross-sectional and correlational in nature and so cannot distinguish the nature of the relationships among the variables. These different school "outcomes" may, of course, in fact be antecedents to different ways of coping, or both coping and the "outcomes" may be the product of some other factor. Studies are needed that have a prospective and longitudinal focus (e.g., Klebanov & Brooks-Gunn, 1992) to allow for the disentanglement of antecedents and consequences and for the detection of possible reciprocal relations between coping and school performance.

A Motivational Perspective on the Outcomes of Academic Coping

Consistent with the general coping literatures, we distinguish short-term from long-term outcomes of academic coping. According to the motivational model, the proximal consequences of children's coping in the academic domain are their engagement versus disaffection with learning activities. And the long-term consequences of this engagement versus disaffection for children are their successful completion of school or early dropout, and in the most general terms, their cognitive, social, and personality development (see Fig. 1).

Engagement versus Disaffection

According to the motivational model, children whose coping is organized, flexible, and benign, who when they run into academic difficulties are likely to strategize, seek information, and contact adults for comfort and help, are more likely to maintain active vigorous interactions with academic material. They are likely to be more fully engaged in learning activities. They show more effort, persistence, concentration, interest, and enthusiasm; they ask more questions, try out new activities, prefer difficult tasks, and actively seek novelty and challenge.

In contrast, children whose coping is disorganized, rigid, or punitive, who in the face of obstacles become confused and try to escape, who perseverate, rely on others, become oppositional, or try to conceal their difficulties, are more likely to become disaffected from school. They are more likely to be passive, withdrawn, anxious, depressed, fearful of novelty; they refrain from asking questions or volunteering in class, they prefer easy tasks, shy away from novelty, and avoid challenge.

Children's engagement versus disaffection in school, as assessed by students themselves, their teachers, or school records (such as absenteeism or effort grades), are central predictors of children's learning and school success, as indexed by school grades and achievement test results (e.g., Skinner, Wellborn, & Connell, 1990). In addition, disaffection is one of the earliest predictors of children's declining performance and eventual early leaving from school (Connell et al., 1993).

Development

Active engagement in learning activities that is full, sustained, and goal directed not only leads to better school grades (e.g., Skinner et al., 1990; Skinner, Zimmer-Gembeck, & Connell, 1995), but should also be advantageous to development. Coping with difficulties and setbacks that is organized, flexible, and benign should lead to the development of a repertoire of actual competencies and should augment beliefs about those competencies. It should contribute positively to cognitive development, in the sense both of learning and of metacognition (Hagen, Barclay, & Newman, 1982). Children should not just acquire specific information about the subjects being studied, but should also become better able to monitor their own learning, recognize when they do not understand something, and decide what the best course of action may be: to study harder, review the material, or go for help.

Mechanisms Through Which Coping Has Its Effects

A final issue critical to the study of the consequences of coping is the consideration of whether coping itself is part of the causal chain in adaptive versus maladaptive development, or whether it is simply a symptom of such development. It is conceivable that a child's suboptimal pattern of coping is primarily the result of dysfunctional child relationships and vulnerabilities in self-system processes, but does not itself contribute directly to the development of maladaptive child outcomes.

To answer this question, research may broaden its focus in order to empirically trace the pathways through which children's patterns of coping contribute to their engagement and subsequent development. We suggest three possible pathways. The first is direct, through the effects of a particular pattern of coping on engagement. For example, as previously mentioned, a helpless pattern of coping preempts a child's active struggles with learning activities. The second pathway, also mentioned briefly before, is the indirect effect of a pattern of coping on encounters with future stressors. Children who are coping in ways that do not allow them to currently grasp concepts and strategies (for example, through concealment) are more likely to encounter difficulties and failures in subsequent learning activities that build upon previous material. Therefore, patterns of coping should predict the occurrence of future stress. Third, patterns of coping should have direct effects on the way the social context, that is, parents and teachers, react to the child. Unfortunately, contexts often react to children's coping in ways that magnify or compound the problem (Skinner & Belmont, 1993). For example, children who become oppositional are more likely to be met with arbitrary force from teachers. Children who conceal their difficulties are more likely to be overlooked by parents. Even "benign" reactions by teachers and parents may serve to remove children from interactions with learning activities. For example, in response to a child's distress, parents may help too much and so complete work that is "delegated" by the child. Or, in response to a child's confusion, teachers may reduce task difficulty but also inadvertently reduce opportunities for learning as well. Hence, the third path by which coping influences development is by shaping the reactions of parents and teachers in ways that affect the child's subsequent motivation and learning.

OPTIMIZATION OF ACADEMIC COPING

Given the importance of academic outcomes, and given the reasonable assumption that how children react to failures and setbacks in school can have an impact on their successful achievement of such outcomes, it may seem surprising to discover that very few studies exist that directly target children's profiles of coping in the classroom. To be sure, there is an enormous literature on interventions designed to promote the same long-term outcomes, namely, school performance, achievement, and completion (Ingraham, 1985). In addition, there are many programs designed to ease school transitions (e.g., Jason, Kurrasaki, Neuson, & Garcia, 1993), to help children manage both anxiety (e.g., Krohne & Laux, 1982) and anger (e.g., Nelson, Hart, & Finch, 1993), and to allow children with learning disabilities to perform up to their full potential (e.g., Borkowski, Carr, Rellinger, & Pressley, 1990; Kurtz & Borkowski, 1984). Although it can be suggested that some of the effects of these interventions may be mediated by changes in children's patterns of coping responses, few, if any, of these studies directly examine the impact of these interventions on coping per se.

Intervention Studies

Even a literature search under the term "coping" reveals, for the most part, only intervention studies in which the term is used to refer generally to the process of dealing with problems, but is neither explicitly defined nor assessed (e.g., Lewis, 1984). The lines of intervention most closely related to coping in school often do not use the term explicitly, but instead target a single way of coping. For example, Kamann and Wong (1993) trained learning disabled children to use adaptive coping self-statements, such as assessing the situation and making a plan, recognizing and controlling negative thoughts, and self-reinforcement. Schunk and Hanson (1985) promoted student's self-efficacy and achievement through the use of peers who modeled "coping." These peers demonstrated initial fears and deficiencies, were hesitant, made errors, and verbalized negative self-statements, but gradually performed better, gained self-confidence, and illustrated how "determined effort and positive self-thoughts can overcome difficulties" (Schunk & Hanson, 1985, p. 314).

An intervention covering a range of strategies for managing frustration was designed by Fagen (1984). He defined coping as "reactions which promote *positive* change in self or environment, i.e., change which maintains or increases self-esteem, prospects for more successful striving, or increased understanding between self and others" (p. 30). The intervention targeted responses aimed at changing the self as well as those aimed at changing the environment (see Table 2 for actual categories).

In this area, most intervention studies have had as their goal to facilitate that cluster of coping strategies that includes problem solving, persistence, direct action, self-instruction, self-regulation, and positive self-statements. These coping strategies have been promoted through such means as attribution retraining, self-efficacy modeling, teaching of problem-solving study skills, cognitive behavior modification techniques, instruction in anxiety reduction procedures, or metacognitive skills training. Although some interventions target skills or behaviors and some target self-perceptions or beliefs (and some target both), in general, intervention techniques have in common that they are individually oriented; that is, the child's behavior has been the immediate target of intervention.

Targets of Intervention

Without directly criticizing these intervention efforts, which as mentioned previously do not typically target coping per se, it can nevertheless be argued that two essential issues in this area remain open questions. The first is the optimal profile of reactions to problems in school (as the target goals of intervention efforts). The second issue is the antecedent conditions, both personal and interpersonal, that impede or promote such patterns of coping. Although, ideally efforts to facilitate children's academic coping would be based on empirical answers to these questions, unfortunately this research base is incomplete. We would argue that there is reason to both question the notion that "approach coping" is always the optimal reaction in academic contexts and to rethink the assumption that the best intervention technique to promote coping is direct instruction, that is, teaching or training individual children to show desired patterns of coping.

Optimal Coping in Academic Contexts

Although there is general agreement that it is difficult to establish a priori the kinds of coping that will be adaptive in any given situation (Lazarus & Folkman, 1984; Roth & Cohen, 1986), nevertheless, in general types of coping classified as "approach" have been consistently better predictors of desirable outcomes in school than avoidance strategies (Causey & Dubow, 1992; see Table 2). However, we interpret the general empirical finding that "approach" coping is usually better than "avoidance" coping as somewhat misleading, because in most studies approach coping included responses that were not only active and toward the stressful situation but were also emotionally positive (such as problem solving or negotiation); more negative approach strategies (such as confrontation or aggression) were typically excluded. And most avoidance coping responses studied were not only active and away from the stressor but usually emotionally negative as well (such as anxious or fearful); emotionally positive avoidance responses, such as decisions that the outcome was not worth the effort, have typically not been included (but see Brandtstaedter & Renner, 1990; Brandtstaedter, Wentura, & Greve, 1993; Heckhausen & Schulz, 1995; Rothbaum, Weisz, & Snyder, 1982, for a discussion of the effectiveness of such strategies).

Hence, optimal coping in academic contexts may not simply be approach coping. In addition to problem solving itself, children also need to know how to move away from learning interactions in order to gather more information, to cooperate, to skip to problems that they know how to solve, to conform, or to get help. Both approach and avoidance coping may be important to successful learning, and the hallmarks of optimal coping responses may turn out to be not their orientation, but their organization, flexibility, and benevolence.

Techniques of Intervention

Since the desired outcomes of coping interventions are changes in children's behavioral, emotional, and cognitive reactions to potentially stressful encounters, it has often been assumed that the most effective way to achieve change is by directly teaching children to use these patterns of behavior or self-statements (e.g., Foersterling, 1985). Underlying these practices is the assumption that the primary reason children show maladaptive reactions to stress is because they have a skill deficit or lack knowledge.

However, in studies of the antecedents of coping, two additional factors continue to surface, often labeled as personal and social resources (Garmezy & Rutter, 1983; Moos & Billings, 1982; Pearlin & Schooler, 1978). This perspective assumes that individuals' belief systems (such as their perceived control) as well as their social relationships have an impact on their coping responses in stressful situations. From this perspective, the target(s) of intervention would be expanded to include both children's belief systems and their social partners. This general viewpoint is consistent with our motivational perspective on optimization of coping.

A Motivational Perspective on Intervention

The motivational view of development makes strong predictions about the targets of intervention in attempts to optimize children's coping. The counterforces against environmental stressors and vulnerable self-system processes are interventions designed to reduce actual neglect, chaos, and coercion in schools and at home, and also designed to bolster children's experiences of themselves as related, competent, and autonomous. This position is summarized in Fig. 3. According to the motivational model, children's belief systems are constructed

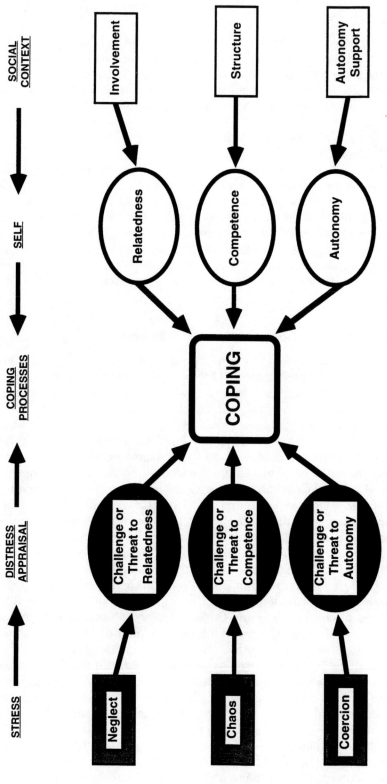

Figure 3. Context and self as coping resources. (Adapted from Skinner & Wellborn, 1994.)

through interactions with the social and physical context, and so it is these interactions or experiences (of relatedness, competence, and autonomy) that are considered to be the prime target of interventions. When these experiences are changed, then resulting changes in children's self-system processes and corresponding coping responses should be obtained. One route by which these interactions can be optimized is by changing the social context of schools (Connell & Ryan, 1984; Connell & Wellborn, 1991; Deci, Connell, & Ryan, 1985; Skinner & Wellborn, 1994).

An additional source of social context for children's schooling is their parents. Although parents rarely participate directly in the school setting itself, their concern for a child's performance in school and their participation in children's schoolwork at home can have a powerful influence on children's coping with problems and setbacks in school (Grolnick & Slowiaczek, 1994; Grolnick, Ryan, & Deci, 1991; Wellborn, 1996; Yoder, 1996). Other participants in the immediate school setting, such as other teachers, principals, bus drivers, and cafeteria workers, may also influence a child's experiences in school (Wellborn, 1991).

Supporting Relatedness, Competence, and Autonomy

What kinds of social contexts can support children's basic needs? First, children's needs for relatedness are met by social contexts that provide involvement. Involvement, a key dimension in theories of parenting and teaching, refers to the communication of warmth, affection, and caring; it includes dedication of time and resources to a child as well as emotional and physical accessibility and availability. When parents and teachers establish warm and trusting relations with their offspring and students, then children will be more likely to feel connected to them and the classroom in general and more able to turn to adults in times of academic difficulty. Interventions to increase communication, belongingness, and genuine affection, for example, by decreasing class size and increasing student–teacher contact, would be expected to result in improvements in students' internal working models of teachers (especially for insecure or alienated students), which would in turn be expected to result in more help-seeking coping on the part of these children.

Second, children have the opportunity to fulfill their need for competence in social contexts that provide structure. Structure, also an important dimension in theories of child rearing and teaching, refers to contingency and consistency; more broadly, it encompasses information provided by social partners about the strategies or routes by which desired outcomes can be reached and undesired outcomes avoided, as well as support for developing the competencies to negotiate these pathways. Structure can be communicated indirectly through rules and norms or taught more directly as strategies for solving academic or interpersonal problems. Provision of structure is central in creating interactions in which students feel able to enact effective strategies. This in turn should prevent them from interpreting failures and setbacks as signs of incompetence, which would allow them to maintain focus, concentration, and active problem solving even in the face of obstacles (Bandura & Schunk, 1981). Curricula and grading systems that allow children to work at their own pace and to continue working on assignments until they have mastered them would be examples of increasing structure. Interventions aimed at teaching teachers and parents how to help children learn and utilize metacognitive strategies (e.g., Borkowski et al., 1990; Kurtz & Borkowski, 1984) and, in general, that focus on the processes and strategies of learning help demystify the steps to mastering new material.

Third, children's needs for self-determination are met in social contexts that provide autonomy support. Autonomy support refers to social partners who allow children the freedom to pursue their own interests and goals, who provide choices and alternatives, who respect the child's rights and wishes, and who acknowledge the child's feelings, even when they are negative (Deci, Schwartz, Sheinman, & Ryan, 1981). Interventions that are designed to increase autonomy support should allow children to experience their interactions with school personnel and materials as more self-determined, which should in turn allow them to react to necessary constraints more cooperatively and to cope in a manner that is more flexible and constructive. Interventions designed to increase children's experience of autonomy include rule systems that are democratically established, in which rules are minimized and their rationales made explicit, curricula in which children are given choices and allowed to follow their interests, and where reward structures are not competitive.

Developmental Windows in Interventions in Coping

It is not the goal of interventions into the academic context to eliminate the "stress" of learning or to create contexts in which children no longer have to "cope." Challenges and obstacles are not only inevitable, they are the building blocks for healthy development. The goal is to prevent children from being overwhelmed by stress, to create optimal challenges, and to help children move through them. "Good stress" and "good coping" are the goals of optimal learning environments (Compas, 1993; Skinner, 1993; Weisz, 1993).

In addition, interventions to optimize involvement, structure, and autonomy support will need to be adapted to children's developmental level (Eccles, Midgley, & Adler, 1984; Haggerty, Sherrod, Garmezy, & Rutter, 1994; Wigfield, Eccles, MacIver, Reuman, & Midgley, 1991; Zeitlin & Williamson, 1994). The kind of parent and teacher behaviors that communicate affection to first graders are obviously not the same behaviors that communicate affection to junior high school students. The metacognitive skills taught to third graders will differ radically from those useful to fifth graders. The choices given to adolescents will be broader than those provided to elementary school children. Also, as children reach adolescence, it may be necessary to change not only their interactions in school, but also to intervene directly into their belief systems. As children's cognitive capacities develop, so too does the scope and inferential power of their self-system processes (e.g., Skinner, 1995). This very development gives children's self-system processes increasing latitude in constructing confirming interpretations of their interactions with the social and physical context. Hence, children's views of school may need to be directly altered, if they are to interpret new interactions as experiences of relatedness, competence, and autonomy.

Development will also inform the timing of interventions. Transition times, such as from kindergarten to first grade, from elementary to middle or junior high school, and from middle school to high school, are obvious points at which interventions designed to optimize coping may influence the success of those transitions (Ingraham, 1985). In addition, several points in cognitive development, specifically third grade, when children begin to form comparative judgments about their academic abilities, and sixth grade, when those perceptions become crystallized, may be important milestones for achieving adaptive transformations in coping. It should not be assumed that single early interventions will be sufficient to "inoculate" children against all future difficulties in school. Both new patterns of coping and new environmental demands emerge. As children develop cognitively, new strategies will be available to them for the first time, such as reframing or focusing on the positive. And the demands of school change as well, as children are asked to deal with increased competition, less individual attention, multiple teacher formats, and more standardized testing.

CONCLUSIONS

Unlike many domains in children's coping, there is no one literature or set of studies examining children's coping in the academic domain. In fact, in many studies of children's reactions to problems in school, no mention of the term "coping" can be found. This makes it impossible to consider any review of the literature in this area as comprehensive or to argue convincingly that any one perspective encompasses all the relevant concepts and empirical referents. However, an attempt was made to use the strengths of a coping framework to build on the few studies that explicitly examine children's academic coping by adding the work on perceived control, helplessness, self-determination, attachment, and help seeking in the classroom. Research was reviewed from the literatures on academic coping and self-perceptions that describe children's experiences of stressors in school, their differential reactions to academic challenges and threats, and the consequences of these ways of coping for school success and satisfaction.

A motivational perspective was used to organize and integrate multiple lines of research that bear on children's coping in school. Using a definition of coping as "action regulation under psychological stress," we derived multiple dimensions of coping (e.g., self vs. context and challenge vs. threat) and from them assembled 36 categories of children's coping in school. It was argued that these patterns included both "syndromes" from the self-perception literature, such as helplessness and rebellion, as well as more specific categories from the coping literature, such as contact seeking and avoidance. This category system included an equal number of positive and negative coping responses, in regulations that were aimed at behavior, emotions, and orientation or outlook.

We argued that these patterns of action have important causal effects on children's learning and development, through their direct effects on engagement and on the reactions of social partners, such as parents and teachers, as well as through their indirect effects on subsequent encounters with more academic stressors. Because these patterns of coping are thought to be a function of children's self-system processes connected to relatedness, competence, and autonomy, intervention implications could be drawn for bolstering these beliefs through interactions with the social and physical environments. Interventions designed to optimize interactions were described that changed the social context by increasing involvement, structure, and autonomy support and by improving children's actions and their interpretations.

Future research on children's coping with stress and challenges in school can take several directions. First, it can consider a broader range of stressful experiences in school. Most research examines how children cope with failure and difficulties in learning new material, situations that the motivational model suggests should impinge on the need for competence. Future work may also wish to analyze how children cope with the pressures and coercion of school rules and practices (which may interfere with the need for autonomy), or how children deal with teachers who are uncaring or even openly hostile (which may impact the need for relatedness).

Second, future studies may wish to consider a broader range of coping responses and especially to focus on the identification of additional positive modes of coping. Especially interesting will be the study of the interaction of different ways of coping as they interfere or supplement each other and as they change over time during the processes of coping. Third, a challenging but important area of research will be the detection of the consequences of different patterns of coping. In these studies, it will be essential to distinguish coping responses from outcomes and to look at their (possible reciprocal) relations over time. Finally, intervention research should be able to reveal much about the individual and social factors that impede or promote positive coping in schools. This research may wish to target teachers, the general school context, and parents, as well as individual children themselves. These studies, if they include multiple ways of coping and a differentiated set of possible consequences, may tell us the most about the complex relations involved in children's coping. It is hoped that this chapter may facilitate discussion among the allied areas in psychology and education that focus on the study of the challenges and stresses children face in school and on intervention attempts to promote children's active efforts to cope with them.

REFERENCES

Ainsworth, M. D. S. (1979). Infant–mother attachment. *American Psychologist, 34*(10), 932–937.

Ainsworth, M. D. S. (1989). Attachment beyond infancy. *American Psychologist, 44*, 709–716.

Alpert-Gillis, L. J., Pedro-Carroll, J. L., & Cowen, E. L. (1989). The Children of Divorce Intervention Program: Development, implementation, and evaluation of a program for young urban children. *Journal of Consulting and Clinical Psychology, 57*, 583–589.

Ames, C., & Ames, R. (1984). *Research on motivation in education: Vol. 1: Student motivation.* San Diego: Academic Press.

Ames, C., & Ames, R. (1985). *Research on motivation in education: Vol. 1. The classroom milieu.* San Diego: Academic Press.

Ayers, T. S., Sandler, I., Bernzweig, J., Harrison, R., Wampler, T., & Lustig, J. (1989). *Handbook for the content analysis of children's coping responses.* Unpublished manuscript, Arizona State University, Tempe.

Baldwin, M. W. (1992). Relational schemas and the processing of social information. *Psychological Bulletin, 112,* 461–484.

Band, E. B., & Weisz, J. R. (1988). How to feel better when it feels bad: Children's perspectives on coping with everyday stress. *Developmental Psychology, 24,* 247–253.

Bandura, A. (1977). Self-efficacy: Toward a unified theory of behavioral change. *Psychological Review, 84,* 191–215.

Bandura, A. (1986). *The social foundations of thought and action: A social cognitive theory.* Englewood Cliffs, NJ: Prentice Hall.

Bandura, A. (1989). Human agency in social cognitive theory. *American Psychologist, 44*(9), 1175–1184.

Bandura, A., & Schunk, D. H. (1981). Cultivating competence, self-efficacy, and intrinsic interest through proximal self-motivation. *Journal of Personality and Social Psychology, 41,* 486–598.

Borkowski, J. G., Carr, M., Rellinger, E., & Pressley, M. (1990). Self-regulated cognition: Interdependence of metacognition, attributions, and self-esteem. In B. Jones & L. Idol (Eds.), *Dimensions of thinking* (pp. 53–92). Hillsdale, NJ: Erlbaum.

Brandtstaedter, J., & Renner, G. (1990). Tenacious goal pursuit and flexible goal adjustment: Explication and age-related analysis of assimilative and accommodative strategies of coping. *Psychology and Aging, 5*(1), 58–67.

Brandtstaedter, J., Wentura, D., & Greve, W. (1993). Adaptive resources of the aging self: Outlines of an emergent perspective. *International Journal of Behavioral Development, 16*(2), 323–349.

Bretherton, I. (1985). Attachment theory: Retrospect and prospect. In I. Bretherton & E. Waters (Eds.), *Growing points of attachment theory and research. Monographs for the Society for Research in Child Development, 50* (Serial No. 209), pp. 3–35.

Cassidy, J. (1988). Child–mother interaction and the self in six-year-olds. *Child Development, 59,* 121–134.

Causey, D. L., & Dubow, E. F. (1992). Development of a self-report measure for elementary school children. *Journal of Clinical Child Psychology, 21*(1), 47–59.

Coleman, M. R. (1992). A comparison of how gifted/LD and average/LD boys cope with school frustration. *Journal for the Education of the Gifted, 15*(3), 239–265.

Compas, B. (1993, April). *An analysis of "good" stress and coping in adolescence.* Paper presented at the 60th meeting of the Society for Research in Child Development, New Orleans, LA.

Compas, B. E. (1987). Coping with stress during childhood and adolescence. *Psychological Bulletin, 101,* 393–403.

Compas, B. E., Banez, G. A., Malcarne, V., & Worsham, N. (1991). Perceived control and coping with stress: A developmental perspective. *Journal of social Issues, 47*(4), 23–34.

Compas, B. E., Malcarne, V. L., & Fondacaro, K. M. (1988). Coping with stressful events in older children and young adolescents. *Journal of Counseling and Clinical Psychology, 56,* 405–411.

Connell, J. P. (1990). Context, self, and action: A motivational analysis of self-system processes across the life-span. In D. Cicchetti & M. Beeghly (Eds.), *The self in transition: From infancy to childhood* (pp. 61–97). Chicago: University of Chicago Press.

Connell, J. P., & Illardi, B. C. (1987). Self-system concomitants of discrepancies between children's and teachers' evaluation of academic competence. *Child Development, 58,* 1297–1307.

Connell, J. P., & Ryan, R. M. (1984). A developmental theory of motivation in the classroom. *Teacher Education Quarterly, 11,* 64–77.

Connell, J. P., & Wellborn, J. G. (1991). Competence, autonomy and relatedness: A motivational analysis of self-system processes. In M. Gunnar & L. A. Sroufe (Eds.), *Minnesota Symposium on Child Psychology* (Vol. 23, pp. 43–77). Chicago: University of Chicago Press.

Crittendon, P. M. (1990). Internal representational models of attachment relationships. *Infant Mental Health Journal, 11,* 259–277.

DeCharms, R. (1968). *Personal causation.* New York: Academic Press.

Deci, E. L., Connell, J. P., & Ryan, R. M. (1985). A motivational analysis of self-determination and self-regulation in the classroom. In C. Ames & R. Ames (Eds.), *Research on motivational analysis of self-determination and self-regulation in the classroom* (pp. 13–52). San Diego: Academic Press.

Deci, E. L., & Ryan, R. M. (1985). *Intrinsic motivation and self-determination in human behavior.* New York: Plenum Press.

Deci, E. L., Schwartz, A. J., Sheinman, L., & Ryan, R. (1981). An instrument to assess adults orientations toward control versus autonomy with children: Reactions on intrinsic motivation and perceived competence. *Journal of Educational Psychology, 73*, 642–650.

Dickey, J. P., & Henderson, P. (1989, February/March). What young children say about stress and coping in school. *Health Education*, 14–17.

Dryfoos, J. G. (1990). *Adolescents at risk. Prevalence and prevention.* New York: Oxford University Press.

Dweck, C. S. (1991). Self-theories and goals: Their role in motivation, personality, and development. In R. a. Dienstbier (Ed.), *Nebraska Symposium on Motivation.* Lincoln: University of Nebraska Press.

Dweck, C. S., & Elliott, E. S. (1983). Achievement motivation. In P. H. Mussen (Series Ed.) & E. M. Hetherington (Vol. Ed.), *Handbook of child psychology: Vol. IV: Socialization, personality, and social development* (pp. 643–691). New York: Wiley.

Dweck, C. S., & Leggett, E. L. (1988). A social–cognitive approach to motivation and personality. *Psychological Review, 95*, 256–273.

Dweck, C. S., & Wortman, C. B. (1982). Learned helplessness, anxiety, and achievement motivation: Neglected parallels in cognitive, affective, and coping responses. In H. W. Krohne & L. Laux (Eds.), *Achievement, stress, and anxiety* (pp. 93–115). New York: Hemisphere Publishing.

Ebata, A. T., & Moos, R. H. (1991, April). *Coping and adjustment in distressed and healthy adolescents. Journal of Applied Developmental Psychology, 12*, 33–54.

Eccles, J. S., Midgley, A., & Adler, T. (1984). Grade-related changes in the school environment: Effects on achievement motivation. In J. G. Nicholls (Ed.), *The development of achievement motivation* (Vol. 3, pp. 283–331). Greenwich, CT: JAI.

Edge, C., & Skinner, E. A. (1997, April). *Coping, control, and the development of children's engagement in school.* Poster presented at the Biennial Meetings of the Society for Research in Child Development, Washington, D.C.

Fad, K. S., & Ryser, G. R. (1993). Social/behavioral variables related to success in general education. *Remedial and Special Education, 14*(1), 25–35.

Fagen, S. A. (1984). Integrating frustration management into the language arts/reading curriculum. *The Pointer, 28*(4), 29–32.

Fanshawe, J. P., & Burnett, P. C. (1991). Assessing school-related stressors and coping mechanisms in adolescents. *British Journal of Educational Psychology, 61*, 92–98.

Foersterling, F. (1985). Attributional retraining: A review. *Psychological Bulletin, 98*, 495–512.

Folkman, S. (1984). Personal control and stress and coping processes: A theoretical analysis. *Journal of Personality and Social Psychology, 46*(4), 839–852.

Fox, N. (Ed.). (1994). The development of emotion regulation: Biological and behavioral considerations. *Monographs of the Society for Research in Child Development, 59*(2–3, Serial No. 240).

Garmezy, N. (1983). Stressors of childhood. In N. Garmezy & M. Rutter (Eds.), *Stress, coping and development in children* (pp. 43–84). New York: McGraw-Hill.

Garmezy, N., & Rutter, M. (Eds.). (1983). *Stress, coping and development in children.* New York: McGraw-Hill.

Grolnick, W. S., & Ryan, R. M. (1989). Parent styles associated with children's self-regulation and competence: A social contextual perspective. *Journal of Educational Psychology, 81*, 143–154.

Grolnick, W. S., Ryan, R. M., & Deci, E. L. (1991). Inner resources for school achievement: Motivational mediators of children's perceptions of their parents. *Journal of Educational Psychology, 83*, 508–517.

Grolnick, W. S., & Slowiaczek, M. L. (1994). Parent's involvement in children's schooling: A multidimensional conceptualization and motivational model. *Child Development, 65*, 237–252.

Hagen, J. W., Barclay, C. R., & Newman, R. S. (1982). Metacognition, self-knowledge, and learning disabilities: Some thoughts on knowing and doing. *Topics in Learning and Learning Disabilities*, April, 19–25.

Haggerty, R., Sherrod, L., Garmezy, N., & Rutter, M. (1994). *Stress, risk, and resilience in children and adolescents.* New York: Cambridge University Press.

Hamack, F. M. (1986). Large school systems; drop-out reports: An analysis of definitions, procedures, and findings. *Teacher's College Record, 87*(3), 324–341.

Harter, S. (1978). Effectance motivation reconsidered: Toward a developmental model. *Human Development, 21*, 36–64.

Harter, S. (1983). Developmental perspectives on the self system. In E. M. Hetherington (Ed.), *Handbook of child psychology: Socialization, personality, and social development* (pp. 275–385). New York: Wiley.

Heckhausen, J., & Schulz, R. (1995). A life-span theory of control. *Psychological Review, 102,* 284–304.

Illardi, B. C., & Bridges, L. J. (1988). Gender differences in self-system processes as rated by teachers and students. *Sex Roles, 18,* 333–343.

Ingraham, C. I. (1985). Cognitive–affective dynamics of crisis intervention for school entry, school transition, and school failure. *School Psychology Reports, 14,* 266–279.

Jason, L. A., Kurrasaki, K., Neuson, L., & Garcia, C. (1993). Training parents in a preventive intervention for transfer children. *The Journal of Primary Prevention, 13,* 213–227.

Kamann, M. P., & Wong, B. Y. L. (1993). Inducing adaptive coping self-statements in children with learning disabilities through self-instruction training. *Journal of Learning Disabilities, 26,* 630–638.

Klebanov, P. M., & Brooks-Gunn, J. (1992). Impact of maternal attitudes, girl's adjustment, and cognitive skills upon academic performance in middle and high school. *Journal of Research on Adolescence, 2*(1), 81–102.

Kliewer, W. (1991). Coping in middle childhood: Relations to competence, type A behavior, monitoring, blunting, and locus of control. *Developmental Psychology, 27,* 689–697.

Knapp, L. G., Stark, L. J., Kurkjian, J. A., & Spirito, A. (1991). Assessing coping in children and adolescents: Research and practice. *Educational Psychology Review, 3*(4), 309–333.

Kopp, C. (1982). Antecedents of self-regulation: A developmental perspective. *Developmental Psychology, 18*(2), 199–214.

Krohne, H. W., & Laux, L. (1982). *Achievement, stress, and anxiety.* New York: Hemisphere Publishing.

Kurtz, B. E., & Borkowski, J. G. (1984). Children's metacognition: Exploring relations between knowledge, process, and motivational variables. *Journal of Experimental Child Psychology, 37,* 335–354.

Lazarus, R. S., & Folkman, S. (1984). *Stress, appraisal, and coping.* New York: Springer.

Levin, H. M. (1986). *Educational reform for disadvantaged students.* Washington, DC: National Education Associates.

Lewis, H. W. (1984). A structured group counseling program for reading disabled elementary students. *The School Counselor, May,* 454–459.

Lynch, M., & Cicchetti, D. (1992). Maltreated children's reports of relatedness to their teachers. *New Directions for Child Development,* 81–107.

Mantzicopoulos, P. (1990). Coping with school failure: Characteristics of students employing successful and unsuccessful coping strategies. *Psychology in Schools, 27,* 138–143.

Mellor-Crummey, C. A., Connell, J. P., & Trachtenberg, S. (1989, April). *Children's coping in social situations.* Paper presented at the Biennial Meetings of the Society for Research in Child Development, Kansas City, MI.

Miller, S., & Green, M. L. (1990). Coping with stress and frustration: Origins, nature, and development: Origins, nature, and development. In M. Lewis & C. Saarni (Eds.), *The socialization of emotions* (pp. 263–314). New York: Plenum Press.

Mischel, H. N., & Mischel, W. (1983). The development of children's knowledge of self-control strategies. *Child Development, 54,* 603–619.

Moos, R. H., & Billings, A, G. (1982). Conceptualizing and measuring coping resources and coping processes. In L. Goldberger & S. Breznitz (Eds.), *Handbook of stress: Theoretical and clinical aspects* (pp. 212–230). New York: Free Press.

Nelson, W. M., Hart, K. J., & Finch, A. J. (1993). Anger in children: A cognitive–behavioral view of the assessment–therapy connection. *Journal of Rational–Emotive and Cognitive-Behavior Therapy, 11,* 135–150.

Nelson-LeGall, S. (1985). Help-seeking behavior in learning. In E. W. Gordon (Ed.), *Review of research in education* (Vol. 12, pp. 55–90). Washington, DC: American Educational Research Association.

Newman, R. (1990). Children's help-seeking in the classroom: The role of motivational factors and attitudes. *Journal of Educational Psychology, 82,* 71–80.

Pearlin, L. I., & Schooler, C. (1978). The structure of coping. *Journal of Health and Social Behavior, 19,* 2–21.

Plante, T. G., & Goldfarb, L. P. (1993). Are stress and coping associated with aptitude and achievement testing among children? A preliminary investigation. *Journal of School Psychology, 31,* 259–266.

Roth, S. & Cohen, L. (1986). Approach, avoidance, and coping with stress. *American Psychologist, 41,* 813–819.

Rothbaum, F., Weisz, J. R., & Snyder, S. S. (1982). Changing the world and changing the self: A two-process model of perceived control. *Journal of Personality and Social Psychology, 42*(1), 5–37.

Rumberger, R. W. (1987). High school dropouts: A review of issues and evidence. *Review of Educational Research, 57,* 101–121.

Rush, S., & Vitale, P. A. (1994). Analysis for determining factors that place elementary students at risk. *Journal of Educational Research, 87,* 325–333.

Rutter, M. (1983). Stress, coping and development: Some issues and some questions. In N. Garmezy & M. Rutter (Eds.), *Stress, coping and development in children* (pp. 1–41). New York: McGraw-Hill.

Rutter, M. (1989). Pathways from childhood to adult life. *Journal of Child Psychology, 30*(1), 23–51.

Ryan, R. M. (1982). Control and information in the intrapersonal sphere: An extension of cognitive evaluation theory. *Journal of Personality and Social Psychology, 43,* 450–461.

Ryan, R. M., & Connell, P. (1989). Perceived locus of causality and internalization: Examining reasons for acting in two domains. *Journal of Personality and Social Psychology, 57,* 749–761.

Ryan, R. M., & Grolnick, W. S. (1986). Origins and pawns in the classroom: Self-report and projective assessments of individual differences in children's perception. *Journal of Personality and Social Psychology, 50,* 550–558.

Schunk, D. H. (1984). Self-efficacy perspective on achievement behavior. *Educational Psychologist, 9,* 48–58.

Schunk, D. H., & Hanson, A. R. (1985). Peer models: influence on children's self-efficacy and achievement. *Journal of Educational Psychology, 77,* 313–322.

Skinner, E. A. (chair). (1993, March). *The search for "good" stress and coping: An analysis of developmentally adaptive stress and coping across the lifespan.* Symposium presented at the biennial Meetings of the Society for Research in Child Development, New Orleans, LA.

Skinner, E. A. (1995). *Motivation, coping and control.* Newbury, CA: Sage.

Skinner, E. A. (1996). A guide to constructs of control. *Journal of Personality and Social Psychology, 71,* 549–570.

Skinner, E. A., Altman, J., & Sherwood, H. (1991a, July). *An analysis of open-ended interviews of children's coping in the domains of academics and friendship.* Paper presented at the biennial meetings of the International Society for the Study of Behavioral Development, Minneapolis, MN.

Skinner, E. A., Altman, J., & Sherwood, H. (1991b). *Coding manual for children's coping in the domains of school and friendship.* Technical report, University of Rochester, New York.

Skinner, E. A., Altman, J., & Sherwood, H. (1993). *An analysis of open-ended interviews of children's coping in the domains of academics and friendship.* Unpublished manuscript.

Skinner, E. A., Altman, J., Edge, K., Sherwood, H., Yoder, R., & Grossmann, S. J. (1997). *A catalog of coping categories.* In preparation.

Skinner, E. A., & Belmont, M. J. (1993). Motivation in the classroom: Reciprocal effects of teacher behavior and student engagement across the school year. *Journal of Educational Psychology, 85,* 571–581.

Skinner, E. A., & Wellborn, J. G. (1992). *Children's coping in the academic domain.* Technical report, University of Rochester, New York.

Skinner, E. A., & Wellborn, J. G. (1994). Coping during childhood and adolescence: A motivational perspective. In D. Featherman, R. Lerner, & M. Perlmutter (Eds.), *Life-span development and behavior* (pp. 91–133). Hillsdale, NJ: Erlbaum.

Skinner, E. A., Wellborn, J. G., & Connell, J. P. (1990). What it takes to do well in school and whether I've got it: The role of perceived control in children's engagement and school achievement. *Journal of Educational Psychology, 82,* 22–32.

Skinner, E. A., Zimmer-Gembeck, M., & Connell, J. (1995, March). *Individual trajectories of perceived control from third to seventh grade: Relations to children's engagement vs. disaffection.* Poster presented at the meetings of the Society for Research in Child Development, Indianapolis, IN.

Special section. (1990). *Journal of Educational Psychology, 82.*

Spirito, A., Stark, L. J., Grace, N., & Stamoulis, D. (1991). Common problems and coping strategies reported in childhood and early adolescence. *Journal of Youth and Adolescence, 20*(5), 531–544.

Stark, L. J., Spirito, A., Williams, C. A., & Guevremont, D. C. (1989). Common problems and coping strategies I. Findings with normal adolescents. *Journal of Abnormal Child Psychology, 17,* 203–212.

Stipek, D., Recchia, S., & McClintic, S. (1992). Self-evaluation in young children. *Monographs of the Society for Research in Child Development, 57*(1, Serial No. 226).

Tero, P. F., & Connell, J. P. (1984, April). *When children think they've failed: An academic coping inventory.* Paper presented at the American Educational Research Association, New Orleans, LA.

Timberlake, E. M., Barnett, L. B., & Plionis, L. B. (1993). Coping with self and academic talent. *Child and Adolescent Social Work Journal, 10.*

United States Department of Education. (1985). *Secretary priorities and concerns for the Department of Education during fiscal year 1986.* Washington, DC: United States Department of Education.

Wade, B. E. (1981). Highly anxious pupils in formal and informal primary classrooms: The relationship between inferred coping strategies and cognitive attainment. *British Journal of Educational Psychology, 51,* 39–49.

Weiner, B. (1979). A theory of motivation for some classroom experiences. *Journal of Educational Psychology, 71,* 3–25.

Weiner, B. (1985). An attributional theory of achievement motivation and emotion. *Psychological Review, 92,* 548–573.

Weiner, B. (1986). *An attributional theory of motivation and emotion.* New York: Springer-Verlag.

Weisz, J. (1993, April). *An analysis of "good" stress and coping in middle childhood.* Paper presented at the 60th meeting of the Society for Research in Child Development, New Orleans, LA.

Weisz, J. R. (1986). Understanding the developing understanding of control. In M. Perlmutter (Ed.), *social cognition: Minnesota Symposium on Child Psychology* (Vol. 18, pp. 219–278). Hillsdale, NJ: Erlbaum.

Wellborn, J. G. (1991). *Engaged and disaffected action: The conceptualization and measurement of motivation in the academic domain.* Unpublished doctoral dissertation, University of Rochester, New York.

Wellborn, J. G. (1996). *Parents as sources of support: A motivational perspective on parental social support and academic coping in early adolescence.* Unpublished manuscript, Vanderbilt University, Nashville.

Wellborn, J. G., Mellor-Crummey, C. A., Connell, J. P., & Skinner, E. A. (1990, August). *A motivational perspective on children's coping in the academic and social domains.* Paper presented at the American Psychological Association, New Orleans, LA.

White, R. W. (1959). Motivation reconsidered: The concept of competence. *Psychological Review, 66,* 297–333.

Wigfield, A., Eccles, J. S., MacIver, D., Reuman, D. A., & Midgley, C. (1991). Transitions during early adolescence: Changes in children's domain-specific self-perceptions and general self-esteem across the transition to junior high school. *Developmental Psychology, 27*(4), 552–565.

Work, W. C., Levinson, H. R., & Hightower, A. D. (1987). *What I usually do: A measure of elementary children's coping strategies.* Unpublished manuscript, University of Rochester, Center for Community Study, Rochester, NY.

Yoder, R. W. (1996). *The effects of parent involvement, structure, and autonomy support on children's help-seeking and problem-solving coping in school.* Unpublished master's thesis. Portland State University, Portland, OR.

Zeitlin, S., & Williamson, G. (1994). *Coping in young children: Early intervention practices to enhance adaptive behavior and resilience.* Baltimore: Brookes.

15

Coping with Childhood Peer Rejection

AUDREY ZAKRISKI, MARLENE JACOBS, and JOHN COIE

Childhood peer rejection has received a great deal of attention in developmental psychopathology and intervention research over the past 10 years. Interest in this phenomenon stems from evidence that childhood peer rejection is related to a variety of negative outcomes in adolescence and adulthood (Kupersmidt, Coie, & Dodge, 1990; Parker & Asher, 1987). Although we have a good understanding of both the outcomes of childhood peer rejection as well as the behaviors that lead children to be rejected by their peers (Coie, Dodge, & Kupersmidt, 1990), much less attention has been focused on the experience of childhood peer rejection and how children cope with being rejected by their peers. We know that rejected children in general are subjected to more aversive interpersonal interactions in school than nonrejected children (Boivin, Cote, & Dion, 1991; Perry, Kusel, & Perry, 1989), and we know that at least some rejected children report experiencing significant amounts of distress with regard to their low peer status (Asher, Hymel, & Renshaw, 1984; Asher, Parkhurst, Hymel, & Williams, 1990; Asher & Wheeler, 1985; Parkhurst & Asher, 1992). Thus, the experience of peer rejection appears to be a stressful one; however, there are currently no studies in the literature that conceptualize peer rejection in a stress and coping framework. There are probably several reasons for this.

First, the early phases of research on peer relations have necessarily been focused on defining peer rejection (Newcomb & Bukowski, 1983; Coie, Dodge, & Coppotelli, 1982), understanding the correlates and precursors of peer rejec-

AUDREY ZAKRISKI • E. P. Bradley Hospital, Brown University School of Medicine, East Providence, Rhode Island 02916.   **MARLENE JACOBS and JOHN COIE** • Department of Psychology, Duke University, Durham, North Carolina 27708.

Handbook of Children's Coping: Linking Theory and Intervention, edited by Wolchik and Sandler. Plenum Press, New York, 1997.

tion (Coie et al., 1990), and understanding the negative outcomes associated with peer rejection (Kupersmidt et al., 1990; Parker & Asher, 1987). Now that this preliminary research has accumulated, it will be possible to focus more on process variables associated with peer rejection, such as how children cope with peer rejection and how coping strategies may be linked to the outcomes of peer rejection.

The second reason is less practical and more theoretical. The stressor of peer rejection is unlike other stressors traditionally discussed in the stress and coping literature (e.g., having one's parents divorce or undergoing aversive medical procedures) in that it has been conceptualized in the literature as being largely brought about by the disliked child rather than as an external phenomenon that impinges on the child's daily life. That is, the stressor of peer rejection is thought to primarily occur because of socially unacceptable behavior on the part of the child experiencing the stressor (Coie et al., 1990; Coie & Kupersmidt, 1983; Dodge, 1983; Putallaz & Gottman, 1981). The general feeling has been that rejected children are the "architects of their own difficulties" (Ladd, 1985, p. 243).

Conceptualizing peer rejection in a stress and coping framework could help move the field from the focus on description and prediction that has dominated research on peer rejection to an understanding of the process of adjustment to peer rejection and to more successful intervention efforts with rejected children. Such a framework would also shift the focus of theory off the individual child and onto the child in social context. That is, to understand the stresses of peer rejection and how children cope with them, we need to adopt a transactional framework for understanding the phenomenon of childhood peer rejection, including the aversive attitudes, behaviors, or characteristics of the rejected child, the peer group's reactions to those qualities, the rejected child's appraisals of the peer group's reactions, coping efforts of the rejected child, and the peer group's reactions to those coping efforts.

Considered in this transactional framework, peer rejection is not viewed as a child characteristic but as a social outcome arising out of transactions between individual children and their relevant peer groups (Coie, 1990). Social status, in general, and peer rejection, in particular, are shared evaluations of a child by a substantial number of members of his or her peer group. The evaluation often is influenced by nonbehavioral factors such as appearance or minority status, but behavior usually is the dominant factor in determining children's evaluations of one another. Some behaviors, such as aggression, are highly predictive of rejection by peers; but rejection, like other evaluations, is made in the context of peer group norms for behavior. So, for example, for some groups, aggression violates the peer group's norms and is related to rejection, whereas for others it is not considered as deviant and is not related to rejection (Wright, Giammarino, & Parad, 1986).

Social rejection is a response of individual children to other individual children, but it also can have group implications as members of the group share their evaluations explicitly and indirectly with one another. These shared negative evaluations probably contribute to the finding that peers treat rejected children less well than they do other children. These are the observable or objective consequences of peer rejection. Not all rejected children receive the same negative treatment from peers, however. There is some evidence that aggressive children who are rejected do not receive as much overt exclusions or abuse from peers as do those who are not aggressive or intimidating. The latter are often victimized by peers. Rejected children perceive the reactions of peers through lenses of varying degrees of clarity; thus, the subjective consequences of rejection do not always bear a direct relation to the objective consequences. A child's awareness of his or her rejected status can lead to important changes in that child. These changes may involve altered self-concepts and emotional states, as well as changes in behavior toward peers. Sometimes the changes in behavior with familiar peers are adaptive and lead to improved status, and in other cases the changes may lead to increased stigmatization and isolation. The nature of these changes in behavior may depend on the emotions evoked and the attributions made about the causes of rejection, as well as the degree of recognition of peer rejection.

In this chapter, we will review the literature on childhood peer rejection and its consequences. We will focus on two types of rejected children—aggressive and nonaggressive—and on evidence that suggests different risk trajectories for these two groups (Rubin, LeMare, & Lollis, 1990). We will next discuss childhood peer rejection from a stress and coping perspective in order to help us better understand the link between the different types of peer rejection and their consequences. This discussion will focus specifically on the different experiences of aggressive– and nonaggressive–rejected children, as recent evidence suggests that these two groups experience peer rejection differently and are likely to have different styles of coping with the stress they experience. We will discuss what is known about developmental trajectories for aggressive– rejected and nonaggressive–rejected children. Finally, we will discuss interventions that have been designed to help children overcome peer rejection and how their reliance on the individual child–skills deficit model of peer rejection has limited their success.

DEFINING PEER REJECTION

Most risk studies of peer rejection use a variation of the method outlined in Coie et al. (1982), which involves dividing children into sociometric status groups based on how strongly they are liked and disliked by the peers in their classroom. Strength of liking and disliking is determined by peer nominations on the items, "Who do you like the most?" and "Who do you like the least?" or by peer ratings on items such as, "How much do you like to play with this person?" or by a combination of both procedures (Asher & Dodge, 1986). Rejected children are strongly disliked by peers. Cutoff points for defining the rejected group are typically set at one standard deviation below the mean for social preference (like most–like least), below the mean for like most, and above the mean for like least. Typically then, less than 15% of all children are identified as experiencing peer rejection.

Aggressive versus Nonaggressive Rejection

Although the three variables that most reliably distinguish rejected from nonrejected children are aggressive, disruptive, and off-task behaviors in the classroom (Coie & Koeppl, 1990), no more than half of all socially rejected children have been observed to be highly aggressive (Coie, 1985; French, 1988). Some have suggested that there are multiple subgroups of rejected children (Cillessen, van IJzendoorn, van Leishout, & Hartup, 1992), but most recent empirical investigations have focused on only two subgroups (Boivin & Begin, 1989; French, 1988).

Whereas one subgroup is clearly aggressive (Coie & Koeppl, 1990), the defining behavioral characteristics of the other group are less clear. Empirically, they have been shown to be significantly less aggressive than both aggressive–rejected and popular children (French, 1988). There is also some evidence that they are more withdrawn (Cillessen, van IJzendoorn, et al., 1992; French, 1988); however, withdrawal is not restricted to the nonaggressive subgroup. Some researchers have attempted to isolate a more homogeneous group from this larger group of nonaggressive–rejected children by selecting children who are high on timidity (Williams & Asher, 1987), withdrawal (Boivin, Thomassin, & Alain, 1988; Cillessen, van IJzendoorn, et al., 1992; French, 1988), or submissiveness (Parkhurst & Asher, 1992). However, others have found that nonaggressive–rejected children share certain beliefs about their peer rejection experiences, suggesting that it may be useful to consider them as one group (Patterson, Kupersmidt, & Griesler, 1990; Zakriski & Coie, 1996).

CONSEQUENCES OF PEER REJECTION

Current interest in peer rejection as a precursor of psychopathology developed from a set of frequently cited studies published in the 1960s and early 1970s (Cowen, Pederson, Babigian, Izzo, & Trost, 1973; Roff, 1960, 1961; Roff, Sells, & Golden, 1972). These studies suggested a relationship between childhood peer relationship problems and poor adjustment in later life. Numerous subsequent studies, with varying degrees of methodological rigor by today's standards, have supported the basic connection between poor peer relations and later adjustment problems. Throughout the 1970s and 1980s, evidence emerged for specific links between peer rejection and criminality, poor school adjustment, school dropout, and other nonspecific mental health problems. These early peer rejection studies have been reviewed by Parker and Asher (1987) and Kupersmidt et al. (1990).

In their review, Parker and Asher (1987) included peer acceptance, aggression, and withdrawal as predictor variables and examined their influence on multiple outcome variables including school dropout, criminality, and adult psychopathology. They concluded that the evidence is strongest for a predictive relationship between peer rejection and school dropout. In addition, they pointed to substantial support for a predictive relationship between peer rejection and criminality. This relationship was less clear-cut, however, given that criminality was even more strongly predicted by childhood aggression and that aggression and rejection are correlated significantly. Finally, they reported that conclusions about the relationship between peer rejection and subsequent psychopathology were limited by methodological problems with studies assessing this outcome, namely their reliance on clinical samples, use of follow-back research designs, and failure to differentiate among specific types of mental health outcomes.

At the time of the Parker and Asher (1987) review, little was known about the separate influences of childhood rejection and aggression on subsequent adjustment. Correlations between these two variables range from .30 to .49, depending on the source of information and the type of aggression (Coie et al., 1990). This fact has led some researchers to hypothesize that only one of them plays a true casual role in the development of antisocial behavior. Parker and Asher (1987) proposed that rejection might act as a "marker" variable for psychopathological processes rather than a casual factor in the process of developing disorder. According to this hypothesis, poor peer status merely reflects social disapproval for the kinds of aggressive behavior that will be labeled as disordered if they continue in later life. Other researchers have suggested that peer rejection stands on its own as a determinant of subsequent disorder, with effects that are separate and independent from those of aggression. In order to tease apart the separate influences of rejection and aggression, more recent studies have included both variables in their predictive models.

Kupersmidt et al. (1990) considered a few studies in which the relative contributions of rejection and aggression were tested. They concluded that peer rejection in elementary school is related to poor school adjustment, school dropout, and delinquent behavior. More specifically, however, they concluded that peer rejection plays a predictive role above and beyond that of aggression in the development of these poor outcomes. Since this review, several new studies have yielded information about the independent predictive nature of early peer rejection. The size of this effect and its clinical significance is illustrated in the following studies.

Coie, Lochman, Terry, and Hyman (1992) followed two large cohorts of third graders into early adolescence. Sociometric data on status and peer-rated aggressive behavior were collected in the third grade. Following the transition to middle school, a representative sample of children were subsequently assessed for evidence of both internalizing and externalizing problems. Taken as a whole, results from this study support the theory that both aggression and rejected status make significant and independent contributions to the prediction of adolescent maladjustment, including psychological disorder, delinquency, substance abuse, and school problems. Using a combined measure of poor adjustment from teacher, parent, and self-report, 62% of rejected–aggressive children exhibited adjustment problems in early adolescence as compared to 40% of nonrejected–aggressive children, 34% of rejected–nonaggressive children, and 18% of nonrejected–nonaggressive children. These figures provided strong support for the additive effects of rejection and aggression in predicting subsequent disorder.

The relative contributions of each factor varied as a function of outcome, however, such that aggression appeared to be the most consistent predictor of externalizing problems across informants, whereas peer rejection appeared to be the most consistent predictor of internalizing problems across informants. The full predictive model of aggression and peer rejection predicted negative outcomes best when the child was the reporter of internalizing problems and the parent was the reporter of externalizing problems. This may prove to be the most useful model because it uses the most accurate sources of information about the two major bands of psychopathology in children (Loeber, Green, & Lahey, 1990; Routh, 1990).

In a follow-up study, the same representative samples were evaluated at two subsequent time points (8th and 10th grade) in order to study the influence of childhood rejection and aggression on the continuity of psychopathology over time (Coie, Terry, Lochman, Lenox, & Hyman, 1995). Once again, results varied as a function of reporting source. According to self-report outcome measures, rejected–aggressive boys showed a pattern of increasing symptomatology (both internalizing and externalizing) as compared to all other boys. Parents of rejected boys reported higher adolescent levels of both externalizing and internalizing symptoms than parents of nonrejected boys. For girls, aggression was a stronger predictor for self-reported externalizing symptoms, while rejection was a stronger predictor for parent-reported externalizing symptoms. Both aggression and rejection predicted parent-rated internalizing symptoms, while neither variable was significant in the prediction of self-reported internalizing symptoms. Thus, it appears that rejected–aggressive boys have the poorest adjustment in adolescence, regardless of sources or type of disorder. For girls, the relationship is more source and symptom specific, resulting in a more complex picture. Nevertheless, both aggression and rejection seem not only to be significant predictors of early adolescent disorder, but seem to be predictive of continued high levels of disorder across the adolescent years.

Lochman and Wayland (1994) also found specific outcome differences between aggressive–rejected children and nonaggressive–rejected children. They followed boys from fourth, fifth, and sixth grade for 5 years and assessed both self-rated and other-rated (observer, teacher, and peer reports) psychopathology. Multiple regression analyses indicated that both rejection and aggression were predictive of externalizing disorder, regardless of source. This finding is consistent with the general conclusion of the Coie et al. (1992) study. Peer rejection did not predict substance abuse when aggression was included in the predictive model. This suggests that the role of peer rejection in the development of substance abuse may be incidental. Finally, in this study self-reported internalizing problems were predicted by both aggression and rejection for African-American boys, but were predicted by rejection only for Caucasian boys. Initial peer rejection was also predictive of subsequent low self-esteem for Caucasian boys, but not for African-American boys. These results suggest that rejection and aggression may operate differently across ethnic groups in a mixed-ethnicity population when predicting to self-reported psychopathology. Similar conclusions were reached in a study by Kupersmidt and Coie (1985). At this point, it is unclear whether the discrepancies can be linked to methodological considerations such as racial bias in sociometric judgments or whether they represent true differences in the phenomena under investigation.

Taken together, the research on peer relations suggests a strong link between childhood rejection and serious negative outcomes including general mental health problems, externalizing symptoms, internalizing symptoms, poor school adjustment and school dropout. Although specificity of outcomes (internalizing and externalizing) and sources of report (self vs. parent vs. teacher) render the findings more complicated, data addressing the joint contributions of rejection and aggression suggest more negative overall outcomes for children who have both problems. Thus, children who experience the stress of peer rejection and are aggressive as well represent a population of youth at great risk.

Rejection Continuity

These longitudinal outcome studies provide a disheartening picture of long-term adjustment for rejected children and one that suggests that most of them do not appear to cope well with the negative treatment they receive from peers. In fact, longitudinal evidence suggests that many rejected children face repeated peer rejection over time (e.g., Coie & Dodge, 1983). After a 1-year period, 45% of rejected children remained rejected. After 2 and 3 years, this figure dropped to 34%, and after 4 years it dropped to 30%. In a study by Coie and Dodge (1983), stability was greater for fifth graders than for third graders. Analyses of behavioral predictors of status change revealed that children who became or remained rejected had relatively low scores as being cooperative and being leaders at the earliest time point and high scores on disrupting and starting fights. These findings suggest that aggression may play a key role in the continuity of rejection over time.

Two other longitudinal studies point to aggression as a significant predictor of rejection continuity (Cillessen, van IJzendoorn, et al., 1992; Vitaro, Tremblay, Gagnon, & Boivin, 1992). Vitaro et al. (1992) found that children who were characterized as aggressive–hyperactive and likely to disturb others were more likely to remain rejected over a 2-year period in early elementary school. Positive sociometric nominations (for boys) were also predictive, and the tendency to start fights (for girls) was also significantly predictive of continuous peer rejection. These findings support the premise that aggressive qualities are predictive of long-term rejection. Similarly, Cillessen, van IJzendoorn, et al. (1992) found that 57% of aggressive–rejected kindergarten and first grade boys were still rejected after the first assessment, whereas only 34% of nonaggressive–rejected children maintained their rejected status. Thus, children who are both aggressive and rejected by peers are more apt to continue to be rejected and to have more serious adjustment problems.

THE EXPERIENCE OF PEER REJECTION

A discussion of children's coping with peer rejection must first begin with an examination of the nature of the stressor they face. This is important because the nature of peer rejection appears to differ for aggressive– and nonaggressive–rejected children. There is a substantial body of research that suggests that nonaggressive–rejected children experience rejection as more stressful than do aggressive–rejected children (Boivin, Poulin, & Vitaro, 1994; Boivin, et al., 1988; Parkhurst & Asher, 1987, 1992). This literature suggests two likely explanations for this difference. One is that nonaggressive and aggressive–rejected children, while both disliked, are treated differently by their peers. It seems that nonaggressive–rejected children experience more active and overt peer dislike than their aggressive–rejected counterparts. A second explanation for the different rejection experiences of aggressive and nonaggressive children is that above and beyond objective differences in peer rejection, nonaggressive–rejected children are more aware of their rejection by peers or are more likely to acknowledge it than aggressive–rejected children. This suggests that nonaggressive–rejected children may have greater access to discomfort and emotional distress associated with peer rejection. There is research support for each of these explanations.

Differences in Peer Treatment

A handful of recent studies have suggested that aggressive–rejected children and nonaggressive–rejected children are treated differently by their peers. Unlike nonaggressive–rejected children, aggressive–rejected children often seem not to get clear feedback that they are disliked. Two factors appear to contribute to this lack of clarity. First, peers might be afraid to give direct evidence of disliking to an aggressive–rejected peer out of fear of retaliation. Some evidence for this comes from a study of instigator and target behavior in male aggressive episodes (Coie, Dodge, Terry, & Wright, 1991). In the face of aggression by aggressive–rejected boys, other boys were generally more likely to submit to these aggressive acts than to stand up for themselves. Aggressive boys in general have also been shown to receive high rates of reinforcement for their aggressive behavior (Patterson, 1982) and to believe that aggressive behavior has positive consequences (Boldizar, Perry, & Perry, 1989; Perry, Perry, & Weiss, 1989). Because their aggressive acts are sometimes not reciprocated or met with resistance and are in fact sometimes rewarded, aggressive–rejected children may not recognize that other children resent their behavior and in fact dislike them.

Research on victimization and peer disregard supports the idea of differential treatment for aggressive– and nonaggressive–rejected children (Boivin et al., 1991; Perry et al., 1989; Schwartz, Dodge, & Coie, 1993). In their sample of third through sixth graders, Perry et al. (1989) found only 25% of aggressive–rejected children to be extremely victimized by their peers, whereas 50% of nonaggressive–rejected children were extremely victimized. Similarly, in their study of first and third graders, Schwartz et al. (1993) found that victims were primarily nonassertive and submissive and rarely initiated proactive aggression. Similarly, Boivin et al. (1991) found that nonaggressive–rejected children were subjected to more active peer disregard (being unable to get others to listen) and passive peer disregard (often left aside) than were aggressive–rejected children, according to peer report. Consistent with their social status, both groups of rejected children were the targets of peer disregard more often than average-status children.

In addition to being subjected to greater peer disregard, nonaggressive–rejected children were more often excluded from peer networks than aggressive–rejected children. While nearly 70% of nonaggressive–rejected children were social isolates, 55% of aggressive–rejected children had two or more relationships and 10% had four or more relationships. Thus, a second reason why peer dislike may be less apparent to aggressive–rejected children is that pockets of social support may counterbalance the evidence of dislike they get from the peer group at large.

In summary, it appears that while aggressive–rejected children are no better liked by their peers, overt evidence of this peer dislike is not usually directed toward them as strongly as it is directed at nonaggressive–rejected children. In addition, although they are disliked by the peer group at large, aggressive–rejected children may belong to peer cliques and receive social support that offsets the impact of their peer rejection. Given that overt evidence of peer dislike differs for aggressive–rejected and nonaggressive–rejected children, it seems quite likely that these two groups of rejected children would perceive their peer rejection differently, experience different levels of distress with regard to their peer rejection, and possibly cope with their peer rejection differently.

Differences in Appraisals of Peer Rejection

In addition to these differences in the transactions involved in peer rejection, there is research suggesting that aggressive– and nonaggressive–rejected children differ in their readiness to acknowledge their own peer rejection. Because acknowledgment of the stressor is an essential component of successful effortful coping (Lazarus & Folkman, 1984), this difference is important to discuss in some detail.

In a classroom-based sociometric study of 591 fourth grade children, Zakriski and Coie (1996) assessed actual social acceptance ("Who do you like most?") and actual social rejection ("Who do you like least?"), as well as perceived social acceptance ("Who likes you the most?") and perceived social rejection ("Who likes you the least?") (Zakriski, Coie, & Wright, 1992). Children's actual social acceptance and rejection scores were subtracted from their perceived social acceptance and rejection scores to assess awareness of social rejection. Although both aggressive–rejected and nonaggressive–rejected children overestimated the number of children who liked them, only aggressive–rejected children underestimated how many peers disliked them. Thus, of these two equally rejected groups of children, only nonaggressive–rejected children seemed to be aware of how many children disliked them.

In this same study, aggressive–rejected, nonaggressive–rejected, and average-status children were interviewed about the status of peers in their classroom to assess whether aggressive–rejected children were generally deficient in their ability to recognize their peers' social preferences or whether they only had difficulty recognizing self-directed social preferences. All subjects were able to discriminate the degree of liking and disliking for other rejected, average, and popular children. The groups also were equally accurate in judging the social acceptance and social rejection of their peers. Together with the findings from the first study, these results suggest that aggressive–rejected children have the skills to accurately assess their own rejection but cannot or do not do so. As pointed out earlier, unclear negative feedback about their own peer rejection or group inclusion may play a role in this phenomenon. However, a laboratory study of rejection awareness suggests that aggressive–rejected children may inaccurately report on their peer social status for reasons other than unclear peer rejection feedback. They inaccurately report on their peer status even when the negative peer feedback is experimentally controlled.

In this study, a subset of the aggressive–rejected, nonaggressive–rejected, and average-status boys from the Zakriski and Coie classroom study were asked to participate in a laboratory study assessing how children interpret standardized negative feedback from peers (Zakriski & Coie, 1996). Fifty-six boys participated in two tasks. First, they were asked to watch videotapes of two children playing a game together in which the protagonist delivered two levels of nonpositive (ambiguous and negative) social feedback about liking to the target child. This was the other-directed condition. Second, they were asked to play the same game successively with two different children who also delivered nonpositive social feedback about liking, but in this case to the subject. This was the self-directed condition. Subjects in the other-directed condition were asked to judge on a seven-point scale how much they thought the child giving the feedback liked the child to whom he was directing the feedback. Then, in the self-directed condition they were asked how much each play partner liked them. Analyses of the liking scores revealed that while all subjects rated self-directed liking higher than other-directed liking, the aggressive–rejected boys did this to a greater degree than either nonaggressive–rejected or average-status boys. This suggests that aggressive–rejected children minimize self-directed peer dislike or are defensive about reporting it, and may distort feedback they receive from peers. Interestingly, the nonaggressive–rejected children were the least affected by social desirability considerations, suggesting that they make more honest assessments of self-directed peer dislike than either aggressive–rejected or average peers.

These conclusions are further supported by additional analyses conducted on children's verbal justifications of their liking ratings (Zakriski & Jacobs, 1995). These responses were given an overall rating by blinded coders to reflect how much liking the response conveyed on a seven-point scale. They were also reliably coded for their use of positive relationship responding [support, intimacy, similarity, association, and positive affect (Furman & Bierman, 1983)], and for negative relationship responding (conflict/competition, detachment, dissimilarity, avoidance, and negative affect), as well as positive and negative distortions. Finally, they were coded for misrepresentation of an explicit liking cue delivered by the protagonists.

Analyses of the coders' overall judgments of the subjects' descriptions of their interactions showed that aggressive–rejected boys described their rejection experience more positively than the nonaggressive–rejected boys did when the feedback was ambiguous. Average boys were also more positive than nonaggressive–rejected boys, suggesting that rather than unusual optimism on the part of the aggressive–rejected boys, nonaggressive boys were being unusually pessimistic. None of the groups differed in their description of the obvious negative feedback.

The analysis of status group differences in the use of positive relationship statements revealed that aggressive–rejected subjects made more positive relationship statements than did nonaggressive rejected children for the ambiguous feedback. None of the groups differed in their use of positive statements to describe the negative feedback. The analyses of negative relationship statements revealed no significant differences between status groups for either the ambiguous or negative feedback.

Finally, we examined subjects' distortions in their perceptions of peer feedback. For the ambiguous rejection feedback, aggressive–rejected children were more likely to make a positive distortion than either the average or the nonaggressive–rejected children. For the negative feedback there were no differences. There were also no group differences in subjects' use of negative distortions to describe the rejection experiences.

In summary, aggressive–rejected children were again more self-favoring, whereas nonaggressive–rejected children were more accurate and, at times, pessimistic. Aggressive–rejected children viewed the interactions more positively and distorted what they experienced to fit their positive perceptions. It is important to note that for the free responses these differences emerged only when the rejection feedback was ambiguous. Of course, social feedback in the real social world is often muted rather than clear-cut, and the ambiguous feedback situation may well be a more accurate representation of the kinds of experiences rejected children face in their day-to-day life.

Emotional Responses to Peer Rejection

In addition to differences in immediate perceptions and encoding of a rejection experience, research suggests that the cognitive and emotional sequelae of rejection differ between aggressive– and nonaggressive–rejected children as well. Research on concurrent loneliness, social satisfaction, self-concept, beliefs about peers, social concerns, and self-referral patterns all points to a distinct difference in the way nonaggressive– and aggressive–rejected children emotionally experience their rejection. Nonaggressive–rejected children report greater feelings of loneliness and social dissatisfaction, are described more often by their peers as sad, and have more negative self-concepts and lower self-esteem than either average-status or aggressive–rejected children (Boivin et al., 1988; Parkhurst & Asher, 1987, 1992; Williams & Asher, 1987). Nonaggressive–rejected children report more negative beliefs about their peers than nonrejected children do (Rabiner & Keane, 1991), and report that they care less about maintaining ongoing interactions with other children (Rabiner & Gordon, 1993). Nonaggressive–rejected children also are significantly more concerned than average-status children about being humiliated or rejected and are significantly more concerned about others' feelings and their relationships with other children (Parkhurst & Asher, 1992).

Aggressive–rejected children, on the other hand, are no more lonely or socially dissatisfied than average-status children and have at least average levels of self-esteem (Boivin et al., 1988; Parkhurst & Asher, 1987, 1992; Williams & Asher, 1987). Aggressive–rejected children report positive beliefs about their relationships with peers (Rabiner & Keane, 1991) and report that they care about maintaining ongoing interactions with other children (Rabiner & Gordon, 1993). Aggressive–rejected children are not more concerned than average-status children about being humiliated or rejected (Parkhurst & Asher, 1992). In studies assessing perceived social competence, aggressive–rejected children overestimate their competence in more domains than either nonaggressive–rejected or average children (Patterson et al., 1990). They also consistently overestimate their social competence (Boivin et al., 1988; Patterson et al., 1990), whereas other rejected children do not.

Both groups of children are disliked by their peers, yet only nonaggressive–rejected children demonstrate a pattern of beliefs and feelings that is consistent with this fact. Aggressive–rejected children demonstrate a pattern of beliefs and feelings that one might expect from a well-liked child. Research on self-referral patterns suggests that not only do aggressive–rejected children report thoughts and feelings more appropriate for a more well-liked child, but under certain conditions they behave as if they think they are well-liked. For example, when offered the opportunity to receive help from a friendship expert, aggressive–rejected children were unlikely to ask for help. Conversely, nonaggressive–rejected children were more likely to ask for help (Asher, Zelis, Parker, & Bruene, 1991).

From these findings, it appears that the two major types of rejected children—nonaggressive– and aggressive–rejected children—have two very different emotional experiences of peer rejection. Nonaggressive–rejected children appear to be cognizant of their rejection and upset by it. Furthermore, they are concerned about their future peer interactions as a result of their past and present experiences of peer rejection and humiliation. Aggressive–rejected children, on the other hand, appear to be either unaware or in denial of their peer rejection. They are not particularly upset by their rejection and expect positive interactions with peers in the future.

These findings raise an important dilemma for the application of a stress and coping framework to peer rejection, particularly in the case of aggressive–rejected children: Can aggressive–rejected children be described as coping with peer rejection if they do not report that their peer relationships are stressful and if we are not even sure that they are aware of their peer rejection? Folkman and Lazarus (1985) define coping as "cognitive and behavioral efforts to manage (master, reduce or tolerate) a troubled person–environment relationship" (p. 152). This definition suggests that an appraisal of the experience as stressful is a necessary part of the coping process.

Closer examination of the behaviors rather than the words of aggressive–rejected children sheds some light on this dilemma. Even though aggressive–rejected children do not openly acknowledge peer rejection as stressful for them, they may still experience it as stressful. In fact, when faced with evidence of peer dislike, they behave in ways that suggest that the experience is stressful for them. Specifically, they minimize or discount the evidence (Zakriski & Coie, 1996; Zakriski & Jacobs, 1995). This seems to be different than appraising it as benign–positive or as irrelevant to them (Folkman & Lazarus, 1985), and provides one possible clue as to how they cope with peer rejection. Their seemingly nonchalant denial of stress may in fact be a very effortful coping strategy designed to alleviate underlying discomfort and distress.

COPING WITH PEER REJECTION

The two coping styles that emerge from our review of the literature on nonaggressive–rejected and aggressive–rejected children's reactions to peer rejection seem similar to styles used to describe children's coping with other stressful experiences, such as aversive medical procedures. Specifically, it seems that the two styles of coping used by aggressive– and nonaggressive–rejected children are theoretically similar to a coping dimension that has alternatively been termed repression versus sensitization (Krohne, 1979), blunting versus monitoring (Miller, 1981; Miller & Green, 1984), and avoidance versus approach (Roth & Cohen, 1986). At its most basic level, this dimension describes the degree to which individuals attend to, process, and deal with stressful circumstances. Repressors–blunters avoid information in threatening situations by distracting themselves or cognitively protecting themselves from sources of danger. Conversely, sensitizers–monitors approach stressful situations, focus their attention on cues that indicate danger, and remain alert for the negative or potentially negative aspects of an experience.

Research on coping with aversive medical procedures suggests that strategies consistent with a blunting style (e.g., selective attention to nonaversive aspects of the procedure, filtering information about the event, distraction from aversive aspects of the procedure) are associated with better adjustment to the procedure (Miller & Green, 1984). However, a coping style or strategy that is effective in one situation may not necessarily be adaptive in another (Compas, 1987). For example, Spivack and Shure (1982) have argued that for coping with interpersonal problems, avoidance and other escape mechanisms are dysfunctional. This difference in the effectiveness of blunting strategies may be, in part, due to the chronicity of the stressor, with blunting being more effective in acute temporary situations and less effective with chronic stressors such as peer rejection. Compas (1987) also argues that the effectiveness of blunting may depend on the amount of personal control a person has in a situation, with blunting being more adaptive in cases where there is little personal control.

If we examine the adaptive tasks of coping with peer rejection, we see that there are significant opportunities for personal control. The first adaptive task appears to be awareness of the peer rejection. The second major task appears to be connecting one's behavior to the peer rejection. The third major adaptive task appears to be developing the motivation to change one's behavior. The fourth and final task appears to be actually changing one's behavior to facilitate better peer relations. Thus, in this instance where there is the possibility of some degree of personal control, blunting may not be a particularly effective strategy. This conclusion is consistent with the finding (Coie et al., 1992) that 62% of aggressive–rejected children versus 34% of nonaggressive–rejected children experience subsequent adjustment problems. In other words, although blunting may be effective for aggressive–rejected children in the short run by reducing the amount of stress they openly experience as a result of their peer rejection, it may put them at greater risk for the more serious long-term consequences of peer rejection.

Blunting as a problem-focused coping mechanism (Folkman & Lazarus, 1980) may be ineffective for aggressive–rejected children in that they are less likely to change their behavior and improve their social status than are nonaggressive–rejected children (Cillessen, van Leishout, & Haselager, 1992) and more likely to suffer negative psychological consequences from being rejected (Coie et al., 1992). However, there may be some adaptive, short-term emotional consequences to blunting as an emotion-focused coping mechanism for aggressive–rejected children. Aggressive–rejected children appear to be regulating the emotional states associated with or resulting from peer rejection in a way that leads to less immediate emotional distress. Whether or not the longer-term emotional consequences are only delayed or exacerbated by this denial is a matter for future research, although the data of Coie et al. (1995) point to the chronic psychological distress that characterizes these antisocial youth during adolescence. In contrast, because nonaggressive–rejected children appear to be less able to deny peer rejection, their vigilance or monitoring may result in more effective problem-focused coping and less effective emotion-focused coping. Recall that nonaggressive–rejected children are less likely than aggressive–rejected children to be chronically rejected, which is consistent with the notion of more effective problem-focused coping. Recall also that nonaggressive–rejected children experience a much higher level of distress due to their peer rejection than aggressive–rejected children, which is consistent with the notion of less effective emotion-focused coping, at least in the short run (Boivin et al., 1988, 1994; Parkhurst & Asher, 1992; Williams & Asher, 1987). It is possible that an accurate reading of their peer status may render them better able to cope with the problem of peer rejection in a way that helps them avoid the extreme long-term negative outcomes faced by aggressive–rejected children.

Unfortunately, most of the evidence of how rejected children cope with their peer rejection is cognitive and emotional rather than behavioral. That is, we have some information about how aggressive– and nonaggressive–rejected children perceive negative feedback and how these perceptions may play a role in their subsequent emotional state and level of self-esteem. We have virtually no information, however, on what rejected children do with their thoughts and feelings about rejection. In order to begin to address the relationship between cognitive–emotional aspects of coping and concrete behavioral strategies, we now turn to a recent study that compared a group of continuously rejected children with a group of initially rejected children who managed to improve their social status over a 2-year period.

Successful versus Unsuccessful Coping with Peer Rejection

The typical approach to studying successful coping is to identify children who have successfully coped with a given stressor and compare them with children who have not (Compas, 1987). This was the goal of a recent study (Jacobs, 1996), which examined the role of behavior, awareness, self-efficacy, and social support in status change. Jacobs (1996) conducted retrospective interviews with 44 sixth grade students and their mothers: 31 children were continuously rejected throughout the fourth and fifth grades, and 13 children were rejected throughout the fourth grade but improved their status by the end of the fifth grade year. While this study did not break down rejected groups into aggressive and nonaggressive subtypes, results shed some light on those mechanisms more generally predictive of status maintenance and change over time.

One of the most interesting findings of this exploratory, hypothesis-generating study was that awareness of rejection in the spring of fourth grade did not predict status change by the spring of fifth grade. This finding highlights our concern that the cognitive and emotional aspects of coping we have described for aggressive– and nonaggressive–rejected children may not map directly onto coping behaviors. One might hypothesize that children who are aware of their social problems would be more likely to make the necessary changes to eliminate them. Results from this study do not support this hypothesis; status awareness alone was not a significant predictor of change. An examination of related variables and their relation to status change, however, may shed light on those processes that mediate the link between children's awareness of their rejected status and their behavioral coping efforts.

First, regression analyses revealed that children's abilities to acknowledge the transactional nature of their peer relationship problems were related to improved status over time. When asked retrospectively about the locus of control for their problems with peer relationships in the fourth grade, "improvers" were more likely to report that their problems were partly due to their own behavior and partly due to the behavior of the peer group. Conversely, children who accepted all blame or placed all blame on the peer group were less likely to improve. Thus, some awareness of one's individual role (in combination with awareness of the peer group's role) in problematic incidents with peers does seem beneficial.

Along the same lines, Jacobs noted that children who labeled their earlier behavior with peers as "annoying" were more likely to improve their social status over time. Similarly, children who retrospectively described themselves as "aggressive" (independent of peer nominations for aggressive behavior) in their interactions with peers were also more likely to improve their social standing. Given what we know about the correlates of peer rejection, it is unlikely that annoying or aggressive behavior per se plays a direct role in status improvement. On the contrary, a host of studies highlights both of these characteristics as strong correlates of peer disapproval and rejection. Jacobs explains this apparent contradiction by hypothesizing that it is not the reported behavior itself, but rather the degree of self-awareness associated with these children's self-reports that is predictive of status change. That is, children who recognize that some of their behavior may have been seen as annoying or aggressive by their peers are more likely to have altered this behavior or found ways to be less aversive to others. Taken together, these findings suggest that the role of awareness in the continuity of status may be more situationally specific than originally thought. That is, it seems that while general awareness of rejected status may not be predictive of improved status over time, more specific behavioral awareness of problematic interpersonal strategies or personality characteristics may be. Children who acknowledge their role in problematic peer circumstances and can recognize their own behavior as aggressive or annoying appear to have improved their status over time. Perhaps these children were able to use this more specific behavioral awareness as a means of pinpointing the causes of their rejection and as a foundation on which to make necessary changes.

These findings suggest that knowing one is rejected by peers by itself does not lead to status change, whereas knowing the impact that one's behavior has on peers and how peers respond to one's behavior or other characteristics may be more important. The role of awareness becomes slightly more complicated, however, when we consider another finding from Jacobs' study. Results indicated that those rejected children who believed they were relatively adept at getting along with other children and who retrospectively rated their fourth grade year as a positive one in terms of getting along with other children were more likely to improve their status over time. This finding is somewhat surprising, because all children were equally rejected in the fourth grade, suggesting that the "improvers" are distorting their previous social status. The finding that improvers were more likely to report they were competent and able in their fourth grade peer interactions suggests that some degree of minimization of one's peer problems, at least in retrospect, may be beneficial. Of course, it is also possible that this positive recall of past peer relationships is a function of the positive affect currently experienced by improvers with regard to their present peer relationships (Isen, 1984).

Regardless of its source, the strong sense of self-efficacy and belief in one's success in the domain of peer relations Jacobs (1996) observed in improvers may serve a function. It also can be reconciled with the apparently contradictory finding that awareness of one's behavioral problems and admission of one's role in peer difficulties are related to status improvement. Jacobs hypothesizes that behavioral awareness (such as acknowledgment of specific behaviors or characteristics that lead to problematic peer relationships) rather than a more general sense of failure and inadequacy (such as labeling oneself as a rejected child) may be more adaptive for rejected children. Perhaps a reluctance to see oneself as rejected in a monolithic sense allows some children to pass through a transient period of peer difficulties without defining themselves as rejected or diminishing their sense of self-efficacy. On the other hand, children who focus on their peer status and think of it as central to their social experiences may begin to fall into the trap of fulfilling the negative prophecies of the peer group. In some sense, then, children who are "overly" aware of their peer problems may begin to define themselves in terms of their rejection and lose their sense of efficacy when attempting to improve problematic peer interactions. Children who are aware of specific, concrete problems but conceptualize them within a broader context of self-efficacy and a positive self-image may, in the long run, be more efficacious troubleshooters.

In addition to their display of a flexible locus of control, acknowledgment of specific problematic behaviors and a generalized belief that they were socially adept, improvers also reported less parental involvement in their social interactions, reported themselves to be more active participants in extracurricular activities, and reported that they were less likely to use aggressive coping styles in response to peer rejection. Taken together, these findings paint a picture of improvers as those children who possess a certain degree of self-awareness about their role in peer difficulties, who believe that they are capable and effective social agents, and who believe that they demonstrate the capacity for proactive and autonomous behavior. Conversely, those children who remained rejected across the fourth and fifth grades can be characterized as more dependent on adult involvement, as less effective social agents, and as being less involved in extracurricular activities that could potentially broaden their interactions with peers.

Thus, although status awareness per se does not appear to be sufficient to cause change, a constellation of factors related to behavioral awareness, self-efficacy, and autonomy do appear to be related to improved status. Perhaps it is not awareness alone, but the combination of awareness and a belief in one's ability to make effective and adaptive changes that is most predictive of status change. This hypothesis awaits further empirical investigation.

Even if future research bears out such a relationship, however, there are serious obstacles to applying such a model to clinical intervention programs. The social psychology literature (and the peer relations literature, in a more limited way) provides a great deal of evidence for the fact that individuals' attempts to change their reputations in a larger social group are often met with disregard or even active disdain. Thus, in addition to overcoming the behavioral difficulties that may contribute to their rejected status, rejected children must face the equally daunting task of overcoming reputational effects associated with peer rejection (see Hymel, Wagner, & Butler, 1990, for a review).

Obstacles to Successful Status Change

Peer group bias toward rejected children provides a serious obstacle to successful coping with peer rejection. Specifically, research by Putallaz and Gottman (1981) and Dodge, Schlundt, Schocken, and Delugach (1983) shows that peers respond more favorably to popular than to unpopular (rejected) children's peer group entry overtures, even when they employ similar strategies. Furthermore, in a study of attributional biases, Hymel (1986) found that positive hypothetical behavior performed by a liked peer was attributed to more stable causes than when it was performed by a disliked peer. In contrast, negative behavior was attributed to more stable causes when performed by a disliked peer. Subjects were also more likely to credit liked peers for positive behavior and minimize their responsibility for negative behaviors. In contrast, disliked peers were viewed as equally responsible for both positive and negative behaviors.

Similarly, in a study of self-reported behavioral responses to hypothetical behaviors of liked and disliked peers (DeLawyer & Foster, 1986), subjects made more active responses to negative behaviors by disliked peers than they did toward liked peers. Also, even when disliked peers performed positive behaviors, they evoked more negative emotional responses from their peers than did more liked peers. A similar pattern of biases has been reported for recall of positive behavior by hypothetical popular and unpopular children (Butler, 1984). Specifically, more positive behaviors were recalled for popular children than unpopular children, even though their rates of positive behaviors were equal. Moreover, in this study, subjects reported expecting more positive than negative future behaviors from popular children and more negative than positive future behaviors from unpopular children.

This pattern of findings suggests that even if rejected children are aware of their rejection, can discern their own role in the rejection transactions, and have the ability to initiate positive change in their behavior, they will most likely be met with resistance from the peer group. For example, Wagner (1986) found that relatively ambiguous hypothetical entry overtures on the part of actual popular children were almost invariably interpreted positively and were accorded more approval from peers. In contrast, the same entry behaviors when performed by unpopular children were almost equally likely to be interpreted as negative and were accorded less approval. None of these studies on reputational bias address whether bias is stronger for aggressive– or nonaggressive–rejected children. However, given what we know about peer reluctance to express rejection directly toward aggressive–rejected children, it seems likely that even if peers hold similar reputational biases toward aggressive– and nonaggressive–rejected children, they may be more likely to behaviorally express these biases to the nonaggressive–rejected children.

Thus, successful coping with peer rejection appears to be a complex problem. For each adaptive task, there are challenges to be faced. Some of the challenges appear to be greater for aggressive–rejected children and some appear to be greater for nonaggressive–rejected children. For example, aggressive–rejected children appear to have greater difficulty acknowledging their trouble with peers, but might meet with less resistance if they were to attempt to change their impact on peers. As a result, they may continue to act in maladaptive ways and miss opportunities for more positive social relationships, but be relatively unaffected by this on an emotional level in the short term. Nonaggressive–rejected children, on the other hand, might be better able to acknowledge their peer difficulties, but meet with more resistance when they attempt to make changes. As a result, they may grow increasingly hopeless and depressed about their prospects for becoming more socially accepted and be less likely to act autonomously on their own behalf to change their social situation.

Analyses using rejected status as a categorical variable in the Jacobs sample revealed that aggressive–rejected children were just as likely to remain rejected as were nonaggressive–rejected children. This underscores the observation that both groups of rejected children face obstacles to status change. Analyses that employed a continuous measure of peer rejection, however, suggest that at this age the more aggressive children may be more likely to improve their social status over time than the less aggressive children. This finding is not consistent with studies of younger children (1st grade) that have linked aggression to the continuity of rejection (Cillessen, van IJzendoorn, et al., 1992; Vitaro et al., 1992). Given the exploratory nature of Jacobs' study, it will be important to study the relationship of aggression, coping style, and status change prospectively to better understand the relationships between these variables.

INTERVENTIONS FOR SOCIALLY REJECTED CHILDREN

Viewed within a stress and coping framework, peer rejection represents a complex set of interactions between the rejected child and the larger social context. Within this framework, intervention should also focus both on the rejected child and the larger social context. However, this has not been the case for intervention research to date. Instead, intervention research has paralleled the risk research reviewed earlier and focused on the individual child and his or her social skills deficits. These intervention programs typically are characterized as positive skill training programs in that they attempt to bolster children's armamentarium of prosocial behaviors (e.g., initiating friendship, participating, communicating, cooperating, being supportive of others, taking others' perspectives, etc.). The implicit assumption underlying this approach is that rejected children are deficient in their enactment of prosocial behaviors when compared to their more socially accepted counterparts, and that increased frequency of such behaviors will lead to increased social status.

In support of the skills deficit hypothesis, there is evidence that low-status children, relative to their more popular classmates, have poorer skills in initiating interactions with other children, establishing friendships, and practicing referential communication (Gottman, Gonso, & Rasmussen, 1975). Furthermore, other studies indicate that rejected children possess deficits in the skills needed to enter a group, to maintain conversations and coordinated play, to deal with teasing and other forms of ambiguous or accidental provocation, and to resolve overt interpersonal conflicts with peers (Coie & Koeppl, 1990; Putallaz, 1983; Putallaz & Shepard, 1990).

Asher (1985) reviewed nine positive skills training programs (Bierman & Furman, 1984; Coie & Krehbiel, 1984; Gottman, Gonso, & Schuler, 1976; Gresham & Nagle, 1980; Hymel & Asher, 1977; Ladd, 1981; LaGreca & Santogrossi, 1980; Oden & Asher, 1977; Siperstein & Gale, 1983), and came to several general conclusions. First, while all nine programs differed in terms of several specific factors such as number of sessions, size of group, and peer dynamics, they all shared a common strategy that was cognitively based and involved some form of direct instruction procedures (either via videos, models, or coaches) and a practice component for the children. Seven out of the nine studies showed evidence of significant sociometric gains for those children involved in the experimental protocol. Furthermore, follow-up analyses suggest that improvement was typically maintained over time, ranging from 1 month to 1 year.

Not all evaluations were positive, however. For example, LaGreca and Santogrossi (1980) found no improvement in target children's status among peers despite significant improvement in targeted behavior and social knowledge. This finding is troubling if social skills and social knowledge are assumed to be the mechanism through which status judgments are formed. In another set of equivocal findings, Hymel and Asher (1977) found gains in social status among target children in the instruction condition, but these gains were no greater than those achieved by children who received no skill training but simply were paired with classmates for play. In this latter case, it appears that mere association with peers in a prosocial setting was as effective as coaching and direct instruction in the use of social skills. This finding also casts doubt on the notion that a child's social status is driven solely by his or her behavior and appropriate enactment of social skills. Finally, Bierman and Furman (1984) had low-accepted children work on a group task along with more socially successful peers. They found that while their prosocial-skills-based intervention did succeed in improving status among the target children, improved status was solely a result of improved judgments from specific play partners, rather than from the peer group as a whole. The only lasting improvements in social status came from children who participated in the group task, regardless of whether or not they received direct instruction in the implementation of social skills. Once again, this finding does not wholly support the skills-deficit hypothesis on which the intervention strategy was based.

Taken together, the prosocial-skill-based intervention programs have had mixed results. Some studies show clear increases in prosocial behavior and status (e.g., Ladd, 1981), while others demonstrate less clear-cut findings. It is important to note that even the most successful programs help between 50 and 60% of the target children, at best (Asher, 1985). This finding raises the inevitable question of why social skills interventions are successful with some children and not others. There are two likely explanations for varying efficacy rates across subjects. First, most intervention programs have not taken into account the specific characteristics of the rejected child. Previous sections of this chapter have emphasized cognitive and behavioral differences among rejected children (especially between aggressive and nonaggressive children), and these distinctions have remained relatively unexplored in intervention studies. Second, the content of most intervention programs has been limited to skills training, which represents only one piece of the rejection phenomenon. Perhaps efficacy rates would be higher if intervention programs broadened their scope and targeted additional areas of the transactional system (e.g., level of awareness of social difficulty and attributional system of the rejected child, along with the expectations and responses of the peer group). It is worth noting that there have been very few published reports of interventions with rejected children over the past 10 years. Whether this is because of the difficulty of doing this kind of research or because of a pervasive impression that basic questions have already been dealt with is unclear.

DIRECTIONS FOR FUTURE INTERVENTION RESEARCH

One approach to better understanding what makes an intervention effective is to examine the characteristics of those programs that did prove to be successful. Ladd's (1981) intervention was extremely successful to the extent that the experimental group's target behaviors and social status improved as a function of the skills training program. What may set this intervention apart from similar protocols is that Ladd specifically chose subjects who received low social preference ratings from peers and showed low levels of the targeted positive behaviors. That is, Ladd handpicked rejected children who showed evidence of specific skill deficits, rather than selecting from a group of rejected children at large. Given the close match between social deficiencies and the content of the program, it is not surprising that his success rate exceeded those of more generic interventions.

While prosocial skills deficits certainly are a major contributor to poor social status in childhood, an even larger contributor for some rejected children is excessively aggressive and disruptive behavior. As described earlier, approximately 50% of rejected children are considered by their classmates to be highly aggressive and/or disruptive. To date, many intervention programs have focused exclusively on prosocial skills training while paying little attention to the sorts of aggressive, disruptive, and off-task behaviors that many rejected children engage in at a high frequency. The rationale for such an approach is that teaching rejected children prosocial skills will indirectly lower their rates of antisocial behavior. It has been conjectured, for example, that rejected children will learn to substitute newly learned prosocial skills for the aggressive or antisocial ones they have used in the past. It is also hypothesized that once rejected children learn how to reinforce positive behavior from their peers, it becomes easier for them to remain engaged in group activities and avoid conflict so that their aggressive and disruptive "triggers" occur less frequently (Coie & Koeppl, 1990). While it is theoretically possible for prosocial skills training to be indirectly linked to decreased negative behaviors, this theory remains untested, because postintervention behavioral observations have focused almost exclusively on the prosocial behaviors being trained in the interventions.

It is possible, then, that the attenuated success rate in prosocial-skills-based programs is due to their failure to address the special needs of aggressive–rejected children. For highly aggressive and disruptive children, improved status may take some time to achieve. Without an intervention component directly aimed toward reducing this negative behavior, a prosocial-skills-based program runs the risk of being continuously sabotaged by the child's reliance on aggressive tactics. Furthermore, aggressive and disruptive behavior have been found to be self-reinforcing, leading rejected children to become ensnared in a cycle of negative behavior and poor status. Until the reinforcers are directly addressed and altered, a prosocial intervention stands little chance of making an impact. In short, a prosocial-skills-based approach may work well for the subset of rejected children who are deficient in those areas. However, children who are rejected primarily as a result of aggressive or disruptive behavior might benefit from an intervention program more closely tailored to their needs.

Lochman, Coie, Underwood, and Terry (1993) conducted such an intervention consisting of social problem solving, positive play training, group-entry skill training, and dealing effectively with strong negative emotions. While the first three components were closely modeled after previously described programs, the last component was designed specifically to target aggressive and antisocial behaviors. Children were taught how to identify and halt impulsive responses and to use self-regulatory statements in order to monitor their behavior. In addition, children were taught to reframe the ways they thought about who "won" in interpersonal conflicts, such that the goal of conflict resolution became self-control rather than dominance.

Lochman et al. (1993) found that their intervention had greatest impact on those rejected children who had been identified as aggressive by their classmates. The finding that aggressive–rejected children responded better than nonaggressive–rejected children provides strong support for the argument that interventions should be tailored to the needs of the population in question rather than assuming that a generic intervention will be equally effective with all rejected children. In the future, researchers need to make finer assessments of rejected children's strengths and weaknesses in order to uncover subsets of children with common behavioral styles, personality characteristics, and intervention needs.

A second strategy for future intervention programs involves the adoption of a broader perspective on the rejection phenomenon. All too often, the topic of rejection is broached with the implicit assumption that a rejected child must be doing something wrong or failing to do the right things in order to remain rejected over time. A transactional framework, on the other hand, acknowledges that there is more to rejected status than problematic behavior. A rejected child's awareness of the problem, attributions about social failure, and social goals also play into the equation. In addition, this framework posits that no single child is fully responsible for his social status. By its very definition, rejection involves the interaction between people and suggests that the peer group plays a large part in preserving a target child's status over time. Therefore, intervention programs may benefit from components geared to the target children's perception of their social experience, beliefs about their ability to improve peer relations, and their motivation to change, on the one hand, and to the expectations and behavioral responses of the peer group on the other.

One example of how to broaden the perspective on rejection in intervention programs involves a focus on rejected children's attributional systems. Goetz and Dweck (1980) have demonstrated that poorly accepted children are more likely to interpret mild peer rejection as a direct result of their own incompetence, and that they are subsequently less likely to persist in efforts to get along well with their peers. Our own research suggests that this is likely to be most true for nonaggressive–rejected children (Zakriski & Coie, 1996). If so, it seems likely that nonaggressive–rejected children could benefit from an intervention designed to help modify self-defeating attributions about their social abilities. More specifically, Ladd (1985) suggests that such rejected children might benefit from learning to attribute their social failures to lack of effort rather than to lack of ability. Such a cognitive shift would help to prevent rejected children from falling into a cycle of learned helplessness and lassitude in which they believe their social success and failure lie somewhere out of their control. A key to this would be to help them understand how their own behavior interacts with peer group exclusionary mechanisms to get them into disfavor with peers. By helping them find strategic moments for demonstrating more socially effective behavior and helping them recognize the possibility of success, they may be induced into greater positive involvement with peers and increased persistence at attempting to solve interpersonal difficulties. Out of these early successes will grow the self-confidence to attempt more difficult peer initiations.

Another potential target for future intervention efforts is the peer group itself. As discussed in the previous section, the peer group can contribute to the rejection cycle in a variety of ways. For instance, rejected children often are viewed as behaving in a manner consistent with their negative reputation, even when that is no longer the case (Hymel et al., 1990). Thus, peer group dynamics can interfere with the change process by ignoring improvements in the target's child's presentation and continuing to respond to that child in the same negative ways. Such a reputation bias is especially likely to occur in instances where change occurs in small and rudimentary steps. Thus, one potentially important intervention strategy might be to prepare rejected children for the types of responses they are likely to receive from their peers in the early stages of intervention. If children are aware of the challenges ahead of them, they might be able to take rebukes, criticisms, or lack of positive reinforcement less personally and be less quick to give up and revert to previous behavior patterns. Furthermore, rejected children might be taught to emphasize self-reinforcement in order to help themselves through the most difficult initial stages of behavioral change. Another approach to this problem might be to enlist the help of the peer group as a whole or of certain critical members of the peer group in intervention efforts with rejected children. Recall that Bierman and Furman (1994) were able to increase rejected children's social status only among intervention play partners. If these play partners were then encouraged to help break the negative reputations of these rejected children by urging others to give them a chance, the success of Bierman and Furman's intervention might become more widespread.

While the peer group often contributes to the problem by continuing to provide negative feedback to rejected children even after they show signs of improvement, another problem arises when they fail to provide appropriate feedback at all. This problem is especially relevant in the case of aggressive–rejected children. As described earlier, these children are commonly unaware of their peer problems and believe that they are far more socially accepted than their actual sociometric status suggests. One reason for their overestimation may be that aggressive children receive subtle support for their behavior in several ways. First, they are often members of peer networks, which may create the illusion of "acceptance" and high positive peer regard. Part of the reason for their inclusion in social networks may be that peers are reluctant to provide highly aggressive children with clear evidence of dislike for fear of retaliation. In addition, peers tend to submit to aggressive behavior. Their submission may unwittingly lead aggressive children to believe that they are more "liked" or "respected." A lack of overt negative feedback coupled with the short-term gratification associated with getting their way increases the likelihood that aggressive children will continue to respond to peers in an instrumental manner. Training the peer group in appropriate ways to provide each other with constructive criticism might be a useful approach to this problem.

CONCLUSIONS

Peer rejection is a serious problem in childhood. It is a stressful experience that has been linked to adolescent maladjustment, including psychological disorder, delinquency, and school problems. Peer rejection has been conceptualized primarily as an individual child problem in risk, behavioral, and intervention research. This focus on the individual child has helped researchers better define the problem of peer rejection and better understand its correlates and consequences. However, as interest in the experience and process of peer rejection has grown, this approach has become limited in its utility. In this chapter, we have drawn together scattered evidence on the nature of children's rejection experiences and the transactions that give rise to these experiences and sustain them. From this picture of rejected children in social context, we have been able to hypothesize about ways children might cope with peer rejection and how these coping efforts might influence their risk trajectory.

We have focused our discussion on the two major subgroups of rejected children—aggressive and nonaggressive—because their experiences of peer rejection are qualitatively different. Aggressive–rejected children are not given clear feedback from their peers that they are disliked, whereas nonaggressive–rejected children are more often the targets of victimization and other forms of peer disregard. In part because of this, aggressive–rejected children are not as aware of their peer difficulties or as troubled by their peer difficulties as are nonaggressive–rejected children. However, even when given clear negative feedback from peers, aggressive–rejected children interpret it more positively than do nonaggressive–rejected children.

From these different experiences of peer rejection, we have hypothesized that aggressive–rejected and nonaggressive–rejected children cope differently with their peer rejection. Cognitive and emotional evidence suggests that aggressive–rejected children are more likely to use avoidance strategies typical of repressors or blunters and nonaggressive–rejected children are more likely to use approach strategies typical of sensitizers or monitors. These different approaches appear to have different costs and benefits for the two groups. Given that aggressive–rejected children are more likely to remain rejected over time and more likely to experience the serious long-term consequences associated with peer rejection, we suggest that their blunting style may be ineffective as a problem-focused coping strategy. It may be more effective as a short-term, emotion-focused coping strategy, because it serves to allow aggressive-rejected children to feel better about themselves and their social situation. In contrast, the monitoring style adopted by nonaggressive–rejected children seems to be less effective as a short-term, emotion-focused coping strategy, because it makes nonaggressive–rejected children acutely aware of their plight with peers. On the other hand, their attention to peer rejection problems may be helpful in problem-focused coping and may be one of the reasons why they are less likely to remain rejected over time.

The conceptualization of peer rejection in a stress and coping framework is an important first step in our understanding of how different children might negotiate the stressful experience of being rejected by their peers. However, coping with peer rejection is clearly not this simple. While our model currently includes only emotional and cognitive coping with rejection, we are much less clear about the role of behavioral strategies. Initially, we have proposed a direct one-to-one mapping of cognitive–emotional coping onto behavioral coping; however, this strategy leaves out one very important component of the transactional picture of peer rejection: the peer group. A child-deficit model of peer rejection would predict that awareness of peer rejection could easily lead to status change. However, we know that rejected children, in general, often face resistance from the peer group to most efforts they make to improve their peer relationships. Given that aggressive–rejected children are treated less negatively by their peers in their everyday interactions than are nonaggressive–rejected children, it is likely that the two groups of rejected children would be met with different levels of resistance to their efforts at status change, as well. As such, nonaggressive–rejected children, while better prepared emotionally and cognitively to initiate changes in their behavior to improve their standing with peers, may meet with more peer group resistance. Because of this, their tendency to approach the problem cognitively and emotionally may be undermined in the behavioral realm.

This discussion of coping with peer rejection is largely speculative. We have drawn upon all available evidence and have presented a clear and cohesive picture of what rejection is like for aggressive and nonaggressive children, and how aggressive–rejected and nonaggressive–rejected children attempt to cope emotionally and cognitively with their experiences. We are less clear about rejected children's behavioral coping efforts and how coping transactions proceed from that point. Data from an exploratory study of coping by Jacobs (1996) underscore our concern about predicting consistency between emotional–cognitive coping and behavioral coping. Jacobs found that status awareness alone was not related to status change in groups of rejected children. However, self-awareness in the form of having an appreciation of the transactional nature of peer rejection was important, as was an ability to act proactively and autonomously on one's own behalf. These factors highlight several issues for future research on coping with peer rejection. First, how do rejected children behave in future encounters with peers who have previously rejected them? How does this change over time? How does this differ for aggressive– and nonaggressive–rejected children? Second, how do rejected children, particularly nonaggressive–rejected children, behave toward children they know do not like them? Third, how do children's attributions of blame for peer relationship problems develop and change in the face of persistent peer rejection? Fourth, what obstacles does the peer group present to rejected children attempting to improve their social situation and how does this differ for aggressive– and nonaggressive–rejected children?

In addition to aiding our understanding of coping with peer rejection, answers to these questions will help better focus intervention efforts with rejected children. To date, the most successful interventions have been helpful with approximately 50–60% of rejected children. Their somewhat limited success most likely has been due to an almost exclusive emphasis on positive social skills, based on the child-deficit model of peer rejection. Key issues to be addressed in future intervention efforts include matching the needs of individual children to the content of the intervention, addressing rejected children's cognitive interpretations of their rejection and attributional systems and targeting peer group reputational biases and the accuracy of peer feedback.

What has emerged from this chapter serves to emphasize the importance of considering the impact of a broad variety of coping mechanisms, both singly and in combination with each other. For example, while self-awareness of peer status alone may not predict subsequent improvements in peer relations, a combination of awareness, an acceptance of personal responsibility, and a peer environment that is conducive to change may well play a role in the improvement of peer status over time. As a developmental phenomena, childhood peer rejection must be viewed from a dynamic perspective that allows for the interlocking effects of many related variables. At this point, there is much to be learned about the unfolding of peer rejection over time, and how children's methods of coping with it may influence its trajectory over time.

REFERENCES

Asher, S. R. (1985). An evolving paradigm in social skill training research with children. In B. H. Schneider, K. H. Rubin, & J. E. Ledingham (Eds.), *Children's peer relations: Issues in assessment and intervention* (pp. 157–171). New York: Springer-Verlag.

Asher, S. R., & Dodge, K. A. (1986). Identifying children who are rejected by their peers. *Developmental Psychology, 22,* 444–449.

Asher, S. R., Hymel, S., & Renshaw, P. D. (1984). Loneliness in children. *Child Development, 55,* 1456–1464.

Asher, S., Parkhurst, J. T., Hymel, S., & Williams, G. A. (1990). Peer rejection and loneliness in childhood. In S. R. Asher & J. D. Coie (Eds.), *Peer rejection in childhood* (pp. 253–273). New York: Cambridge University Press.

Asher, S. R., & Wheeler, V. A. (1985). Children's loneliness: A comparison of rejected and neglected peer status. *Journal of Consulting and Clinical Psychology, 53,* 500–505.

Asher, S. R., Zelis, K. M., Parker, J. G., & Bruene, C. M. (1991). *Self-referral for peer relations problems among aggressive and withdrawn low-accepted children.* Paper presented at the biennial meeting of the Society for Research in Child Development, Seattle, WA.

Bierman, K. L., & Furman, W. (1984). The effects of social skills training and peer involvement on the social adjustment of preadolescents. *Child Development, 55,* 151–162.

Boivin, M., & Begin, G. (1989). Peer status and self-perception among early elementary school children: The case of the rejected children. *Child Development, 60,* 591–596.

Boivin, M., Cote, L., & Dion, M. (1991). *The self-perceptions and peer experiences of aggressive–rejected and withdrawn–rejected children.* Paper presented at the eleventh biennial meeting of the International Society for the Study of Behavioral Development, Minneapolis, MN.

Boivin, M., Poulin, F., & Vitaro, F. (1994). Depressed mood and peer rejection in children. *Development and Psychopathology, 6,* 483–498.

Boivin, M., Thomassin, L., & Alain, M. (1988). *Peer rejection and self-perceptions among early elementary school children: Aggressive rejectees vs. withdrawn rejectees.* Paper presented at the NATO Advanced Study Institute: Social Competence in Developmental Perspective, Savoie, France.

Boldizar, J. P., Perry, D. G., & Perry, L. C. (1989). Outcome values and aggression. *Child Development, 60,* 571–579.

Butler, L. J. (1984). *Preadolescent children's differential processing of social information in the peer group.* Unpublished doctoral dissertation, University of Waterloo, Waterloo, Ontario.

Cillessen, A. H. N., van IJzendoorn, H. W., van Leishout, C. F. M., & Hartup, W. W. (1992). Heterogeneity among peer rejected boys: Subtypes and stabilities. *Child Development, 63,* 893–905.

Cillessen, A. H. N., van Leishout, C. F. M., & Haselager, G. J. T. (1992). Children's problems caused by consistent rejection in early elementary school. In J. B. Kupersmidt (Chair), *Longitudinal research in child psychopathology: Peer rejection and children's behavior adjustment.* Symposium conducted at the Centennial Convention of the American Psychological Association, Washington, DC.

Coie, J. D. (1985). Fitting social skills intervention to the target group. In B. H. Schneider, K. H. Rubin, & J. E. Ledingham (Eds.), *Children's peer relations: Issues in assessment and intervention* (pp. 141–156). New York: Springer-Verlag.

Coie, J. D. (1990). Toward a theory of peer rejection. In S. A. Asher & J. D. Coie (Eds.), *Peer rejection in childhood* (pp. 365–401). New York: Cambridge University Press.

Coie, J. D., & Dodge, K. A. (1983). Continuities and changes in children's sociometric status: A five-year longitudinal study. *Merrill-Palmer Quarterly, 29,* 261–282.

Coie, J. D., Dodge, K. A., & Coppotelli, H. (1982). Dimensions and types of social status: A cross-age perspective. *Developmental Psychology, 18,* 557–570.

Coie, J. D., Dodge, K. A., & Kupersmidt, J. B. (1990). Peer group behavior and social status. In S. R. Asher & J. D. Coie (Eds.), *Peer rejection in childhood* (pp. 17–59). New York: Cambridge University Press.

Coie, J. D., Dodge, K. A., Terry, R., & Wright, V. (1991). The role of aggression in peer relations: An analysis of aggression episodes in boys' play groups. *Child Development, 62,* 812–826.

Coie, J. D., & Koeppl, G. K. (1990). Adapting intervention to the problems of aggressive and disruptive rejected children. In S. R. Asher & J. D. Coie (Eds.), *Peer rejection in childhood* (pp. 309–337). New York: Cambridge University Press.

Coie, J. D., & Krehbiel, G. (1984). Effects of academic tutoring on the social status of low-achieving, socially rejected children. *Child Development, 55,* 1465–1478.

Coie, J. D., & Kupersmidt, J. B. (1983). A behavioral analysis of emerging social status in boys' groups. *Child Development, 54,* 1400–1416.

Coie, J. D., Lochman, J. E., Terry, R., & Hyman, C. (1992). Predicting adolescent disorder from childhood aggression and peer rejection. *Journal of Consulting and Clinical Psychology, 60,* 783–792.

Coie, J. D., Terry, R., Lenox, K., Lochman, J., & Hyman, C. (1995). Childhood peer rejection and aggression as predictors of stable patterns of adolescent disorder. *Development and Psychopathology, 7,* 699–714.

Compas, B. E. (1987). Coping with stress during childhood and adolescence. *Psychological Bulletin, 101,* 393–403.

Cowen, E. L., Pederson, A., Babigian, H., Izzo, L. D., & Trost, M. A. (1973). Long-term follow-up of early detected vulnerable children. *Journal of Consulting and Clinical Psychology, 41,* 438–446.

DeLawyer, D. D., & Foster, S. L. (1986). The effects of peer relationship on the functions of interpersonal behaviors in children. *Journal of Consulting and Clinical Psychology, 15,* 127–133.

Dodge, K. A. (1983). Behavioral antecedents of per social status. *Child Development, 54,* 1386–1399.

Dodge, K. A., Schlundt, D. G., Schocken, I., & Delugach, J. D. (1983). Social competence and children's sociometric status: The role of peer group entry strategies. *Merrill-Palmer Quarterly, 29,* 309–336.

Folkman, S., & Lazarus, R. S. (1980). An analysis of coping in a middle-aged community sample. *Journal of Health and Social Behavior, 21,* 219–239.

Folkman, S., & Lazarus, R. S. (1985). If it challenges it must be a process: Study of emotion and coping during three stages of a college examination. *Journal of Personality and Social Psychology, 48,* 150–170.

French, D. C. (1988). Heterogeneity of peer rejected boys: Aggressive and nonaggressive subtypes. *Child Development, 59,* 976–985.

Furman, W., & Bierman, K. L. (1983). Developmental changes in young children's conceptions of friendship. *Child Development, 54,* 549–556.

Goetz, T. E., & Dweck, C. S. (1980). Learned helplessness in social situations. *Journal of Personality and Social Psychology, 39,* 246–255.

Gottman, J., Gonso, J., & Rasmussen, B. (1975). Social interaction, social competence, and friendship in children. *Child Development, 46,* 709–718.

Gottman, J., Gonso, J., & Schuler, P. (1976). Teaching social skills to isolated children. *Journal of Abnormal Child Psychology, 4,* 179–197.

Gresham, F. M., & Nagle, R. J. (1980). Social skills training with children: Responsiveness to modeling and coaching as a function of peer orientation. *Journal of Consulting and Clinical Psychology, 48,* 718–729.

Hymel, S. (1986). Interpretations of peer behavior: Affective bias in childhood and adolescence. *Child Development, 57,* 431–445.

Hymel, S., & Asher, S. A. (1977). *Assessment and training of isolated children's social skills.* Paper presented at the biennial meeting of the Society for Research in Child Development, New Orleans, LA.

Hymel, S., Wagner, E., & Butler, L. (1990). Reputational bias: View from the peer group. In S. R. Asher & J. D. Coie (Eds.), *Peer rejection in childhood* (pp. 253–273). New York: Cambridge University Press.

Isen, A. M. (1984). Toward understanding the role of affect in cognition. In Wire & Srull (Eds.), *Handbook of social cognition* (Vol. 3, pp. 179–236). Hillsdale, NJ: Fervlbaum.

Jacobs, M. R. (1996). *A developmental perspective on peer rejection: Mechanisms of stability and change.* Unpublished doctoral dissertation, Duke University, Durham, NC.

Krohne, H. W. (1979). Parental child-rearing behavior and the development of anxiety and coping strategies in children. In I. G. Sarason & C. D. Speilberger (Eds.), *Stress and anxiety* (Vol. 7, pp. 233–245). Washington, DC: Hemisphere.

Kupersmidt, J. B., & Coie, J. D. (1985). *The prediction of delinquency and school-related problems from childhood peer status.* Unpublished manuscript, Duke University, Durham, NC.

Kupersmidt, J. B., Coie, J. D., & Dodge, K. A. (1990). The role of peer relationships in the development of disorder. In S. R. Asher & J. D. Coie (Eds.), *Peer rejection in childhood* (pp. 274–305). New York: Cambridge University Press.

Ladd, G. W. (1981). Effectiveness of a social learning method for enhancing children's social interaction and peer acceptance. *Child Development, 52,* 171–178.

Ladd, G. W. (1985). Documenting the effects of social skills training with children: Process and outcome assessment. In B. H. Schneider, K. H. Rubin, & J. E. Ledingham (Eds.), *Children's peer relations: Issues in assessment and intervention* (pp. 243–269). New York: Springer-Verlag.

LaGreca, A. M., & Santogrossi, D. (1980). Social skills training with elementary school students: A behavioral group approach. *Journal of Consulting and Clinical Psychology, 48,* 220–227.

Lazarus, R. S., & Folkman, S. (1984). *Stress, appraisal, and coping.* New York: Springer.

Lochman, J. E., Coie, J. D., Underwood, M. K., & Terry, R. (1993). Effectiveness of a social relations intervention program for aggressive and nonaggressive rejected children. *Journal of Consulting and Clinical Psychology, 61,* 1053–1058.

Lochman, J. E., & Wayland, K. K. (1994). Aggression social acceptance and race as predictors of negative adolescent outcomes. *Journal of the American Academy of Child and Adolescent Psychiatry, 33,* 1026–1035.

Loeber, R., Green, S. M., & Lahey, B. B. (1990). Mental health professionals' perceptions of the utility of children, parents, and teachers as informants on childhood psychopathology. *Journal of Consulting and Clinical Psychology, 19,* 136–143.

Miller, S. M. (1981). Predictability and human stress: Toward clarification of evidence and theory. In L. Berkowitz (Ed.), *Advances in experimental social psychology* (Vol. 14, pp. 203–255). New York: Academic Press.

Miller, S. M., & Green, M. L. (1984). Coping with stress and frustration: Origins, nature, and development. In M. Lewis & C. Saarni (Eds.), *The socialization of emotions* (pp. 263–314). New York: Plenum Press.

Newcomb, A. F., & Bukowski, W. M. (1983). Social impact and social preference as determinants of children's peer groups status. *Developmental Psychology, 19,* 856–867.

Oden, S., & Asher, S. R. (1977). Coaching children in social skills for friendship-making. *Child Development, 48,* 495–506.

Parker, J. G., & Asher, S. R. (1987). Peer relations and later personal adjustment: Are low-accepted children "at risk"? *Psychological Bulletin, 102,* 357–389.

Parkhurst, J. T., & Asher, S. R. (1987). The social concerns of aggressive–rejected children. In J. D. Coie (Chair), *Types of aggression and peer status: The social functions and consequences of children's aggression.* Symposium conducted at the biennial meeting of the Society for Research in Child Development, Baltimore.

Parkhurst, J. T., & Asher, S. R. (1992). Peer rejection in middle school: Subgroup differences in behavior, loneliness, and interpersonal concerns. *Developmental Psychology, 28,* 231–241.

Patterson, C. J., Kupersmidt, J. B., & Griesler, P. C. (1990). Children's perceptions of self and of relationships with others as a function of sociometric status. *Child Development, 61,* 1335–1349.

Patterson, G. R. (1982). *A social learning approach: Coercive family processes.* Eugene, OR: Castalia.

Perry, D. G., Kusel, S. J., & Perry, L. C. (1989). Victims of peer aggression. *Developmental Psychology, 24,* 807–814.

Perry, D. G., Perry, L. C., & Weiss, R. J. (1989). Sex differences in the consequences that children anticipate for aggression. *Developmental Psychology, 25,* 312–319.

Putallaz, M. (1983). Predicting children's sociometric status from their behavior. *Child Development, 54,* 1417–1426.

Putallaz, M., & Gottman, J. M. (1981). An interactional model of children's entry into peer groups. *Child Development, 52,* 986–994.

Putallaz, M., & Shepard, B. H. (1990). Social status and children's orientation to limited resources. *Child Development, 61,* 2022–2027.

Rabiner, D. L., & Gordon, L. (1993). Relations between children's self-concepts and social interaction strategies; differences between rejected and accepted boys. *Social Development, 2,* 83–94.

Rabiner, D. L., & Keane, S. P. (1991). *Children's beliefs about peers in relation to their social status.* Paper presented at the biennial meeting of the Society for Research in Child Development, Seattle, WA.

Roff, M. (1960). Relations between certain preservice factors and psychoneurosis during military duty. *Armed Forces Medical Journal, 11,* 152–160.

Roff, M. (1961). Childhood social interactions and young adult bad conduct. *Journal of Abnormal and Social Psychology, 63,* 333–337.

Roff, M., Sells, S. B., & Golden, M. M. (1972). *Social adjustment and personality development in children*. Minneapolis: University of Minnesota Press.

Roth, S., & Cohen, L. J. (1986). Approach, avoidance, and coping with stress. *American Psychologist, 41,* 813–819.

Routh, D. K. (1990). Taxonomy in developmental psychopathology. In M. Lewis & S. M. Miller (Eds.), *Handbook of developmental psychopathology* (pp. 53–62). New York: Plenum Press.

Rubin, K. H., LeMare, L. J., & Lollis, S. (1990). Social withdrawal in childhood: Developmental pathways to peer rejection. In S. R. Asher & J. D. Coie (Eds.), *Peer rejection in childhood* (pp. 217–249). New York: Cambridge University Press.

Schwartz, D., Dodge, K. A., & Coie, J. D. (1993). The emergence of chronic victimization in boys' play groups. *Child Development, 64,* 1755–1772.

Siperstein, G. N., & Gale, M. E. (1983). Improving peer relationships of rejected children. Paper presented at the biennial meeting of the Society for Research in Child Development, Detroit, MI.

Spivack, G., & Shure, M. B. (1982). The cognition of social adjustment: Interpersonal cognitive problem-solving thinking. In B. B. Lahey & A. E. Kazdin (Eds.), *Advances in clinical child psychology* (Vol. 5, pp. 323–372). New York: Plenum Press.

Vitaro, F., Tremblay, R. E., Gagnon, C., & Boivin, M. (1992). Peer rejection from kindergarten to grade 2: Outcomes, correlates, and prediction. *Merrill-Palmer Quarterly, 38,* 382–400.

Wagner, E. (1986). *Bias in preadolescent children's responses to ambiguous social information about peers.* Unpublished doctoral dissertation, University of Waterloo, Waterloo, Ontario.

Williams, G. A., & Asher, S. R. (1987). *Peer and self-perceptions of peer rejected children: Issues in classification and subgrouping.* Paper presented at the biennial meeting of the Society for Research in Child Development, Baltimore.

Wright, J. C., Giammarino, M., & Parad, H. (1986). Social status in small groups: Individual–group similarity and the social "misfit." *Journal of Personality and Social Psychology, 50,* 523–536.

Zakriski, A. L., & Coie, J. D. (1996). A comparison of aggressive–rejected and nonaggressive–rejected children's interpretations of self-directed and other-directed rejection. *Child Development, 67,* 1048–1070.

Zakriski, A. L., Coie, J. D., & Wright, J. C. (1992). The accuracy of children's sociometric self-perceptions. In J. B. Kupersmidt (Chair), *Multiple sources of information about children's peer relationships.* Symposium conducted at the Conference on Human Development, Atlanta, GA.

Zakriski, A. L., & Jacobs, M. R. (1995). A process analysis of rejection awareness in late elementary school children. In M. Derosier & A. H. N. Cillessen (Chairs), *Children's social self-perceptions: Developmental links to social, behavioral, and emotional adjustment.* Symposium conducted at the biennial meeting for the Society for Research in Child Development, Indianapolis, IN.

16

Staying out of Harm's Way
Coping and the Development
of Inner-City Children

PATRICK H. TOLAN, NANCY G. GUERRA, and
LUISA R. MONTAINI-KLOVDAHL

INTRODUCTION

Staying out of harm's way is the daily goal of many children living in the inner city. In this case, "harm" is not limited to physical assault or violence, but encompasses a myriad of everyday urban threats. By the time children reach adolescence, they often have navigated a lifetime of fear and hopelessness, making choices requiring cognitive sophistication, moral clarify, and social deftness beyond that of any child and most adults. They have been exposed to harm caused not only by crime and violence, but by drugs, teenage pregnancy, abuse, neglect, poverty, and racism. The joys of childhood are often lost or compromised to the perils of the streets. Rather than trying to maximize positive outcomes, children and families are often preoccupied with simply staying out of harm's way.

Consider a scene from the recent movie, "Boyz N the Hood," that chronicles the lives of four young boys growing up in South Central Los Angeles. In a seemingly ironic act of childhood play, the boys, football in hand, set out to view a dead body in a nearby vacant lot. They are confronted by a group of menacing adolescents, and one of the adolescents says, "Throw me the football . . . I'm not going to steal it, I got enough money to buy a hundred footballs," in a voice that is both threatening and friendly. Quickly contemplating what to do

PATRICK H. TOLAN • Department of Psychiatry and Psychology, University of Illinois at Chicago Medical School, Chicago, Illinois 60612.   NANCY G. GUERRA • Department of Psychology, University of Illinois at Chicago, Chicago, Illinois 60680.   LUISA R. MONTAINI-KLOV-DAHL • Department of Psychiatry, University of California at San Francisco, San Francisco, California 94560.

Handbook of Children's Coping: Linking Theory and Intervention, edited by Wolchik and Sandler. Plenum Press, New York, 1997.

with his prized football, the young boy tosses it to the adolescent, who laughs and tosses the ball to his group, clearly planning to keep it. As the boys follow the adolescents, they must quickly decide what to do. Should they try to get the football back and risk further harm or accept their imposed fate? In an instant, the boy's older brother intervenes and is beaten up for his efforts. The boy not only loses his prized football but his older brother is also hurt.

In such situations, children must marshal cognitive, emotional, physical, and moral resources to respond to a finely woven texture of ambiguous cues. Choosing the best response requires simultaneous consideration of the complex elements of the situation. A wrong response could lead to dire consequences, and few responses will lead to complete escape from harm. As this scene illustrates, inner-city life is distinguished by constant exposure to high levels of potentially harmful and often life-threatening circumstances against a background of chronic poverty and few opportunities for positive engagement. In this setting, children and families face a barrage of stressful events and circumstances that make it harder simply to survive, let alone experience the carefree moments of childhood necessary for optimal development. Although most children still find time to play and enjoy themselves and ultimately lead healthy and productive lives, coping is first and foremost a matter of staying out of harm's way by anticipating adversities and getting through dangerous moments with minimal costs (Garbarino, Kostelny, & Dubrow, 1991). This coping orientation may result in responses that are momentarily adaptive but are ultimately ineffective; they are harmful in the long run in terms of personal well-being and quality of life. Thus, the stressors faced and the nature of coping for inner-city children are qualitatively different from those faced by most children in the United States at this time.

The purpose of this chapter is to examine the stressors and coping mechanisms affecting children's development in the inner city and to suggest a framework for their study and application. Figure 1 illustrates the components of the suggested framework. As can be seen, this framework focuses on qualities of stressors imposing on children. Rather than being distinguished by a single type of stressor, there is a need to consider the multiple stressors of inner-city life. Also, we list a dimensional structure of coping strategies derived from our studies of inner-city youth (Tolan, Gorman-Smith, Chung, & Hunt, 1996). We distinguish the adaptive function of coping from its long-term effectiveness (Tolan, Montaini, & Gorman-Smith, 1996). This distinction is important because of the constraints the inner city imposes on the impact of individual coping methods. Also, as we describe in this chapter, Fig. 1 represents coping as one part of a support, resource, and coping process that affects functioning. These processes are theorized as part of a larger framework of the individual within a family within a neighborhood and community (see Tolan & Gorman-Smith, 1997; Tolan & Guerra, 1994; Tolan, Guerra, & Kendall, 1995). In order to present this framework clearly, we first briefly examine the dimensions empirically derived from the characteristics of the inner city that negatively impact children's development. Next, we present a specific organization of types of stressors in this setting. This is followed by a discussion of coping theory and research in relation to this population and summarization of a recently tested model. We draw on data from three recent studies we have conducted

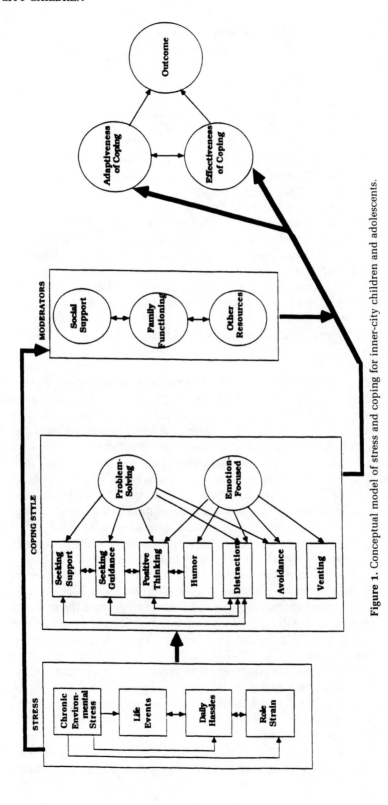

Figure 1. Conceptual model of stress and coping for inner-city children and adolescents.

to suggest a framework for evaluating coping of inner-city children. We then note the ancillary issue of the role of the family in understanding child coping. Finally, we discuss the implications of this model for interventions in this setting.

THE INNER CITY AS A DEVELOPMENTAL SETTING

About 9% of the 17.2 million children in families living below the poverty line live in inner-city neighborhoods (urban communities with at least 40% poverty) (Bane & Ellwood, 1989; Lindsey, 1994). As recent epidemiological and survey data indicate, inner-city children are more likely than other children to achieve below expected levels in school and/or not complete high school (Kozol, 1992), display elevated rates of aggression and psychopathology (Tolan, Henry, Guerra, VanAcker, Huesmann, & Eron, 1996), engage in serious criminal behavior (National Institute of Justice, 1992), die from intentional injury (Centers for Disease Control, 1992), become teenage parents (National Commission on Children, 1991), and have difficulty obtaining and maintaining regular employment (Jencks, 1992). For the sake of illustration, we have listed some of the levels of risk elevation for inner-city children and families in Table 1. Thus, children growing up in this setting have elevated risk by almost every marker of maladjustment.

The risk seems to be attributable to influences other than simply individual or family limitations (Tolan & Gorman-Smith, 1997). For example, in a recent analysis comparing family relations and parenting characteristics as predictors of antisocial behavior, we found that in inner-city neighborhoods, parenting and family relations characteristics have no significant impact on outcome once stress levels are considered. However, in other poor urban communities (but not inner city), family relations and parenting characteristics mediate stress impact on child antisocial behavior (Gorman-Smith, Tolan, & Henry, in press). Similarly, many studies have presented data that suggest extreme poverty imperils family functioning and exacerbates any individual differences in risk (e.g., Connell, Spencer, & Aber, 1994; Sampson & Laub, 1994; see McLoyd, 1990, for a meticulous analytic review of these processes).

The poor economic base has resulted from the transformation of the US economy from a manufacturing to service and technical base. Manufacturing jobs have been steadily moving out of central cities, and most technical and service firms have not located in these neighborhoods. Furthermore, many inner-city residents lack the training needed to enter technical and service positions. This combination of lack of skills and difficulty in finding and reaching jobs in the suburbs has contributed to spiraling rates of unemployment for urban families and has seriously limited opportunities for adolescents and young adults. Children face limited economic opportunities with little hopes of finding well-paying and satisfying jobs at local employers when they are ready to enter the job market (Jencks, 1992).

This deterioration of the economic base and associated job loss has also been accompanied by an exit of the working and middle class, resulting in a loss of economic support for schools and other community institutions and a rapid deterioration in housing. Many children live in substandard housing and attend boarded-up schools with inadequate supplies and demoralized teachers. For example, in the Chicago public schools, approximately 5700 children come to school each day and find they have no teacher (Kozol, 1992). The exit of the middle class has also reduced opportunities for children to interact with economically successful persons of their own ethnicity and backgrounds.

Accompanying the loss of an economic base and the exit of middle-class residents has been the increasing concentration of social problems. High rates of teenage pregnancy, single parents, substance use, violence, and gang activity create a pervasive experience that engenders an ecology of isolation, despair, and danger (Wilson, 1987). This concentration, in light of the depleted economic opportunities and the resulting deterioration of social institutions, has led to economic, social, and psychological isolation and alienation of these neighborhoods from the mainstream society. As part of this alienation, the attraction and plausibility of conventional accomplishments and conventional avenues to success fades, and standard markers of success are often equated with being "white" and abandoning one's ethnic identity.

With all of these negative forces at work, inner cities tend to be more violent than other communities, and such violence is more likely to be ubiquitous. Violent crime rates in central cities are twice that of cities outside metropolitan areas and four times that of rural areas (Federal Bureau of Investigation, 1992). Surveys indicate that more than half of inner-city youth have witnessed a violent attack in the previous year, and even more children report staying inside their home due to fear of violence (Attar, Guerra, & Tolan, 1994). A child living in the inner city is more likely to die from violence than almost any other cause (Federal Bureau of Investigation, 1992). Thus, inner-city children are exposed to more violence as witnesses and victims, and this violence becomes more normative (Anderson, 1991). However, although violent events are more common, they are also unpredictable. This combination of commonality and unpredictability can lead to symptoms such as emotional numbness and a preoccupying vigilance that are characteristic of posttraumatic stress disorder (Garbarino et al., 1991).

The conditions in the inner city thus create formidable impediments to healthy development and are sources of high levels of stress that would strain the coping skills of almost anyone. In order to examine these conditions from a stress and coping perspective, it is useful to consider these conditions as sources of stress and to relate them to more common forms of stress. These social structure sources that characterize and differentiate the inner city can be considered stable environment features affecting all residents and therefore different from most stressors that are usually defined as specific events or experiences that happen to individuals. However, as others have argued, conditions of extreme poverty, economic inequities, racism, and oppression can act much like stressors in impeding development and requiring responses to cope (Anderson, 1991). In the following section, we discuss four distinct types of stress that result from these extreme setting characteristics.

A TYPOLOGY OF STRESS IN THE INNER CITY

A number of different schema have been proposed for characterizing stress exposure in disadvantaged urban settings (e.g., Anderson, 1991; Peters & Massey, 1983; Pierce, 1975). A particular feature of many of these is that they incorporate the distinct experience of ethnic minority groups. Synthesizing these typologies, we propose that the nature and impact of stress for inner-city children is best understood by distinguishing at least four types of stress: (1) chronic environmental stress, (2) life events, (3) daily hassles, and (4) role strain. This organization differentiates stress type both by its specific impact and required coping tasks. The typology also permits examination of how conditions of chronic environmental stress relate to increased levels of the other types of stressors in this setting.

Chronic environmental stress is defined as stress due to a background level of specific characteristics of the environment that impose coping requirements (Anderson, 1991). Conditions described in the previous section such as large-scale unemployment, violence, and widespread social problems are prime examples of chronic environmental stress in the inner city. Other corollaries of inner-city life that are chronic environmental stress include limited access to society's resources and both subtle and obvious discrimination. Chronic environmental stress is experienced by all inner-city residents and is largely uncontrollable. Harm is caused via the constant presence of the specific stressors rather than as time-limited events. Because such stress becomes part of the "background noise" of the community, it has been referred to as mundane extreme environmental stress (Peters & Massey, 1983; Pierce, 1975). Although not absolutely required, usually such stress is differentiated from the other three types by being a feature of ethnic and class group membership and/or residence (McLoyd, 1990). It has been argued that this type of stress is particularly detrimental to ethnic minority groups living in central cities because the chronic environmental stressors of poverty, danger, and widespread social problems are added to racism and oppression, which are pervasive in society. For instance, Anderson (1991) proposed that this type of stress represents a substantial and persistent constraint on the ability of African-American families to work, live, and survive in the United States. Coping strategies must include accommodating to, "transcending" (growing), or overcoming these general impediments. Similarly, these pervasive and routine conditions may seriously constrain the effects that coping can have. Not only can the efficacy of direct action and problem solving be blunted if chronic environmental stress is present, but such conditions may promote short-term oriented coping that results in detrimental long-term outcomes (Garbarino et al., 1991). For example, denying oneself the fun of socializing with friends rather than staying in to study to achieve in school is a different choice in an environment in which living long enough to complete school is questionable and the quality of the school is poor enough to make adequate education unlikely.

Life events are defined as the stressful events and life transitions that, by their occurrence, cause distress to the person experiencing them. Most studies that include tallies of stressful events focus on a variety of life events, including temporary economic disruptions, death of a family member, and property loss (Tolan, Miller, & Thomas, 1988). Life events are distinguished by their time-limited nature and variation in their occurrence from the ongoing conditions. Life events also can be distinguished from the minor irritations due to daily hassles. However, induced transitions that represent a change in life circumstance, such as moving to a new apartment building, can also have stressful effects akin to life events (see Felner, Farber, & Primavera, 1983). Although there can be distinctions made between these two types of stress, the shared characteristic of a discrete onset with a substantial impact on life leads us to include them in a single category (Tolan et al., 1988).

Although all children may experience life events stress (Compas, Worsham, & Ey, 1992), inner-city children are likely to experience more of these events than other children. For example, in a study we recently conducted with urban elementary school children (Attar et al., 1994), nearly 50% of the children surveyed reported a loss of a friend or family member, significant health problems in the family, or witnessing violence in the preceding year. When we divided the sample based on neighborhood distress, children from the most distressed neighborhoods experienced rates of life events stress that were twice as high as children from the moderately distressed neighborhoods, although all children experienced rates that were four to six times higher than that reported in other studies of suburban children (Dubow, Tisak, Causey, Hryshko, & Reid, 1991).

In addition to the increased prevalence of stressful life events, there is also reason to believe that inner-city children are more vulnerable to the impact of stressful events. Studies have shown that lower-socioeconomic-status persons are more vulnerable to negative effects of job loss than those in the middle class (McLoyd, 1990). Also, compared to white males, African-American males report more physical and psychological problems and more family problems following loss of employment (Buss & Redburn, 1983). Similar relations of race to psychological symptoms were greater for those living in lower-socio-economic-status neighborhoods (Kessler & Neighbors, 1986). Thus, it may be that both the greater frequency of events and the greater impact of these events increases the harmful consequences for inner-city residents (Kessler, 1979; Neff, 1985). In some cases, this increased impact is related to the status of being both poor and minority (Kessler & Cleary, 1980; Ulbrich, Warheit, & Zimmerman, 1989). However, all of these studies have been of adults, and so the actual validity of this presumed "double effect" for children is an important area for future study. Assuming these effects are not limited to adults, it seems that not only do inner-city children face extreme levels of life event stressors, but it seems likely that they are also likely to be more adversely affected by such events. This may be due to having fewer resources to facilitate coping, the rapidity and constancy of stressful events, or the reduced impact of individual coping on outcome (Anderson, 1991; McLoyd, 1990).

Daily hassles are minor stressors that are part of day-to-day life. In many cases, daily hassles have been found to be the most significant predictors of distress in children and youth (Felner et al., 1983; Tolan et al., 1988). Daily hassles are considered harmful because they detract from feelings of well-being and interfere with productive activity. In addition, it has been argued that chronic environmental stress, high levels of stressful life events, and limited resources and support make it more difficult for children to manage daily hassles.

Two common complications of daily hassles for inner-city residents are the exacerbation of daily hassles due to racism and how the community problems make managing normal minor disruptions more difficult. For children of the inner city, racism may be experienced in the form of an insult or personal humiliation, disruption of a simple interaction or completion of a daily task, greater constraints in coping with normal stress, or the exacerbation of a daily hassle. For example, approaching a teacher about schoolwork or a dispute about a grade, a daily hassle for most children in most communities, can be overwhelming if this teacher's behavior is motivated by prejudice. Similarly, a common minor hassle can be exacerbated by community characteristics. For example, needing to go out to purchase milk late at night becomes a substantial problem if there is no store nearby or it is simply too dangerous to go out at night. In either case, common effective coping responses for otherwise minor hassles may be inadequate, seem irrelevant, or actually increase risk for harm or humiliation. The response needed not only requires more effort but also more sophisticated strategies for everyday problems.

Role strain is defined as stress due to one's inability to fulfill socially ascribed roles (Pearlin, 1983). Originally, role strain was seen to be caused by personal inadequacies, such as severe psychopathology, that kept one from fulfilling the ascribed responsibilities of one's social position. For example, a man's alcoholism could cause role strain if it prevented fulfillment of his role as the family breadwinner. However, it is also clear that role strain can result from contextual factors that limit access to legitimate social roles or undermine effectiveness (McLoyd, 1990; Wilson, 1987). Because of diminished resources, many inner-city residents experience limited access and blocked opportunities for meeting social role demands (Gorman-Smith, Tolan, Zelli, & Huesmann, 1996).

Furthermore, members of ethnic minority groups can experience role strain because of conflict between the values of their culture and those of mainstream society (Anderson, 1991; Ogbu, 1985). This conflict creates stress because attempts to fulfill mainstream role demands may require individuals to compromise, disregard, or fail to achieve the role demands of their own culture. For example, the valuing of family loyalty in Mexican culture can conflict with the mainstream culture's emphasis on autonomy support and therefore increase risk (Florsheim, Tolan, & Gorman-Smith, 1996; Gorman-Smith, Tolan, & Henry, in press). Further, an inner-city child of this culture who focuses on achievement at school as a means of attaining higher economic and social status may be forsaking cultural values requiring duty and loyalty to his or her family (Laosa, 1979). The consequences of individual achievement may be disaffection from family members as well as the literal move to a higher-socioeconomic neighborhood. The lack of occasion to capitalize on this achievement because of low employment opportunity or the implausibility of attending college may result in further role strain. The cultural conflicts and setting characteristics can cause role strain because they prevent the fulfillment of role demands because of external constraints (Anderson, 1991).

Role strain also can be accentuated for inner-city children by conflicts due to social class differences. For example, for children who are both minority and poor, concerns over group identity may be more salient (Boykin, 1979; Spencer, Dobbs, & Swanson, 1988). Thus, any activity focused on diminishing group identity may create role strain (e.g., involvement with others not from the neighborhood or accomplishing high achievement in school or other activity that may lead to leaving the neighborhood). This role strain is not just a situational or event stress; it can influence outcome by modifying development processes. The meaning of developmental tasks such as achieving autonomy as well as apparent support (or lack of it) for the inner-city child's management of cultural conflict can lower esteem and security (Spencer et al., 1988). What elsewhere is a positive expectable developmental task can be a problem for inner-city, ethnic minority children. Role strain can thus insidiously impose onerous harm to inner-city children.

COPING THEORY AND INNER-CITY CHILDREN

The multiple stressors occurring at high rates and chronically afflicting inner-city children impose sizable constraints on which coping methods can be used and what effects they will have. Most contemporary models of coping emphasize coping as a process rather than a specific disposition. The efficacy of a response depends on the stress, the context, and the resources available (Billings & Moos, 1981; Folkman & Lazarus, 1988). Unfortunately, there has been continuing interpretation of direct problem solving as better than less direct or more emotion-focused methods (Compas et al., 1992). The equation of coping effectiveness with any immediate reduction in distress can be misleading. Although it is important to consider the context, stress level, and resources available in evaluating the efficacy of a given method of coping, such assessment does not account for long-term implications. Reduction of distress or removal of an immediate stressor is desirable, but it is not synonymous with long-term benefit. This distinction is particularly important when considering inner-city children. To understand coping in this setting, it is important to distinguish among different aspects of coping impact (effectiveness vs. adaptiveness) and to differentiate coping impact from coping style.

Coping Impact: Effectiveness versus Adaptiveness

Effectiveness can be defined as the extent to which a coping method is likely to prevent or curtail a given stressor, or limit its impact on long-term adjustment if the occurrence of the stressor is beyond individual control. *Adaptability* can be defined as the extent to which a coping method reduces distress immediately regardless of its effect on the continuation or reoccurrence of the stressor or its effect on long-term outcomes. An adaptive coping response may serve to remove or curtail the stressor or may simply provide escape. Adaptability and effectiveness may have some relation, but they are not synonymous, particularly for inner-city children. For example, when faced with economic hardship, an inner-city teenager may quit school to get a job. This is adaptive because it relieves the economic distress, but it is not effective since it is unlikely to bring sufficient and dependable income to ward off economic distress for very long. Also, it makes obtaining a productive career unlikely.

Another useful distinction between coping effectiveness and adaptability is the extent to which the functional impact is to improve or maintain successful role functioning such as achievement, health behaviors, or social status. Adaptability is the extent to which the coping serves to aid some more subjectively determinable status such as well-being, distress, satisfaction, or perceived efficacy. It is an important aspect of effectiveness that the evaluation is based on the extent to which coping promotes obtaining socially sanctioned goals. In some cases, effective responses based on mainstream social goals may not be adaptive for inner-city children. For example, working hard in school may be effective in increasing financial success, but it may carry costs such as alienation from peers. One goal of coping research should be to identify coping strategies that are both effective and adaptive for inner-city children and adolescents.

For inner-city children, the ever-present threat of danger and harm can require forsaking effectiveness for adaptability (Garbarino et al., 1991). If control over long-term outcomes is low, the effectiveness of a given coping response may be difficult to predict and the danger of not adapting to immediate situational demands can overwhelm these more distal concerns. Also, because the most likely effect one can have is to prevent, minimize, or postpone harm rather than to solve a problem or increase one's approximation to some goal, the salient concern of the child may be to adapt, with any effectiveness concerns experienced as abstract or irrelevant. For many inner-city children, gang membership is an adaptive way to cope with danger, avoid being victimized, and create a buffer against the unpredictable harm around them. However, this protection often extracts a high cost in terms of school failure, imprisonment, and injury.

Coping Style

Understanding the coping of inner-city children also requires consideration of issues related to evaluating coping styles. In addition to developing a sound typology of coping styles for this population, there is need to consider how best to measure the impact of styles and the relation of style to impact. Coping style can be defined as the preferred method or methods of coping when facing a given stressor. The fact that people respond with a variety of methods to any given stressor suggests that stylistic differences can be important dimensions for understanding the relation between coping and adjustment. For example, the use of avoidant strategies has been shown to relate to poorer outcome for adolescents compared to other styles (Ebata & Moos, 1991), but the relations of style to distress and behavior also have been shown to differ depending on the type of stress (Wills, 1986).

Although there may be a relation between style and effectiveness, it is not a one-to-one relation and it is not consistent across settings and stressors (Tolan, Montaini, & Gorman-Smith, 1996). For example, we found the effectiveness rating of a given style of coping ranged from .00 to .40 in magnitude depending on which two stressors were compared. In addition, the range of coping responses in a person's repertoire or the fit of response to the stressor faced may be important determinants of coping impact.

For inner-city children, coping style may depend less on individual differences and more on situational demands (Slavin, Rainer, McCreary, & Gowda, 1991). It may be more useful to understand what types of stress elicit what types of coping and how effective different responses are for a given set of stressors. For example, the use of avoidant strategies has been shown to increase as control decreases (Altshuler & Ruble, 1989; Band & Weisz, 1988). Given conditions of chronic environmental stress, it seems likely that inner-city children are less able to exert control over stressors and may be more likely to rely on avoidant strategies, regardless of individual tendencies. This style may be adaptive but not effective in the long run. Thus, the available typologies of children's coping styles have not been well-tested, and even less attention has been paid to their applicability for inner-city children.

A Model for Differentiating Coping Styles of Inner-City Youth

Although there is extensive study of coping in children and adolescents, there has been limited investigation of coping of inner-city youth. A survey of the existing studies finds some variation in the number of types of coping identified and the labeling of the different types found (see Tolan, Gorman-Smith, et al., 1996, for a fuller discussion of these issues). Our review of the literature suggested several possible models to apply, but none were empirically demonstrated to be superior to the others or to be particularly applicable to inner-city youth. For example, as has occurred in adult studies, some studies of adolescents and children differentiate coping as either emotion focused or problem solving (Compas, 1987). Others have suggested three factors, differentiating approach (problem solving) from avoidance (emotion focused) and appraisal (Moos & Billings, 1982). One can find instances of up to 12 to 15 factors (Patterson & McCubbin, 1987; Phelps & Jarvis, 1994). Sandler, Tein, and West (1994) have recently reported a factor analytic test of alternative theoretical models of children's coping. Although the children studied were not from urban poor backgrounds, the confirmed model had categories similar to those found in studies of urban youth (Phelps & Jarvis, 1994; Wills, 1986). The four types were derived from ten subscales and are labeled active, avoidant, distraction, and social support seeking. Distraction was distinguished from avoidant, in that the former involved engaging in some alternative activity, while the latter involved purposely not thinking about a problem (Ayers, 1991; Sandler et al., 1994). Others have also suggested a similar set of four factors (Kurdek & Sinclair, 1988; Phelps & Jarvis, 1994). In addition to these types, one can also find some cross-study evidence for differentiating seeking support from seeking guidance and for differentiating positive thinking or optimism from other problem-solving and appraisal methods (see Tolan, Gorman-Smith, et al., 1996, for a review). These seven types of coping (active problem solving, avoidance, distraction, support seeking, seeking guidance, positive thinking) may be basic dimensions or may fit some fewer dimensions in accord with competing theoretical views (Compas et al., 1992; Sandler et al., 1994). However, there has been no clear direction about which alternative model is the dimensional structure most useful for conceptualizing and measuring coping reported by inner-city youth.

As a first step in testing alternative models, we applied a carefully developed questionnaire about coping preferences (the A-COPES) (Patterson & McCubbin, 1987) to see which of several competing models provide the best fit to the data. Responses from 309 11- to 16-year-old adolescents drawn from inner-city neighborhoods of two large midwestern cities were used. The sample comprised 51% males and 49% females, 60% African American, 22% Hispanic, and 18% Caucasian. We first attempted to extract two-, three-, and seven-factor solutions from the data. A two-factor solution based on the Folkman and Lazarus (1988) distinction of problem-solving versus emotion-focused styles accounted for only 21% of the variance and the content of items loading on each factor was not coherent across items. Similarly, a three-factor solution based on the Moos and Billings (1982) approach (problem-focused or approach behaviors, emotion-focused, and appraisal/avoidance) explained only 26% of the variance and had little conceptual coherence.

The scree plot of an exploratory factor analysis suggested that eight-factors accounting for 42% of the item variance was optimal. However, all but one of the items on the eighth factor loaded at least well on other factors. The content of each of seven remaining factors was consistent with the types listed above as identified across studies, with one exception: there was not a specific problem-solving scale. Several scales correlated in a manner that suggested there was an underlying emotion-focused component. Finally, humor emerged as a separate factor (Phelps & Jarvis, 1994). These results led to the identification of seven first-order factor scales: Seeking Support, Seeking Guidance, Positive Thinking, Venting, Distraction, Avoidance by Substance Use, and Humor.

Table 1 lists the items loading on each scale and other basic scale characteristics. This model was then replicated (χ^2 (116) = 352.78, p = .08, (RMSR) = .09) using data collected 1 year later from a subsample of the samples used for the exploratory analysis (see Tolan, Gorman-Smith, et al., 1996, for details). Sample size prevented testing the factor structure by group. Correlation coefficients between scales differed little by ethnic group, gender, or age. However, some differences were found in relative reliance on some types of coping. Post hoc, Bonferroni-corrected means comparisons suggested that African Americans reported more use of Support Seeking and Seeking Guidance than non-Hispanic whites and Hispanics; non-Hispanic whites reported more use of Avoidance than the other two groups; while Hispanics reported less use of Venting than the other two ethnic groups. The single significant gender differ-

Table 1. Characteristics of the Seven First-Order Coping Scales

1. *Seeking Support M* = 3.21 *SD* = .86 (α = .73, Eigenvalue = 7.35, 13.6% of variance)
   .69 Go along with parents requests and rules
   .72 Do things with your family
   .64 Try to reason with parents and talk things out; compromise
   .72 Talk to your mother about what bothers you
   .55 Apologize to people
2. *Venting M* = 2.78 *SD* = .89 (α = .72, Eigenvalue = 4.16, 7.7% of variance)
   .69 Blame others for what is going wrong
   .71 Let off steam by complaining to family members
   .68 Get angry and yell at people
   .68 Say mean things to people; be sarcastic
   .63 Let off steam by complaining to your friends
3. *Avoidance by Substance Use M* = 1.50 *SD* = .81 (α = .73, Eigenvalue = 2.57, 4.8% of variance)
   .80 Drink beer, wine, or liquor
   .76 Use drugs (not prescribed by a doctor)
   .80 Smoke
4. *Distraction M* = 2.98 *SD* = .89 (α = .69, Eigenvalue = 2.35, 4.3% of variance)
   .71 Play video games
   .73 Do a strenuous physical activity
   .66 Work on a hobby you have
   .55 Get more involved in activities at school
   .54 Get a job or work harder at one
5. *Positive Thinking M* = 3.51 *SD* = .84 (α = .63, Eigenvalue = 1.95, 3.6% of variance)
   .64 Try to improve yourself (get body into shape, get good grades, etc.)
   .61 Try to think of the good things in your life
   .54 Try to see the good things in a difficult situation
6. *Seeking Guidance M* = 2.24 *SD* = .80 (α = .64, Eigenvalue = 1.63, 3.0% of variance)
   .70 Talk to teacher or counselor at school about what bothers you
   .58 Talk to a minister/priest/rabbi
   .63 Talk to your father about what bothers you
   .79 Pray
7. *Humor M* = 3.20 *SD* = 1.12 (α = .64, Eigenvalue = 1.52, 2.8% of variance)
   .9 Try to be funny and make light of it all
   .60 Joke and keep a sense of humor

ence was that males reported more use of Distraction. A trend was noted for females to report more use of Seeking Guidance and less of Humor. Age comparisons showed that the younger group (11–13) showed higher use of Seeking Support and a lower use of Avoidance. Also, the 14-year-old group showed more Venting than either those younger or older than this age.

When we then applied higher-order confirmatory factor analysis to test a problem-solving versus emotion-focused three-factor model (approach, avoidance, and appraisal model) and a four-factor model (problem solving, emotion focused, support seeking, and distraction), we found the best-fitting model by conventional criteria was the two-factor model of problem-solving and emotion-focused dimensions (χ^2 = 368.76, p = .05, RMSR = .07). Notably, the scales loading on the Problem-Solving factor were not just items reflecting direct action, but also included seeking aid and guidance from others, hence the label Problem Solving rather than Problem Focused. Also, some of the measured scales loaded on both factors (e.g., Positive Thinking, Avoidance,

Distraction). However, the latent factors did not correlate significantly otherwise ($r = .10$). The relation between these two underlying dimensions is represented by their simultaneous contributions to some of the measured scales.
This may reveal a fine but important distinction in understanding the relations
among coping styles. Many reflect multiple underlying dimensions. Fig. 2 illustrates that model.

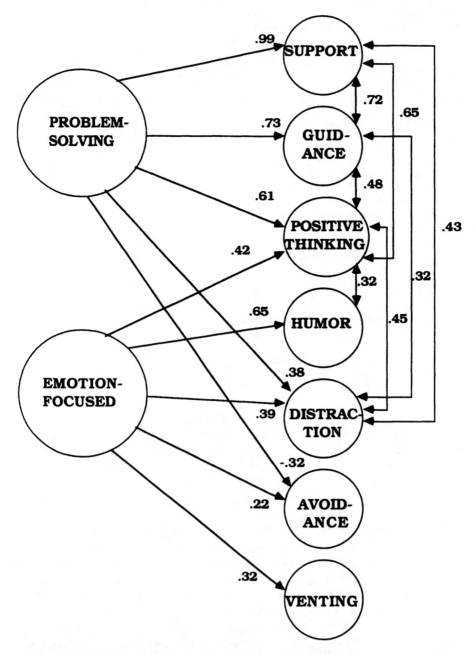

Figure 2. Confirmatory factor analysis model for coping: Higher-order two-factor model.

This model was developed from a dispositional questionnaire that inventoried the relative reliance on a list of different coping responses and emphasized general preference. The value of the model for evaluating situation-specific coping responses was tested in a second study by Tolan, Montaini, and Gorman-Smith (1996) that used interviews of inner-city adolescent males and tapped specific coping responses to specific stressors. These interviews asked subjects about experience of a standardized list of 38 stressors in the last year. When subjects reported experiencing a given stressor, they were then asked what they did "to deal with it, to make themselves feel better, or to make it better" (Tolan & Gorman-Smith, 1990). The sample comprised 315 13- to 15-year-old inner-city young adolescent males and their families. Seventy-five percent of the sample came from families living below the poverty level and 62% were from single-parent families. The sample was 53% African American and 47% Latino (primarily Mexican-Americans). Coping responses were coded for style using the seven categories of Tolan, Gorman-Smith, et al. (1996). They were also coded independently for effectiveness, using a four-point scale that focused on the extent to which the coping ended a stressor or prevented its reoccurrence. In addition, a range of coping score was calculated that represented the number of different types of coping used (0–7).

The most frequently used coping methods were distraction (used 39.7% of the time) and positive thinking (used 24.6% of the time). The least frequently used method was avoidance by substance use. The range of styles used was normally distributed and the median score was 3. These characteristics are consistent with the trends found in the dispositional questionnaire study (Tolan, Gorman-Smith, et al., 1996).

Three specific questions were addressed concerning inner-city children's and adolescents' coping. First, we examined the consistency of style or type of coping used across different types of stressors. Second, we examined the relation of effectiveness to extent of use of each style. Stressors were 38 items categorized into life events, daily hassles, and developmental and induced life transactions (changes in life circumstance) (see Tolan et al., 1988). The latter two categories included items that would fit chronic environmental stress and role strain under the stress categorization offered in this chapter. Third, we examined whether styles used and effectiveness were independent contributors to explaining distress and behavior (see Tolan et al. 1996 for details of data analyses). In regard to the first question, the results indicated that there was substantial variation in the type of coping used for responding to different stressors within a given category and even more variation in coping across types of stressors by a given respondent. In fact, the data suggested that an individual's coping methods were not very consistent across stressors. Distraction was used more and emotional venting was used less when facing induced transitions in life circumstances (e.g., parental unemployment). Traumatic events were responded to with seeking support, seeking guidance, and distraction more than other types of coping. Also, positive thinking and emotional venting were used more for this type of stressor than other types. Despite these large and more consistent differences due to stress type, there were significant differences among individuals in type of response used when facing a similar type of stress (see Tolan et al. 1996). Thus, there appears to be differential reliance on coping methods depending on the type of stress faced and this difference seems more substantial than that attributable to individual differences. However, for each type of stress there was evidence of a significant difference among youth in their tendency to use a given coping style. These results suggest that stressor plus individual proclivity need to be considered in evaluating coping styles of inner-city youth.

The Relation of Effectiveness to Style

Examining the relation of coping effectiveness and style, we found that there was substantial variation in the rating of effectiveness for a given coping style depending on the stress type. For example, responses coded as positive thinking were scored as significantly more effective for developmental transitions than other types of stress. Responses coded as support seeking were rated as significantly more effective when in response to daily hassles than support seeking used with traumatic life events or induced life transitions.

To evaluate whether effectiveness and style made independent contributions to explaining functioning, we entered both in regression analyses predicting distress (self-reported depression) and behavior problems (antisocial behavior). In these analyses coping type was entered as number of types reported (range of coping responses). Less effective coping and smaller range of coping were related to higher depression. Only range of coping predicted antisocial behavior. However, in both cases, the variance explained by the model was small (5% for each outcome). This level of explained variance is consistent with a finding from a previous study of coping as a main effect for inner-city youth (Davis, 1990). This level of relation suggests that coping style and effectiveness may be better considered as one part of a stress, coping, and support model than as the primary determinants of inner-city children's adaptation or outcome.

This study suggests that for inner-city children, the coping methods used and their effectiveness are heavily dependent on the type of stress faced. In addition, the study provides evidence that style and effectiveness are two related but distinct dimensions of coping. These findings, however, do not address questions about the role of coping in a stress–support–coping model for inner-city children.

The Interaction of Stress Type, Support, and Coping Dimensions

In a third study, Blitz, Tolan, and DelBoca (1995) evaluated the moderating role of coping for different types of stressors. This study was prompted by the consistent finding that among inner-city youth coping is weakly correlated with symptom levels, once previous status or other competing predictors are considered (Davis, 1990). It may be that a focus on coping as a main effect will lead to a picture of coping as an insignificant consideration in evaluating functioning. As we have suggested here, among inner-city children the situational constraints, levels and complexity of stressors, and the limited efficacy of commonly effective coping methods could lead to coping methods having low correlation to functioning. In this study, we evaluated the relation of coping style and effectiveness to outcome as a function of stressor type, support available, and locus of control.

Subjects were 161 African-American (51% males, 49% females), 11- to 15-year-old inner-city children from two large midwestern cities. This is a subsample of the subjects used to develop and test the seven factor/two-dimension model of coping in the first study (Tolan, Gorman-Smith, et al., 1996). Two interviews were conducted at 1-year intervals to prospectively evaluate the moderating impact of coping effectiveness (rated 1 to 5), coping style (the seven factors), and social support (network size, peer vs. overall network, network density). In addition, locus of control (internal/external) was also considered as a moderator. Subjects reported stress experience on a standardized stress questionnaire (Tolan et al., 1988) and completed a coping disposition questionnaire. Coping effectiveness was tapped by asking subjects to report likely responses to eight common interpersonal dilemmas. Responses were coded for extent to which they would resolve the problem or prevent further occurrence. Coping range was also computed. The fourfold differentiation of type of stress used in the other two studies was applied here: normal expectable developmental transitions, induced transitions that change life circumstance, life events, and daily hassles (Tolan et al., 1988), because this differentiation was originally based on a conceptual distinction of the likely impact on functioning and the types of coping likely to be required by each of these four types of stress (see Tolan et al., 1988; Tolan, Cromwell, & Brasswell, 1986, for a fuller discussion). This differentiation varies from that espoused in this chapter. Thus, the direct transferability to the framework suggested here may be limited.

This study was intended to test how coping interacts with support and stress type (three-way interactions) in determining later functioning among inner-city children, applying moderated regression analysis (Aiken & West, 1991). All analyses were carried out prospectively, controlling for the status on the dependent variable at time one. The focus of moderated regression analysis is on how two- and three-way moderator interactions relate to differential status on dependent variables.

In moderated regression, significant bivariate correlations between the primary independent variable (stress) and the dependent variable are expected, while nonsignificant bivariate correlations between the moderator variable and the outcome are expected. This occurred for each instance in these data. Stress levels correlated to subsequent levels of distress and behavior problems, controlling for previous levels. Correlations ranged from .04 to .36, depending on the type of stress and whether the outcome was distress or behavior problems. All relations were statistically significant except for the relation of development transitions to behavior problems. Similarly, controlling for previous stress level, distress and behavior problems predicted later stress level for all four types of stress ($r = .25$ to .38). Most time-one moderator variables had correlations to the time-two criterion variables that were close to zero ($r = -.07$ to .18). Thus, from a traditional analytic perspective, coping effectiveness and range, social support, and locus of control would seem to be of little use in understanding subsequent symptomology.

However, when considered as interacting moderators with specific relations for each type of stress, several significant relationships emerged. For example, locus of control, size of peer network, and coping effectiveness each moderate the impact of developmental stress on subsequent internalizing problems (distress). Similarly, the relation of daily hassles to distress was moderated by each of these three variables. Further, although behavior problems were more likely when there was more developmental stress, that relation was moderated by an internal locus of control, greater coping effectiveness, and a larger social support network.

When interactions between support and coping as moderators of the stress–outcome relation were tested, two of the eight showed significant interaction terms. Coping range, in interaction with network size, moderated the level of later behavior problems among subjects experiencing higher levels of daily hassles. Apparently, among these subjects, a restricted range of coping and a smaller support network led to more behavior problems. The second significant relation was for the interaction of coping effectiveness and network size as moderators of the relationship between level of developmental transitions and further behavior problems. Among subjects with higher rates of developmental transitions, those with more support and more effective coping report less subsequent distress. Thus, the role of coping seems to interact with social support levels when higher levels of stress are occurring.

Overall, these results suggest that coping effectiveness can play a role in moderating stress impact on symptomology among inner-city children. However, it appears this is limited to daily hassles and developmental transitions. Perhaps the major implication of this study is to illustrate that the role of coping is complex and depends on the type and level of stress being faced, as well as other characteristics such as prior functioning and support available.

Implications for Coping of Inner-City Children and Adolescents

This set of studies started with identifying seven types of coping that represent two underlying dimensions (problem solving and emotion focused). The specific types of coping in this model are consistent with several other studies, although not replicating results of any one study (e.g., Compas et al., 1992). Notably, several of the seven factors load on both underlying dimensions, suggesting that during adolescence some coping responses have problem-solving as well as emotion-focused functions. The second study showed that the coping methods used vary considerably by stress faced, although there were some consistent differences in individuals' preferred methods. Also, the effectiveness of coping varied by stress type. The third study placed coping effectiveness and range of types used within a multivariate model as moderators of stress experienced and support available and comoderators with support. Coping range may interact with good support to help lessen the impact of daily hassles, while effectiveness may interact with support level to ease normal developmental transitions. These initial analyses highlight the need to evaluate context, stressor type, and coping range and effectiveness in understanding the development of inner-city children and youth.

FAMILY AND DEVELOPMENTAL INFLUENCES

In addition to the issues of setting constraints, stress types and levels, and coping dimensions and characteristics, understanding inner-city children also requires consideration of the role of the family and developmental aspects of coping (Gorman-Smith, Tolan, & Henry, in press). Although these factors are essential in understanding coping of children from any setting, there are issues in each area that are particularly relevant for inner-city children.

Family as Buffer

Among the family characteristics that have been cited as mitigating the stress of inner-city life for children are family resourcefulness, adaptability, and structure (McAdoo, 1982), the development of reliable and effective social ties (McAdoo, 1982), and protective parenting styles (Clark, 1983; Ogbu, 1985). Staples (1978) notes that historically, African-American families have provided their members with a sanctuary that buttresses against pervasive oppression and racism (Mason, Cauce, Gonzales, Hiraga, & Grove, 1994). Another commonly cited form of buffering is the extended family and informal kin networks (Massey, Scott, & Dornbusch, 1975). Compas et al. (1992) suggest that a well-functioning family may protect an inner-city child from the deleterious effects of stress, although they note this has not been carefully evaluated.

Parent practices have demonstrated a relation to stress impact, although there have been few specific studies of buffering effects of inner-city children. Most studies of this sample have focused on the adjacent question of how poor family practices can result from inner-city conditions or can mediate poverty effects on antisocial behavior (Dodge, Pettit, & Bates, 1994; McLoyd, Jayaratne, Ceballo, & Borquez, 1994). Bradley et al. (1994) showed that responsive, accepting, and stimulating parental care promoted resilience among low-birthweight premature children living in poverty. However, direct examples of stress buffering are yet to be produced.

There is a particular need to understand how family coping relates to adolescent coping (Tolan et al., 1995). There are studies of non-inner-city youth that may be relevant. Hardy, Power, and Jaedicke (1993) report that family support was related to a more restricted range of types of coping used and more reliance on avoidance when in uncontrollable situations. Also, as family control increased, the use of aggressive coping decreased. In another study, Tolan (1988) found that high stress and low family cohesion interacted to predict antisocial behavior. However, a needed additional step is to test the effects of family characteristics on adolescent coping and to focus on multiple outcomes.

Family Coping

In addition to the buffering and refuge from harm that families can provide, inner-city families may enhance the coping of children by teaching them strategies for survival, methods of mutual support, and by fighting myths of society (Massey et al., 1975). Also, the individual coping of children usually occurs within constraints of family functioning and as part of family functioning. For example, Peters (1976) found that most parents of African-American children reported they expected their child to encounter racism by age 6, but felt uncertain about how to prepare the child or how to help him or her cope with it. Although it was clear that parents saw racism as an inevitable stressor, they also reported fears about influencing the children to be overly self-conscious about race and racism. Their primary strategy was to delay the encounter as long as possible. Thus, effectiveness was compromised because the stress could not be prevented or prepared for adequately. Coping for both families and children becomes oriented toward minimizing actual and potential harm.

Parental Distress

Impaired parental functioning can result from the same high level of difficult stressors that children face, and so can limit parents' ability to aid children with their coping (McLoyd, 1990). Since seeking support and guidance from family is a highly used coping response of inner-city youth, parental distress and impairment are important considerations in evaluating and attempting to aid children's coping. Parental distress can be due to marital conflict, parental psychopathology, or other stressors. For example, Pearlin (1983) reported a correlation between level of life stress events and parental role strain. Coping responses of acquiring social support, mobilizing family to seek help, and passive appraisal showed a moderating effect on maternal distress. However, acquiring social support was the only response that related to lower problems in boys, and this same response related to increased problems for girls. McLoyd et al. (1994) demonstrated that economic distress can disrupt parental practices. Similar results were reported by Myers, Taylor, Alvy, Arrington, and Richardson (1992). They found that high family stress related to maternal psychological distress and both predicted behavior problems in inner-city children. Family involvement in shared recreational activities seemed to moderate stress effects for boys but exacerbated problems for girls. No family coping method offered protection against risk. Reframing the problem related to more behavior problems, and activity seeking helped boys but hurt girls.

IMPLICATIONS FOR FURTHER RESEARCH

As we noted at the outset of this chapter, children growing up in the inner city face elevated levels of stressful life events and daily hassles against a background of ongoing chronic environmental problems and role strain. In this context, much of their coping must be oriented toward avoiding harm or minimizing potential damage. The stressful situations often demand judgmental acuity that is beyond what is reasonable to expect of a child, and the consequences of inept responding can be deadly. All of this occurs with fewer resources, less adult supervision, and less control than other children have. Thus, the process of coping can be less direct, with the impact of a given response more dependent on circumstance and timing. The overall impact can be that coping is experienced less as an active controlling of stress and more as managing fate and capitalizing on any good luck one might encounter (Rothbaum, Weisz, & Snyder, 1982).

We have attempted to synthesize existing research and theory to suggest that if coping is a matter of staying out of harm's way, then the existing coping typologies may not be appropriate. However, as there are only a limited number of studies that specifically target coping of inner-city youth, the proposed framework is as dependent on rational evaluation as empirical support. Nevertheless, we propose a conceptual model, which identifies four major types of stress and seven common coping styles, that differentiates adaptiveness and effectiveness of coping and focuses on coping as a moderator of other risk influences. Some preliminary studies suggest that children's coping may be only a small part of what determines their outcome, and its effect may depend on the type of stress, the support and resources available, and other setting characteristics. This promising but thin strain highlights the need for more research examining this topic. Three particular areas of immediate need can be identified.

First, there is a need to cross-validate or delimit the coping schema reported in Tolan and colleagues (Tolan, Gorman-Smith, et al., 1996; Tolan et al., 1996) and Blitz et al. (1995). More generally, there is a need to determine if this model can be replicated with other inner-city and other non-inner-city samples. In addition to these validity analyses, the initial results suggest that it would be advisable for studies of coping of inner-city youth to include evaluation of stress types, differentiated along dimensions suggested here: chronic environmental stress, role strain, life events and transitions, and daily hassles.

Second, there is a need to link child and adolescent coping to family functioning and family coping (Tolan & Gorman-Smith, 1997). We suggest this will best be done if investigations move from a perspective that views inner-city families as lacking skills or motivations of families in higher socioeconomic levels to one of families struggling to prevail in a hostile and unpredictable environment (Mason et al., 1994). This would not ignore effects of deficits, but would shift our focus to issues of coping for the majority of families living in these settings. Accordingly, there is a need to evaluate children's coping as a component of and perhaps a reflection of the family struggle (Tolan & Gorman-Smith, 1997). Most prominently, there is a need for studies that can test for the buffering effects of good family functioning. Although not a direct test of this, our comparison of family functioning and stress effects on antisocial behavior suggests families may not be able to buffer stress effects in the inner-city (Gorman-Smith et al., in press).

Another area of needed research is to determine the relation of adaptive coping to effective coping. We have suggested that for children in the inner city, coping that is adaptive in the short term may not be effective in the long term. It would be important to determine if this holds empirically, and if so to determine under what circumstances short-term adaptive responses can be effective in the long term. Establishing this connection may provide a great deal of direction about how coping-based interventions might aid inner-city youth. One potential link is to try to relate preferred styles (e.g., distraction, support seeking) as part of a process leading to more effective coping. For example, children and adolescents can be trained to seek support from prosocial and more dependable peers and adults, making this adaptive style more effective. By developing the effectiveness of a naturally preferred coping method, coping can go beyond merely maintaining adaptation and escaping harm.

The third area of needed additional research is bringing contextual factors such as violence, economic deprivation, and inadequate schools into coping models (Gorman-Smith et al., 1996). How do inner-city children cope with unsafe neighborhoods and inadequate schools? How does the presence of a good school, a neighborhood block watch, or a rising level of gang tensions affect coping methods used and their effects? These events and setting characteristics are rarely included in models of coping, but their relevance to understanding inner-city children's coping is obvious. In particular, such studies will provide needed specificity about practical issues in applying a coping perspective.

IMPLICATIONS FOR INTERVENTION

Most coping interventions for children emphasize cognitive training, education, and/or more effective use of social support (Dahlquist, 1992). Not surprisingly, most focus on a specific stressor (e.g., medical problems, parental divorce). Thus, the source of the need to cope can be directly ascertained and the goal fully specified. Also, the preferred effect of coping is to minimize the harmful impact or remove the stressor (Compas et al., 1992). However, it is not clear what strategies would provide such effects for inner-city youth. Most obviously, moving out of the inner city or obtaining massive economic reforms are the two "coping" responses that fit common criteria for effective coping and toward which interventions might be directed. However, these are obviously not realistic options for most inner-city children. Similarly, interventions that are meant to manage stressors beyond the child's control (e.g., parental divorce, serious illness, or death) may not be appropriate for children in the inner city. These approaches are usually focused on a single event or life transition for a targeted audience. Helping with coping in the inner city may require understanding how multiple coping methods with multiple stressors are organized. For example, how should skills to face precipitous but common life events be taught along with skills to minimize the demoralization and dangers of chronic environmental stress? Thus, although there are some analogous areas of intervention research and technology that can be drawn from, their applicability to the inner-city setting and its stressors is yet to be determined.

Although there are few interventions that focus exclusively on improving coping with the stressors of inner-city life, one can find elements of common coping intervention strategies in many existing interventions. Many of the preventive interventions frequently evaluated in inner-city settings have intended effects that could enhance coping (Guerra, 1994). Many of the social skills training and social problem-solving programs used in schools and community agencies are designed to increase effective responding to social dilemmas and the situational stressors of daily life (Tolan & Guerra, 1994). For example, conflict management programs often teach children methods of weighing the utility of alternative responses to challenges from others or temptations to break rules. Generating alternative solutions and weighing consequences seem to be likely to aid coping (Goldstein & Pentz, 1984; Guerra, Huesmann, & Hanish, 1995). Similarly, cognitively oriented programs that increase the ability to empathize with or see the perspective of others should also aid problem-solving skills and effective coping (Crick & Dodge, 1994). However, these programs have not been developed to specifically aid coping with the stressors of inner-city life. Similarly, there seems much promise in programs designed to enhance self-esteem, cultural pride, and political sophistication (Tolan & Guerra, 1994). They are likely to lead to more careful and planful responding to issues of safety, access to resources, and self-regard (Tolan & Guerra, 1994). It seems likely that such programs will increase the use of effective rather than adaptive coping responses. Manhood development programs and other approaches that use culture-based ethical guidance to cope with the daily stresses of inner-city life seem promising (Tolan & Guerra, 1994). However, tests of their effects as well as empirical tests of theorized models of how they aid coping and development are needed.

In addition to the aforementioned need to focus on children's coping as part of a family, it could be that family skills training interventions can also enhance coping by either reducing parental stress, family discord, and dysfunction or improving family coping skills (Tolan & Guerra, 1994). For example, it would be useful to determine if family interventions designed to improve parenting, family relations, or family problem-solving skills would improve child coping skills. Alternatively, it may be useful to shift family interventions for inner-city families to focus on coping methods in addition to improving parenting and family organization skills (Tolan & McKay, 1996).

However, we think these interventions are likely to have limited effects unless they are directly informed by recognition of the social characteristics of the inner city and the resulting orientation to limiting potential harm. It may be that the individual's coping should not be the primary target. Political and other societal-level interventions may be the better focus. Policies and activities that can decrease the economic and social isolation of the central cities and improve substandard conditions of basic resources such as housing, schools, and health care may be needed as a basic prerequisite for coping interventions to have a substantial impact on the elevated prevalence of the multiple problems facing inner-city youth. These programs are also likely to directly enhance children's coping by lessening the level of chronic environmental stress and role strain. By enabling children and families to redirect their coping resources toward daily hassles and life events that occur, such interventions may directly lead to more effective coping.

Interventions directed at simply improving children and families' coping or ability to escape harm, whether large scale or small scale, general or targeted, preventive or remedial, may not have a large impact on inner-city children in the absence of political and societal-level interventions. In analytic parlance, the interventions may not produce main effects, but rather may serve as moderators of an imposing fate. Just as children of the inner city come to concentrate their efforts on staying out of harm's way, without large-scale improvement in the safety, opportunity, and support these children receive, interventions may be limited to helping them delay pending harm rather than escaping or removing it.

ACKNOWLEDGMENT

Support for this work was provided by NIMH grants (RO1 MH48248 and R18 MH48034) and the University of Illinois Great Cities Institute Faculty Scholars Program. Correspondence should be addressed to the first author at the Institute for Juvenile Research, Department of Psychiatry, University of Illinois at Chicago, 907 S. Wolcott Avenue, Chicago, IL 60612.

REFERENCES

Aiken, L. S., & West, S. G. (1991). *Multiple regression: Testing and interpreting interactions.* Newbury Park, NJ: Sage.

Altshuler, J. L., & Ruble, D. N. (1989). Developmental changes in children's awareness of strategies for coping with uncontrollable stress. *Child Development, 60,* 1337–1349.

Anderson, L. P. (1991). Acculturative stress: A theory of relevance to black Americans. *Clinical Psychology Review, 11,* 685–702.

Attar, B. K., Guerra, N. G., & Tolan, P. H. (1994). Neighborhood disadvantage, stressful life events, and adjustment in urban elementary school children. *Journal of Consulting and Clinical Psychology, 23,* 391–400.

Ayers, T. S. (1991). *A dispositional and situational assessment of children's coping: Testing alternative theoretical models.* Unpublished doctoral dissertation, Arizona State University.

Band, E. B., & Weisz, J. R. (1988). How to feel better when it feels bad: Children's perspectives on coping with everyday stress. *Developmental Psychology, 24,* 247–253.

Bane, M. J., & Ellwood, D. T. (1989). One fifth of the nation's children: Why are they poor? *Science, 245,* 1047–1053.

Billings, A. G., & Moos, R. H. (1981). The role of coping responses and social resources in attenuating the stress of life events. *Journal of Behavioral Medicine, 4,* 139–157.

Blitz, C. C., Tolan, P. H., & DelBoca, F. K. (1995). *A prospective analysis of behavioral adjustment, stressful life events, and moderators for high-risk urban minority youth.* Unpublished doctoral dissertation, University of Illinois at Chicago.

Boykin, A. W. (1979). Black psychology and the research process: Keeping the baby but throwing out the bath water. In A. W. Boykin, A. J. Frankling, & J. F. Yates (Eds.), *Research directions of black psychologists* (pp. 25–53). New York: Sage.

Bradley, R. H., Whiteside, L., Mundfrom, D. J., Casey, P. H., Kelleher, K. J., & Pope, S. K. (1994). Early indications of resilience and their relation to experiences in the home environments of low birthweight, premature children living in poverty. *Child Development, 65,* 346–360.

Buss, T., & Redburn, F. S. (1983). *Mass unemployment: Plant closings and community mental health.* Beverly Hills, CA: Sage.

Centers for Disease Control. (1992). Behaviors related to unintentional and intentional injuries among high school students—United States, 1991. *Morbidity and Mortality Weekly Report, 41,* 760–765.

Clark, R. (1983). *Family life and school achievement: Why poor black children succeed or fail.* Chicago: University of Chicago Press.

Compas, B. E. (1987). Coping with stress during child and adolescence. *Psychological Bulletin, 101,* 393–403.

Compas, B. E., & Worsham, N. L. (1991, April). *When mom or dad has cancer: Developmental differences in children's coping with family stress.* Paper presented at the conference of the Society for Research on Child Development, Seattle, WA.

Compas, B. E., Worsham, N. L., & Ey, S. (1992). Conceptual and developmental issues in children's coping with stress. In A. M. LaGreca, L. J. Siegel, J. L. Wallander, & C. E. Walker (Eds.), *Stress and coping in child health* (pp. 4–24). New York: Guilford Press.

Connell, J. P., Spencer, M. B., & Aber, J. L. (1994). Educational risk and resilience in African-American youth: Context, self, action, and outcomes in school. *Child Development, 65,* 493–506.

Crick, N. R., & Dodge, K. R. (1994). A review and reformulation of social information-processing mechanisms in children's social adjustment. *Psychological Bulletin, 115,* 74–101.

Dahlquist, L. M. (1992). Coping with aversive medical treatments. In A. M. LaGreca, L. J. Siegel, J. L. Wallander, & C. E. Walker (Eds.), *Stress and coping in child health* (pp. 345–376). New York: Guilford Press.

Davis, L. A. (1990). *A stress and coping framework for the delinquency of high-risk African-American adolescents.* Unpublished doctoral dissertation, DePaul University, Chicago, IL.

Dodge, K. A., Pettit, G. S., & Bates, J. E. (1994). Socialization mediators of the relationship between socioeconomic status and child conduct problems. *Child Development, 65,* 649–665.

Dubow, E. F., Tisak, J., Causey, D., Hryshko, A., & Reid, G. (1991). A two-year longitudinal study of stressful life events, social support, and social problem-solving skills: Contributions to children's behavioral and academic adjustment. *Child Development, 62,* 583–599.

Ebata, A., & Moos, R. H. (1991). Coping and adjustment in distressed and healthy adolescents. *Journal of Applied and Developmental Psychology, 12,* 33–54.

Federal Bureau of Investigation. (1992). *Uniform crime reports.* Washington DC: U.S. Government.

Felner, R. D., Farber, S. S., & Primavera, J. (1983). Transitions and stressful life events: A model for primary prevention. In R. D. Felner, L. A. Jason, J. N. Moritsugu, & S. S. Farber (Eds.), *Preventive psychology: Theory, research and practice* (pp. 199–215). New York: Pergamon.

Florsheim, P., Tolan, P. H., & Gorman-Smith, D. (1996). Family processes and risk for externalizing behavior problems among African-American and Hispanic boys. *Journal of Consulting and Clinical Psychology, 64,* 1222–1230.

Folkman, S., & Lazarus, R. S. (1980). An analysis of coping in a middle-aged community sample. *Journal of Health and Social Behavior, 21,* 219–239.

Folkman, S., & Lazarus, R. S. (1988). *Manual for the ways of coping questionnaire, research edition.* Palo Alto: Consulting Psychologists Press.

Garbarino, J., Kostelny, K., & Dubrow, N. (1991). What children can tell us about living in danger. *American Psychologist, 46,* 376–383.

Goldstein, A. P., & Pentz, M. A. (1984). Psychological skill training and the aggressive adolescent. *School Psychology Review, 13,* 311–323.

Gordon, R. (1983). An operational definition of prevention. *Public Health Reports, 98,* 107–119.

Gorman-Smith, D., Tolan, P. H., & Henry, D. (in press). The relation of community and family to risk among urban poor adolescents. To be published in P. Cohen, L. Robins, & C. Slomskowski (Eds.), *Where and when: Influence of historical time and place on aspects of psychopathology.* Hillsdale, NJ: Erlbaum.

Gorman-Smith, D., Tolan, P. H., Zelli, A., & Huesmann, L. R. (1996). The relation of family functioning to violence among inner-city minority youth. *Journal of Family Psychology, 10,* 115–129.

Guerra, N. G. (in press). Intervening to prevent childhood aggression in the inner-city. In J. McCord (Ed.), *Growing up violent: Contributions of inner city life.* Cambridge: Cambridge University Press.

Guerra, N. G., Huesmann, L. R., & Hanish, L. (1995). The role of normative beliefs in children's social behavior. In N. Eisenberg (Ed.), *Review of personality and social psychology: Social development* (Vol. 15, pp. 140–158). Thousand Oaks, CA: Sage.

Hardy, D. F., Power, T. G., & Jaedicke, S. (1993). Examining the relation of parenting to children's coping with everyday stress. *Child Development, 64,* 1829–1841.

Jencks, C. (1992). *Rethinking social policy.* Cambridge, MA: Harvard University Press.

Kessler, R. (1979). Stress, social status and psychological distress. *Journal of Health and Social Behavior, 20,* 259–272.

Kessler, R., & Cleary, P. (1980). Social class and psychological distress. *American Sociological Review, 45,* 463–478.

Kessler, R., & Neighbors, H. (1986). A new perspective on the relationships among race, social class, and psychological distress. *Journal of Health and Social Behavior, 27,* 1078–115.

Kozol, J. (1992). *Savage inequalities.* New York: Harper Perennial.

Kurdek, L. A., & Sinclair, R. J. (1988). Adjustment of young adolescents in two-parent nuclear, stepfather, and mother-custody families. *Journal of Consulting and Clinical Psychology, 56,* 91–96.

Laosa, L. (1979). Social competence in childhood: Toward a developmental, socioculturally relativistic paradigm. In M. Kent & J. Rolf (Eds.), *Primary prevention of psychopathology: social competence in children* (pp. 301–340). Hanover, NH: University Press of New England.

Lazarus, R. S., & Folkman, S. (1984). *Stress, appraisal and coping.* New York: Springer.

Lindsey, D. (1994). *The welfare of children.* New York: Oxford University Press.

Mason, C. A., Cauce, A. M., Gonzales, N., Hiraga, Y., & Grove, K. (1994). An ecological model of externalizing behaviors in African-American adolescents: No family is an island. *Journal of Research on Adolescence, 4,* 639–655.

Massey, G. C., Scott, M., & Dornbusch, S. M. (1975). Racism without racists: Institutional racism in urban schools. *The Black Scholar, 7,* 3–10.

McAdoo, H. P. (1982). Stress absorbing systems in black families. *Family Relations, 31,* 479–488.

McLoyd, V. C. (1990). The impact of economic hardship on black families and children: Psychological distress, parenting, and socioemotional development. *Child Development, 61,* 311–346.

McLoyd, V. C., Jayaratne, T. E., Ceballo, R., & Borquez, J. (1994). Unemployment and work interruption among African-American mothers: Effects on parenting and adolescent socio-emotional functioning. *Child Development, 65,* 562–589.

Moos, R. H., & Billings, A. G. (1982). Conceptualizing and measuring coping resources and process. In L. Goldberger & S. Breznitz, S. (Eds.), *Handbook of stress: Theoretical and clinical aspects* (pp. 212–230). New York: Free Press.

Myers, H. F., Taylor, S., Alvy, K. T., Arrington, A., & Richardson, M. A. (1992). Parental and family predictors of behavior problems in inner-city black children. *American Journal of Community Psychology, 20,* 557–576.

National Commission on Children. (1991). *Beyond rhetoric: A new American agenda for children and families.* Final report. Washington, DC: Author.

National Institute of Justice. (1992, August). *Community policing in Seattle: A model partnership between citizens and police.* Washington, DC: Author.

Neff, J. A. (1985). Race and vulnerability to stress: An examination of differential vulnerability. *Journal of Personality and Social Psychology, 49,* 481–491.

Ogbu, J. (1985). A cultural ecology of competence among inner-city blacks. In M. B. Spencer, G. K. Brookins, & W. R. Allen (Eds.), *Beginnings: The social and affective development of black children* (pp. 45–66). Hillsdale, NJ: Erlbaum.

Patterson, J. M., & McCubbin, H. I. (1987). Adolescent coping style and behaviors: Conceptualization and measurement. *Journal of Adolescence, 10,* 163–186.

Pearlin, L. I. (1983). Role strain and personal stress. In H. Kaplan (Ed.), *Psychosocial stress* (pp. 76–91). New York: Academic Press.

Peters, M. F. (1976). *Nine black families: A study of household management and childrearing in black families with working mothers.* Ann Arbor, MI: University Microfilms.

Peters, M. F., & Massey, G. (1983). Mundane extreme environmental stress in family stress theories: The case of black families in white America. *Marriage and Family Review, 6,* 193–218.

Phelps, S. B., & Jarvis, P. A. (1994). Coping in adolescence: Empirical evidence for a theoretically based approach to assessing coping. *Journal of Youth and Adolescence, 23,* 359–371.

Pierce, C. (1975). The mundane extreme environment and its effect on learning. In S. G. Brainard (Ed.), *Learning disabilities: Issues and recommendations for research* (pp. 41–64). Washington, DC: National Institute of Education.

Rothbaum, F., Weisz, J., & Snyder. (1982). Ideas of secondary control. *Journal of Personality and Social Psychology, 42*, 5–37.

Sampson, R. J., & Laub, J. H. (1994). *Urban poverty and the family context of delinquency: A new look at structure and process in a class study. Child Development, 65*, 523–540.

Sandler, I. N., Tein, J.-Y., & West, S. G. (1994). *Coping, stress and the psychological symptoms of children of divorce: A cross-sectional and longitudinal study.* Unpublished manuscript.

Slavin, L. A., Rainer, K. L., McCreary, M. L., & Gowda, K. K. (1991). Toward a multicultural model of stress process. *Journal of Counseling and Development, 70*, 156–163.

Spencer, M. B., Dobbs, B., & Swanson, D. P. (1988). African American adolescents: Adaptational processes and socio-economic diversity in behavioral outcomes. *Journal of Adolescence, 11*, 117–137.

Staples, R. (1978). *The black family: Essays and studies.* Belmont, CA: Wadsworth.

Tolan, P. H. (1988). Socioeconomic, family, and social stress correlates of adolescents' antisocial and delinquent behavior. *Journal of Abnormal Child Psychology, 16*, 317–332.

Tolan, P. H., Cromwell, R. E., & Brasswell, M. (1986). The application of family therapy to juvenile delinquency: A critical review of literature. *Family Process, 25*, 619–649.

Tolan, P. H., & Gorman-Smith, D. (1990). *The Chicago Stress and Coping Interview.* Technical Report. Chicago: University of Illinois.

Tolan, P. H., & Gorman-Smith, D. (in press). Families and the development of urban children. In O. Reyes, H. Walberg, & R. Weissberg (Eds.), *Interdisciplinary perspectives on children and youth* (pp. 67–91). Newberry Park, CA: Sage.

Tolan, P. H., Gorman-Smith, D., Chung, K., & Hunt, M. (1996). *Styles of coping of inner-city youth.* Manuscript submitted for publication.

Tolan, P. H., Montaini, L., & Gorman-Smith, D. (1996). *Stress type and individual differences in coping.* Manuscript available from author.

Tolan, P. H., & Guerra, N. G. (1994). *What works in reducing adolescent violence: An empirical review of the field.* Monograph prepared for the Center for the Study and Prevention of Youth Violence. Boulder: University of Colorado.

Tolan, P. H., Guerra, N. G., & Kendall, P. G. (1995). A developmental–ecological perspective on antisocial behavior in children and adolescents: Toward a unified risk and intervention framework. *Journal of Consulting and Clinical Psychology, 63*, 579–584.

Tolan, P. H., Henry, D., Guerra, N. G., VanAcker, R., Huesmann, L. R., & Eron, L. (1996). *Patterns of psychopathology in inner city children I: Gender, ethnicity, age, and location trends.* Manuscript submitted for publication.

Tolan, P. H., & McKay, M. M. (1996). Preventing serious antisocial behavior in inner-city children: An empirically based family prevention program. *Family Relations, 45*, 148–155.

Tolan, P. H., Miller, L., & Thomas, P. (1988). Perception and experience of types of social stress and self-image among adolescents. *Journal of Youth and Adolescence, 17*, 147–163.

Ulbrich, P. M., Warheit, G. J., & Zimmerman, R. S. (1989). Race, socioeconomic status, and psychological distress: An examination of differential vulnerability. *Journal of Health and Social Behavior, 30*, 131–146.

Wills, T. A. (1986). Stress and coping in early adolescence: Relationships to substance abuse in urban school samples. *Health Psychology, 5*, 503–529.

Wilson, W. J. (1987). *The truly disadvantaged: The inner city, the underclass, and public policy.* Chicago: University of Chicago Press.

17

Stress and Coping in an Ethnic Minority Context
Children's Cultural Ecologies

NANCY A. GONZALES and LAUREN S. KIM

Because ethnic minority children are disproportionately exposed to stressful life conditions such as family poverty, diminished community resources, and racial discrimination, minority children as a group are assumed to be at increased risk for mental health problems. This assumption derives apparent support from the numerous social problems that are reported to occur to a greater extent within some minority communities: school dropout, teenage parenthood, alcohol and substance use, juvenile delinquency, and youth violence. In fact, however, very little is known about the mental health status of ethnic and racial minority children in the United States, including why some minority children may be at greater risk than others for poor mental health.

If minority children are at increased risk for mental health problems, it is plausible, and generally assumed, that this heightened vulnerability is almost exclusively a function of poverty. Under this hypothesis, if the effects of socioeconomic status were empirically controlled in studies that compare majority and minority youths, ethnic group differences in mental health status should be eliminated. However, it is also possible that minority status itself constitutes an independent risk factor because it exposes children to a number of challenging life conditions: Minority youths may experience both subtle and overt forms of racism and discrimination and conflicts that arise when they are caught between cultures that have differing values and norms (Phinney, Lochner, & Murphy, 1991). Such ethnicity-linked stressors may complicate development to varying degrees for minority youths at all socioeconomic lev-

NANCY A. GONZALES and LAUREN S. KIM • Department of Psychology, Arizona State University, Tempe, Arizona 85287-1104.

Handbook of Children's Coping: Linking Theory and Intervention, edited by Wolchik and Sandler. Plenum Press, New York, 1997.

els. On the other hand, it is also possible that some ethnic minority children are less vulnerable to psychological distress because of ethnic-specific coping mechanisms or cultural influences that protect them from the negative effects of stress. Such protective mechanisms may have evolved for some groups in response to cumulative indignities endured as minorities, or may stem from traditional cultural values that are maintained even as ethnic individuals acculturate to the dominant culture (Spencer, 1990).

This chapter explores the foregoing possibilities through a review and analysis of the literature on the mental health status of ethnic minority children and adolescents. First, we provide a brief demographic profile of the four major ethnic and racial groups identified as distinct categories in the United States. For each group, we then provide a critical review of epidemiological data on the prevalence of emotional and behavioral difficulties for children under the age of 18, followed by a summary of the literature on risk and protective factors.* Consistent with a life stress theoretical perspective, we give specific attention to studies regarding the nature and impact of stress experienced by ethnic minority children and to the literature on children's coping. The chapter closes with a review of culturally sensitive preventive interventions for minority youth.

DEFINING AND STUDYING ETHNICITY

For purposes of this review, the term "ethnic minority" refers to a citizen of the United States who is African American, Hispanic, American Indian or Alaska Native, or Asian American or Pacific Islander.† These four racial and ethnic categories represent approximately 25% of the US population and 32% of the population under the age of 20 (US Bureau of Census, 1994). We present and analyze empirical findings for children and adolescents from all four groups, rather than focusing on any single group. This not only allows us to compare commonalities inherent to the "minority experience," but also highlights important distinctions among the groups.

In reviewing this diverse literature, we are confronted by several limitations. First, there is an insufficient database from which to conduct a critical analysis for any one ethnic group. Data are particularly scarce for the American Indian/Alaska Native and Asian/Pacific Island populations. Second, re-

---

*Owing to a lack of sufficient data to conduct separate analyses by age, this review will not be developmentally oriented. The term "adolescent" will be used when referring specifically to children over 12 and when the contrast between children and adolescents is specifically highlighted. At other times, the general term "children" or "youths" will be used inclusively to refer to all individuals under the age of 18.

†These categories and terms are used because that is how they are defined by the U.S. Census Bureau and because much of the literature has also divided them in this way. However, while the terms were chosen to be descriptively accurate, they do not necessarily reflect terms that are generally used or preferred by each group (i.e., non-Hispanic Caucasian). For example, the term "Latino" is the more widely preferred term for Hispanics. Also, these groups are each comprised of many subgroups that represent important regional, historical, and national distinctions. When distinctions have been made in the literature (i.e., Japanese-American vs. Korean-American), the specific terms will be used.

searchers have used markedly different approaches to study the various ethnic groups, including ethnic group-specific (within-group) studies, cross-ethnic (between-group) research, and studies based on multiethnic samples. Although some argue that one methodology is better than the other, we take the position that each strategy yields important information about particular groups. However, this does complicate analysis.

Third, cross-ethnic research is often difficult and potentially hazardous to interpret. One justifiable concern is the risk that it will simply support damaging racial and ethnic stereotypes rather than provide useful information about minority populations. Such is inevitably the case when studies report ethnic and racial group differences, yet fail to examine factors that might account for such differences. Further, there is often little evidence to support the assumed cross-ethnic or cross-language equivalence of standard research measures (Knight & Hill, in press). For this reason, measurement in equivalence must be considered as an alternative explanation for findings regarding ethnic differences. Finally, in research with ethnic minority populations, social class remains very difficult to disentangle from minority status. Researchers frequently only study "poor minorities," ignoring the social class variability that exists within groups. Further, most comparative studies confound socioeconomic background with ethnicity, making it difficult to isolate the relative influences of these two factors (Laosa, 1990). As these limitations apply to many of the studies reviewed in the following sections, they will not be noted each time they arise. Nevertheless, they remain important issues for consideration throughout.

MENTAL HEALTH STATUS OF ETHNIC MINORITY CHILDREN AND ADOLESCENTS

Although other social indicators (i.e., academic failure, substance use, teenage parenthood, self-esteem) are relevant to children's psychological well-being, space limitations required that we specifically limit our epidemiological review to the two most commonly studied child mental health outcomes: children's behavior problems and depression. Thus, while some relevant data will be presented for other child outcomes throughout the chapter, the literature relevant to these outcomes is not systematically reviewed.

Epidemiological studies provide the best method of estimating the prevalence of mental health problems in selected populations. Estimates of child mental health disorders (without regard for ethnicity) fall between 17 and 24% within the general population (Costello, 1989). Unfortunately, prevalence data often are not reported separately for distinct ethnic groups in the epidemiological literature. Accordingly, conclusions regarding ethnic group differences in mental health must also be based on nonrandom community surveys and clinic-based studies (i.e., treated cases), which are subject to a number of biases. The latter are particularly problematic because they are biased by ethnic differences in help-seeking behavior, service availability, and referral practices (Sue, Fujino, Hu, Takeuchi, & Zane, 1991). Of necessity, however, the following review includes community surveys and clinic-based studies as evidence for the relative prevalence of mental health disorders within each of the four ethnic groups.

African-American Mental Health

Demographic Profile

The African-American population is a culturally diverse group representing individuals whose ancestors were brought as slaves from different African countries, as well as newer emigrants from Africa and the West Indies. African Americans are the largest ethnic minority group, comprising approximately 12% of the general population and 15% under the age of 20 (US Bureau of Census, 1995). Relative to the nonblack population, African Americans are poor, young, and urban. It is estimated that over 30% of the youth in the US central cities are African American (Myers, 1989).

Epidemiological Profile

A few school-based surveys have reported significantly higher depression scores for African Americans, and African American males in particular, relative to non-Hispanic Caucasian adolescents (Garrison, Jackson, Marsteller, McKeown, & Addy, 1990; Schoenbach, Kaplan, Wagner, Grimson, & Miller, 1983). A national probability survey also found that the suicide rate increased more rapidly in the past decade for black males, aged 15 to 19, than for white males or black females (Shaffer, Gould, & Hicks, 1994). However, other studies have failed to find higher rates of depression for African-American adolescents (Gibbs, 1986; Roberts & Sobhan, 1992), and the suicide rate remains higher for non-Hispanic Caucasians. Moreover, studies reporting higher rates of depression for African-American adolescents have been limited by sampling biases, including disproportionately lower recruitment rates and substantially lower scores on socioeconomic variables for African Americans. In contrast to these studies, Roberts and Sobhan (1992) examined ethnic differences in depression based on a random probability survey of US households. While depression scores for African-American adolescents were higher than for non-Hispanic Caucasian adolescents, these differences were not significant.

Several studies have reported higher rates of externalizing problems, including aggression and antisocial behavior, among African-American adolescents (e.g., Wells et al., 1992), school-aged children (e.g., Guerra, Huesmann, Tolan, Acker, & Eron, 1995), and preschoolers (e.g., Duncan, Brooks-Gunn, & Klebanov, 1994; Leadbetter & Bishop, 1994) relative to non-Hispanic Caucasians and other ethnic groups. However, notwithstanding the consistency of these findings, there are reasons to suspect they are not an accurate representation of true differences in the general population. First, many studies have failed to account for gender, which may interact with ethnicity to produce differential estimates of prevalence. Duncan et al. (1994) conducted a study with a preschool sample of inner-city children born to adolescent mothers. While African-American males were reported by their mothers to have significantly more behavior problems compared to Puerto Rican children, African-American females were not.

Second, most of the studies reporting higher rates of antisocial behavior have been conducted exclusively with low-income African-American samples. Studies using more representative samples have not reported higher rates for African-American youth. Windle (1990) used data from the National Longitudinal Survey of Youth to examine rates of alcohol and substance use and antisocial behavior for African-American, Hispanic, and non-Hispanic Caucasian adolescents. No ethnic differences in delinquency were found for the males in the sample, and African-American and Hispanic females reported significantly lower levels of alcohol-related delinquency than non-Hispanic Caucasian females. Barnes, Farrell, and Banerjee (1994) also reported lower levels of both drinking and deviant behavior for African-American adolescents relative to Caucasian adolescents in a large, representative household survey.

Moreover, few studies have controlled for socioeconomic and contextual confounds when conducting comparisons with African-American adolescents. Peeples and Loeber (1994) examined rates of delinquent behavior for a sample of roughly 500 first, fourth, and seventh grade boys attending public schools. African-American boys were six times more likely to engage in delinquency than the "other" children comprised primarily of non-Hispanic Caucasians. Along with this disparity in child behavior, however, the findings revealed an even greater disparity between the two groups on neighborhood characteristics in that African-American youths were 20 times more likely to live in underclass neighborhoods. When African-American and Caucasian youths not living in underclass neighborhoods were compared, there were no differences in rates of delinquency. These findings are similar to Vega, Khoury, Zimmerman, Gil, and Warheit (1993), who surveyed over 2000 adolescents and reported significantly higher rates of "caseness" (determined by clinical cutoff scores) for African Americans relative to non-Hispanic and Hispanic adolescents, which disappeared when group comparisons were restricted to individuals at higher family income levels.

In both of the foregoing studies, however, at the lower levels of neighborhood and income status, respectively, race differences in symptomatology and caseness remained. Thus, as suggested by previous research with adults (Kessler & Neighbors, 1986), it is possible that race and socioeconomic status interact as risk factors to place disadvantaged African-American children at substantially greater risk for poor mental health.

Conclusion

Notwithstanding the problems associated with sampling bias, the empirical evidence does suggest that African-American youths in high-risk, urban environments, particularly males, are at greater risk for behavioral difficulties. Our review also suggests that researchers should be cautious about generalizing the problems of high-risk neighborhoods to all African-American communities. The sampling strategy, location, and choice of comparison group are all factors that may produce marked differences in prevalence estimates. We found no evidence for increased prevalence of behavioral or emotional problems, while a few studies were suggestive of decreased problem rates, for African-American youths within less disadvantaged homes. However, as few studies have included African-American youths in less disadvantaged homes and neighborhoods, conclusions about their mental health status must await further research.

Hispanic-American Mental Health

Demographic Profile

The Hispanic population is a diverse group, with Mexican Americans representing the largest subgroup (64%), followed by Puerto Ricans (11%), Central and South Americans (13%), Cubans (5%), and other Hispanics (7%). Though the various Hispanic subgroups share many cultural traits, including the Spanish language, they also differ in ways that may impact their risk for psychological difficulties. Such differences include migration patterns, socioeconomic status, family size, education, and rates of intermarriage with other groups (Laosa, 1990). Hispanics are the second largest and fastest growing minority population. They comprise approximately 10% of the US population and 13% under the age of 20 (US Bureau of Census, 1995). The Hispanic group is also one of the youngest, with 30% of its population under 15 years of age compared to 19% of all other Americans. Like African Americans, a large proportion of Hispanics reside in urban communities.

Epidemiological Profile

Some studies have found higher rates of depressive symptoms for Hispanic children relative to non-Hispanic Caucasians. Emslie, Weinberg, Rush, Adams, and Rintelman (1990) surveyed 3294 African-American, non-Hispanic Caucasian, and Hispanic high school students and found significantly more Hispanic females reporting moderate to severe levels of depression (31.2% vs. 18.1% for the sample) on the Beck Depression Inventory. Knight, Virdin, and Roosa (1994) and Gonzales, Gunnoe, Samaniego, and Jackson (1995) reported higher scores on the Child Depression Inventory (CDI) (Kovacs, 1982) for Mexican-American preadolescents and adolescents, respectively, relative to Non-Hispanic Caucasians. However, Knight et al. (1994) found no differences in parent reports of child depression. Further, although Mexican-American children obtained significantly higher scores on the CDI, they did not have higher scores on other measures that are known to covary with depression. Thus, CDI scores may not have an equivalent scalar meaning for Mexican Americans.

There is also substantial intragroup variability when attempts are made to derive prevalence estimates for the subgroups referred to collectively as Hispanic. In a random household survey of non-Hispanic Caucasian, African-American, and Hispanic adolescents, Roberts and Sobhan (1992) divided the Hispanic group into Mexican American and "other Hispanics." Mexican-American adolescents reported significantly higher rates of depressive symptoms and were more likely to be diagnosed with depression than all other groups, even after adjusting for age, gender, and household income. However, other studies have assessed general psychological distress and have found no differences between Hispanic and non-Hispanic Caucasians or among Hispanic subgroups (Dornbusch, Mont-Reynaud, Ritter, Chen, & Steinberg, 1991). For example, Vega et al. (1993) reported no differences in the percentage of non-Hispanic Caucasian and Hispanic adolescents meeting criteria for caseness (combined internalizing and externalizing scores) and no differences among Cuban, Nicaraguan, Colombian, Puerto Rican, or "other" Hispanics.

Evidence regarding behavior problems for Hispanics is also inconsistent. Some studies report no differences between Hispanic and non-Hispanic Caucasian samples (Barrera, Li, & Chassin, 1995; Knight et al., 1994), while other studies report that Hispanics are more likely to engage in deviant activity (Chavez, Oetting, & Swaim, 1994). However, some studies have utilized school-based samples, which may be biased by ethnic differences in school attendance and dropout. Dropout rates are substantially higher for some Hispanic subgroups, particularly Mexican Americans and Puerto Ricans (Bernal, Saenz & Knight, 1991; Malgady, Rogler, & Constantino, 1990).

Intragroup variability within Hispanic populations may also result from differences in generation and acculturation status. For example, Buriel, Calzada, and Vasquez (1982) examined differences between first-, second-, and third-generation Mexican Americans and found that third-generation adolescents engaged in significantly more delinquent behaviors than earlier generations. Vega et al. (1995) compared problem rates between foreign-born and US-born Hispanic adolescents (Cuban and Puerto Rican) and found that US-born adolescents had higher symptomatology scores and a higher percentage who met criteria for caseness. More acculturated Hispanic youths have also been shown to have higher rates of teenage pregnancy, school dropout, and alcohol and substance use relative to less acculturated youths (Laosa, 1990; Szapocznik & Kurtines, 1980). Together, these findings suggest that the effects of acculturation should be included when examining factors that influence the mental health status of Hispanic youths.

Conclusion

Overall, the epidemiological evidence supports few strong conclusions for Hispanic youths. The limited evidence indicates that Mexican Americans may be at greater risk for depression when compared to African Americans, non-Hispanic Caucasians, and "other Hispanics." However, given the potential measurement equivalence problems, these findings must be regarded as tentative. Preliminarily, it also seems that some subgroups of US-born or more acculturated Hispanics may be at higher risk for delinquency and other problem behaviors.

Asian/Pacific Island-American Mental Health

Demographic Profile

The groups that make up the Asian/Pacific Islander category are quite diverse. Asian Americans constitute approximately 95% of the population, representing 28 ethnic groups, including persons of Chinese, Japanese, Filipino, Asian Indian, Korean, and Vietnamese ancestry (Asian and Pacific Islander Center for Census Information and Services, 1992). Some of the Asian American groups (i.e., Chinese, Japanese, and Filipinos) began immigrating to the United States more than 100 years ago, but a vast majority (65.6%) are recent immigrants. Although their numbers are small, Pacific Islanders consist of approximately 30 different ethnic groups from the Pacific Island region. Although Asian/Pacific Island Americans represent only 3% (7.9 million) of the total US population, this population increased in size by 95% between 1980 and 1990 (Ong & Hee, 1992). The Asian/Pacific Island group is the youngest of the four ethnic and racial groups, with an estimated 32% of this population under 19 years of age (US Bureau of the Census, 1990).

Epidemiological Profile

We found no studies that assessed mental health indicators for younger Asian/Pacific Island children. However, two studies found fewer psychological symptoms and less deviance among Asian American adolescents when compared to African-American, Hispanic, and non-Hispanic Caucasian adolescents (Dornbusch et al., 1991; Wells et al., 1992). Studies of treated cases provide a similar view of decreased risk for Asian adolescents. Among adolescents utilizing treatment services within Los Angeles County, Asian/Pacific Island youths are significantly less likely to receive a psychiatric diagnosis (Bui & Takeuchi, 1992). These findings are also consistent with the "model minority" view of the Asian/Pacific Island population and with epidemiological evidence on social indicators such as school dropout, teenage pregnancy, and drug and alcohol use for which Asian adolescents consistently demonstrate lower rates (Liu, Yu, Chang, & Fernandez, 1990).

However, studies that have examined intragroup variability have highlighted significant differences among various subgroups in the extent and type of problems they experience (Kim & Chun, 1993). This research suggests that immigration status, length of stay in the United States, and socioeconomic status influences adjustment. Psychological difficulties and suicide rates tend to be higher for those individuals and subgroups who have migrated more recently and, within specific subgroups, foreign-born youths relative to those born in the United States (Liu et al., 1990). Moreover, recent studies have identified Southeast Asian refugees as a subgroup at markedly increased risk for psychological problems, including posttraumatic stress disorder and depression (e.g., Hinton, Chen, and Tran, 1993; Kinzie, Sack, Aryelle, Clarke & Ben, 1989).

Conclusion

Examined as a single group, it appears that Asian/Pacific Island adolescents may experience fewer mental health problems relative to the general population. However, without epidemiological studies, informed estimates of prevalence are not possible for this group. Also, specific subgroups of recent immigrants may be at increased risk, particularly those who settled in the United States as refugees under highly stressful circumstances.

American Indian/Alaska Native Mental Health

Epidemiological Profile

The bulk of psychological research with American Indian and Alaska Native youth has focused on either alcohol and substance abuse or adolescent suicide, both of which are significant problems for these groups. The rate of alcoholism is estimated to be as high as two to three times the national average, although the rate varies widely among tribes (Oetting & Beauvais, 1991). Indian and Native adolescents also have the highest suicide rate in the United States (Yates, 1987).

The limited information on the mental health status of the American Indian/Alaska Native populations comes primarily from studies of children referred to Indian Health Services. Mental health referral rates have been reported to range from 20 to 25% (Yates, 1987), which is higher than non-Indian referral rates. However, these findings may be biased because they are based on small-scale tribal studies and prevalence rates vary from one tribe to another (Yates, 1987).

Prevalence estimates based on global referral rates also mask large differences between younger children and adolescents. Beiser and Attneave (1982) compared national data on the use of outpatient mental health services by American Indian/Alaska Native children in 1974 to national data on non-Indian children who received services in 1969. Though these authors acknowledged the limitations of such comparisons, their findings revealed a striking developmental pattern. Whereas American Indian/Native and non-Indian children were at roughly equal risk for entering the treatment system between the ages of 5 to 9, referral rates showed a steady rise for American Indian/Native children between the ages of 10 to 14. By ages 15 to 19, American Indian/Native males were 3.5 times more likely and females were 5.4 times more likely to seek services relative to same-gender, non-Indian adolescents.

Conclusion

There is a definite need for research on the mental health status of American Indian and Alaska Native populations. Problems such as suicide and both alcohol and substance abuse are known to be high, yet few studies have examined prevalence rates for mental health outcomes. Preliminary findings, based exclusively on mental health referral rates, suggest that American Indian/Alaska Native adolescents experience more mental health problems than younger Indian/Native children and, possibly, more than non-Indian adolescents.

CHILDREN'S CULTURAL ECOLOGIES, LIFE STRESS, AND MENTAL HEALTH

The foregoing review provides evidence that some ethnic minority youths are at greater risk for poor mental health. The literature also highlights problems of particular concern for some groups. However, this body of research is marked by methodological limitations that prohibit encompassing conclusions. These include bias in selection of research populations, lack of information about the cross-ethnic equivalence of measures, and failure of many studies to account for gender differences and intragroup variability. Further, nearly all of the available studies have been conducted with adolescents, rather than younger children. Given this fact, the ensuing discussion is also most relevant for adolescents.

The preceding review also revealed substantial variability within each racial and ethnic group in their pattern and extent of symptomatology. These differences were shown to relate to a number of contextual variables, including socioeconomic status, area of residence, and immigration and acculturation status. Along with ethnicity and race, these contextual variables represent dimensions of cultural diversity that significantly shape the context of development for minority youth. Together, we believe, they also help to account for differences in mental health outcomes and related social problems between and within diverse groups and subgroups.

In their writing on African-American adolescent development, Bell-Scott and Taylor (1989) urge researchers to acknowledge the impact that minority adolescents' "multiple ecologies" have on their life experiences and developmental trajectories. Their arguments echo those of Bronfenbrenner (1989) and a growing body of research that illustrates the importance of a cultural–ecological framework for understanding the development and psychological well-being of ethnic minority group individuals. Consistent with this view and with the preceding literature review, we propose a stress–mental health process model in which "cultural ecology" plays a central role as a mediator of the impact of ethnicity on child and adolescent mental health. That is, we propose that there are at least four cultural ecological variables, identified in the extant research with ethnic minority populations and outlined in greater detail in the following sections, that help to describe the conditions under which ethnic minority status places children at increased risk for poor mental health.

The model, which is presented in Fig. 1, is similar to the general framework used in stress-related research (Lazarus & Folkman, 1984), but differs by including variables with specific relevance to minority populations. The model posits that ethnic minority status (see Fig. 1), is related to poor mental health because it is frequently associated with at least four context-shaping conditions: (1) low socioeconomic status, (2) high-risk neighborhood context, (3) migration and acculturation, and (4) racism and discrimination. These variables represent cultural ecological conditions because they have pervasive effects on an individual's life experiences, including day-to-day experiences within primary developmental contexts (family, peers, school), the behaviors and values that are encouraged within these contexts, and their relation to the larger society. Further, these conditions combine in unique ways to impact the mental health of particular ethnic groups by differentially predisposing them to a wide range of stressful life events and by influencing the coping responses employed in response to these events. Finally, conditions and resources in one's environment, particularly within the family, play both mediating and moderating roles as protective factors.

In the following subsections, we review research relevant to each of the

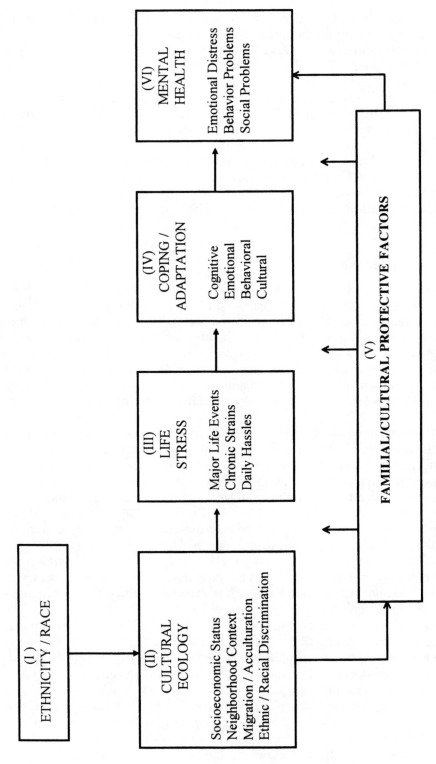

Figure 1. Cultural ecological stress process model for ethnic minority children.

four cultural ecological variables included in the model. The first three dimensions were specifically highlighted as mental-health-relevant variables in the foregoing epidemiological review. The final contextual variable, racism and discrimination, is also included because it is frequently cited as an important, context-shaping dimension of life and a major source of stress for minority group individuals (Spencer, 1990). While these four crosscutting variables are discussed as distinct aspects of children's lives, they are all interrelated. Family poverty, for example, is highly related to residence in high-risk neighborhoods and to immigrant status. Further, while these broad constructs are relevant in varying degrees for all minority groups, it is likely that some dimensions (e.g., poverty, acculturation difficulties) may have a more powerful effect on the stress process and mental health of one group (e.g., low-acculturation Mexican Americans), while having little or no effect for another cultural group (e.g., high-acculturation Japanese Americans).

Socioeconomic Status

Poverty, not race or ethnicity, is the greatest predictor of mental health for children of all ages and ethnic categories (Rutter, 1983). Poverty is also closely related to race and ethnicity in the United States. With few exceptions (e.g., Cuban Americans, some Asian-American subgroups), minority children have substantially lower socioeconomic status than the general US population. According to the most recent census information, child poverty rates were 43% for African Americans, 40% for Hispanics, 61% for American Indian/Alaska Natives, 16% for Asian Pacific Americans, and 12% for non-Hispanic Caucasians.

Poverty-related risks have been well-documented in the literature for both minority and nonminority populations. Children living in poverty are more likely to live in single-parent families, to experience less effective parenting, poor parental mental health, more conflictual family relations, and a large number of extrafamilial environmental stressors (e.g., Brody, Stoneman, Flor, McCrary, Hastings, & Convers, 1994; Felner et al., 1995; McLoyd, 1990). McLoyd (1990) argues that poverty "diminishes the capacity for supportive, consistent, and involved parenting and renders parents more vulnerable to the effects of negative life events" (p. 312). She argues further that parental psychological distress mediates the relations between poverty and negative socioemotional development in children because it is associated with greater interparental conflict and more punitive and coercive parenting behaviors.

There is little doubt among researchers that socioeconomic differences account for a large proportion of variance in mental health status that exists between groups. When ethnic differences in children's psychological and social problems are found in the literature, the most economically disadvantaged groups (e.g., African American, Hispanic, American Indian/Alaska Native) and subgroups (e.g., Mexican American, Southeast Asian) are invariably included among those with the most problems. Some studies have also shown that ethnic differences are attenuated and in some cases eliminated when socioeconomic status is controlled. However, our review also revealed that socioeconomic differences may not explain all of the variance between groups. For example, the most pronounced ethnic differences in psychological functioning are found among members of the lowest social classes; these differences are not consistently eliminated when socioeconomic variables are controlled (Peeples & Loeber, 1994; Vega et al., 1993). Thus, it may be necessary to include other contextual variables to fully explain why some groups are at greater risk than others for poor mental health.

Neighborhood Context

Along with being generally poorer, ethnic minority families are also more likely to reside in the most disadvantaged neighborhoods where opportunities for social, economic, and educational development are severely limited (i.e., inadequate schools, deteriorated housing, insufficient youth programs) and where they may be exposed to unusually high levels of stress.

Community Impoverishment

According to the 1990 Census, only 15% of poor blacks and 20% of poor Hispanics reside in nonpoverty areas (poverty rate less than 20%) compared to nearly 70% of poor whites. Further, whereas nearly 40% of all blacks live in extreme poverty areas (poverty rate 40% or more), this figure is less than 7% for whites. American Indian and Alaska Native communities also suffer from severe impoverishment, with unemployment rates around 30% for most reservations and as high as 90% for some tribes (Berlin, 1987).

Several studies have shown a direct relationship between neighborhood disadvantage and a number of child and adolescent problems, including depression, poor cognitive development, academic underachievement, teenage pregnancy, juvenile delinquency, and aggression (Aber, 1994; Brooks-Gunn, Duncan, Kato & Klebganov, 1991; Dornbusch et al., 1991; Guerra et al., 1995; Peeples & Loeber, 1994). Further, in some cases, neighborhood characteristics have been shown to predict child outcomes over and above variations in these outcomes explained by family socioeconomic status.

Urban Stress

Among the impoverished neighborhoods in which disadvantaged, minority families reside, inner-city neighborhoods are a particularly difficult context. Inner-city neighborhoods expose children to a number of stressful and dangerous conditions (urban crowding, crime, drugs, gangs, violence) that may not be present in suburban or rural contexts (Attar, Guerra, & Tolan, 1994). Neighborhood crime and delinquent youth groups (i.e., gangs) threaten the personal safety of family members and exert a strong influence on children's behaviors and attitudes through direct modeling, pressure, and encouragement to engage in deviant activity (Guerra et al., 1995; Sampson & Laub, 1994). Exposure to community violence is also an issue of great concern. Within the country's largest cities, as many as 26–39% of children report that they have seen a person shot, 29–35% have witnessed a stabbing, and 24% report that they have witnessed a murder (Fitzpatrick & Boldizar, 1993). Epidemiological data also indicate that African-American males are at highest risk for violent assault and homicide; the lifetime risk of violent death has been estimated to be 1 in 27 for African-American males compared to 1 in 117 for African-American females and 1 in 205 for white males (Hammond & Yung, 1993).

As discussed in chapter 16 (this volume), the effects of violence exposure and victimization are severe. These experiences have been related to increased aggression, delinquency, and gang involvement (Guerra et al., 1995; Hammond & Yung, 1993). Violence-exposed children also report lower self-esteem, excessive fear and worry about death, and a decline in cognitive performance (Bell & Jenkins, 1991; Freeman, Mokros, & Poznanski, 1993). In the most extreme cases, exposure to traumatic violence is linked to serious psychological symptomatology, particularly depression and posttraumatic stress disorder (Fitzpatrick & Boldizar, 1993).

In sum, there is little doubt that poor, inner-city neighborhoods place a disproportionate number of minority youths at greater risk for problematic emotional and behavioral outcomes. However, most of this literature has focused on African-American and, to a lesser extent, Hispanic youths, who represent the largest demographic groups in the inner city. Little is known about Asian/Pacific Island or American Indian/Alaska Native youths living in large urban centers.

Migration and Acculturation Experiences

Acculturation refers to the process of change that occurs when culturally distinct groups and individuals come into contact with another culture (Berry & Kim, 1988). This process begins with migration for immigrant groups, but is expected to continue for several generations. Acculturation is also expected to occur for nonimmigrant groups, such as Native Americans/Alaska Natives and African Americans, as a function of their dual cultural existence in the United States.

Cultural change occurs on a number of dimensions for acculturating individuals. It may include the gradual incorporation of cultural beliefs, values, behaviors, and language of the dominant society, as well as changes in one's loyalty and sense of belonging to the host culture and to one's culture of origin (Rogler, Cortes, & Malgady, 1991). Acculturation is also expected to have an impact on mental-health-relevant variables including stressful life events, help-seeking behavior, individual coping styles, and subjective feelings of distress (Vega et al., 1993).

Differences in exposure to acculturative stress have been proposed as one explanation for varying mental health outcomes among individuals within a given cultural group (Berry & Kim, 1988). The acculturative stress perspective suggests that individuals experience a number of stressors during the acculturation process as a result of conflicts that arise between the individual's ethnic culture and the dominant culture. Similar stressors have been identified for American Indian/Alaska Native, Asian/Pacific Island, and Hispanic children (Chavez, Moran, Reid, & Lopez, 1995; Clarke, Sack, & Goff, 1993; Dinges & Duong-Tran, 1993; Vega et al., 1993). These have included migration-induced strains for recent arrivals, as well as cultural conflicts that occur at varying stages of acculturation for both immigrant and nonimmigrant groups.

Migration Strain

Even when it is viewed as a positive experience (i.e., search for economic opportunities, political freedom), migration represents a major disruption for children and families. It disrupts attachments to social support systems that are left behind in one's country of origin at the same time that it imposes on the migrant the difficult task of incorporation into the social and economic structure of a new culture (Rogler et al., 1991). The first several years after migration are expected to be especially stressful, particularly for individuals who are culturally and racially dissimilar to the indigenous population. Migration is also expected to be more difficult for those who enter a new culture at the lowest levels of its social stratification system (Kunz, 1981).

Children may experience difficulty adjusting to life in a new culture if they have been exposed to severe levels of stress during the migration process. The experiences and problems reported within certain refugee populations underscore the importance of this issue. Southeast Asian children, during their forced migration and resettlement, endured traumatic war-related stressors, painful separations from family members, and difficult experiences in refugee camps (Clarke et al., 1993). The literature suggests that these stressful events, combined with the stress of having to adapt to life in a new country, account for the increased prevalence of psychiatric problems reported for Southeast Asian children (e.g., Abe, Zane, & Chun, 1994).

However, while this research has identified a small but important subset of youths at increased risk for psychological difficulties, there is little evidence to support a link between migration-induced stress and psychological distress for immigrant youths whose experiences are less severe. On the other hand, as newly arrived immigrant children represent an understudied population, their risk for mental health problems has yet to be adequately assessed.

Bicultural Conflict

The uprooting experiences of migration are accompanied by a more extended process of adjustment during which acculturating individuals must learn the language, behavioral norms, and values characteristic of the host society (Rogler et al., 1991). Language difficulties present an immediate strain for children who do not speak English (Chavez et al., 1995). Minority children (both immigrant and nonimmigrant) may also experience conflicts with peers or teachers when they become aware that their own cultural values or behaviors are not understood or valued within the dominant culture (Phinney et al., 1991). Because children often acculturate more rapidly than parents and older relatives, conflicts may also develop within the family. Conflicts may occur as children adopt values and beliefs that are different from those of their parents. Intergenerational acculturative conflict has been reported as a problem for Hispanic, American Indian/Alaska Native, and Asian/Pacific Island families

(Chavez et al., 1995; Rick & Forward, 1992; Yates, 1987). Further, clinical accounts suggest that intergenerational acculturative conflict may lead to serious problems for youths because it disrupts family relations and leads children to reject their parents as socializing agents (Szapocznik & Kurtines, 1980).

However, while theoretical discussions have consistently identified a common set of stressors for acculturating children and their families, the psychological and behavioral effects of acculturative stress have rarely been examined. Most of the evidence for the negative effects of intergenerational acculturative conflict, for example, comes from clinical samples and anecdotal observations. Only very recently have researchers begun to assess acculturative stressors for children within the general population and to relate these to mental health outcomes. For example, Vega and colleagues (1993) examined the link between delinquency and two dimensions of culturally linked stress for Cuban and Puerto Rican adolescents; whereas "language conflicts" were related to delinquency for both US-born and foreign-born adolescents, "perceptions of discrimination" and "perceptions of a closed society" were only significant for US-born adolescents. Dinges and Duong-Tran (1993) found "loss of cultural support," a dimension of acculturative stress reported among American Indian/Alaska Native adolescents, to be associated with depression, substance abuse, and suicidality.

Despite some preliminary findings, studies of the effects of acculturative stress are as yet too few to support strong conclusions. Whether acculturation produces significantly higher levels of stress and the extent to which this stress accounts for clinically significant differences in child and adolescent mental health has yet to be determined. Also unknown are those factors that predispose some children within different cultural groups to higher rates of acculturative stress than others. The process of acculturation and its relation to both stress and mental health are likely to vary, depending on a wide array of mitigating factors, such as whether an individual migrates to a bicultural, ethnic, or mainstream community; the rate at which family members acculturate; conditions surrounding migration; and the country from which each group migrated (Rogler et al., 1991). Continued research is needed to shed light on these complex issues.

Ethnic and Racial Discrimination

Many minority youths are also exposed to environmental conditions that include prejudice and discrimination. According to Spencer (1990), ethnic minorities live with either a sense of invisibility (e.g., absence from school materials and other media), or, worse, with a preponderance of negative images and stereotyped attitudes about their cultural group. In addition, minority youth may confront social inequalities, blocked opportunities, or other structural barriers.

When asked to report about these experiences, ethnic minority youths indicate that they perceive prejudice and that they have been the target of discrimination and stereotyping within their schools and the larger community (Gonzales et al., 1995; Vega et al., 1993). Caucasian youths may also experience discrimination and hostility when they interact with other ethnic groups. However, these events take on particular importance in the lives of those groups that are stigmatized within the larger society. While negative stereotypes are associated with African-American, Hispanic, and Indian/ Native youths, positive attitudes (or at least more balanced perceptions) are typically associated with non-Hispanic Caucasians. These youths are therefore less likely to experience the chronic stress and problems associated with an implied group deviance (Spencer & Markstrom-Adams, 1990). Although generally positive, Asian American-linked stereotypes may also provide a significant source of stress for those who feel pressured to live up to the "achieving Asian" stereotype (Liu et al., 1990).

Spencer (1990) argues that racial and ethnic stereotypes combine with the lack of status, political power, and economic opportunity for some minority groups to produce problematic behavioral outcomes. In support, perceived discrimination has been associated with deviant behavior for African-American and Hispanic youths (Gonzales et al., 1995; Vega et al., 1993). Biafora et al. (1993) also found a strong relationship between racial mistrust and deviant behavior for African-American, Haitian, and Caribbean Island black adolescent males.

However, while there is widespread agreement that many ethnic minority youths are subject to social inequalities and racist attitudes, ethnic and racial discrimination represent the least-studied sources of stress for children and adolescents. This is due, in part, to difficulties in operationalizing this source of life stress. Also, it is possible that racial discrimination does not constitute a risk context for minority youths on its own, but interacts with other aspects of the environment, such as family and community poverty, to threaten optimal development.

COPING AND RESILIENCE OF ETHNIC MINORITY CHILDREN

Ethnic group differences on mental health indicators are not purely a function of variance in stress exposure. Whereas some children are hard hit by the stressful events in their lives, others will show resilient outcomes (Wyman, Cowen, Work, & Parker, 1991). Indeed, ethnic minority communities provide numerous examples of resiliency. Migrant children somehow manage to adjust to life in a new cultural environment. Among the poorest Native American communities are examples of tribes with markedly lower rates of child and adolescent mental health problems (Yates, 1987). As a group, Asian-American youths consistently have fewer mental health and social problems when compared to non-Hispanic Caucasians. A few studies have also shown Hispanic and African-American youths to be less vulnerable to the negative effects of stress when compared to non-Hispanic Caucasians (Barrera et al., 1995; Dornbusch et al., 1991).

An important step in the development of culturally relevant and effective prevention programs is the identification of factors that can account for such examples of resiliency. Accordingly, we next review the coping literature, followed by a discussion of familial and cultural influences that are thought to be protective for minority children (see Fig. 1).

Coping Strategies of Minority Youth

Coping has been defined as "cognitive and behavioral efforts to manage specific external and/or internal demands that are appraised as taxing or exceeding the resources of the person" (Lazarus & Folkman, 1984, p. 142). This definition has three important features. First, it is process oriented in that it refers to a person's thoughts and behaviors as the situation unfolds. Second, coping is determined by the person's interpretation ("appraisal") of the demands for that particular situation. Third, coping refers to efforts to manage a situation, rather than the actual success or outcome of these efforts. As reviewed in Chapter 1 (this volume), theoretically and empirically derived models have been developed to account for the relevant dimensions of children's coping. This literature has shown that some coping strategies are more effective than others at producing optimal mental health outcomes. However, the literature on ethnic minority children's coping is limited by three broad gaps.

First, there is a dearth of empirical studies (we found only five) that examine the coping strategies of children under the age of 18 from one or more ethnic groups. Overall, these studies revealed more similarities than differences in coping strategies across ethnic groups. When asked to respond to hypothetical stressors or when asked to endorse items from a list of possible coping responses, African-American and Mexican-American children and adolescents have been shown to give response patterns that are similar to those of non-Hispanic Caucasian youths (e.g., Halstead, Johnson, & Cunningham, 1993).

A few studies have also noted some modest differences between groups. In a study of African-American, Mexican-American, and Caucasian urban adolescents, Munsch and Wampler (1993) found African Americans to report more reliance on "seeking alternative rewards" as a coping strategy. In a study of pregnant and parenting adolescents, Mexican-American adolescents chose more avoidant responses than non-Hispanic Caucasian adolescents (Codega, Pasley, & Kreutzer, 1990). Also, two studies have shown Mexican Americans to be somewhat more likely than Caucasians to endorse religious coping (Codega et al., 1990; Copeland & Hess, 1995). However, while these initial studies provide important groundwork on minority children's coping, they did not examine the link between coping and mental health outcomes. Consequently, there is no way to evaluate whether similar coping strategies produce similar outcomes across groups, or whether the few noted differences are of relevance to psychological well-being.

Second, researchers have not specifically examined children's coping with respect to the unique types of stressors to which minority youths are exposed. This is an important issue, since there is reason to question whether traditional coping models will apply as well to the uncontrollable, relentless, and extreme events that characterize the environments of some minority youths. Neighborhood violence and crime, for example, are stressful circumstances that may not respond in predictable ways to problem-focused or emotion-focused coping. Avoidant coping, a strategy typically associated with poor adjustment, may serve some adaptive function for youths under these circumstances. It is also likely that minority youths employ many subtle, complex, and context-specific (i.e., "streetwise") strategies to cope with the demands of their environments.

Future studies should attempt to identify these strategies and to include them, along with culturally relevant stressors, in stress process research with minority samples.

Finally, it may also be important to examine children's coping with ethnicity-linked stress from an ethnic- or race-based cultural framework—that is, with some appreciation for the impact that ethnicity or race may have on children's appraisals of these events and on their evaluation of coping options and desired outcomes. For example, children's responses to ethnicity-linked stress (i.e., acculturative stress, discrimination) are likely to be influenced by their understanding of what it means to be a member of their ethnic or racial group. Ethnic identity may therefore be an important aspect of coping for minority individuals. To illustrate, the next section briefly outlines coping-related adaptive responses described in the acculturation and ethnic identity literatures.

Cultural Adaptation as Coping

Researchers have identified a variety of coping responses, or "cultural adaptations," that individuals may adopt as they appraise and respond to ethnicity-linked stress (Berry & Kim, 1988; Phinney et al., 1991; Oetting & Beavais, 1991). These alternatives can generally be summarized as follows: (1) *assimilation* (to the majority culture), (2) *separation* (from the majority culture), (3) *deculturation* or marginalization (rejection of both), and (4) *biculturalism* or integration. Deculturation is generally viewed as the most problematic adaptation, whereas biculturalism and a strong ethnic or racial identity have both been described as a source of resilience for ethnic minority individuals (LaFromboise, Coleman, & Gerton, 1993).

Biculturalism, or bicultural competence, connotes the capacity to operate with ease in two cultural contexts while maintaining a sense of pride in one's own origins and distinctive identity. Research has shown that bicultural adolescents have higher self-esteem and interpersonal sensitivity, more cognitive and problem-solving flexibility, and a lower incidence of behavior problems and substance abuse than monoculturally oriented adolescents (La Fromboise et al., 1993; Phinney et al., 1991). However, biculturalism may not be equally possible for all minority youth. Structural factors such as social boundaries, discrimination, and poverty may block these pathways for a given individual or group (Tajfel, 1978).

For some individuals, stereotype vulnerability, or the need to consistently disavow group-based negative feedback, will have important consequences for the adaptive coping strategies that they use (Crocker & Major, 1989). For example, attribution of negative life events to racial discrimination or to barriers in the social system may constitute an important coping resource for some minority youths (Barbarin, 1993). In support, African-American adolescents consistently report that they are more external in their control beliefs. Moreover, external locus of control is not related to low self-esteem or poor mental health for this group (Myers, 1989).

In an effort to protect one's sense of self in the context of damaging ethnic stereotypes, some minority youths may also respond with separation, racial mistrust, or active defiance of the mainstream culture and its values (Oyserman & Saltz, 1993). On one hand, it is important to understand that these responses may be "adaptive" in the sense that they help to assuage negative self-evaluations for disparaged groups (Biafora et al., 1993). However, despite some possible short-term benefits, these responses are ultimately maladaptive for those youths who withdraw from activities that provide greater access to the reward structures of the dominant society or engage in problem behaviors that increase their risk for long-term difficulties (Myers, 1989). For example, Fordham and Ogbu (1987) suggest that African-American youths often reject academic achievement because it is seen as irrelevant to success within their own community and it is viewed among their peers as a form of "acting white." Indeed, a variety of adolescent behavioral outcomes (i.e., violence, alcohol and substance use, adolescent pregnancy, gang membership) may be environmentally motivated responses that enable youths to achieve lifestyle and identity goals that are valued by their peer reference group (Dembo, Williams, & Schmeidler, 1993). Conventional paths for achieving such goals, such as those supported by the dominant culture or by traditional ethnic culture, may be perceived by some adolescents as less attainable or desirable. Thus, to understand how minority children cope with life's adversities, it may be necessary to consider the cultural meanings attached to those stress events and coping options that they encounter within their immediate environments.

Familial/Cultural Protective Factors: Moderators of Risk for Minority Youth

Protective factors are variables that modify, or moderate, the impact of risk factors (i.e., stressful life events) on mental health outcomes for individuals exposed to the risks in question. That is, the existence of protective resources (i.e., Fig. 1, family protective factors) will deter or significantly alter the process by which stress-inducing environments lead to life stress and related mental health problems. It is possible for these protective factors to alter the extent or severity of stress exposure (e.g., decrease exposure to violence), influence the type of coping strategies that are used in response to stress (e.g., prepare children to cope with racism), or moderate the effectiveness of coping on children's mental health (e.g., provide resources such as social support that may enhance children's coping efforts).

In our review, we found many references to protective factors for minority youths, particularly the stress-buffering qualities of ethnic minority families and traditional ethnic cultures. However, there is as yet little empirical evidence that these variables actually operate as moderators of stress for minority youths. Nevertheless, the following section will briefly describe a few frequently cited protective factors, along with relevant empirical findings where available.

Family Bonds

Strong family bonds, particularly between parents and children, are expected to provide an important source of protection for children. This is expected to be true for most children and adolescents, but may be especially true for ethnic minority groups which are often described as being more family centered (Garcia-Coll, Meyer, & Brillon, 1995).

Focusing on urban, African-American families, Mason, Cauce, Gonzales, and Hiraga (1995) examined the moderating effects of both a strong mother–child bond and father absence (lack of parent–child bond) on the relationship between delinquent peer association and problem behavior. Over a 1-year time period, African-American adolescents who associated with deviant peers were less likely to engage in delinquent behavior if they had a father figure in the home or a strong relationship with their mother.

The work of Barrera and colleagues (1995) demonstrates the importance of positive family relations as a source of protection for Hispanic adolescents. Barrera et al. (1995) examined the effects of life stress and family conflict on the emotional and behavioral adjustment of non-Hispanic Caucasian and Hispanic (primarily Mexican American) families. They found no differences in stress exposure between the two groups, but they did find a significant interaction between life stress and ethnicity. Whereas life stress led to increased family conflict and, in turn, increased psychological distress for non-Hispanic Caucasian youths, the relation between life stress and family conflict was significantly smaller for Hispanics. Consequently, at similar levels of stress, Hispanic adolescents displayed fewer emotional and behavioral symptoms. Traditional Hispanic family values are discouraging of family conflict and may therefore represent an important protective resource for Hispanic families during times of stress (Marin & Marin, 1991).

Extended Kin

Ethnic minority children may also receive added protection against life stress when they can rely on the support of extended kin networks. The extended family, a structure that is common to many ethnic minority groups, has been described as a "problem-solving and stress-coping system that addresses, adapts, and commits available family resources to normal and nonnormal transitional and crisis situations" (Harrison, Wilson, Pine, Chan & Buriel, 1990, p. 351). Though the relation between extended kin and children's mental health has rarely been examined, two studies have shown that minority adolescents (Hispanic and African American) are more likely to rely on extended family members for support relative to non-Hispanic Caucasians (Levitt, Guacci-Franco & Levitt, 1993; Munsch & Wampler, 1993).

Ethnic/Racial Socialization

Ethnic or racial socialization may also represent an important resource for minority youths (Harrison et al., 1990). Ethnic socialization may be accomplished by deliberate teaching or may be transmitted through tacit socialization, and it may be performed by parents, ethnic role models, or by the larger ethnic community.

Ethnic or racial socialization serves a variety of functions (Garcia-Coll et al., 1995). First, it instills a positive orientation toward one's own group as a means of promoting ethnic or racial pride and biculturalism (Bowman & Howard, 1985; Harrison et al., 1990). Second, ethnic socialization strategies can prepare children to cope with racism, prejudice, and discrimination. Studies have shown that some minority parents, especially African Americans, directly talk to their children about these issues (Bowman & Howard, 1985; Phinney & Chavira, 1996).

A third function of ethnic socialization is to promote children's internalization of culturally prescribed values (Garcia-Coll et al., in press). For example, in many Asian cultures, ethnic socialization has as its primary goal the "proper development of character" and may include the socialization of behavior patterns and values that promote conventional developmental paths. Emphasis is placed on academic achievement and effort as the means by which to achieve personal advancement, gain access to societal institutions, achieve higher social status, wealth, and family respect, and to overcome discrimination (Lum & Char, 1985).

Socialization of cultural values and maintenance of traditional practices may also be protective for African-American, Hispanic, and American Indian and Alaska Native youths. Among the various tribal communities, for example, suicide rates are reported to be higher in dislocated tribes where members are unable to practice their traditional lifestyle and lower on reservations where traditional practices are maintained and children attend school within the tribal community (May, 1987).

Religion/Spirituality

Religion and spirituality have also been important in the lives of many ethnic minority groups (Garcia-Coll et al., 1995). For African Americans, for example, the black church has played a central role, facilitating mutual support and responsibility for the moral socialization of children and offering a spiritual understanding of life's struggles that may promote effective coping. To date, two studies have shown church or religious involvement to be protective against delinquency for African-American adolescents (Barnes et al., 1994; Zimmerman & Maton, 1992). However, as with most of the protective factors mentioned here and in the extant literature, additional research is needed to empirically demonstrate the moderating influence of religion as it relates to minority children's mental health.

CULTURALLY SENSITIVE PREVENTION PROGRAMS FOR ETHNIC MINORITY YOUTH

The final section provides a summary of empirically validated, culturally sensitive preventive interventions for ethnic minority youths. Interventions are included if they were explicitly designed or modified to be used with specific ethnic groups, or if they were evaluated with a predominantly minority sample; they targeted mental-health-related outcomes in general rather than specific behaviors such as substance use, academic achievement, or health behaviors; and they reported data on the effectiveness of the program in a clinical trial that included a comparison with a control group. A total of five family-focused interventions and three coping skills interventions that met these criteria were identified in the literature.*

Family-Based Interventions

Of the five family-based interventions, four were parent-focused (i.e., parenting) interventions that targeted African-American and Hispanic children in low-income, urban environments. These programs had similar goals of providing parents with child-rearing and family management skills and facilitating strong parent–child bonds. First, the Gutelius Child Health Supervision Project (Gutelius, Kirsch, MacDonald, Brooks, & McErlean, 1977) provided long-term intensive parent support services, with a general focus on parenting, to low-income African-American teenage mothers of young infants. Program evaluation data collected 5 to 6 years after the intervention indicated fewer behavioral problems in the program children compared to no-treatment controls. Schweinhart, Berrueta-Clement, Barnett, Epstein, and Weikart (1985) evaluated a parent support group intervention with low-income mothers of 123 4-year-old African-American children at risk for failing in school. The Perry Preschool Project targeted school readiness and cognitive development by facilitating parental involvement in the child's education. Program mothers attended 2.5-hour meetings, five days per week for 7.5 months during each of the 2 years of the program. Though the program was not specifically intended as a mental health intervention, longitudinal follow-up showed improvement on a number of relevant indicators. A significantly greater proportion of children in the treatment group attended college (38% vs. 21%), had lower detention and arrest rates (31% vs. 51%), and fewer teenage pregnancies relative to an IQ-matched control group.

The Houston Parent Child Development Center (Johnson & Walker, 1987) is a primary prevention program for infants and parents designed to promote social and intellectual competence in low-income Mexican-American children. Program evaluation involved children between 1 and 3 years of age whose mothers attended approximately 25 1.5-hour sessions over the course of 2 years. During the first year, topics included child development, parenting skills, and home-learning strategies. The second year involved topics related to maintaining a healthy family life such as child management and homemaking. Program mothers reported fewer child behavior problems than control group mothers 5 to 8 years after the program ended. This finding was corroborated with teacher ratings of classroom behavior.

Myers et al. (1992) designed the Effective Black Parenting Program for inner-city African-American parents of young first and second grade children. This 15 week, 3 hour/week program is a culturally adapted, cognitive–behavioral parenting skill training program that incorporates a component on "pride

---

*All articles for the section on interventions, and for the chapter as a whole, were identified through the Psych-Lit database system. Because of the difficulties in conducting such a broad search, some studies may have been missed if they did not use key words that would identify them as being relevant to ethnic minority children in general or to any of the specific ethnic groups that were reviewed.

in blackness," with an emphasis on positive communications about ethnicity, ethnic self-disparagement, and ways to help children cope with racism. Pre- and postchanges on parental acceptance/rejection, family relationships, child behavior problems, and social competencies were found in the treatment group, which showed greater gains than the control group on all but the social competence measures. Reductions in parental rejection and child behavior problems were maintained at 1 year follow-up.

The fifth family based program is somewhat different from the others because it focuses on substance abuse and mental health and targets the whole family as the unit of intervention. The Family Effectiveness Training Program (FET) (Szapocznik et al., 1989) is one of the most extensive prevention efforts with Hispanic families (mostly Cuban and Puerto Rican) and is designed to reduce behavior problems in general and adolescent substance use in particular. FET is based on research that identified a constellation of family behaviors, including intergenerational acculturative conflict, that characterizes families with substance-abusing adolescents. A structural family therapy format is used to address these family processes and is combined with group workshops for adolescents to facilitate coping and bicultural adaptation. Changes in alcohol knowledge, attitudes, and behaviors have been reported for program participants. Participants have also shown significantly greater improvements than control families, posttreatment and at 6-month follow-up, on independent measures of structural family functioning, adolescent self-concept, and problem behaviors.

The above programs provide evidence for family-based programs to reduce the incidence of emotional and behavioral problems among African-American and Hispanic children. The strongest evidence of effectiveness is provided by the three early-intervention parenting programs that have targeted low-income mothers of infants in high-risk settings. These programs have demonstrated impressive effects into childhood and early adulthood. It should be noted, however, that these programs involved long-term (e.g., 2 years), intensive efforts. Though parenting and family (FET) interventions of shorter duration demonstrated modest short-term effects for school-age children and adolescents, these programs will require continued follow-up. Future evaluations should include larger and more varied samples and randomized designed that were not used in some cases.

Evaluation data are also needed for other parenting and family interventions that have been used with minority populations. Two programs, which have yet to present formal outcome data, deserve specific mention as promising examples of culturally sensitive interventions. First, the Raising Successful Children Program (RSC) (Dumka, Roosa, Michaels, & Suh, 1995), is a parenting intervention for low-income, inner-city children (primarily African American and Hispanic). RSC was based on the extant literature linking specific parenting strategies and social learning theory to child mental health and on input from families in the target community about their cultural beliefs systems and preferences. Second, Tolan and McKay (1996) developed a 22-week family intervention program to prevent antisocial behavior and increase the rate of high school completion among urban, minority children. Their Metropolitan Area Child Study Program is based on an empirically driven theoretical model for strengthening critical family processes related to the emergence of antisocial behavior.

Child-Focused Coping Skills Interventions

Coping skills approaches have also been used with minority children within high-stress, low-income neighborhoods. For example, Shure and Spivak (1982) implemented their cognitive problem-solving skills intervention with a sample of African-American school-aged children. The program involved two 12-week sessions over a 2-year period and was designed (1) to teach alternative solutions to peer and authority problems, and (2) to anticipate potential consequences to an interpersonal act. Results showed significant improvement in behavior problems for program participants at posttest and 6-month follow-up compared to a control group.

Schinke, Jansen, Kennedy, and Shi (1994) designed an intervention using puppets to reduce high-risk behavior among African-American children between the ages of 6 and 16. The puppets were life-size and ethnically representative, and the skits addressed problems such as drugs, violence, and peer pressure. Follow-up data showed that program group participants differed from the control group in their knowledge of and positive intentions about violence and drug use. However, evidence for behavior change was not presented.

Cuento therapy is a widely used intervention that uses Puerto Rican role models to foster ethnic identity, self-concept, and adaptive coping behavior (Malgady et al., 1990). The authors of this intervention assert that it provides a culturally grounded method of dealing with stressors such as minority status, bilingualism, and bicultural conflict. *Cuento* therapy was found to be effective at improving cognitive abilities and lowering trait anxiety and aggression in treatment children (grades K–3) relative to control children at posttreatment and at 1-year follow-up (Constantino, Malgady, & Rogler, 1986). This program also produced decreased anxiety and improvements in self-concept and pride in being Puerto Rican among eighth and ninth grade students relative to controls; however, these effects varied as a function of grade level, gender, and father presence in the home.

Few coping interventions have targeted mental health or general well-being for minority children. Of those that have, program effects have only been demonstrated for at most 1-year follow-up and the demonstrated gains have been modest. Nevertheless, these short-term effects lend some support for the use of coping interventions to reduce the incidence of behavior problems and emotional distress among African-American and Hispanic children. Further, though we found few coping interventions that met our criteria for inclusion in this review, there are, in fact, many others reported in the literature that have either not been evaluated or that only target alcohol and substance use. These interventions have included a variety of ethnic groups, including American Indian/Alaska Native and some Asian-American groups. Most of these programs have been culturally tailored to provide general training in specific coping skills along with an emphasis on bicultural adaptation as a desired goal. Data are needed on the effectiveness of these programs.

LINKING RESEARCH, CULTURE, AND PRACTICE

Cultural sensitivity and a sound empirical basis are both critical considerations when developing interventions for diverse populations. The concept of
cultural sensitivity refers to the process of taking into consideration ethnicity
and culture when treating people of color (McGoldrick, Pearce, & Giordano,
1982). It involves understanding and respecting the experiences, values, and
beliefs of the target ethnic group and attempts to maximize available family and
community resources. Cultural sensitivity also requires attention to program
presentation and format to provide an experience that is comfortable and appealing to participants (Dumka et al., 1995). The above programs included
several components that meet these goals, such as inclusion of ethnic program
leaders and role models, use of available community supports (i.e., local
churches and schools), input from the community on curriculum design, provision of services in Spanish, and inclusion of culturally meaningful materials
and content.

With respect to the second consideration, the link between the empirical
literature and the interventions that we reviewed was not clear. Most programs
addressed many of the putative mediators and moderators highlighted in the
current chapter. For example, the focus on parenting with the low-income
minority families is consistent with the bulk of evidence that suggests that
poverty and, in turn, parenting are primary contributors to poor mental health
for ethnic minority children. Many programs also addressed culturally relevant
stressors, such as acculturative stress and discrimination, and some interventions were designed to promote bicultural adaptation. However, while some
programs clearly articulated links to the theoretical and empirical literature
relevant to these issues, others did not. Lack of empirical grounding was most
evident for "cultural" program aspects and is likely due to lack of sufficient
empirical data on those processes that are thought to be unique to the ethnic
minority experience or to specific ethnic groups. Empirical data on the effects
of culture-specific risk factors such as acculturation and discrimination, or on
culture-specific models of processes such as parenting and coping, currently
lag far behind theoretical speculation on these issues. Additional research is
therefore needed to address these gaps.

In sum, the preceding review leaves little doubt that many ethnic minority
children are exposed, within distinct cultural ecologies, to a variety of stressful
experiences. Family poverty, high-risk neighborhoods, acculturation and immigration difficulties, and ethnic and racial discrimination all create notable, if
not uniform, strains for minority group children and adolescents. As a result,
many ethnic minority children are at increased risk for emotional and behavioral difficulties and for a number of social problems that have become pat-
terned outcomes within many minority communities (Spencer, 1990). However,
our review also suggests that these patterns do not apply to all ethnic individuals or even to all individuals within a specific ethnic group or subgroup. A
greater understanding of this fact and of the risk and protective factors that
account for varying mental health outcomes between and within ethnic groups
should facilitate continued development and refinement of culturally sensitive
and effective prevention programs for minority children and adolescents.

REFERENCES

Abe, J., Zane, N., & Chun, K. (1994). Differential responses to trauma: Migration-related discriminants of post-traumatic stress disorder among Southeast Asian refugees. *Journal of Community Psychology, 22*, 121–135.

Aber, J. L. (1994). Poverty, violence and child development: Untangling family and community level effects. In C. A. Nelson (Ed.), *Threats to optimal development: The Minnesota Symposium on Child Psychology* (Vol. 29, pp. 229–272). Hillsdale, NJ: L. Erlbaum Associates.

Asian and Pacific Islander Center for Census Information and Services. (1992). *Asian and Pacific Islander American profile series.* San Francisco: Author.

Attar, B., Guerra, N. G., & Tolan, P. G. (1994). Neighborhood disadvantage, stressful life events, and adjustment in urban elementary school children. *Journal of Clinical Child Psychology, 23*, 394–400.

Barbarin, O. (1993). Coping and resilience: Exploring the inner lives of African American children. *Journal of Black Psychology, 19*, 478–492.

Barnes, G. M., Farrell, M. P., & Banerjee, S. (1994). Family influences on alcohol abuse and other problem behaviors among black and white adolescents in a general population sample. *Journal of Research on Adolescence, 4*, 183–201.

Barrera, M., Jr., Li, S. A., & Chassin, L. (1995). Effects of parental alcoholism and life stress on Hispanic and non-Hispanic Caucasian adolescents: A prospective study. *American Journal of Community Psychology, 23*, 479–507.

Beiser, M., & Attneave, C. L. (1982). Mental disorders among Native American children: Rates and risk periods for entering treatment. *American Journal of Psychiatry, 139*, 193–198.

Bell, C. C., & Jenkins, E. J. (1991). Traumatic stress and children. *Journal of Health Care for the Poor and Underserved, 2*, 175–184.

Bell-Scott, P., & Taylor, R. L. (1989). Introduction: The multiple ecologies of Black adolescent development. *Journal of Adolescent Research, 4(2)*, 119–124.

Berlin, I. N. (1987). Effects of changing Native American cultures on child development. *Journal of Community Psychology, 15*, 299–306.

Bernal, M. E., Saenz, D. S., & Knight, G. P. (1991). Ethnic identity and adaptation of Mexican American youths in school settings. *Hispanic Journal of Behavioral Sciences, 13*, 135–154.

Berry, J. W., & Kim, U. (1988). Acculturation and mental health. In P. Dasen, J. W. Berry, & N. Sartorius (Eds.), *Health and cross-cultural psychology: Towards application* (pp. 207–236). London: Sage.

Biafora, F. A., Jr., Warheit, G. J., Zimmerman, R. S., Gil, A. G., Apospori, E., & Taylor, D. (1993). Racial mistrust and deviant behavior among ethnically diverse black adolescent boys. *Journal of Applied Social Psychology, 23*, 891–910.

Bowman, P. J., & Howard, C. (1985). Race related socialization, motivation and academic achievement: A study of black youth in three generation families. *Journal of the American Academy of Child Psychiatry, 24*, 1134–1141.

Brody, G. H., Stoneman, Z., Flor, D., McCrary, D., Hastings, L., & Convers, O. (1994). Financial resources, parent psychological functioning, parent co-caregiving, and early adolescent competencies in rural two-parent African-American families. *Child Development, 65*, 590–605.

Bronfenbrenner, U. (1989). Ecological systems theory. *Annals of Child Development, 6*, 187–249.

Brooks-Gunn, J., Duncan, G. J., & Klebanov, P. K. (1993). Do neighborhoods influence child and adolescent development? *American Journal of Sociology, 99(2)*, 353–392.

Bui, K. V., & Takeuchi, D. T. (1992). Ethnic minority adolescents and the use of the community mental health care system. *American Journal of Community Psychology, 20*, 403–417.

Buriel, R., Calzada, S., & Vasquez, R. (1982). The relationship of traditional Mexican-American culture to adjustment and delinquency among three generations of Mexican-American male adolescents. *Hispanic Journal of Behavioral Sciences, 4(1)*, 41–55.

Chavez, E. L., Oetting, E. R., & Swaim, R. C. (1994). Dropout and delinquency: Mexican American and Caucasian non-Hispanic youth. *Journal of Clinical Child Psychology, 23*, 47–55.

Chavez, D. V., Moran, V. R., Reid, S. L., & Lopez, M. (in press). Acculturative stress in children: A modification of the SAFE scale. *Hispanic Journal of Behavioral Sciences.*

Clarke, G., Sack, W. H., & Goff, B. (1993). Three forms of stress in Cambodian adolescent refugees. *Journal of Abnormal Child Psychology, 21*, 65–77.

Codega, S. A., Pasley, B. K., & Kreutzer, J. (1990). Coping behaviors of adolescent mothers. *Journal of Adolescent Research, 5,* 34–53.

Constantino, G., Malgady, R. G., & Rogler, L. H. (1986). Cuento therapy: A culturally sensitive modality for Puerto Rican children. *Journal of Consulting and Clinical Psychology, 54*(5), 639–645.

Copeland, E. P., & Hess, R. S. (1995). Differences in young adolescents' coping strategies based on gender and ethnicity. *Journal of Early Adolescence, 15,* 203–219.

Costello, E. J. (1989). Developments in child psychiatric epidemiology. *Journal of the American Academy of Child and Adolescent Psychiatry, 28,* 836–841.

Crocker, J., & Major, B. (1989). Social stigma and self-esteem. The self-protective properties of stigma. *Psychological Review, 96,* 608–630.

Dembo, R., Williams, L., & Schneidler, J. (1994). Psychosocial, alcohol, other drug use, and delinquency differences between urban black and white male high risk youth. *International Journal of the Addictions, 29(4),* 461–483.

Dinges, N. G., & Duong-Tran, Q. (1993). Stressful life events and co-occurring depression, substance abuse and suicidality among American Indian and Alaska Native adolescents. *Culture, Medicine, and Psychiatry, 16,* 487–502.

Dornbusch, S. M., Mont-Reynaud, R., Ritter, R. L., Chen, A., & Steinberg, L. (1991). Stressful events and their correlates among adolescents of diverse backgrounds. In M. E. Colten & S. Gore (Eds.), *Adolescent stress: Causes and consequences* (pp. 111–130). New York: Aldine de Gruyter.

Dumka, L. E., Roosa, M. W., Michaels, M. L., & Suh, K. W. (1995). Using research to develop prevention programs for high risk families. *Family Relations, 44,* 78–86.

Duncan, G. J., Brooks-Gunn, J., & Klebanov, P. K. (1994). Economic deprivation and early childhood development. *Child Development, 65,* 296–318.

Emslie, G. J., Weinberg, W. A., Rush, A. J., Adams, R. M., & Rintelman, J. W. (1990). Depression symptoms by self-report in adolescence: Phase I of the development of a questionnaire for depression by self-report. *Journal of Child Neurology, 5,* 114–121.

Felner, R. D., Brand, S., DuBois, D. L., Adan, A. M., Mulhal, P. R., & Evans, E. G. (1995). Socioeconomic disadvantage, proximal environmental experiences, and socioemotional and academic adjustment in early adolescence: Investigation of a mediated effects model. *Child Development, 66,* 774–792.

Fitzpatrick, K.M., & Boldizar, J.P. (1993). The prevalence and consequences of exposure to violence among African American youth. *Journal of the American Academy of Child and Adolescent Psychiatry, 32,* 424–430.

Fordham, S., & Ogbu, J. U. (1987). Black student's school success: Coping with the "burden of acting white." *Urban Review, 18,* 176–206.

Freeman, L. N., Mokros, H., & Poznanski, E. O. (1993). Violent events reported by normal urban school-aged children: Characteristics and depression correlates. *Journal of the American Academy of Child and Adolescent Psychiatry, 32,* 419–423.

Garcia-Coll, C. T., Meyer, E. C., & Brillon, L. (in press). Ethnic and minority parenting. In M. H. Bornstein (Ed.), *Handbook of parenting* (Vol. 2). Hillsdale, NJ: Erlbaum.

Garrison, C. Z., Jackson, K. L., Marsteller, F., McKeown, R., & Addy, C. (1990). A longitudinal study of depressive symptomatology in young adolescents. *Journal of the American Academy of Child and Adolescent Psychiatry, 29,* 581–585.

Gibbs, J. (1986). Assessment of depression in urban adolescent females: Implications for early intervention strategies. *American Journal of Social Psychiatry, 6,* 50–56.

Gonzales, N. A., Gunnoe, M. L., Samaniego, R., & Jackson, K. (1995). *Validation of a multicultural event schedule for adolescents.* Paper presented at the Biennial Conference of the Society for Community Research and Action, Chicago, IL.

Guerra, N. G., Huesmann, L. R., Tolan, P. H., VanAcker, R., & Eron, L. D. (1995). *Journal of Consulting and Clinical Psychology, 63,* 518–528.

Gutelius, M. F., Kirsch, A. D., MacDonald, S., Brooks, M. R., & McErlean, T. (1977). Controlled study of child health supervision: Behavioral results. *Pediatrics, 60,* 294–304.

Halstead, M., Johnson, S. B., Cunningham, W. (1993). Measuring coping in adolescents: An application of the ways of coping checklist. *Journal of Clinical Child Psychology, 22,* 337–344.

Hammond, R., & Yung, B. (1993). Psychology's role in the public health response to assaultive violence among young African-American men. *American Psychologist, 48,* 142–154.

Harrison, A. O., Wilson, M. N., Pine, C. J., Chan, S. Q., & Buriel, R. (1990). Family ecologies of ethnic minority children. *Child Development, 61,* 347–362.

Hinton, W. L., Chen, Y. C., Du, N., & Tran, C. G. (1993). Disorders in Vietnamese refugees: Prevalence and correlates. *Journal of Nervous and Mental Disease, 181,* 113–122.

Johnson, D. L., & Walker, T. (1987). Primary prevention of behavior problems in Mexican American children. *American Journal of Community Psychology, 15*(4), 375–385.

Kessler, R., & Neighbors, H. (1986). A new perspective on the relationships among race, social class, and psychological distress. *Journal of Health and Social Behavior, 27,* 107–115.

Kim, L. S., & Chun, C. (1993). Ethnic differences in psychiatric diagnosis among Asian American adolescents. *Journal of Nervous and Mental Diseases, 181,* 612–617.

Kinzie, J. D., Sack, W., Aryelle, R., Clarke, G., & Ben, R. (1989). A three year follow-up of Cambodian young people traumatized as children. *Journal of the American Academy of Child and Adolescent Psychiatry, 28,* 501–504.

Knight, G. P., & Hill, N. (in press). Measurement equivalence in research involving minority adolescents. In V. McLoyd & L. Steinberg (Eds.), *Research on minority adolescents: Conceptual, methodological and theoretical issues.* Hillsdale, NJ: Erlbaum.

Knight, G. P., Virdin, L., & Roosa, M. (1994). Socialization and family correlates of mental health outcomes among Hispanic and Anglo-American families. *Child Development, 65,* 212–224.

Kovacs, M. (1982). *The Children's Depression Inventory: A self-rated depression scale for school age youngsters.* Unpublished manuscript, University of Pittsburgh.

Kunz, E. F. (1981). Exile and resettlement: Refugee theory. *International Migration Review, 15,* 42–51.

La Fromboise, T. D., Coleman, H. L. K., & Gerton, J. (1993). Psychological impact of biculturalism: Evidence and theory. *Psychological Bulletin, 114,* 395–412.

Laosa, L. M. (1990). Psychosocial stress, coping, and development of Hispanic immigrant children. In F. C. Serafica, A. J. Schuebel, R. K. Russell, P. D. Isaac, & L. Myers (Eds.), *Mental health of ethnic minorities* (pp. 42–65). New York: Praeger.

Lazarus, R. S., & Folkman, S. (1984). *Stress, appraisal, and coping.* New York: Springer.

Leadbetter, B. J., & Bishop, S. J. (1994). Predictors of behavior problems in preschool children of inner-city Afro-American and Puerto Rican adolescent mothers. *Child Development, 65,* 638–648.

Levitt, M. J., Guacci-Franco, N., & Levitt, J. L. (1993). Convoys of social support in childhood and early adolescence: Structure and function. *Developmental Psychology, 29,* 811–818.

Liu, W., Yu, E., Chang, C., & Fernandez, M. (1990). The mental health of Asian American teenagers: A research challenge. In A. Stiffman & L. Davis (Eds.), *Ethnic issues in adolescent mental health* (pp. 92–112). Newbury Park, CA: Sage.

Lum, K., & Char, W. F. (1985). Chinese adaptation in Hawaii: Some examples. In W. Tsent & D. Y. H. Wu (Eds.), *Chinese culture and mental health* (pp. 215–226). Orlando, FL: Academic Press.

Malgady, R. G., Rogler, L. H., & Constantino, G. (1990). Hero/heroine modeling for Puerto Rican adolescents: A preventive mental health intervention. *Journal of Consulting and Clinical Psychology, 58,* 469–474.

Marin, G., & Marin, B. V. (1991). *Research with Hispanic populations.* Newbury Park, CA: Sage.

Mason, C. A., Cauce, A. M., Gonzales, N. A., & Hiraga, Y. (1995). Adolescent problem behavior: The effect of peers and the moderating role of father absence and the mother–child relationship. *American Journal of Community Psychology, 22,* 723–743.

May, P. A. (1987). Suicide and self-destruction among American-Indian youths. *American Indian and Alaska Native Mental Health Research, 1*(1), 52–69.

McGoldrick, M., Pearce, J. K., & Giordano, J. (1984). *Ethnicity and Family Therapy.* New York: Guilford Press.

McLoyd, V. C. (1990). Socialization and development in a changing economy. *American Psychologist, 44,* 293–302.

Munsch, J., & Wampler, R. S. (1993). Ethnic differences in early adolescents coping with school stress. *American Journal of Orthopsychiatry, 63,* 633–646.

Myers, H. F. (1989). Urban stress and mental health in Afro-American youth: An epidemiologic and conceptual update. In R. Jones (Ed.), *Black adolescents* (pp. 123–152). Berkeley, CA: Cobb & Henry.

Myers, H. F., Alvy, K. T., Arrington, A., Richardson, M. A., Magana, M., Huff, R., Main, M., & Newcomb, M. D. (1992). Impact of the effective black parenting program on parental practices and child behaviors. *Journal of Community Psychology, 20*, 132–147.

Oetting, E. R., & Beauvais, F. (1991). Orthogonal cultural identification theory: The cultural identification of minority adolescents. *The International Journal of the Addictions, 25*, 655–685.

Ong, P., & Hee, S. J. (1992). The growth of the Asian Pacific American population: Twenty million in 2020. In *The state of Asian Pacific America: Policy issues to the year 2020* (pp. 11–24). Los Angeles: Asian American Public Policy Institute and UCLA Asian American Studies Center.

Oyserman, D., & Saltz, E. (1993). Competence, delinquency, and attempts to attain possible selves. *Journal of Personality and Social Psychology, 65*, 360–374.

Peeples, F., & Loeber, R. (1994). Do individual factors and neighborhood context explain ethnic differences in juvenile delinquency? *Journal of Quantitative Criminology, 10*, 141–157.

Phinney, J. S., & Chairra, V. (1996). Parent ethnic socialization and coping with problems related to ethnicity. *Journal of Adolescent Research, 50*, 31–39.

Phinney, J. S., Lochner, B. T., & Murphy, R. (1991). Ethnic identity development and psychological adjustment in adolescence. In A. Stiffman & L. Dairs (Eds.), *Advances in adolescent mental health, Vol. V: Ethnic Issues* (pp. 53–72). Greenwich, CT: JAI Press.

Rick, K., & Forward, J. (1992). Acculturation and perceived intergenerational differences among Hmong youth. *Journal of Cross-Cultural Psychology, 23*(1), 85–94.

Roberts, R. E., & Sobhan, M. (1992). Symptoms of depression in adolescence: A comparison of Anglo, African, and Hispanic Americans. *Journal of Youth and Adolescence, 21*, 639–651.

Rogler, L. H., Cortes, D. E., & Malgady, R. G. (1991). Acculturation and mental health status among Hispanics. *American Psychologist, 46*, 585–597.

Rutter, M. (1983). Stress, coping, and development: Some issues and some questions. In N. Garmezy & M. Rutter (Eds.), *Stress, coping and development in children* (pp. 1–41). New York: McGraw-Hill.

Sampson, R. J., & Laub, J. H. (1994). Urban poverty and the family context of delinquency: A new look at structure and process in a classic study. *Child Development, 65*, 541–561.

Schinke, S., Jansen, M., Kennedy, E., & Shi, Q. (1994). Reducing risk-taking behavior among vulnerable youth: An intervention outcome study. *Family Community Health, 16*(4), 49–56.

Schoenbach, V. J., Kaplan, B. J., Wagner, E. H., Grimson, R. C., & Miller, F. T. (1983). Prevalence of self-reported depressive symptoms in young adolescents. *American Journal of Public Health, 73*, 1281–1287.

Schweinhart, L. J., Berrueta-Clement, J. R., Barnett, W. S., Epstein, A. S., & Weikart, D. P. (1985). Effects of the Perry Preschool Program on youths through age 19: A summary. *Topics in Early Childhood Education, 5*(2), 26–35.

Shaffer, D., Gould, M., Hicks, R. C. (1994). Worsening suicide rate in Black teenagers.

Shure, M. B., & Spivak, G. (1982). Interpersonal problem solving in young children: A cognitive approach to prevention. *American Journal of Community Psychology, 10*(3), 341–357.

Spencer, M. B. (1990). Development of minority children: An introduction. *Child Development, 61*, 267–269.

Spencer, M. B., & Markstrom-Adams, C. (1990). Identity processes among racial and ethnic minority children in America. *Child Development, 61*, 290–310.

Sue, S., Fujino, D. C., Hu, L., Takeuchi, D. T., & Zane, N. (1991). Community mental health services for ethnic minority groups: A test of the cultural responsive hypothesis. *Journal of Consulting and Clinical Psychology, 59*(4), 433–540.

Szapocznik, J., & Kurtines, W. (1980). Acculturation, biculturalism, and adjustment among Cuban Americans. In A. Padilla (Ed.), *Acculturation: Theory, models, and some new findings* (pp. 139–159). Boulder, CO: Westview.

Szapocznik, J., Santisteban, D., Rio, A., Perez-Vidal, A., Santisteban, D., & Kurtines, W. M. (1989). Family effectiveness training: An intervention to prevent drug abuse and problem behaviors in Hispanic adolescents. *Hispanic Journal of Behavioral Sciences, 11*(1), 4–27.

Tajfel, H. (1978). *The social psychology of minorities.* New York: Minority Rights Group.

Takeuchi, D. T., Bui, K. V., & Kim, L. (1993). The referral of minority adolescent to community mental health centers. *Journal of Health and Social Behavior, 34*, 153–164.

Tolan, P. H., & McKay, M. M. (1996). Preventing anti-social behavior in inner-city children. *Family Relations, 45,* 148–155.

US Bureau of the Census. (1994). Population and housing summary Tape File 1C.

US Bureau of the Census. (1994). Census of population and housing subject summary tape file 17. US Department of Commerce, Washington, DC.

US Bureau of the Census. (1995). *Race and Hispanic origin: 1995.* Census Profile Number 2, September 1995. Washington, DC: Government Printing Office.

Vega, W. A. Khoury, E. L., Zimmerman, R. S., Gil, A. G., & Warheit, G. J. (1995). Cultural conflicts and problem behaviors of Latino adolescents in home and school environments. *Journal of Community Psychology, 23,* 167–178.

Wells, E. A., Morrison, D. M., Gillmore, M. R., Catalano, R. F., Iritani, B., & Hawkins, J. D. (1992). Race differences in antisocial behaviors and attitudes and early initiation of substance use. *Journal Drug Education, 22,* 115–130.

Windle, M. (1990). A longitudinal study of antisocial behaviors in early adolescence as predictors of late adolescent substance use: Gender and ethnic group differences. *Journal of Abnormal Psychology, 99,* 86–91.

Wyman, P. A., Cowen, E. L., Work, W. C., & Parker, G. R. (1991). Developmental and family milieu correlates of resilience in urban children who have experienced major life stress. *American Journal of Community Psychology, 19,* 405–425.

Yates, A. (1987). Current status and future directions of research on the American Indian child. *American Journal of Psychiatry, 144*(9), 1135–1142.

Zimmerman, M. A., & Maton, K. I. (1992). Life-style and substance use among male African-American urban adolescents: A cluster analytic approach. *American Journal of Community Psychology, 20,* 121–138.

V

Conclusion

18

Preventing the Negative Effects of Common Stressors
Current Status and Future Directions

MARK W. ROOSA, SHARLENE A. WOLCHIK, and IRWIN N. SANDLER

The prevention research cycle has been described in many ways (e.g., Bloom, 1979; Coie et al., 1993; Cowen, 1982; Heller, Price, & Sher, 1980; Mrazek & Haggerty, 1994; Price, 1983, 1987; Price & Lorion, 1989; Sandler, Gersten, Reynolds, Kallgren, & Ramirez, 1988). Most of these approaches to prevention research include: (1) a generative stage in which researchers seek to develop a theory of the causal processes that place a particular group of children at heightened risk of adverse developmental outcomes; (2) a program development stage in which behavior change technology is utilized to design programs to change putative causal processes identified in the theory; (3) a field trial stage in which experimental trials are used to test whether the programs are effective in changing the putative causal processes and the targeted outcomes; and (4) an innovation diffusion stage in which a standardized program is implemented on a large scale in a wide range of naturalistic community settings (see Fig. 1).

Research that describes the processes of adaptation to stress is part of the generative stage of prevention research. The central goal of this stage has been to identify risk and protective processes that determine whether and to what degree a major stressor may impact a child (Lorion, Price, & Eaton, 1989; Rutter, 1990, 1994). Most major stressors do not directly impact children's developmental trajectories (Rutter, 1990). Instead, the occurrence of a major stressor

MARK W. ROOSA • Department of Family Resources and Human Development and Program for Prevention Research, Arizona State University, Tempe, Arizona 85287-1108. SHARLENE A. WOLCHIK and IRWIN N. SANDLER • Department of Psychology and Program for Prevention Research, Arizona State University, Tempe, Arizona 85287-1108.

Handbook of Children's Coping: Linking Theory and Intervention, edited by Wolchik and Sandler. Plenum Press, New York, 1997.

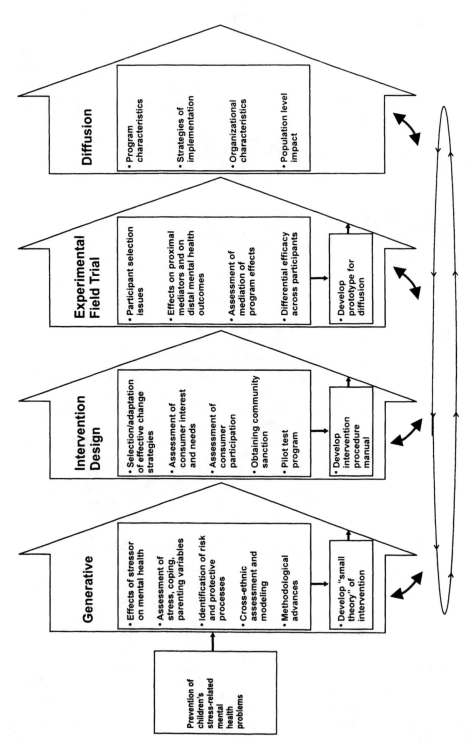

Figure 1. The four phases of the prevention research cycle.

often sets in motion a process, or series of processes, including multiple small-er stressors, that impact a child and/or the child's environment. These pro-cesses are proximal to the child and have a more direct impact on development than more distal major stressors. Knowledge of the proximal processes or caus-al sequences through which a major stressor threatens healthy development, of the processes that prevent or reduce the negative impact of a major stressor, and the interplay among these processes provides an important foundation for the development of successful preventive interventions (e.g., Mrazek & Haggerty, 1994; Price, 1987).

The generalized stress process model shown in Fig. 2 provides an organiz-ing structure for illustrating some of the types of theoretical causal processes that are of interest to prevention researchers. Earlier chapters in this volume have described a wide variety of major stressors that threaten children's devel-opmental outcomes. The model shows two major classes of processes that influence how these stressors impact children's outcomes: moderating pro-cesses and mediating processes. Mediators and moderators can be characteris-tics of the child, the child's family, or the larger environment that determine the degree to which a stressor may impact child outcomes (Garmezy, 1985; Masten & Garmezy, 1985).

Moderators alter the strength of the relation between exposure to a stressor and outcomes. A stressor may have little or no effect in the presence of a moderator, but may greatly increase or decrease the likelihood of negative outcomes in the absence of a moderator (or vice versa). For instance, the pres-ence of social support from adults has been shown to reduce the negative effects of life stress for children in divorced families (Wolchik, Ruelhman, Braver, & Sandler, 1989). Thus, social support is considered a protective factor. As shown in Fig. 2, protective factors are moderators that reduce the strength of the relation of a stressor to developmental outcomes, while vulnerability fac-tors are moderators that increase the strength of this relation. Typically, re-searchers identify moderators by finding variables that interact with stressors to influence adaptation (Rutter, 1985, 1990). In general, moderators themselves are not influenced by the occurrence of the stressor.

Unlike moderators, mediators are affected (degraded or enhanced) by the

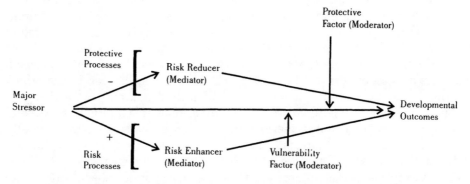

Figure 2. The stress process model showing mediation and moderation effects.

presence or strength of major stressors. Mediators in turn are related to mental health outcomes, either in a positive or negative direction. For instance, positive parenting behaviors such as warmth or consistent discipline are positively related to child mental health. However, these parenting qualities can be reduced by exposure to high levels of stress and the diminished quality of parenting can increase a child's likelihood of developing mental health problems (e.g., Roosa, Tein, Groppenbacher, Michaels, & Dumka, 1993). Like moderators, mediators are more proximal to the child, and their influences are direct or at least more direct, than those of major stressors. A risk reducer (e.g., parental warmth) is a mediator that has a positive impact on developmental outcomes, but exposure to the major stressor degrades the quality of this variable. In contrast, a risk enhancer (e.g., parental hostility) is a mediator that has a negative impact on developmental outcomes and is increased by exposure to the stressor.

Stressful events are a common mediator of most major stressors. That is, the occurrence of a major stressor often sets in motion a number of negative life events for a child. Increased exposure to stressful events can impact other aspects of the child's environment (e.g., parent–child relationships, family functioning), as well as impacting the child's physical or mental health. In the absence of protective processes, such a sequence of events can contribute to mental health problems, problems in relationships with peers, or problems in school.

A major advantage of the stress process model is that it reminds us to look for factors and processes that contribute to children's positive outcomes (or protect children from negative outcomes), as well as the more common strategy of finding factors or processes that increase the likelihood of negative outcomes. Furthermore, using this model to guide or interpret research contributes to the development of a theory of intervention (Price, 1987). A theory of intervention is a "small theory" of the processes leading to poor or optimal outcomes under adverse conditions (Lipsey, 1990). There are several important advantages to using a small theory approach to develop and evaluate preventive interventions (e.g., Coie et al., 1993; Grych & Fincham, 1992; West, Sandler, Pillow, Baca, & Gersten, 1991). First, it provides a theoretical framework to guide program design by identifying putative mediating or moderating variables that, if changed, should improve children's long-term adjustment. Second, it specifies and tests proximal outcomes that the program is intended to affect. Such information is useful in program redesign by helping to differentiate between aspects of the intervention that were too poorly implemented to have any impact versus aspects of the intervention that were well implemented but did not generate the theoretically expected effects. Third, this approach provides a rigorous test for the underlying theory about processes that affect children's mental health outcomes. Most identified risk and protective processes arise from correlational studies in which plausible alternative explanations cannot be ruled out. Experimentally induced changes on theoretically specified mediators and targeted outcomes provide a stronger test of the hypothesis that these variables are causally related to outcomes.

The chapters in this volume clearly show that there has been differential progress across major stressful conditions in understanding the processes that affect adaptation from a stress process perspective and in applying this knowledge to the development of interventions that promote healthy adaptation. In some areas, there has been very little research or thinking about the risk condition in terms of the stress process model, although there may be other very rich research literatures. In other areas, there is a solid generative base, but these findings have not been used to develop and evaluate preventive interventions. In a few areas, there is both a rich generative literature and a flourishing tradition of theory-based interventions. In only one area do we find evidence that the prevention research cycle has reached the diffusion stage.

In this chapter, we review the state of preventive intervention development in each topic area covered in this volume. Each topic area is evaluated in terms of its use of a stress process model and progress through the prevention research cycle. Our goal is to identify commonalities and uniquenesses in developing stress process theory-based preventive interventions, testing the efficacy of these interventions, and disseminating the interventions in naturalistic settings. After reviewing the state of prevention research in each area, we discuss the lessons and challenges that future prevention research using the stress process model must address.

AREAS WITH MINIMAL GENERATIVE RESEARCH FOUNDATIONS USING THE STRESS PROCESS MODEL

Although there are rich research literatures on teenage pregnancy and parenting, children who experience peer rejection, and child maltreatment, very little of this research is based on the stress process model. Given the inherently stressful nature of these conditions, the lack of research from this perspective is surprising. For instance, Langfield and Pasley (Chapter 9, this volume) found a great deal of support for the argument that teenage pregnancy/parenting is highly stressful, but they report minimal research that examined whether stress in teenage pregnancy or parenting was related to pregnancy performance, the teenage mother's mental health, the quality of her parenting, or her child's development. Similarly, although there is research examining the relation of a major stressor—poverty—to the risk for teenage pregnancy, researchers have not examined whether stressful life events play a role in increasing the risk for teenage pregnancy or influence pregnancy outcomes. Researchers have described some stressful experiences associated with teenage motherhood, have identified ethnicity or culture as a moderator of responses to teenage pregnancy or parenting, and have investigated the role of social support as a potential protective factor. However, this latter research appears to be descriptive and not necessarily theoretically driven. For instance, researchers have reported that social support was related to more positive parenting behavior by teenage mothers, but it was not clear whether this was due to a stress-buffering relation (moderation) or to other processes such as modeling of effective parenting practices by supporters. Langfield and Pasley reported that many programs designed to prevent teenage pregnancies lack a theoretical base and may ignore the research literature as well. Tests of the mediating or moderating effects of stressful life events and other relevant variables on child developmental outcomes, pregnancy performance, and maternal mental health for teenage mothers would move the generative research base forward and provide a foundation for theory-guided intervention development. Langfield and Pasley also noted the need to use developmentally appropriate measures of social support and measures of stressful life events that adequately capture the experiences of pregnant or parenting teenagers to contribute to progress in the development of a stress process research foundation in this area.

Similarly, research on the developmental impact of child maltreatment, although often theoretically driven, generally has not used the stress process model (Haugaard, Reppucci, & Feerick, Chapter 3, this volume). Some research has shown that stressful conditions increase the likelihood of child maltreatment (Sameroff & Chandler, 1975). Haugaard et al. use theory and research to identify several correlates of the effects of child abuse on child outcomes; however, apparently little has been done to determine which of these variables might be mediators. Thus, there is little empirical work on which to build stress theory-based preventive interventions that seek to prevent either child maltreatment or its effects on child mental health. However, the authors provide a list of individual and family characteristics related to better adjustment that could guide the search for mediators or moderators, which then would serve as the foundation for the next generation of interventions. Of course, legal and ethical issues make research on child maltreatment more challenging than research in many other areas. Even with these additional challenges, reframing what we learn from clinical practice with this population into a stress process model should strengthen the foundation for developing theory-based preventive interventions. In addition, retrospective studies with children who have been abused and neglected as well as with their families may identify potential moderators and mediators of this stressor.

Zakriski, Jacobs, and Coie (Chapter 15, this volume) argue that "conceptualizing peer rejection in a stress and coping framework could help move the field from the focus on description and prediction that has dominated research on peer rejection to an understanding of the process of adjustment to peer rejection and to more successful intervention efforts." The authors' discussion of the limited research on the nature of the stressor of peer rejection and children's appraisals of it represents an important initial step in applying the stress process model to this risk situation. Further, research on how peer-rejected children appraise episodes of peer rejection highlights the importance of distinguishing between aggressive and nonaggressive rejected children in future applications of the stress process model. Aggression may be an important moderator of the peer rejection experience that needs to be taken into account in both generative research and the development of interventions. A unique challenge to intervention developers with this risk group is the need to work with targeted children's peer group as well as those who are rejected by their peers in order that behavior changes are accepted by the community of peers.

Although none of these research areas include an extensive stress process generative research base, numerous prevention efforts have been implemented. However, apparently none of these have been guided by stress process theory or research. Further, the efficacy of these preventive interventions has not been convincingly demonstrated. There is reason to believe that well-conceived, systematic research programs based on the stress process model would provide rich generative research bases on which preventive interventions could be developed in each of these areas. The authors of each of these chapters have articulated several research questions that can provide guidance for the development of more extensive generative research bases and, eventually, stress process based preventive interventions.

AREAS WITH REASONABLE GENERATIVE BASES BUT NO EVALUATED STRESS-BASED PREVENTION PROGRAMS

The review of research on the influences of parental illness on children's mental health (Worsham, Compas, & Ey, Chapter 7, this volume) reveals a newly evolving literature. Furthermore, much of the recent research has used a stress process model and some potential mediators and moderators of the influence of parental illness on children's mental health have been identified (e.g., child gender, child developmental level, coping efforts, marital adjustment, parenting). In particular, reports of the moderating roles of child gender and developmental level highlight the importance of these and other fundamental demographic variables in research on the stress process model for this and probably other risk situations. Research on the impact of parental illness on children's adjustment probably would benefit from efforts to operationalize what it is about parental illness that children find stressful and thereby to quantify exposure to stressful life events. Although several preventive interventions have been developed for this population, none of these have been guided by the stress process model, and apparently none have been adequately evaluated. Despite the fact that the stress process model has been applied to this research area only recently, it appears that there may be a sufficient research foundation to guide the development of first-generation, theoretically based preventive interventions.

Research on the complex impact of disasters on children's mental health (Saylor, Belter, & Stokes, Chapter 13, this volume) has identified several correlates of children's adjustment (e.g., parental mental health, family functioning, sources of stress) and studied the impact of some potential moderators of children's adjustment (e.g., gender, age, ethnicity). The identification of several features of the disaster experience (e.g., degree of exposure, perceived threat to life, loss or separation from family members) that are related to children's adjustment provides important information that future research might build on by developing more comprehensive assessments of the nature of disaster related stress. The reliance on zero-order correlations or analysis of variance in much of the research in this area has precluded determining whether the variables related to child adjustment are mediators, moderators, or spurious correlates because of their relations to other, more direct influences on children's adjustment. Although interventions have been developed based on the empirical literature, to date stress-process-based preventive interventions have not been rigorously evaluated. Most interventions appear to be based on providing children with a variety of sources of social support and providing triage services to direct those most in need to mental health services.

Both research on and interventions for children who experience disasters are different phenomena than any other area reviewed in this volume. Disasters are immediate, acute events that usually impact large numbers of people simultaneously. Thus, research and intervention have to take place within a limited, externally imposed time frame, a restriction not applicable to other major stressors. The emphasis of most intervention programs is on returning families and communities to some semblance of normality as soon as possible and making referrals for those who may face adjustment problems. Interventions, therefore, are brief. Although little evidence has been developed for the efficacy of these interventions, an effort has been made to record intervention components that seem effective and to share them among agencies providing services during disasters. In addition to rigorous evaluations of these interventions, more theory-driven research that tests the nature of the relations of key variables to adjustment would help in the development of stress-based theory-guided interventions that might be useful to children.

RESEARCH AREAS WITH EVALUATED STRESS-BASED INTERVENTIONS

The daily challenges faced by inner-city children can be overwhelming, as Tolan, Guerra, and Montaini-Klovdahl (Chapter 16, this volume) remind us. In addition to living in a state of chronic high stress, inner-city children may be more vulnerable to the effects of stress primarily due to a lack of resources. Furthermore, the stresses these children face threaten their health and lives, as well as their mental health, unlike most other stressful situations reviewed in this volume. While focusing on inner-city children's coping behaviors, Tolan et al. make an important distinction between coping effectiveness and adaptability. They argue that inner-city children may develop coping responses that are effective in the short term, but which may threaten their long-term well-being. Furthermore, because the stressors these children face are pervasive and overwhelming, interventions that target only children, or only children and their families, may not be sufficient (e.g., Coie et al., 1993; Sameroff & Fiese, 1989; Yoshikawa, 1994). As Tolan and his colleagues note, interventions may need to be broadened not only to the community as a whole, but they may need to include changes in public policy and social institutions.

Although relatively few studies have explicitly used the stress process model to study inner-city children and their developmental outcomes, several potential mediators or moderators of adjustment to life in the inner city have been identified (e.g., coping, social support, parenting, family functioning, family conflict), and a reasonable foundation for developing interventions exists. In fact, a number of programs for inner-city children and/or their families that target one or more of these mediators or moderators have been developed and intensively evaluated. In a recent review, Yoshikawa (1994) discusses programs that have shown significant positive and cost-effective impacts on inner-city children over periods ranging from a few years to over a decade. Yoshikawa argues that successful programs for this at-risk group need to begin early in children's lives, be extensive, and target multiple risk factors in multiple settings. Thus, although much work remains to understand contextual influences on inner-city children's lives and to intervene at the social policy and institutional levels, several programs have demonstrated that psychosocial interventions based on the stress process model can make a difference in inner-city children's lives.

A factor that contributes to the challenge of research on and interventions for inner-city children concerns the ethnic diversity of inner-city communities. In fact, ethnic minority groups are overrepresented among those at risk for poor developmental outcomes in general, although few of the chapters in this volume seemed to take ethnicity into consideration. Interpreting generative research with ethnic minority populations is complicated because of the common problem of confounding ethnicity and social class and the common practice of assuming that measures developed with middle-class European Americans are reliable and valid when used with low-income and/or minority groups (Gonzales & Kim, Chapter 17, this volume). Ethnicity is a critical variable to consider in stress process research and stress theory-based interventions because it can be a source of stress (e.g., acculturation, racism, discrimination) or serve as a stress buffer. Further, if ignored, ethnicity can be an obstacle to participation in preventive interventions or to program effectiveness. That is, if prevention programs are not designed to be attractive to members of minority groups or if programs or staff are not culturally sensitive, it may be difficult to recruit or retain minority participants or to induce members of minority groups to see how program goals apply to them.

Gonzales and Kim also identify four cultural ecology variables (family poverty, high-risk neighborhood context, migration and acculturation experiences, and racism and discrimination) that may account for much of the diversity within ethnic groups and help explain why minority status is often shown to be related to children's adjustment problems. The authors also argue that cultural sensitivity, taking ethnicity and culture into consideration in research and intervention, is as important as a sound empirical foundation for the development of effective preventive interventions. Gonzales and Kim identify several culturally sensitive family or child-focused programs that targeted mediators identified by stress process research and that have been shown to be effective. Interestingly, all of these programs appear to target low-income and/or inner-city families or children. Developing culturally sensitive versions of preventive interventions for the other at-risk groups reviewed in this volume is an area needing further attention.

Cultural issues beyond those represented by ethnicity also may be important to prevention researchers. Greenberg, Lengua, and Calderon (Chapter 11, this volume) reviewed the literature on deafness and children's adjustment. These authors introduce the intriguing notion that the experience of a major chronic stressor may produce a culture and that this culture can contribute greatly to healthy developmental outcomes. In addition, Greenberg et al. introduce a heuristic stress process model of influences on the mental health of deaf children that takes many contextual factors into consideration as potential mediators. The notion of a culture being created by those who experience a major stressor and many aspects of the model these authors present may apply to many other groups as well (e.g., pregnant and parenting teenagers, inner-city children, children with chronic illnesses). The PATHS curriculum, based on their model, has been shown to produce the desired changes in targeted mediators and in developmental outcomes for this population.

Hammen (Chapter 5, this volume) reviews a rich generative research base that builds on the stress process model and identifies several potential mediators or moderators of adjustment for children of depressed parents (e.g., child social competence, quality of parenting, family conflict, family cohesion). One would think that this research foundation would provide considerable guidance to those interested in the development of theory-based preventive interventions. However, apparently only one stress process theory-guided prevention program has been developed. As Hammen noted, because parental behavior is the major source of risks to the child's mental health, prevention programs will need to deal with parent–child and other family relationships and help children understand a depressed parent's behavior.

As Hammen points out, the fundamental challenge to providing preventive services for children of depressed parents involves identifying those children who are at risk, especially among children of parents with chronic, subclinical forms of depression. Prevention of problems resulting from major stressors that are not marked by some public event (e.g., divorce), are not easily observable, or do not have clear beginnings (e.g., parental mental illness, parental substance abuse) present prevention program developers with considerable challenges. In particular, how can members of the target population be identified and recruited into preventive interventions without violating their legal or ethical rights (cf. Roosa, Michaels, Groppenbacher, & Gersten, 1993)? The mechanics of developing research and theory about how parental depression impacts children's developmental outcomes and using this research base to develop preventive interventions may be easier to deal with than the practical and ethical challenges of gaining access to this target population.

Skinner and Wellborn (Chapter 14, this volume), in their chapter on children's coping with academic problems, outline an intriguing heuristic model of the role of motivation in children's coping when faced with a variety of types of stressors. Through this model, which integrates perspectives from the coping, emotion regulation, and behavior regulation literatures, the authors challenge us to examine more closely the relations among children's stress, self-perceptions, appraisals of threat, coping responses, and social context. In addition, Skinner and Wellborn call our attention to a broader array of positive coping responses than are commonly used in the literature. This model should be valuable for stimulating and guiding research and contributing to an empirical foundation for future interventions in many areas. Interestingly, although apparently there is relatively little stress-focused generative research on children's coping with academic problems, Skinner and Wellborn report that at least a few interventions have attempted to change children's coping behavior to improve their responses to academic problems.

Grych and Fincham (Chapter 6, this volume) identify several factors or processes that contribute to the likelihood of negative mental health outcomes for children whose parents divorce. Interparental conflict and changes that occur as a result of the divorce appear to be risk enhancers, while the quality of the parent–child relationship appears to be a risk reducer. Social support from parents and other adults, certain cognitive processes, and particular coping efforts appear to be protective factors. Aspects of child temperament also may be either protective or vulnerability factors. Although there may be little hope of changing children's temperaments, program developers may need to be sensitive to such individual differences when deciding on which approaches may be most successful for particular children. These findings provide a foundation for the development of preventive interventions: increasing the magnitude of risk reducers, introducing protective factors in children's lives, or reducing the magnitude of risk enhancers should be related to a reduced risk of negative outcomes for children of divorce.

Some stress-based preventive interventions for children of divorce and/or their families (generally custodial parents) have been developed and evaluated. These programs have focused on reducing postdivorce interparental conflict, improving parent–child relationships, helping children seek social support, and/or improving children's coping processes. Promising evaluation results from some of these programs support the utility of developing programs on the basis of the empirical literature. An important issue that emerges from these interventions is whether it is more effective to design interventions for children only, for parents only, or for both children and parents.

There is also a considerable body of research using a stress process model to understand how children cope with chronic illnesses (Kliewer, Chapter 10, this volume). Children's appraisal processes and coping behavior are two child characteristics that researchers have shown to be significantly associated with adjustment. Furthermore, research on children with chronic illness has identified family characteristics (e.g., conflict, cohesion, rigidity) that influence children's coping or adjustment. Kliewer reported that there have been at least four stress-based interventions for children with chronic illness. These have included family-focused interventions, stress management training, and social support building approaches. To date, however, the evaluation results have been somewhat mixed. Kliewer identifies a problem in intervention studies that is fairly common in other areas as well: "Most of these studies approach intervention with strong empirical justification, but fail to adequately specify or test the mediators they propose are responsible for changes in physical or psychological functioning" (see also Grych & Fincham, Chapter 6, this volume).

Research with bereaved children (Lutzke, Ayers, Sandler, & Barr, Chapter 8, this volume) also has identified several child (e.g., locus of control, self-esteem) and contextual (e.g., parent–child relations, family cohesion) characteristics that are potential mediators of children's adjustment to the death of a parent. Despite what appears to be a substantial research base, only one stress-process-based intervention has been developed and evaluated. Evaluation results from this prevention program were mixed (the intervention was successful based on parents' reports but not based on children's reports). The reasons for these mixed results probably are quite complex, but this example illustrates the value of multireporter evaluations of prevention programs targeting children.

Research on the adjustment of children of alcoholics (Chassin, Barrera, & Montgomery, Chapter 4, this volume) may be one of the few research areas that has identified more moderators of risk than mediators. Potential moderators include genetic factors (e.g., temperament), family conflict, ethnicity, self-esteem, perceived control, and social support. In addition, stressful life events, children's coping behavior, alcohol expectancies, and the quality of parenting apparently mediate children's risk for poor adjustment. As the authors note, the few interventions for children of alcoholics based on the stress process model have targeted children's coping skills, self-esteem, or alcohol expectancies. Unfortunately, few of these programs have been rigorously evaluated and the results are, at best, mixed.

Researchers who develop interventions for children of alcoholics face a challenge similar to those who focus on children of depressed parents. How can children of alcoholics in the general population be identified and recruited into interventions without violating their legal or ethical rights (Roosa et al., 1993)? Research showing the potential harm from labeling those who would participate in such interventions makes the provision of prevention services for this population particularly challenging (Burke & Sher, 1990). Chassin et al. suggest that universal programs designed to enhance children's coping skills within existing school-based substance abuse prevention programs may be a way of intervening with children of alcoholics without the risk of stigma inherent in more targeted programs.

INTERVENTION RESEARCH THAT HAS REACHED THE DISSEMINATION STAGE

Research on children's responses to stressful medical procedures is the most advanced of the research areas reviewed in this volume in terms of progress along the prevention research cycle (Peterson, Oliver, 7 Saldana, Chapter 12, this volume). This research is different from that reviewed in other chapters in some important dimensions: (1) this is the only major stressor reviewed that is often anticipated and planned for; (2) in most cases, children are exposed to this stressor for a very limited amount of time; and (3) the primary outcomes of interest are short-term, not long-term, adjustment. This also is one of the few areas in which the major stressor has diminished in stressfulness over time as medical procedures have evolved.

Researchers have identified children's coping, knowledge, and preparation and parental support as important to children's adjustment to medical procedures. Perhaps more so than in many other areas, researchers have highlighted the importance of children's developmental level to their response to stressful medical procedures. Preventive interventions have used modeling via films or puppets, preparation training, distraction, and parent training to modify key risk-reducing factors. Most interventions have shown at least some success, although evaluations have not been planned to identify which aspects of multiple component interventions contributed to positive outcomes.

Interventions to prepare children for stressful procedures are commonly used in most hospitals today. However, the diffusion of these interventions apparently has been unplanned and unstudied. The adoption of components of the successful interventions probably has occurred because of the perceived needs of patients and hospital staffs. Important questions for future research include the assessment of the components of the interventions that have been widely adopted, the extent to which they have been adapted, and the extent to which common preparation programs facilitate adjustment to medical procedures.

CROSSCUTTING ISSUES FOR FUTURE RESEARCH

In the previous sections we highlighted key aspects of research and intervention development in each major stressor reviewed in this volume. Although each body of literature has unique characteristics, there are several themes that are relevant across topics. In this section, we discuss the ideas, challenges, and methodologies that are potentially important to the successful progress of prevention research across a variety of stressors.

One common issue involves the lack of attention to identifying what it is about a major stressor that is stressful and operationalizing how stressful the phenomenon is for a particular child. Attention to these basic issues is needed to identify moderating and mediating processes. The most common way of identifying mediators and moderators is to compare children who have adjusted well to those who have adjusted poorly after exposure to a major stressor on personal or contextual characteristics that are related to their adjustment. However, we cannot accurately identify mediators and moderators unless we can determine that children who have adjusted differently have had similar exposure to stressful experiences (Rutter, 1990). Without measuring how much stress children experience, researchers are in danger of simply identifying correlates of adjustment, only some of which may be mediators, and overlooking potential moderators altogether. Interventions have a greater likelihood of success to the degree that they target factors that play a role in the transmission of risk to the child's development. One approach to assessing risk exposure is tailor-made life event measures that specifically operationalize the smaller stressors that occur in the context of major stressors (e.g., Sandler, Wolchik, Braver, & Fogas, 1986).

Perhaps because of the lack of risk-specific stress measures, much of the research reviewed identified potential mediators based on zero-order correlations between potential mediators and outcomes. A mediator needs to be correlated to both the level of stress experienced and the measure of adjustment, but more importantly, a mediator must be shown to account for at least some of the relation between a major stressor and children's adjustment. Similarly, potential moderators have been identified by using analysis of variance to look for differences on outcome variables across groups defined on the basis of demographic characteristics or intrapersonal and interpersonal factors. However, significant differences on outcomes across groups is not enough to establish moderation. Specific procedures have been outlined for assessing whether mediation or moderation exists (Baron & Kenny, 1986). The development of theoretically guided preventive interventions requires researchers to move beyond the descriptive stage to systematically testing theoretical models of causal relations.

One of the advantages of using the stress process model to guide the development of interventions is the clear identification of the mediators or moderators that can be targeted for change to produce subsequent change in adjustment. Therefore, program evaluation should involve assessment of both whether the intervention succeeded in bringing about the intended changes in targeted mediators or moderators and, if this step was successful, whether these changes resulted in positive changes in adjustment. This latter step provides an experimental test of the theory of the intervention as well as a measure of intervention efficacy (Price, 1987). Failure to clearly specify the mediators or moderators targeted for change or to examine if the desired changes in the mediating or moderating variables did in fact occur during intervention undermines our ability to determine what accounts for program effects on mental health outcomes or to improve intervention programs.

In their chapter, Eisenberg, Fabes, and Guthrie (Chapter 2, this volume) place coping theory and research within the larger context of research and theory on emotion regulation. This broader perspective, in conjunction with the motivational model presented by Skinner and Wellborn (Chapter 14, this volume), should be useful to both generative researchers and intervention developers in a wide variety of areas. Focusing on emotion regulation forces us to take developmental issues into account, issues that too often are neglected as researchers focus on a single, narrow age group. Second, the focus on emotion regulation also encourages us to examine children's appraisals of stressful situations and the role that appraisals may play both in coping responses and adjustment. More attention to the cognitive processes that precede and mediate coping responses as well as increased attention to how children's development may moderate these cognitive processes could contribute to the development of more effective interventions.

The various research literatures reviewed differed considerably in the relative amount of attention that has been given to the study of the child's family or larger social context as influences on children's outcomes. For major stressors that potentially are more controlled by the child (e.g., child chronic illness, peer rejection, academic stress), a research bias toward children's own capacity to cope and adjust may be appropriate. In other cases in which the major stressors are largely beyond their control, research also must focus on features of children's larger social contexts. For instance, research on disasters must focus on potential mediators or moderators of children's outcomes such as parent and family coping styles and family, community, and school supportiveness to truly understand why children adjust differently after such events. Similarly, research on children's adjustment in inner-city communities must look beyond the children and their characteristics to understand why some children are resilient and others are not (cf. Baldwin, Baldwin, & Cole, 1990; Masten, Morison, Pellegrini, & Tellegen, 1990). Children's individual characteristics as well as parent, family, community, and cultural factors are all likely to play important roles as mediators or moderators of children's motivation, appraisals, coping, and outcomes for most major stressors (e.g., Furstenberg & Hughes, 1995; O'Donnel & Tharp, 1990). Further, in most cases interventions are less likely to be successful if they focus solely on children (Sameroff & Fiese, 1989).

Another recurring theme involved the lack of communication between generative researchers using a stress process model and program developers (cf. Price, 1987). This is unfortunate because "successful interventions are viewed as being theory driven, including both theories of the problem and theories of the interventions" (Consortium on the School-Based Promotion of Social Competence, 1994, p. 287; see also Coie et al., 1993; Cowen, 1982; Lorion, 1983, 1985; Lorion et al., 1989). There may be many reasons for the gulf between those who conduct generative research and develop theory and those who develop interventions. First, rarely are the same people involved in both generative research and intervention development (Price, 1987). Instead, there often are differences between these two groups in disciplinary backgrounds (e.g., psychology vs. social work or medicine), and therefore in the journals they read and in which they publish, work environments (e.g., universities vs. hospitals, schools, or agencies), and mandates (e.g., rigorous science and publication vs. meeting the immediate needs of clients or institutions). Second, very little formal training is available in how to develop theory-based preventive interventions (Mrazek & Haggerty, 1994) and relatively few published examples of the developmental process are available to serve as models (see Dumka, Roosa, Michaels, & Suh, 1995; Roosa, Gensheimer, Ayers, & Short, 1990; Sandler et al., 1988; West et al., 1991, for exceptions). Systematic efforts at increasing cross-disciplinary communication and training opportunities are needed to reduce the size of this gulf and to improve the quality, and likely success, of the next generation of preventive interventions.

Interestingly, researchers in quite diverse literatures have identified, albeit with different degrees of supportive evidence, many of the same or similar potential mediators and moderators of children's adjustment (e.g., social support, coping behavior, appraisals, family functioning, parenting behavior). Such replication across risk factors should be comforting and should provide clear guidance to researchers in newly emerging fields of inquiry using the stress process model. The fact that children's coping behavior, quality of parenting and home environment, and support from family, community, and school are significantly associated with children's outcomes when exposed to major stressors could increase the speed with which new stress-based interventions are developed. Researchers in areas that are in the initial stages of the prevention research cycle can learn a great deal from their predecessors in other areas without having to cover all the steps taken by more pioneering intervention developers. However, it is critical that the unique characteristics of each major stressor are given adequate attention.

On the other hand, several studies have documented that children rarely experience developmental difficulties after exposure to a single risk factor (e.g., Rutter, 1979; Sameroff, 1987; Sameroff, Seifer, Barocas, Zax, & Greenspan, 1987; Werner & Smith, 1992). Only children who have experienced several risk factors are highly likely to develop mental health problems. Furthermore, it is not uncommon for major stressors to co-occur (Dryfoos, 1991). For instance, low-income inner-city children are more likely than middle-class peers to have chronic illnesses or parents with serious illnesses, experience child maltreatment, and have teenage pregnancies. Given the commonality of many risk and protective processes across major stressors and the co-occurrence of many major stressors, it may be time to challenge the wisdom of continuing to study stress and coping and developing preventive interventions on a risk factor by risk factor basis (Mrazek & Haggerty, 1994; Rutter, 1994). Developing universal interventions for young children that focus on the most common and benign protective processes across risk factors may provide a means of accessing all high-risk children including the hard-to-reach populations (e.g., children of depressed parents, children of alcoholics). Selective prevention programs could be offered to children who are at high risk because of exposure to multiple risk factors. Such an approach may be less threatening to children and parents and may increase the cost-benefit ratio of preventive interventions, because only the highest risk cases would be provided with more extensive targeted prevention services (Emery, 1991; Pillow, Sandler, Braver, Wolchik, & Gersten, 1991; Reid, 1991). Screening also can increase the likelihood of success in preventive interventions and increase the power of program evaluations (Pillow et al., 1991). Both the question of single risk factor prevention programs versus universal prevention programs and the value of screening for prevention programs deserve more systematic investigation.

SUMMARY

Earlier chapters in this volume carefully documented the rich and exciting advances in research on several major stressors that can threaten normal child development. Progress in research on these topics varied considerably. Research in some areas remains primarily descriptive, while in several areas of research there is a reasonable amount of generative research that has been guided by the stress process model and mediators and moderators of stress have been identified. In some areas, stress process models have been used to develop preventive interventions, although relatively few interventions have been rigorously evaluated. Although considerable challenges have been identified that will require systematic attention before the potential for prevention science can be realized fully, we are optimistic about the future of preventive interventions for children. Clearly, there is a need for more rigorous research on risk and protective processes to strengthen theories of how major stressors place some children at risk. Similarly, systematic attention is needed on how to move beyond the generative stage of the prevention research cycle to the rigorous evaluation of prevention programs. This effort will require more and improved training in prevention science, more and better cross-disciplinary communication of research and theory developments, more multidisciplinary research efforts, and the allocation of the financial resources to take the expensive step of program development and evaluation. Recent policy initiatives in prevention research training and funding (NIMH, 1996) may provide the necessary tools and resources for advancing prevention program development and evaluation.

REFERENCES

Baldwin, A. L., Baldwin, C., & Cole, R. E. (1990). Stress-resistant families and stress-resistant children. In J. Rolf, A. S. Masten, D. Cicchetti, K. H. Nuechterlein, & S. Weintraub (Eds.), *Risk and protective factors in the development of psychopathology* (pp. 287–280). New York: Cambridge University Press.

Baron, R. M., & Kenny, D. A. (1986). The moderator–mediator distinction in social psychological research: Conceptual, strategic, and statistical considerations. *Journal of Personality and Social Psychology, 51,* 1173–1182.

Bloom, B. L. (1979). Prevention of mental disorders: Recent advances in theory and practice. *Community Mental Health Journal, 15,* 179–191.

Burk, J. P., & Sher, K. J. (1990). Labeling the child of an alcoholic: Negative stereotyping by mental health professionals and peers. *Journal of Studies on Alcohol, 51,* 156–163.

Coie, J. D., Watt, N., West, S. G., Hawkins, D., Asarnow, J., Markman, H., Ramey, S., Shure, M., & Long, B. (1993). The science of prevention: A conceptual framework for some directions for a national research program. *American Psychologist, 48,* 1013–1022.

Consortium on the School-Based Promotion of Social Competence. (1994). The school-based promotion of social competence: Theory, research, practice, and policy. In R. J. Haggerty, L. R. Sherrod, N. Garmezy, & M. Rutter (Eds.), *Stress, risk, and resilience in adolescents: Processes, mechanisms, and interventions* (pp. 354–385). New York: Cambridge University Press.

Cowen, E. L. (1982). The wooing of primary prevention. *American Journal of Community Psychology, 8,* 258–284.

Dryfoos, J. G. (1991). *Adolescents at risk: Prevalence and prevention.* New York: University of Oxford Press.

Dumka, L. E., Roosa, M. W., Michaels, M. L., & Suh, K. (1995). Using theory and research in the development of interventions for high risk families. *Family Relations, 44,* 78–86.

Emery, R. E. (1991). Mediational screening in theory and practice. *American Journal of Community Psychology, 19,* 853–857.

Furstenberg, F. F., Jr., & Hughes, M. E. (1995). Social capital and successful development among at-risk youth. *Journal of Marriage and the Family, 57,* 580–592.

Garmezy, N. (1985). Stress resistant children: The search for protective factors. In J. Stevenson (Ed.), *Recent research in developmental psychopathology: Journal of Child Psychology and Psychiatry Book Supplement No. 4.* (pp. 213–233). Oxford, England: Pergamon Press.

Grych, J. H., & Fincham, F. D. (1992). Interventions for children of divorce: Toward greater integration of research and action. *Psychological Bulletin, 111,* 1–20.

Heller, K., Price, R., & Sher, K. J. (1980). Research and evaluation in primary prevention. Issues and guidelines. In R. H. Price, R. F. Ketterer, B. C. Bader, & J. Monahan (Eds.), *Prevention in mental health. Research, policy, and practice* (Vol. I, pp. 285–313). Beverly Hills, CA: Sage.

Lipsey, M. W. (1990). Theory as method: Small theories of treatments. In L. Sechrest, E. Perrin, & J. Bunker (Eds.), *Research methodology: Strengthening causal interpretations of nonexperimental data* (pp. 33–51) (DHHS Publication No. 90-3454). Washington, DC: US Department of HHS, Agency for Health Care Policy and Research.

Lorion, R. P. (1983). Environmental approaches to prevention: The danger of imprecision. *Prevention in Human Services, 4,* 193–205.

Lorion, R. P. (1985). Evaluating preventive interventions: Guidelines for the serious social change agent. In R. D. Feiner, L. Jason, J. Moritsugu, & S. S. Farber (Eds.), *Preventive psychology: Theory, research, and practice in community intervention* (pp. 251–272). New York: Pergamon Press.

Lorion, R. P., Price, R. H., & Eaton, W. W. (1989). The prevention of child and adolescent disorders: From theory to research. In D. Shaffer & M. M. Silverman (Eds.), *Prevention of mental disorders, alcohol and other drug use in children and adolescents* (OSAP Prevention Monograph-2) (pp. 55–96) (DHHS Publication No. (ADM) 90-1646). Washington, DC: US Government Printing Office.

Masten, A. S., & Garmezy, N. (1985). Risk, vulnerability, and protective factors in developmental psychopathology. In B. B. Lahey & A. E. Kazdin (Eds.), *Advances in clinical child psychology* (Vol. 8, pp. 1–52). New York: Plenum Press.

Masten, A. S., Morison, P., Pellegrini, D., & Tellegen, A. (1990). Competence under stress: Risk and protective factors. In J. Rolf, A. S. Masten, D. Cicchetti, K. H. Nuechterlein, & S. Weintraub (Eds.), *Risk and protective factors in the development of psychopathology* (pp. 236–256). New York: Cambridge University Press.

Mrazek, P. J., & Haggerty, R. J. (1994). *Reducing the risks for mental disorders: Frontiers for preventive intervention research.* Washington, DC: National Academy Press.

NIMH. (1996). *A plan for prevention research for the National Institute of Mental Health: A report* to the National Advisory Mental Health Council (NIH Publication No. 96-4093). Washington, DC: US Government Printing Office.

O'Donnell, C. R., & Tharp, R. G. (1990). Community intervention guided by theoretical development. In A. S. Belleck, M. Hersen, & A. E. Kazdin (Eds.), International handbook of behavior modification and therapy (2nd ed., pp. 251–266). New York: Plenum Press.

Pillow, D., Sandler, I., Braver, S., Wolchik, S., & Gersten, J. (1991). Theory based screening for prevention: Focusing on mediation processes in children of divorce. American Journal of Community Psychology, 19, 809–836.

Price, R. H. (1983). The education of a prevention psychologist. In R. D. Felner, L. A. Jason, J. N. Moritsugu, & S. S. Farber (Eds.), Preventive psychology: Theory research and practice (pp. 290–297). New York: Pergamon Press.

Price, R. H. (1987). Linking intervention research and risk factor research. In J. A. Steinberg & M. M. Silverman (Eds.), Preventing mental disorders: A research perspective (pp. 48–56). Washington, DC: US Government Printing Office.

Price, R. H., & Lorion, R. P. (1989). Prevention programming as organizational reinvention: From research to implementation. In D. Shaffer, I. Phillips, & N. B. Enzer (Eds.), Prevention of mental disorders, alcohol, and other drug use in children and adolescents (OSAP Prevention Monograph-2) (pp. 97–123) (DHHS Publication No. (ADM) 90-1646). Washington, DC: US Government Printing Office.

Reid, J. B. (1991). Mediational screening as a model for prevention research. American Journal of Community Psychology, 19, 867–872.

Roosa, M. W., Gensheimer, L. K., Ayers, T., & Short, J. L. (1990). Development of a preventive intervention for children in alcoholic families. Journal of Primary Prevention, 11, 119–141.

Roosa, M., Michaels, M., Groppenbacher, N., & Gersten, J. (1993). The validity of children's self-reports of family drinking problems. Journal of Studies on Alcohol, 54, 71–79.

Roosa, M. W., Tein, J., Groppenbacher, N., Michaels, M., & Dumka, L. (1993). Mothers' parenting behavior and child mental health in families with a problem drinking parent. Journal of Marriage and the Family, 55, 107–118.

Rutter, M. (1979). Protective factors in children's responses to stress and disadvantage. In M. W. Kent & J. E. Rolf (Eds.), Primary prevention in psychopathology. Vol. 3: Social competence in children (pp. 49–74). Hanover, NH: University Press of New England.

Rutter, M. (1985). Resilience in the face of adversity: Protective factors and resistance to psychiatric disorder. British Journal of Psychiatry, 147, 598–611.

Rutter, M. (1990). Psychosocial resilience and protective factors. In J. Rolf, A. S. Masten, D. Cicchetti, K. H. Nuechterlein, & S. Weintraub (Eds.), Risk and protective factors in the development of psychopathology (pp. 181–214). New York: Cambridge University Press.

Rutter, M. (1994). Stress research: Accomplishments and tasks ahead. In R. J. Haggerty, L. R. Sherrod, N. Garmezy, & M. Rutter (Eds.), Stress, risk, and resilience in adolescents: Processes, mechanisms, and interventions (pp. 354–385). New York: Cambridge University Press.

Sameroff, A. J. (1987). Transactional risk factors and prevention. In J. A. Steinberg & M. M. Silverman (Eds.), Preventing mental disorders: A research perspective (pp. 74–89). Washington, DC: US Government Printing Office.

Sameroff, A. J., & Chandler, M. (1975). Reproductive risk and the continuum of caretaking casualty. In F. Horowitz, M. Hetherington, S. Scarr-Salapatek, & G. Siegel (Eds.), Review of child development research (Vol. 4, pp. 187–244). Chicago: University of Chicago Press.

Sameroff, A. J., & Fiese, B. H. (1989). Conceptual issues in prevention. In D. Schaffer, I. Philips, & N. B. Enzer (Eds.), Prevention of mental disorders, alcohol and other drug use in children and adolescents (pp. 23–52) (Office of Substance Abuse Prevention Monograph-2, DHHS Publication No. ADM 90-1646). Washington, DC: US Government Printing Office.

Sameroff, A. J., Seifer, R., Barocas, R., Zax, M., & Greenspan, S. (1987). IQ scores of 4-year-old children: Social environmental risk factors. Pediatrics, 79, 343–350.

Sandler, I. N., Gersten, J. C., Reynolds, K., Kallgren, C., & Ramirez, R. (1988). Using theory and data to plan support interventions: Design of a program for bereaved children. In B. Gottleib (Ed.), Marshalling social support: Formats, processes, and effects (pp. 53–83). Beverly Hills, CA: Sage.

Sandler, I. N., Wolchik, S. A., Braver, S. L., & Fogas, B. S. (1986). Significant effects of children of divorce: Toward the assessment of risky situations. In S. M. Auerbach & A. L. Stolberg (Eds.),

Crisis intervention with children and families (pp. 65–83). New York: Hemisphere Publishing Corporation.

Werner, E. E., & Smith, R. S. (1992). *Overcoming the odds: High risk children from birth to adulthood.* Ithaca, NY: Cornell University Press.

West, S. G., Sandler, I. N., Pillow, D., Baca, L., & Gersten, J. C. (1991). The use of structural equation modeling in generative research: Toward the design of a preventive intervention for bereaved children. *American Journal of Community Psychology, 19,* 459–480.

Wolchik, S. A., Ruelhman, L. S., Braver, S. L., & Sandler, I. N. (1989). Social support of children of divorce: Direct and stress buffering effects. *American Journal of Community Psychology, 17,* 485–501.

Yoshikawa, H. (1994). Prevention as cumulative protection: Effects of early family support and education on chronic delinquency and its risks. *Psychological Bulletin, 115,* 28–54.

Index